ATLAS OF TUMOR PATHOLOGY

Third Series
Fascicle 25

TUMORS OF THE TESTIS, ADNEXA, SPERMATIC CORD, AND SCROTUM

by

Thomas M. Ulbright, M.D.
Professor of Pathology & Laboratory Medicine and
Director of Anatomic Pathology
Indiana University School of Medicine
Indianapolis, Indiana

Mahul B. Amin, M.D.
Director of Surgical Pathology
Emory University Hospital and
Associate Professor of Pathology and Urology
Emory University School of Medicine
Atlanta, Georgia

Robert H. Young, M.D., FRCPath
Pathologist and Director of Surgical Pathology
Massachusetts General Hospital
Professor of Pathology
Harvard Medical School,
Boston, Massachusetts

Published by the
ARMED FORCES INSTITUTE OF PATHOLOGY
Washington, D.C.

Under the Auspices of
UNIVERSITIES ASSOCIATED FOR RESEARCH AND EDUCATION IN PATHOLOGY, INC.
Bethesda, Maryland
1999

Accepted for Publication
1997

Available from the American Registry of Pathology
Armed Forces Institute of Pathology
Washington, D.C. 20306-6000
ISSN 0160-6344
ISBN 1-881041-46-8

ATLAS OF TUMOR PATHOLOGY

EDITOR
JUAN ROSAI, M.D.

Department of Pathology
Memorial Sloan-Kettering Cancer Center
New York, New York 10021-6007

ASSOCIATE EDITOR
LESLIE H. SOBIN, M.D.

Armed Forces Institute of Pathology
Washington, D.C. 20306-6000

EDITORIAL ADVISORY BOARD

EDITORS' NOTE

The Atlas of Tumor Pathology has a long and distinguished history. It was first conceived at a Cancer Research Meeting held in St. Louis in September 1947 as an attempt to standardize the nomenclature of neoplastic diseases. The first series was sponsored by the National Academy of Sciences-National Research Council. The organization of this Sisyphean effort was entrusted to the Subcommittee on Oncology of the Committee on Pathology, and Dr. Arthur Purdy Stout was the first editor-in-chief. Many of the illustrations were provided by the Medical Illustration Service of the Armed Forces Institute of Pathology, the type was set by the Government Printing Office, and the final printing was done at the Armed Forces Institute of Pathology (hence the colloquial appellation "AFIP Fascicles"). The American Registry of Pathology purchased the Fascicles from the Government Printing Office and sold them virtually at cost. Over a period of 20 years, approximately 15,000 copies each of nearly 40 Fascicles were produced. The worldwide impact that these publications have had over the years has largely surpassed the original goal. They quickly became among the most influential publications on tumor pathology ever written, primarily because of their overall high quality but also because their low cost made them easily accessible to pathologists and other students of oncology the world over.

Upon completion of the first series, the National Academy of Sciences-National Research Council handed further pursuit of the project over to the newly created Universities Associated for Research and Education in Pathology (UAREP). A second series was started, generously supported by grants from the AFIP, the National Cancer Institute, and the American Cancer Society. Dr. Harlan I. Firminger became the editor-in-chief and was succeeded by Dr. William H. Hartmann. The second series Fascicles were produced as bound volumes instead of loose leaflets. They featured a more comprehensive coverage of the subjects, to the extent that the Fascicles could no longer be regarded as "atlases" but rather as monographs describing and illustrating in detail the tumors and tumor-like conditions of the various organs and systems.

Once the second series was completed, with a success that matched that of the first, UAREP and AFIP decided to embark on a third series. A new editor-in-chief and an associate editor were selected, and a distinguished editorial board was appointed. The mandate for the third series remains the same as for the previous ones, i.e., to oversee the production of an eminently practical publication with surgical pathologists as its primary audience, but also aimed at other workers in oncology. The main purposes of this series are to promote a consistent, unified, and biologically sound nomenclature; to guide the surgical pathologist in the diagnosis of the various tumors and tumor-like lesions; and to provide relevant histogenetic, pathogenetic, and clinicopathologic information on these entities. Just as the second series included data obtained from ultrastructural (and, in the more recent Fascicles, immunohistochemical) examination, the third series will, in addition, incorporate pertinent information obtained with the newer molecular biology techniques. As in the past, a continuous attempt will be made to correlate, whenever possible, the nomenclature used in the Fascicles with that proposed by the World Health Organization's International Histological Classification of Tumors. The format of the third series has been changed in order to incorporate additional items and to ensure a consistency of style throughout. Close cooperation between the various authors and their respective liaisons from the editorial board will be emphasized to minimize unnecessary repetition and discrepancies in the text and illustrations.

To its everlasting credit, the participation and commitment of the AFIP to this venture is even more substantial and encompassing than in previous series. It now extends to virtually all scientific, technical, and financial aspects of the production.

The task confronting the organizations and individuals involved in the third series is even more daunting than in the preceding efforts because of the ever-increasing complexity of the matter at hand. It is hoped that this combined effort—of which, needless to say, that represented by the authors is first and foremost—will result in a series worthy of its two illustrious predecessors and will be a suitable introduction to the tumor pathology of the twenty-first century.

Juan Rosai, M.D.
Leslie H. Sobin, M.D.

Tumors
of the
Testis, Adnexa,
Spermatic Cord,
and Scrotum

Atlas
of
Tumor Pathology

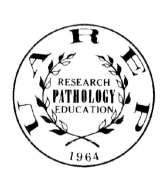

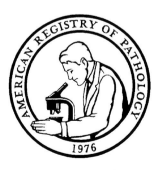

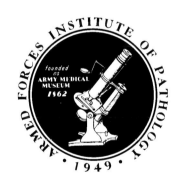

ACKNOWLEDGMENTS

We have tried to create in this publication a resource for both the usual and unusual lesions that may be encountered in the testis and adjacent tissues, including the scrotum. Although the scope of the Fascicles has changed since their initial inception, as noted by the editors in their introduction, we have attempted to continue the "atlas" tradition of these works by including in many instances several illustrations of the various entities discussed. If this work has at least in part accomplished our goal, it is, in a very real sense, because of the willingness of the pathology community to share material with us. We have acknowledged many of the contributors in the figure legends, but omissions have undoubtedly occurred, and we offer our sincere apologies for any unintended oversights. We are indebted to all those who donated case material for our use, several of whom deserve special mention. Dr. Stewart Cramer (Rochester, New York) contributed may beautiful lantern slides of gross specimens and Dr. Deborah Gersell (St. Louis, Missouri) rummaged through the archives of Barnes Hospital for similar photographs. Dr. Mark A. Weiss of Cincinnati, Ohio, and Dr. Stacey E. Mills of Charlottesville, Virginia, kindly provided a number of illustrations from their *Atlas of Genitourinary Tract Disorders*. Despite the many contributions from other institutions, the single greatest number of cases is from the Urologic Services of Indiana University Medical Center and the Massachusetts General Hospital. We are grateful to the chiefs of service, Dr. John P. Donohue and Dr. W. Scott McDougal, and their colleagues for this case material and for what we have learned from them about the clinical aspects of these cases over the years, and for their invariably cooperative attitude and appreciation of pathology. Similar comments pertain to our colleagues in Radiation Medicine and Medical Oncology. Dr. Judith A. Ferry of the Massachusetts General Hospital contributed greatly to the section dealing with hemato-poietic neoplasms and we are most appreciative for this input. Michael Goheen, Susan Cooper, and Nancy Maguire at Indiana University and Stephen Conley and Michelle Forestall of the Massachusetts General Hospital provided superb assistance with photography. Judy Surber, Charlott Shellhouse, Beth Reeves, Terri Steinke, and Marlene Fairbanks provided outstanding secretarial help. We are also deeply appreciative for the support and patience of our families during the many late nights at the office and library.

We are indebted to the two anonymous reviewers who carefully read our manuscript and made a number of helpful suggestions. The editorial staff of the Atlas of Tumor Pathology was most helpful and capable in the production of the work and showed great tolerance with the last minute tinkering of the authors and what must have seemed endless requests to add another just published paper to the references. One of the authors (TMU) is grateful to Indiana University for providing him a 6-month sabbatical during which time initial drafts of several of the chapters were written. The editor of the third series Fascicles, Dr. Juan Rosai, brought new meaning to the word patience in his tolerance of the authors' tardiness in submitting the final manuscript to him and we are most thankful to him for this.

We would be remiss if we did not acknowledge that our work is very much placed upon that of our predecessors, not only the prior authors of the Fascicles, but the numerous individuals who have contributed significantly to our knowledge of testicular pathology. Although we have tried to incorporate as much "new" information as possible concerning the entities discussed, the foundation of this work was built by many astute pathologists over numerous years.

This Fascicle is the first of two that are the successors to the 1952 first series Fascicle *Tumors of the Male Sex Organs* by Drs. Frank J. Dixon and Robert A. Moore and the 1973 second series Fascicle, *Tumors of the Male Genital System* by Drs. F. K. Mostofi and Edward B. Price. The efforts of the authors of those two works is noted with respect and we are honored to follow in their footsteps. The first Fascicle was published 6 years after one of the seminal contributions to testicular pathology, "Tumors of the Testis. A Report on 922 Cases," published in *Military Surgeon* 1946;99:573–93. In large measure, that paper set the stage for the contemporary classification of testicular tumors, and the major contribution of the senior author of that paper, Dr. Nathan B. Friedman, to testicular pathology is acknowledged.

Finally, we would like to thank the overseer of this Fascicle, Dr. Robert E. Scully. Not only did he offer numerous helpful comments to us while the work was in progress, but he generously allowed us to "plunder" his wonderful collection of testicular tumor pathology. The latter was amassed over his more than 50 years of study of this area since his initial work, conducted while still a resident, that resulted in the first of his many publications on testicular pathology in 1946 (see reference 114, page 99). With admiration for his seminal role in the pathology of the gonads, and with respect and affection, we dedicate this work to him.

Thomas M. Ulbright, M.D.
Mahul B. Amin, M.D.
Robert H. Young, M.D., FRCPath

Permission to use copyrighted illustrations has been granted by:

American Society of Clinical Pathologists:
Am J Clin Pathol 1956;26:1303–13. For figure 8-83.
Testicular Tumors, 1990. For figures 3-3, 3-4, 3-18, 3-29, 3-41, 4-46, 4-76, 4-100C, 4-101, 5-8, 5-16, 5-17, 5-18, 6-38, 6-40, 6-56, 7-16, 7-26, 7-27, 7-52, 7-79, 8-8, 8-12, 8-21, 8-30 through 8-33, 8-35, 8-36, 8-43, 8-47, 8-90.

Blackwell Scientific:
Int J Androl 1981;4:153–62. For figure 2-3.

Churchill-Livingstone:
Uropathology, 1989. For figure 1-7.

Fundacion Puigvert:
Atlas de Patologia de los Tumores Urogenitales, 1991. For figure 8-22.

John Wiley & Sons:
Am J Anat 1963;112:35–51. For figure 1-10.

Lippincott-Raven:
Am J Surg Pathol 1991;15:66–74. For figure 8-68.
Atlas of Genitourinary Tract Disorders, 1988. For figures 9-11, 9-17A, 9-27, and 9-28.
Diagnostic Surgical Pathology, 1994. For figure 4-25.

Massachusetts Medical Society:
N Engl J Med 1966;274:928–30. For figure 8-47.

Mosby:
Urologic Surgical Pathology, 1997. For figures 1-5 and 8-86.

Oxford University Press:
Cunningham's Textbook of Anatomy, 12th ed., 1981. For figure 1-6.

W.B. Saunders:
Atlas of Surgical Pathology of the Male Reproductive Tract, 1997. For figures 7-70, 7-73, 9-17B,C.
Semin Urol 1984;2:217–29. For figures 1-21 and 1-22.

Williams & Wilkins:
J Urol 1963;90:220–9. For figure 8-5.
J Urol 1983;130:423–7. For table 9-3.
Medical Embryology and Human Development—Normal and Abnormal, 2nd ed., 1969. For figures 1-1 through 1-4.

Contents

1. Testicular Tumors: General Considerations 1
   Introduction 1
   Embryology, Anatomy, and Histology 1
      Embryology 1
      Anatomy 4
      Histology 7
   Classification 15
   Patterns of Spread and Metastasis in Testicular Cancer 18
   Staging 20
   Gross Examination 20
   Frozen Section Examination 23
   Cytologic Examination 23
   Epidemiology 23
      Cryptorchidism 27
      Bilateral Testicular Germ Cell Tumors 29
      Familial Testicular Cancer 29
      Intersex Syndromes 30
      Infertility 30
   General Clinic Aspects 31
2. Germ Cell Tumors: Histogenetic Considerations and Intratubular Germ Cell Neoplasia . 41
   Histogenesis 41
   Intratubular Germ Cell Neoplasia 45
      Intratubular Germ Cell Neoplasia, Unclassified Type 45
      Other Forms of Intratubular Germ Cell Neoplasia 53
3. Germ Cell Tumors: Seminomas 59
   Typical Seminoma 59
   Spermatocytic Seminoma 85
4. Germ Cell Tumors: Nonseminomatous 103
   Embryonal Carcinoma 103
   Yolk Sac Tumor (Endodermal Sinus Tumor) 119
   Choriocarcinoma and Other Rare Forms of Trophoblastic Neoplasia 138
   Teratoma 147
   Monodermal and Highly Specialized Tumors 160
      Carcinoid 160
      Primitive Neuroectodermal Tumor 163
      Other Monodermal Teratomas 164
5. Mixed Germ Cell, Regressed Germ Cell, and Germ Cell-Sex Cord- Stromal Tumors 175
   Mixed Germ Cell Tumors 175
   Regression of Testicular Germ Cell Tumors ("Burnt-out" Germ Cell Tumors) 181
   Germ Cell-Sex Cord-Stromal Tumors 184

Gonadoblastoma 185

Unclassified Germ Cell-Sex Cord Stromal Tumors 188

6. Sex Cord-Stromal Tumors 193

Sertoli-Stromal Cell Tumors 193

Sertoli Cell Tumors 193

Large Cell Calcifying Sertoli Cell Tumor 202

Sertoli-Leydig Cell Tumor 209

Leydig Cell Tumor 210

Granulosa-Stromal Cell Tumors 219

Adult-Type Granulosa Cell Tumor 219

Juvenile-Type Granulosa Cell Tumor 222

Tumors in the Fibroma-Thecoma Group 226

Sex Cord-Stromal Tumors, Mixed and Unclassified 227

Immunohistochemistry of Sex Cord-Stromal Tumors 229

7. Miscellaneous Primary Tumors of the Testis, Adnexa, and Spermatic Cord,
Hematopoietic Tumors and Secondary Tumors 235

Miscellaneous Primary Tumors of the Testis, Adnexa, and Spermatic Cord 235

Ovarian-Type Epithelial Tumors 235

Benign Tumors of the Rete Testis 239

Carcinoma of the Rete Testis 240

Adenomatoid Tumor 243

Malignant Mesothelioma 247

Desmoplastic Small Round Cell Tumor 253

Papillary Cystadenoma of the Epididymis 254

Carcinoma of the Epididymis 255

Retinal Anlage Tumor 256

Soft Tissue Tumors 259

Benign or Locally Aggressive Tumors 259

Sarcomas 265

Other Rare Primary Tumors 271

Hematopoietic Tumors 272

Malignant Lymphoma 272

Multiple Myeloma and Plasmacytoma 277

Leukemia, Including Granulocytic Sarcoma 279

Secondary Tumors 281

8. Tumor-Like Lesions of Testis, Paratestis, and Spermatic Cord 291

Leydig Cell Hyperplasia and Extraparenchymal Leydig Cells 291

Sertoli Cell Nodules 292

Testicular "Tumor" of the Adrenogenital Syndrome 293

Steroid Cell Nodules with Other Adrenal Diseases 297

Adrenal Cortical Rests 298

Torsion, Infarcts, and Hematomas of Testis 299

The Testicular Appendages and Walthard Nests 302

Orchitis and Epididymitis 304

Bacterial Orchitis 304

Viral Orchitis 304

Granulomatous Orchitis, Infectious 305

Granulomatous Orchitis, Idiopathic 306

Granulomatous Epididymitis 308

Sarcoidosis 309

Malakoplakia 309

Rosai-Dorfman Disease (Sinus Histiocytosis with Massive Lymphadenopathy) 313

Hydrocele-Related Changes and Miscellaneous Other Abnormalities of the Tunica
    Vaginalis 314

Inflammatory Pseudotumor (Pseudosarcomatous Myofibroblastic Proliferation;
    Proliferative Funiculitis) 315

Fibrous Pseudotumor, Fibromatous Periorchitis, Nodular Periorchitis 317

Meconium Periorchitis 319

Mesothelial Hyperplasia 319

Sclerosing Lipogranuloma 321

Abnormalities Related to Sexual Precocity/Idiopathic Hypertrophy 321

Hyperplasia and Miscellaneous Other Benign Lesions of the Rete Testis 322

Cysts 323

Cystic Dysplasia 326

Microlithiasis 326

Spermatocele 327

Sperm Granuloma 329

Vasitis Nodosa 331

Splenic-Gonadal Fusion 331

Tumor-Like Aspects of Normal Histology 333

Miscellaneous Other Lesions 334

9. The Scrotum 343

Introduction 343

Normal Anatomy and Histology 343

Malignant Epithelial Tumors 345

Squamous Cell Carcinoma 345

Basal Cell Carcinoma 349

Paget's Disease 350

Merkel Cell Carcinoma 352

Miscellaneous Malignant Tumors of Skin Adnexal Type 352

Malignant Mesenchymal Tumors 352

Leiomyosarcoma 352

Liposarcoma 353

Malignant Fibrous Histiocytoma 353

Malignant Lymphoma 353

Malignant Melanoma 353

Benign Tumors 353

Benign Epithelial Tumors 354

Benign Mesenchymal Tumors 354

Secondary Tumors 358

Tumor-Like Lesions 358

   Condyloma Acuminatum 358

   Verruciform Xanthoma 358

   Porokeratosis of Mibelli 359

   "Idiopathic" Scrotal Calcinosis and Epidermoid Cysts 360

   Sclerosing Lipogranuloma (Paraffinoma) 361

   Post-Traumatic Spindle Cell Nodule 363

   Scrotal Hamartoma Including "Accessory Scrotum" 363

   Fibrous Hamartoma of Infancy 364

   Smooth Muscle Hamartoma of Dartos 364

   Isolated Exophytic Elastoma 364

   Scrotal Fat Necrosis 364

   Scrotal Edema 364

   Polymorphic Reticulosis of Genital Skin 366

   Inflammatory and Infectious Diseases 366

   Fournier's Gangrene 366

Index 375

TUMORS OF THE TESTIS, ADNEXA, SPERMATIC CORD, AND SCROTUM

1
TESTICULAR TUMORS: GENERAL CONSIDERATIONS

INTRODUCTION

Since the publication of the last Fascicle that discussed the testis in 1973, great advances have been made in the field of testicular oncology. There is now effective treatment for almost all testicular germ cell tumors (which constitute most testicular neoplasms), whereas in 1973 seminoma was the only histologic type that could be effectively treated after metastases had developed. The elegant studies of Skakkebaek and his associates (2,3,10,13–17) have established that most germ cell tumors arise from morphologically distinctive intratubular malignant germ cells. This work supports a common pathway for the different morphologic types of germ cell tumors and reaffirms the approach to nomenclature of the World Health Organization (WHO) (9). The past two decades have seen the advent of immunohistochemistry in surgical pathology, and testicular germ cell tumors have been the subject of many studies that have resulted in important findings that are diagnostically helpful in some situations. Cytogenetic and deoxyribonucleic acid (DNA) ploidy studies have provided new insights into possible relationships between different morphologic types of germ cell tumors (1,4–8,11,12). Despite these advances, from a practical viewpoint, routine light microscopy remains the bedrock for evaluation of germ cell tumors and other testicular neoplasms. Progress has also been made in the field of sex cord–stromal tumors, with recognition of several new variants within this group (see chapter 6), and many clinicopathologic studies have significantly increased our knowledge of a number of miscellaneous primary, secondary, and hematopoietic neoplasms (see chapter 7). As in any area of diagnostic pathology, the possibility that a mass lesion may represent a non-neoplastic process should be borne in mind, particularly in certain situations, and peculiar non-neoplastic microscopic lesions may also simulate neoplasia (chapter 8). Finally, this Fascicle also includes consideration of scrotal pathology (chapter 9).

EMBRYOLOGY, ANATOMY, AND HISTOLOGY

Several thorough reviews of the embryology (18,21,23,29,32,34,36,37), anatomy (26,29,34, 39), and histology (20,35,38) of the testis may be consulted for more detailed information than the summaries provided here.

Embryology

The primordial and undifferentiated gonad is first detectable at about 4 weeks of gestational age when paired condensations of mesenchyme are identified at either side of the midline, between the mesenteric root and the mesonephros (fig. 1-1, left). These so-called genital or gonadal ridges, at the maximum point of their development, extend from the sixth thoracic to the second sacral segments of the embryo. They are covered by layers of thickened, proliferated celomic epithelium, some of which subsequently migrate into the underlying mesenchyme to develop into the primitive sex cords (fig. 1-1, right). By 6 weeks of development, germ cells have migrated into the developing gonad following a pathway from their initial site of formation in the caudal portion of the wall of the yolk sac, close to the allantois, along the wall of the hindgut and the dorsal root of the mesentery, and from there to the adjacent gonads (fig. 1-2). Such cells are distinctive and recognizable by their high content of placental-like alkaline phosphatase (PLAP) and glycogen. This migration is accomplished by ameboid movement of the germ cells, with the role of an undefined chemotactic factor controversial. It is hypothesized that the

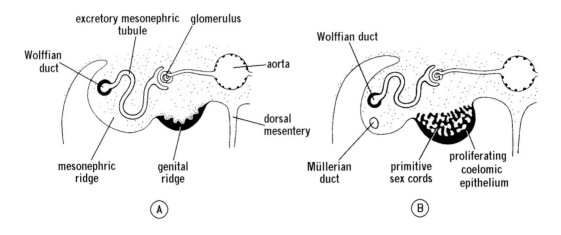

Figure 1-1
EMBRYOLOGY OF TESTIS

Left: At 4 weeks, the genital ridges are apparent as mesenchymal condensations with a covering of coelomic epithelium that has proliferated.

Right: At 6 weeks, there is ingrowth of the coelomic epithelium with extension into the mesenchyme to form the primitive sex cords. (Fig. 11-13 from Langman J. Medical embryology and human development—normal and abnormal, 2nd ed., Baltimore: Williams & Wilkins, 1969:164.)

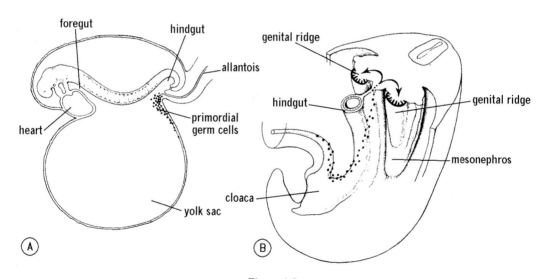

Figure 1-2
EMBRYOLOGY OF TESTIS

Left: At 3 weeks, the primordial germ cells form in the wall of the yolk sac.

Right: At 6 weeks, the primordial germ cells migrate to the wall of the hindgut, along the dorsal mesenteric root, and into the genital ridges. (Fig. 11-14 from Langman J. Medical embryology and human development—normal and abnormal, 2nd ed., Baltimore: Williams & Wilkins, 1969:165.)

occurrence of extragonadal germ cell tumors is explained by the arrested migration of some germ cells to involve such sites as the pineal region, the anterior mediastinum, the sacrococcygeal area, and possibly the retroperitoneum.

In subsequent development, a longitudinal groove forms between the gonadal ridge and the more lateral mesonephric body resulting in a separation of these structures. Under the influence of XY chromosome-containing germ cells,

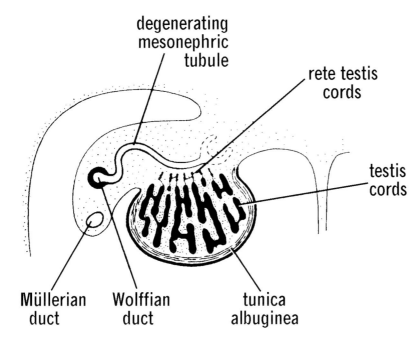

degenerating mesonephric tubule

rete testis cords

testis cords

Müllerian duct

Wolffian duct

tunica albuginea

Figure 1-3
EMBRYOLOGY OF TESTIS
At 8 weeks of gestation, the tunica albuginea surrounds the developing testis, and the rete testis cords intermingle with mesonephric tubules at the hilum. (Fig. 11-15A from Langman J. Medical embryology and human development—normal and abnormal, 2nd ed. Baltimore: Williams & Wilkins, 1969:165.)

continued proliferation of the sex cord epithelium occurs, and by day 42, the developing testis becomes distinct from a developing ovary by virtue of its more prominent sex cord proliferation. It is felt that a testis determining factor, controlled by a gene on the distal short arm of the Y chromosome (31), is responsible for the organization of the indifferent gonad into a testis in males. A key step in the process is the formation of precursors of Sertoli cells, without which the gonad would develop along ovarian lines (28). With continued proliferation, the sex cords penetrate deep into the medulla of the testis and form the testis or medullary cords. These testis cords are, therefore, composed of a dual population of cells: one derived from the primitive sex cords and destined to form the Sertoli cells of the seminiferous tubules and one representing the migrated germ cells that become the spermatogonia of the testis. At this stage (day 42) the anlage of the tunica albuginea is apparent at the periphery of the embryonic testis as a layer of flattened cells. With further development, the testis cords lose their original connection with the surface epithelium, and the tunica albuginea becomes better defined (fig. 1-3). With the formation of distinct testis cords, a third cellular component of the developing testis becomes apparent as the primitive stromal component that occupies the area between the cords. The interstitial (Leydig) cells differentiate from this stromal component, becoming apparent at about 8 weeks. They are particularly prominent between the fourth and sixth months of gestation, only to regress following birth and to reappear at puberty.

Near the hilum of the developing testis, the testis cords break up into a network of very small strands of cells that intermingle with mesonephric cells. The rete testis forms out of these components, although the relative contribution of the sex cords and mesonephros to its structure remains controversial (30). During subsequent development, the rete testis cords merge with portions of the regressing mesonephric tubules and establish the basis for subsequent continuity between the seminiferous tubules and the excretory duct of the mesonephros (wolffian duct) (fig. 1-4). Continued growth of the testis cords, now designated seminiferous cords, results in a looped configuration, with the ends of the loops developing into the narrow tubuli recti. The seminiferous cords remain solid until spermatogenesis begins at puberty at which time lumens develop within the cords to produce seminiferous tubules. At this time, continuity is established between the tubuli recti and the tubules of the rete testis.

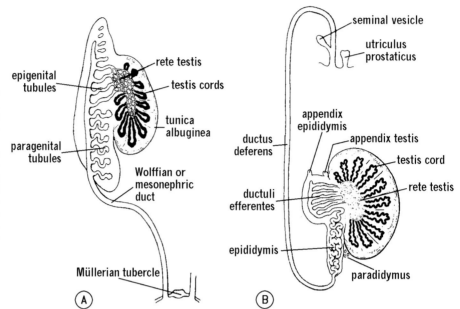

Figure 1-4
EMBRYOLOGY OF TESTIS
Left: By 4 months of gestation, the rete testis cords have merged with the epigenital tubules of the mesonephros.
Right: Diagram of the mature testis after descent showing the relationships of various structures. (Fig. 11-18 from Langman J. Medical embryology and human development—normal and abnormal, 2nd ed. Baltimore: Williams & Wilkins, 1969:169.)

The initially elongated configuration of the developing testis becomes contracted to a more adult-like ovoid form by about 8 weeks of gestation; at this time the testis extends from the diaphragm to the site of the abdominal inguinal ring. During subsequent development, the testis attains a position in the iliac fossa near the internal inguinal ring until descent, which normally begins at the seventh month. The excretory ducts of the testis develop as some of the mesonephric tubules (epigenital tubules) establish continuity with the cords of the rete testis to become the efferent ductules (fig. 1-4). Just caudal to the efferent ductules, the mesonephric or wolffian duct, under the trophic influence of testosterone, becomes briefly elongated and convoluted, forming thereby the body and tail of the epididymis, while the efferent ductules form the head (fig. 1-4). The remaining portion of the mesonephric duct forms the ductus (vas) deferens. Vestigial remnants of the cranial portion of the mesonephric duct may persist as the appendix epididymis (figs. 1-4, 1-5). Mullerian-inhibiting substance, a glycoprotein produced by the fetal Sertoli cells, causes the mullerian (paramesonephric) duct to regress as early as day 51. A small remnant of the mullerian duct often persists on the anterior-superior surface of the testis, near the head of the epididymis, as the appendix testis (figs. 1-4, 1-5).

Descent of the testis begins at about 7 months' gestation, at which time the gonad occupies a retroperitoneal position in the iliac fossa. As the testes move caudally toward the embryonic scrotal swellings, two outpouchings of the peritoneal cavity, the vaginal processes, protrude through the inguinal canal into the twin scrotal sacs. Both testes follow this pathway, but remain retroperitoneal, and localize within the scrotum. Obliterative changes subsequently occur in the upper portions of the vaginal processes, whereas the caudal-most portions of these processes continue to invest the testes as the tunicae vaginalis. Incomplete obliteration of the processus vaginalis permits the intrascrotal leakage of peritoneal fluid and the formation of a hydrocele.

Anatomy

The adult testis is normally located in one of two testicular compartments within the scrotal sac. It is ovoid, has an average weight of 19 to 20 g (22), and measures approximately 4–5 x 2.5 x 3 cm. It is surrounded, over most of its area, by a peritoneal sac, the tunica vaginalis. The external surface of the tunica albuginea is lined by peritoneal-derived mesothelium that constitutes the visceral layer of the tunica vaginalis (fig. 1-6). A small amount of serous fluid may be present in the space of the tunica vaginalis. The tunica albuginea is a tough, fibrous coating which invests

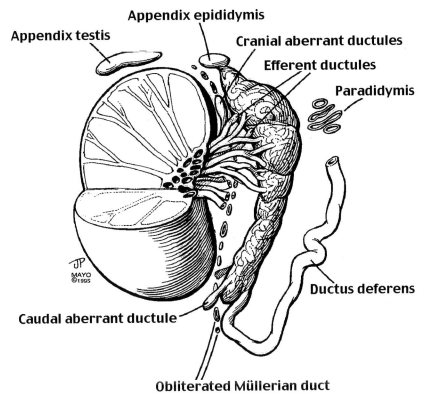

Appendix testis

Appendix epididymis

Cranial aberrant ductules

Efferent ductules

Paradidymis

Ductus deferens

Caudal aberrant ductule

Obliterated Müllerian duct

Figure 1-5
ANATOMY OF TESTIS
Diagram of testicular anatomy, with vestigial embryonic remnants. Note the appendix testis, the appendix epididymis, the aberrant ductules, and the paradidymis. The efferent ductules of the epididymis enter the testis at the hilum. (Fig. 12-1 from Bostwick DG. Spermatic cord and testicular adnexa. In: Bostwick DG, Eble JN, eds. Urologic surgical pathology. St. Louis: Mosby, 1997:646–73.)

the testis. The epididymis is closely applied to the testis, with the epididymal head being present superomedially and the tail posterolaterally (fig. 1-5).

The testicular parenchyma is homogeneous and light tan, consisting of densely packed seminiferous tubules arranged in poorly defined lobules separated by thin fibrous septa. The terminal portion of the seminiferous tubules empty into the tubuli recti (or straight tubules) that then connect with the tubules of the rete testis at the testicular hilum. Although a portion of the rete testis tubules intermingles with the structures of the testicular parenchyma near the hilum, the majority of the rete testis is surrounded by an intratesticular extension of dense fibrous tissue of the tunica albuginea at the testicular hilum; this combination of rete testis and fibrous tissue constitutes the mediastinum testis (fig. 1-6). The rete testis tubules anastomose with 15 to 20 efferent ductules (or ductuli efferentes) that penetrate the tunica albuginea and coil to form the head of the epididymis (figs. 1-4, 1-5). These tubules are in continuity with the epididymal duct of the body and tail, which in turn drains into the vas (ductus) deferens. The vas deferens exits the scrotum through the inguinal canal as one of the structures of the spermatic cord. Vestigial tubular structures include the appendix testis (figs. 1-4, 1-5), derived from the regressed mullerian duct; the appendix epididymis (figs. 1-4, 1-5), derived from the cranial portion of the mesonephric duct; the ductuli aberrantes (vas aberrans of Haller) (fig. 1-5), derived from mesonephric remnants; and the paradidymis (figs. 1-4, 1-5), derived from the caudal portion of the mesonephric tubules (the paragenital tubules).

The major arterial supply to the testis is derived from the testicular artery, which most commonly originates from the aorta, slightly inferior to the renal artery. It passes through the inguinal ring with the other structures of the spermatic cord. As the testicular artery approaches the testis, it gives off two branches to supply the head (the anterior epididymal artery) and the body and tail (the posterior epididymal artery) of the epididymis, often further subdivides into two or three branches, and penetrates the tunica albuginea of the posterior testis (fig. 1-7). These branches then run along the surface of the testis,

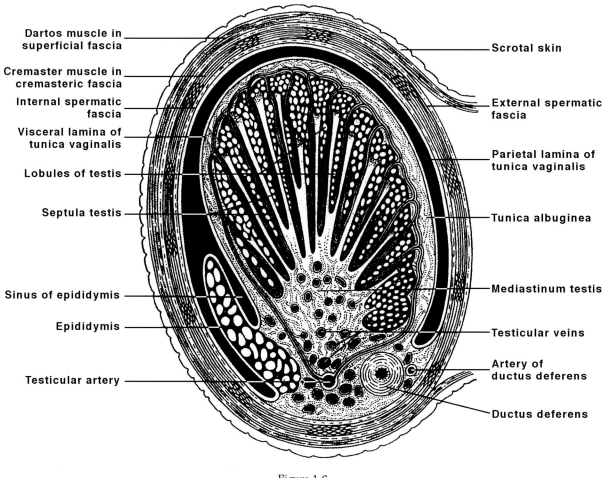

Figure 1-6
ANATOMY OF TESTIS
Cross sectional diagram of testicular anatomy at the level of the mediastinum testis. There is accentuation of the space between the parietal and visceral layers of the tunica vaginalis. (Fig. 8.38 from Romanes GJ, ed. Cunningham's textbook of anatomy, 12th ed. Oxford: Oxford University Press, 1981:555.)

giving off penetrating branches at intervals (centripetal arterial branches) to supply the testicular parenchyma (fig. 1-7). They cannot be visualized through the tunica albuginea, and since there is a risk of vascular damage to the testis when performing testicular biopsies in this area, these procedures are usually performed at the anterosuperior aspect of the testis, an area less likely to contain a surface arterial branch. The artery of the vas deferens provides a second source of blood to the testis. It is derived as a branch of the superior vesical artery, supplies the vas deferens, and may anastomose with the main testicular artery or the posterior epididymal branch of the testicular artery.

The venous drainage of the testis occurs through a series of small veins that interconnect and exit the testis as four to eight branches at the mediastinum. Other small veins may run beneath the tunica albuginea and connect with the venous branches at the mediastinum testis. These venous structures then form a convoluted mass of veins, the pampiniform plexus, that invests the testicular artery (fig. 1-7). Eventually, anastomoses occur and reduce the number of veins to one on the right side and one or two on the left side. The right testicular vein usually empties into the inferior vena cava slightly below the ostium of the right renal vein. The left testicular vein(s) most commonly drains into the left renal vein.

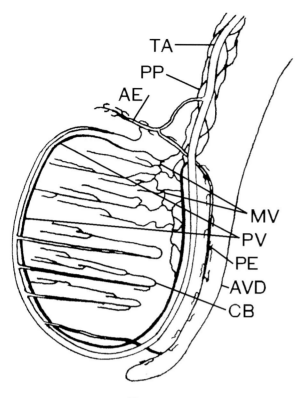

Figure 1-7
VASCULAR SUPPLY OF TESTIS

Schematic diagram of the arterial supply and venous drainage of the testis. See the text for details. Abbreviations: AE - anterior epididymal artery; AVD - artery of the vas deferens; CB - centripetal artery branch; MV - mediastinal venous plexus; PE - posterior epididymal artery; PP - pampiniform venous plexus; PV - peripheral veins; TA - testicular artery. (Fig. 22-2 from Wheeler JE. Anatomy, embryology and physiology of the testis and its ducts. In: Hill GS, ed. Uropathology, New York: Churchill-Livingstone, 1989:935–54.)

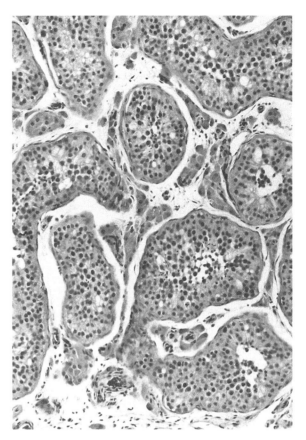

Figure 1-8
NORMAL HISTOLOGY OF ADULT TESTIS

Clusters of Leydig cells, small vessels, and spindle-shaped stromal cells are present in the interstitium between seminiferous tubules showing active spermatogenesis with germ cells and Sertoli cells.

The difference in the venous drainage between the right and left testis, with an increased hydrostatic pressure on the left side due to its right-angle anastomosis with the renal vein, is a frequently cited explanation for the predominance of left-sided varicocele when that disorder is unilateral.

Histology

The visceral layer of the tunica vaginalis consists of a layer of flattened mesothelium on a supporting basement membrane that is applied to the external aspect of the dense fibrous tissue of the tunica albuginea. Ducts, nerves, and vessels enter and exit the testis at the posterior aspect, where the tunica albuginea is thickened

and forms the mediastinum testis. Thin fibrous septa project from the inner aspect of the tunica albuginea (sometimes known as the tunica vasculosa because of its prominent vascularity), across the parenchyma to the mediastinum testis to subdivide the testis into lobules consisting of one to four convoluted seminiferous tubules. An average testis is subdivided into 200 to 300 such lobules, with a total testicular content of 400 to 600 seminiferous tubules, each 30 to 80 cm long. Lennox and colleagues (27) have estimated the total combined length of seminiferous tubules in both testes at 300 to 980 m. Small blood vessels, lymphatics, scattered macrophages, testosterone-producing interstitial (Leydig) cells, and spindle-shaped stromal cells are present between the seminiferous tubules (fig. 1-8).

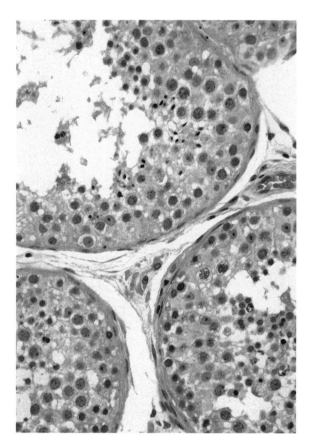

Figure 1-9
NORMAL HISTOLOGY OF TESTIS
Portions of three seminiferous tubules with Sertoli cells, spermatogonia, primary spermatocytes with mitotic figures, spermatids, and spermatozoa.

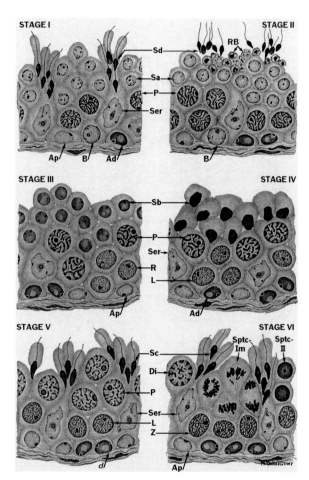

Figure 1-10
SPERMATOGENESIS
Drawing of different cell types in the seminiferous tubules during different stages of spermatogenesis. Note Sertoli cells (Ser); type A spermatogonia (Ap and Ad); type B spermatogonia (B); primary spermatocytes in stages of meiosis (R - resting, L - leptotene, Z - zygotene, P - pachytene, Di - diplotene, Sptc Im - division); secondary spermatocytes (Sptc II); spermatids (Sa, Sb, Sc, and Sd), and residual bodies (RB). (Fig. 3 from Clermont Y. The cycle of the seminiferous epithelium in man. Am J Anat 1963: 112:35–51.)

Each seminiferous tubule is surrounded by a thin layer of connective tissue and a well-defined basement membrane that separate the seminiferous epithelium from the underlying connective tissue, the lamina propria of the testis. Three to five layers of flattened, contractile cells with features of smooth muscle (myoid cells) are present in the lamina propria. Actin and desmin can be demonstrated in these cells, and it is felt that they play a critical role in the movement of spermatozoa into the ductal system of the testis. The seminiferous epithelium is composed of two basic cell types: the Sertoli cells and the various spermatogenic cells (fig. 1-9).

Sertoli cells are roughly triangular, columnar, or elongated and extend the entire thickness of the seminiferous epithelium, from the basement membrane to the luminal surface (fig. 1-10). In hematoxylin and eosin–stained preparations, Sertoli cells have an ill-defined, lightly eosinophilic cytoplasm, a nucleus with fine chromatin, and a moderate-sized, round nucleolus. Notches in the nuclear membrane are common (fig. 1-10) (19). By electron microscopy, Sertoli cells have extremely intricate cytoplasmic processes (fig. 1-11) that completely surround the adjacent spermatogenic cells. A distinctive ultrastructural feature in human Sertoli cells of postpubertal subjects is the presence of long, spindle-shaped inclusions in

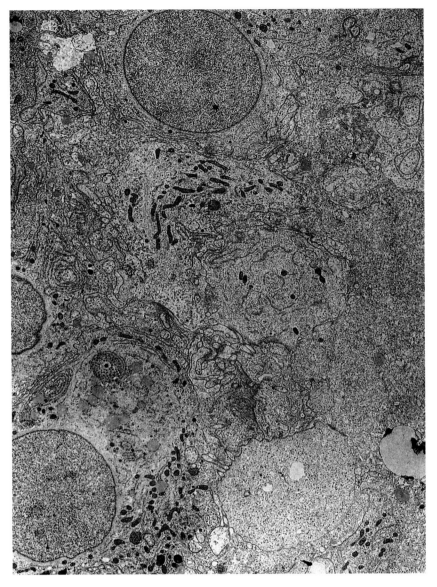

Figure 1-11
SERTOLI CELLS
Electron micrograph of Sertoli cells showing intricate, interdigitating cytoplasmic processes. Cell at bottom left has numerous lipid droplets and annulate lamellae (X5,500).

the basal and perinuclear aspect of the cytoplasm, known as Charcot-Böttcher filaments or inclusion bodies (fig. 1-12). Adjacent Sertoli cells are joined by long tight junctions where the membranes undergo fusion; this resultant structure is considered to be responsible for the maintenance of a blood-testis barrier (35). Lipid droplets and a well-developed smooth endoplasmic reticulum are consistent with the steroid hormone–synthesizing capacity of Sertoli cells (fig. 1-12). Sertoli cells, in addition to providing a "nurturing" function for the maturing germ cell population, are also phagocytic and may contain fragments of degenerated germ cells.

The spermatogonia are the first cells of spermatogenesis and occupy a basal position in the seminiferous tubules adjacent to the basement membrane. Two types of spermatogonia are described: type A, which serve as self-renewing stem cells and type B, derived from mitotic division of type A spermatogonia but which later differentiate, after additional mitotic divisions, to more mature spermatogenic cells, primary spermatocytes (19). Type A spermatogonia have an ovoid nucleus, one or two nucleoli adjacent to the nuclear membrane, a finely granular chromatin, and generally pale cytoplasm (fig. 1-10). Type B spermatogonia have a more round nucleus, clumps

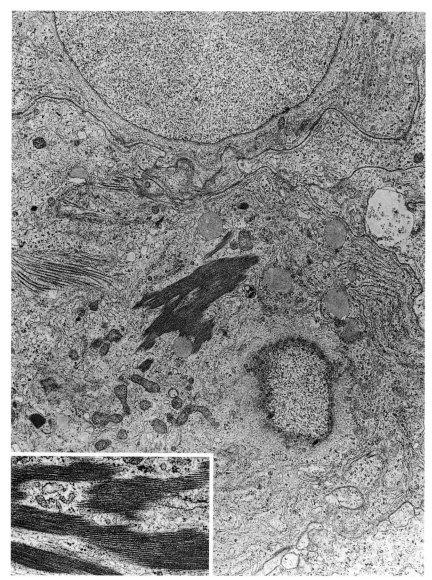

Figure 1-12
SERTOLI CELL
Sertoli cell with prominent, juxtanuclear Charcot-Böttcher filaments, cytoplasmic lipid droplets, and cisternae of smooth and rough endoplasmic reticulum (X13,000). Inset shows characteristic parallel arrangement of Charcot-Böttcher filaments (X38,750).

of peripheral nuclear chromatin, and a single, central nucleolus (fig. 1-10) (19). The primary spermatocytes are tetraploid cells that occupy the cell layers just luminal to the basal layer of spermatogonia and participate in meiotic division to give rise to the distinctive, filamentous chromatin patterns of a prolonged prophase (fig. 1-10). The product of the first meiotic division of a primary spermatocyte is the secondary spermatocyte, which contains a diploid amount of DNA but a haploid number of chromosomes. These cells are rarely observed in sections because they rapidly undergo a second meiotic division to form the haploid spermatids, the

early forms of which they closely resemble. The early spermatid is recognized on the luminal aspect of the primary spermatocyte layer as a round cell with finely granular, pale chromatin, and a nuclear diameter of about 6 μm (fig. 1-10). Spermatids gradually transform, in the process of spermiogenesis, into spermatozoa as the nuclear chromatin condenses and the nucleus becomes oval to pear shaped (fig. 1-10). A given cross-section of a seminiferous tubule may not show complete spermatogenesis because of the wave-like pattern of maturation that occurs within the seminiferous tubules. Examination of many cross-sections is therefore necessary before a

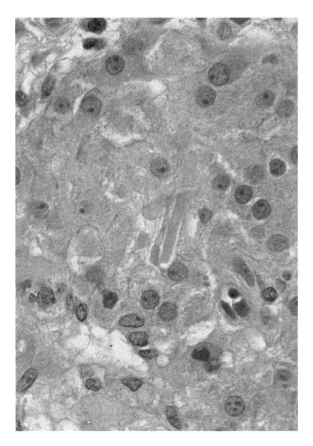

Figure 1-13
LEYDIG CELLS

Cluster of Leydig cells in the testicular interstitium. Note the round, eccentrically placed nuclei, round nucleoli, and abundant eosinophilic cytoplasm. There are rod-shaped, intracytoplasmic Reinke crystals with surrounding retraction artifact (center).

conclusion concerning pathologic maturation arrest is indicated, and some investigators have concluded that "maturation arrest" is actually an artifact of this pattern in patients with hypospermatogenesis (24).

The interstitium of the testis comprises the space between the seminiferous tubules, and is occupied by blood vessels, lymphatics, loose connective tissue, mast cells, and Leydig cells. Leydig cells are normally scant in number from just after the neonatal period to puberty, at which time Leydig cell proliferation occurs and large numbers of them are present. Leydig cells characteristically occur in clusters and vary from round or polygonal to ovoid. They have a round nucleus with a central nucleolus and eosinophilic, sometimes vacuolated cytoplasm

that, in postpubertal patients, often contains lipochrome pigment (fig. 1-13). In addition, rod-shaped crystals (crystals of Reinke), measuring up to 20 µm in length, may be identified in some Leydig cells (fig. 1-13). These crystals have characteristic geometric configurations on ultrastructural examination (fig. 1-14) and apparently contain protein and lipid substances, but their precise functional significance, if any, remains unclear. Large numbers of vesicles of smooth endoplasmic reticulum, mitochondria with tubular cristae, and lipid droplets, characteristics of steroid hormone–producing cells, occupy the cytoplasm of Leydig cells (fig. 1-14). Leydig cells synthesize testosterone and other steroid hormones. In addition to occurring in the interstitium between seminiferous tubules, Leydig cells may also be seen in the testicular mediastinum, within the tunica albuginea, and in the paratesticular soft tissues, including those associated with the epididymis and vas deferens. Such "ectopic" Leydig cells are often identified in close association with small nerves (fig. 1-15) (25).

The straight tubules (tubuli recti) are lined by a cuboidal epithelium and lack the Sertoli cells characteristic of seminiferous tubules. They run a short distance to empty into the branching channels of the rete testis that, for the most part, are invested by the dense connective tissue of the mediastinum testis (fig. 1-16), although occasional tubules of the rete testis are present among the seminiferous tubules adjacent to the testicular mediastinum. The tubules of the rete testis are lined by an epithelium varying from cuboidal to columnar, with frequently grooved nuclei. Occasional tufts of the underlying connective tissue of the mediastinum testis project as epithelial-lined papillae into the lumens of the rete testis and are known as the chordae retis. The tubules of the rete testis empty into the efferent ductules, a group of 8 to 12 tubular channels that are interposed between the rete testis and the epididymal tubules (fig. 1-17). These tubules comprise part of the head of the epididymis and are lined by pseudostratified, columnar epithelium with foci of interspersed cuboidal epithelium, a pattern that produces a characteristic undulating luminal surface. Intracytoplasmic lipofuscin occurs in the epithelium of the efferent ductules. A small amount of circular smooth muscle is closely applied to the

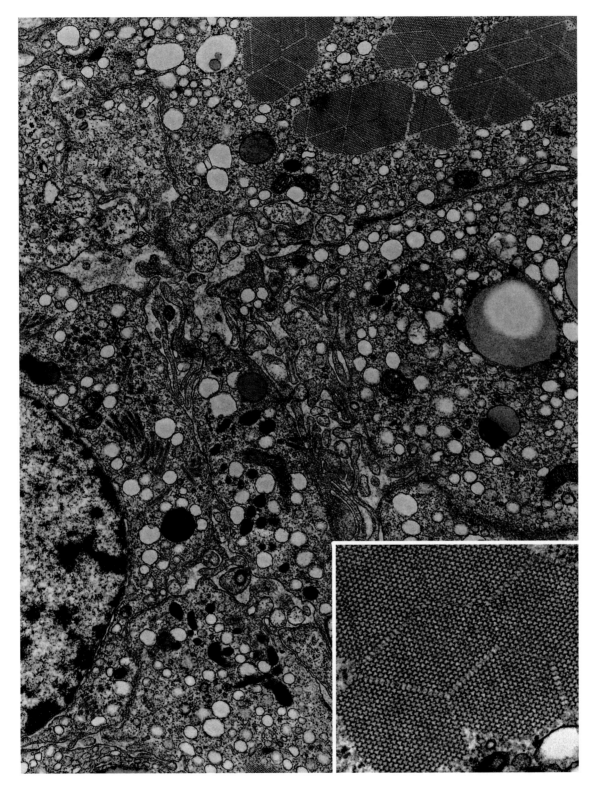

Figure 1-14
LEYDIG CELLS

A cluster of Leydig cells shows prominent vesicles of smooth endoplasmic reticulum, lipid droplets, lysosomes, and characteristic geometric patterns of Reinke crystals (X16,500). Inset shows the striking periodicity of the Reinke crystals (X52,500).

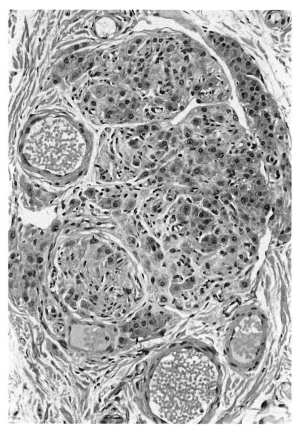

Figure 1-15
LEYDIG CELLS
Clusters of Leydig cells are normally present in the paratesticular soft tissues, usually associated with small nerves.

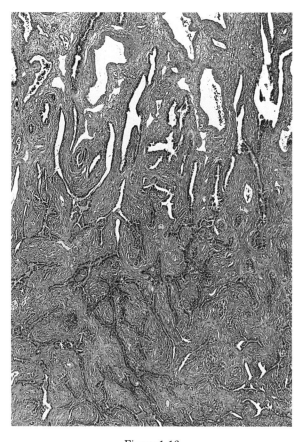

Figure 1-16
RETE TESTIS
Branching tubules of the rete testis are set in the dense, hypocellular fibrous stroma of the mediastinum testis.

basal aspect of the epithelium of the efferent ductules, and is separated from it only by a basement membrane and scant connective tissue.

The efferent ductules empty into a highly convoluted tubule, the ductus epididymis, that forms the body and tail of the epididymis. Cross sections of the convoluted epididymal duct produce multiple profiles often referred to as epididymal tubules. These epididymal tubules are lined by two layers of cells: a basal layer of smaller cells with spherical nuclei and a luminal layer of tall, columnar cells (the principal cells) with elongate nuclei. Unlike the efferent ductules, the epididymal tubules have a smooth luminal surface that is punctuated by long stereocilia (fig. 1-18, left), long branching microvilli that are artifactually aggregated in routine histologic preparations. A small amount of concentrically arranged smooth muscle cells invests

this highly convoluted epididymal duct. Cribriform arrangements of the epithelium may sometimes occur (fig. 1-19). Periodic acid-Schiff (PAS)–positive, intranuclear inclusions are present in the principal cells as well as the epithelium of the vasa deferentia and seminal vesicles. Other findings in the normal epididymis include cytoplasmic lipofuscin granules, foci of Paneth cell–like metaplasia (fig. 1-20) (27a,32a), intranuclear cytoplasmic inclusions, and focal moderate to severe nuclear atypia (fig. 1-18, right) (33). The epididymal duct in turn joins the ductus (vas) deferens at the tail of the epididymis. The epithelium of the ductus deferens is similar to that of the epididymal duct, and stereocilia are visible along its luminal surface. Thick layers of smooth muscle comprise the wall of the ductus deferens: an innermost longitudinally oriented layer, a middle circular layer, and an outermost longitudinal

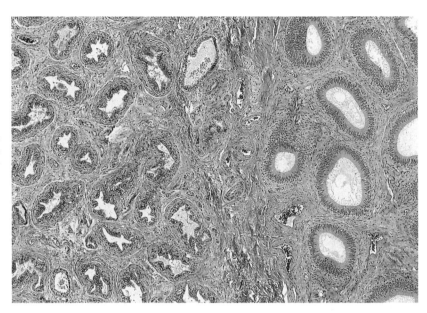

Figure 1-17
EPIDIDYMIS
The efferent ductules (left) have an undulating luminal surface unlike the straight luminal border of the epididymal tubules (right).

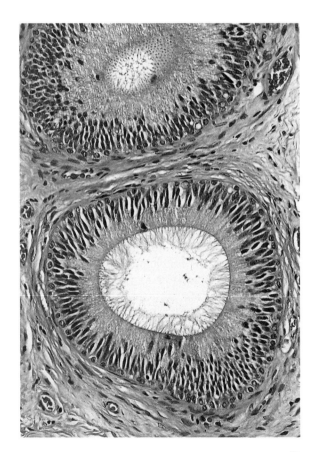

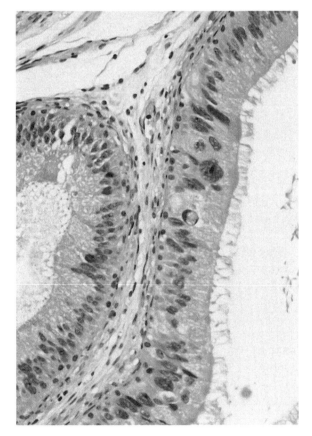

Figure 1-18
EPIDIDYMIS
Left: Epididymal tubules lined by an innermost layer of tall columnar cells with luminal stereocilia and a much less conspicuous layer of basal cells.
Right: Focal nuclear atypia, a normal variant.

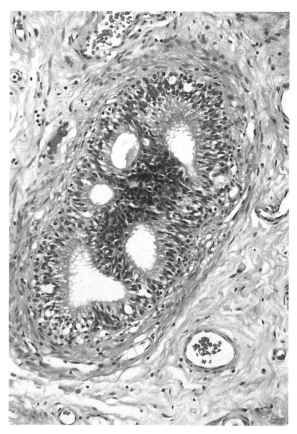

Figure 1-19
EPIDIDYMIS
Cribriform pattern of the epithelium, a normal variant.

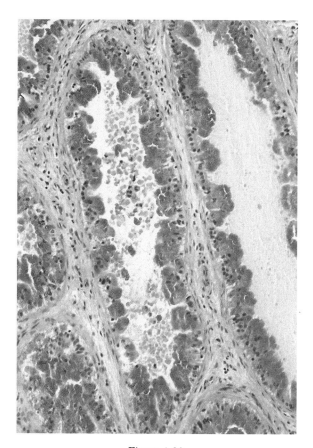

Figure 1-20
EPIDIDYMIS
Paneth cell-like metaplasia of the epithelium, a normal variant.

layer. These are applied closely to the epithelium of the ductus with only a thin layer of connective tissue separating them.

CLASSIFICATION

Table 1-1 provides a classification of testicular neoplasms and also non-neoplastic lesions that may, either clinically or pathologically, mimic neoplasms. There is a lack of uniformity in the classification of testicular germ cell tumors, with two major systems currently in widespread use, one formulated by the WHO and the other proposed by the British Testicular Tumour Panel (BTTP). The classification of testicular germ cell tumors used here (Table 1-1) is a modification of the WHO classification which, in turn, is derived largely from the work of Friedman and Moore (45), Dixon and Moore (41,42), Melicow (46), and Mostofi and Price (48). The fundamental tenet of

this classification is that all of the different morphologic types of germ cell tumor are derived from neoplastic germ cells that differentiate along various pathways. The close association of virtually all of the morphologic types of germ cell tumor (except for spermatocytic seminoma) with the lesion designated "intratubular germ cell neoplasia, unclassified" (see chapter 2) provides convincing support for this viewpoint.

The classification system of the BTTP (49) represents a modification of that originally proposed in 1964 by Collins and Pugh (40). A comparison of some of the entities in the WHO-based system and the equivalent British nomenclature is provided in Table 1-2. In the British system testicular neoplasms are classified as either seminoma or teratoma, with further subdivision of the teratoma category into undifferentiated, intermediate, and trophoblastic. These two basic

Table 1-1

CLASSIFICATION OF TESTICULAR AND PARATESTICULAR TUMORS AND TUMOR-LIKE LESIONS

Germ Cell Tumors
 Precursor lesions
  Intratubular germ cell neoplasia, unclassified
  Intratubular germ cell neoplasia, specific types
 Germ cell tumors of one histologic type
  Seminoma
   Variant: with syncytiotrophoblast cells
  Spermatocytic seminoma
   Variant: with sarcomatous component
 Embryonal carcinoma
 Yolk sac tumor (endodermal sinus tumor)
 Trophoblastic tumors
  Choriocarcinoma
  Placental site trophoblastic tumor
  Unclassified
 Teratoma
  Mature teratoma
   Variant: dermoid cyst
  Immature teratoma
  Teratoma with a secondary malignant
   component (specify)
  Monodermal teratoma
   Carcinoid
   Primitive neuroectodermal tumor
   Others
 Germ cell tumors of more than one histologic type
  Mixed germ cell tumors (specify individual
    components and estimate their amount as
    percentage of the tumor)
   Polyembryoma
   Diffuse embryoma
 Regressed ("burnt out") germ cell tumors
  Scar only
  Scar with intratubular germ cell neoplasia
  Scar with minor residual germ cell tumor
   (teratoma, seminoma, or other)

Germ Cell –Sex Cord–Stromal Tumors
 Gonadoblastoma
 Unclassified

Sex Cord–Stromal Tumors
 Sertoli-stromal cell tumors
  Sertoli cell tumor
   Variants: large cell calcifying
       sclerosing
  Sertoli-Leydig cell tumor
  Leydig cell tumor

 Granulosa-stromal cell tumors
  Granulosa cell tumor
   Variants: adult
        juvenile
  Tumors in the fibroma-thecoma group
 Mixed
 Unclassified

Tumors of the Rete Testis
 Adenoma/Adenofibroma/Cystadenoma
 Carcinoma

Miscellaneous (including unclassified tumors and
  tumors of uncertain cell type)

Paratesticular Tumors (including tumors of
  spermatic cord)*
 Tumors of ovarian epithelial type
 Adenomatoid tumor
 Malignant mesothelioma
 Desmoplastic small round cell tumor
 Epididymal cystadenoma
 Epididymal carcinoma
 Melanotic neuroectodermal tumor (retinal
  anlage tumor)
 Benign (or locally aggressive) soft tissue-type tumors
  Fibromatous tumors
  Vascular tumors
  Aggressive angiomyxoma
  Angiomyofibroblastoma
  Calcifying fibrous pseudotumor
  Others
 Malignant soft tissue-type tumors
  Rhabdomyosarcoma
   Embryonal
    Variant: spindle cell
   Alveolar
   Others
  Liposarcoma
   Well-differentiated
   Pleomorphic/round cell
   Others
  Leiomyosarcoma
  Others
 Miscellaneous

Hematopoietic Tumors
 Lymphoma
 Plasmacytoma
 Leukemia and granulocytic sarcoma

Secondary Tumors

* Some of these tumors may rarely be primary in the testis.

Table 1-1

CLASSIFICATION OF TESTICULAR AND
PARATESTICULAR TUMORS AND TUMOR-LIKE LESIONS (Continued)

Tumor-Like Lesions
    Leydig cell hyperplasia
    Sertoli cell nodules
    Testicular tumor of the adrenogenital syndrome
    Steroid cell nodules with other disorders
    Adrenal cortical rests
    Torsion/infarct (of testis, of appendix testis, of
        appendix epididymis)
    Hematoma/hematocele
    Testicular appendages and Walthard nests
    Orchitis/epididymitis
        Infectious (bacterial, viral, granulomatous)
        Idiopathic granulomatous
        Granulomatous epididymitis
        Sarcoidosis
        Malakoplakia
    Rosai-Dorfman disease (sinus histiocytosis with
        massive lymphadenopathy)
    Hydrocele-related changes

Inflammatory pseudotumor (proliferative funiculitis)
Fibrous pseudotumor
Meconium periorchitis
Mesothelial hyperplasia
Sclerosing lipogranuloma
Abnormalities related to sexual precocity
Idiopathic hypertrophy
Hyperplasia of the rete testis
Epidermoid cyst
Other cysts (parenchymal, rete, of tunics, epididymal)
Cystic dysplasia
Microlithiasis
Spermatocele
Sperm granuloma
Vasitis nodosa
Splenic-gonadal fusion
Others

Table 1-2

COMPARISON OF NOMENCLATURE OF THE WHO-BASED SYSTEM
AND THE BRITISH TESTICULAR TUMOUR PANEL (BTTP) CLASSIFICATION*

Modified WHO Classification	BTTP Classification
Tumors of One Histologic Type	———
Seminoma	Seminoma
Spermatocytic seminoma	Spermatocytic seminoma
Embryonal carcinoma	Malignant teratoma, undifferentiated (MTU)
Yolk sac tumor	Yolk sac tumour (pure neoplasms only)
Teratoma	
Mature	Teratoma, differentiated (TD)
Immature	TD
With a sarcomatous or carcinomatous component	Malignant teratoma, intermediate (MTI)
Choriocarcinoma (pure)	Malignant teratoma, trophoblastic (MTT)
Mixed Germ Cell Tumors	———
Embryonal carcinoma and mature and/or immature teratoma	MTI
Yolk sac tumor and mature and/or immature teratoma	MTI
Seminoma and teratoma	Combined tumor (seminoma and TD)
Seminoma and embryonal carcinoma	Combined tumor (seminoma and MTU)
Choriocarcinoma and embryonal carcinoma	MTT
Choriocarcinoma and teratoma	MTT
Choriocarcinoma and seminoma	Combined tumor (MTT and seminoma)

*Adapted from references 47 and 50.
From: Ulbright TM, Roth LM. Testicular and paratesticular neoplasms. In: Sternberg SS, ed. Diagnostic surgical pathology. New York: Raven Press, 1994:1885-1947.

categories are based on the concept of Willis (52) that seminomas are of germ cell origin but the other tumor types are derived from displaced embryonic blastomeres that escaped developmental organization. The association of intratubular germ cell neoplasia with both seminoma and "teratoma" of the British system, however, contradicts the blastomere theory of histogenesis of the latter. While histogenetic correctness is important in formulating a system of classification, meaningful clinicopathologic distinctions between entities remain of paramount concern. Mostofi (47) has pointed out that with the use of the British system there is a loss of information correlating certain histologic features with specific serum tumor markers and a tendency for "lumping" entities that may have different biologic behaviors. For instance, in the British system, malignant teratoma intermediate encompasses both tumors composed of embryonal carcinoma and teratoma as well as those composed of yolk sac tumor and teratoma. It is, however, worthwhile categorizing these entities separately, given the close association of yolk sac tumor with elevations of serum alpha-fetoprotein (51), the apparent increased aggressiveness of embryonal carcinoma (43), and the possible negative correlation of yolk sac tumor elements with occult metastases in clinical stage I patients (44). Furthermore, comparison of the effectiveness of various therapies is hindered if a uniform system of classification is not used. For these reasons, the modified WHO system is recommended by us and is widely accepted by urologists and oncologists in the United States and numerous other countries.

PATTERNS OF SPREAD AND METASTASIS IN TESTICULAR CANCER

The tunica albuginea is a difficult barrier for testicular cancers to penetrate. Most testicular neoplasms extend into the paratesticular structures by way of the mediastinum testis, but even this is seen uncommonly, with only 10 to 15 percent of malignant testicular tumors involving either the epididymis or spermatic cord (59). Extension into the rete testis is, however, common, being seen in about 80 percent of seminomas in one series (63). Involvement of scrotal skin is an unusual and late event.

Most of the information regarding the distribution of metastases is derived from studies of patients with testicular germ cell tumors, which represent the overwhelming majority (approximately 95 percent) of primary malignant tumors of the testis. However, malignant tumors other than germ cell tumors appear to have similar metastatic patterns (58). Metastases occur via either lymphatic or hematogenous routes. Seminoma tends to spread by lymphatics, with hematogenous metastases usually occurring late in the clinical course. Choriocarcinoma, on the other hand, has a proclivity for early dissemination through blood-borne routes, although nodal metastases also occur. The other nonseminomatous germ cell tumors may show both lymphatic and hematogenous patterns of dissemination, with early cases tending to have mainly lymphatic-based metastases, although recent studies suggest that childhood yolk sac tumor is an exception, with a proclivity for hematogenous metastases (57).

The sites of lymph node metastases depend upon the side of testicular involvement and the presence or absence of paratesticular extension. Neoplasms of the right testis tend to first metastasize to the interaortocaval, retroperitoneal lymph nodes at about the level of the second lumbar vertebral body (59), although precaval and right paracaval involvement may also occur (fig. 1-21). Donohue (55) has noted an essential absence of both suprahilar nodal involvement and left para-aortic involvement below the inferior mesenteric artery in early retroperitoneal metastases from right-sided tumors. The left testis tends to first produce retroperitoneal nodal metastases in the left para-aortic region, an area between the left ureter, left renal vein, aorta, and origin of the inferior mesenteric artery (fig. 1-22) (59). Left pre-aortic involvement is also common, but there is an absence of right paracaval and precaval involvement. Unlike right-sided lesions, early left-sided tumors may produce occasional suprahilar nodal metastases (55). Because of this tendency for selective site involvement in early stage disease, limited retroperitoneal dissections, tailored according to the side of the primary tumor, may now be offered to patients. Limited dissections have allowed a greater number of patients to retain the ability to ejaculate than when more extensive retroperitoneal dissections were performed (54,56).

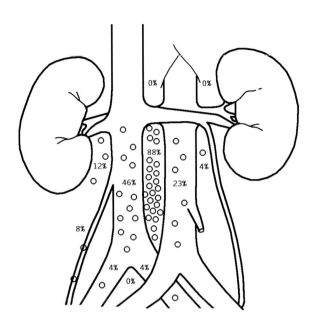

Figure 1-21
PATTERN OF
RETROPERITONEAL METASTASES

This diagram shows the distribution of retroperitoneal metastases in early stage II (B) nonseminomatous germ cell tumors from right-sided testicular lesions. The majority of metastases occur in the interaortocaval and precaval areas. There is an absence of suprahilar involvement and left para-aortic involvement below the level of the inferior mesenteric artery. (Fig. 2 from Donohue JP. Metastatic pathways of nonseminomatous germ cell tumors. Semin Urol 1984;2:217–29.)

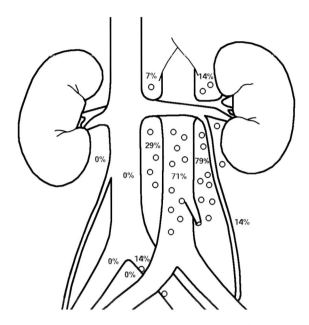

Figure 1-22
PATTERN OF
RETROPERITONEAL METASTASES

This diagram shows the distribution of retroperitoneal metastases in early stage II (B) nonseminomatous germ cell tumors from left-sided testicular lesions. The majority of the metastases occur in the left para-aortic and preaortic areas. There is an absence of precaval, right paracaval, and right iliac involvement. (Fig. 5 from Donohue JP. Metastatic pathways of nonseminomatous germ cell tumors. Semin Urol 1984;2:217–29.)

With more advanced disease, widespread retroperitoneal involvement occurs. Suprahilar involvement occurs with right-sided lesions, and contralateral spread is seen. The likelihood of suprahilar spread increases greatly for left-sided lesions, as does interaortocaval and contralateral (precaval) involvement (55). As the volume of retroperitoneal tumor increases, retrograde metastases develop and iliac and inguinal nodal areas may become involved. Inguinal nodal involvement may also be seen as a consequence of extension of the primary tumor to the scrotal skin or prior inguinal or scrotal surgery. A transscrotal surgical approach in a patient with a possible testicular tumor is therefore contraindicated because of the consequent increase in the potential metastatic field. Involvement of the epididymis may lead to external iliac node involvement. Cephalad dissemination eventually develops, with the occurrence of mediastinal and supraclavicular nodal involvement. In rare cases, mediastinal or supraclavicular metastases may occur in the absence of clinical retroperitoneal involvement (60). If supraclavicular involvement occurs, it is the left supraclavicular area that is affected in 85 percent of the cases (61).

Distant organ metastases are usually the consequence of hematogenous spread, although gastrointestinal tract involvement may result from direct spread of retroperitoneal metastases (62). In an autopsy study of patients with testicular germ cell tumors, 89 percent had pulmonary involvement, 73 percent had liver metastases, 31 percent had brain metastases, and 30 percent had bone metastases (53). In a clinical study, gastrointestinal involvement by metastases from testicular germ cell tumors occurred in only 3.6 percent of the patients (62). Choriocarcinoma is particularly prone to produce brain metastases and seminoma to produce bone metastases (53). The latter are also commonly seen with malignant Sertoli cell tumors.

Table 1-3

COMPARISON OF HISTOLOGIC TYPES OF PRIMARY TESTICULAR GERM CELL TUMORS AND THE TYPES IDENTIFIED IN METASTASES AT AUTOPSY (PRECHEMOTHERAPY DATA)*

| Primary Tumor | Autopsy Findings | | | |
	Seminoma (%)	Embryonal Carcinoma (%)	Teratoma (%)	Choriocarcinoma (%)
Seminoma (N = 23)	74	26	4	9
Embryonal carcinoma (N = 74)**	4	96	8	5
Teratoma (N = 16)**	0	63	63	25
Mixed germ cell tumors (N = 74)	0	80	42	30
Choriocarcinoma (N = 7)	0	0	0	100

*Data from: Dixon FJ, Moore RA. Testicular tumors: a clinicopathologic study. Cancer 1953;6:427–54.
**Pure or with seminoma.

An interesting and important aspect of testicular germ cell tumors is the marked tendency of metastatic lesions to show a different histology from that seen in the primary tumor. This observation antedates the utilization of chemotherapy, as is shown in Table 1-3.

STAGING

Several different systems (Table 1-4) for the staging of testicular tumors are in use, and there is a need for a single, consensus approach. Most staging systems are roughly based on the original work of Boden and Gibb (64) who divided the stages into purely testicular, retroperitoneal, and extraretroperitoneal. Unfortunately, the further modification of these stages, with the creation of subdivisions, has not been uniform, and different institutions have different approaches. While such a situation may not hinder intrainstitutional work, the comparison of prognoses with different forms of therapy between institutions is made difficult because of this lack of uniformity. In some institutions there are entirely separate systems for the staging of seminomatous versus nonseminomatous tumors (67). It is also important to clearly distinguish the methods employed to arrive at the assignment of a given stage, i.e., whether based on clinical-diagnostic methods alone, surgical assessment, postsurgical pathologic evaluation, retreatment staging, or autopsy evaluation (67). With the continued refinement of radiologic and other clinical methods for the evaluation of the extent of disease, there is now less discrepancy between clinical and pathologic stages. Nonetheless, such discrepancies remain common (71,72). For instance, in a study of nonseminomatous germ cell tumors, Klepp et al. (68) noted that 27 percent of patients with clinical stage I disease had retroperitoneal metastases at operation. It, therefore, is imperative that the method of staging be specified so that meaningful comparisons are possible.

We advocate adoption of the TNM staging system of the American Joint Committee on Cancer (AJCC) and the International Union Against Cancer (UICC) (63a,66a). This staging system is displayed in Table 1-4, with elaboration of each T, N, and M category, and further modification based on serologic information (S). T, N, M, and S categories are then grouped into stages 0 to III, as shown. More widespread use of this method, or at least its conjoint use in studies that also employ other staging systems, will be helpful in the assessment of interinstitutional results. Some authorities, however, feel that while the AJCC/UICC method provides a useful approach for nonseminomatous germ cell tumors, it is not as useful in determining meaningful staging subdivisions in patients with seminoma (75).

GROSS EXAMINATION

Orchiectomy specimens should be received fresh and dissected promptly. Many of the diagnostic problems in testicular neoplasia (especially

Table 1-4

STAGING SYSTEMS FOR TESTICULAR CANCER

TNM System[†] (AJCC and UICC)*			Stage Grouping for AJCC/UICC System	
pTx -	Unknown status of testis		Stage 0 -	Tis, N0, M0, S0
pT0 -	No apparent primary (includes scars)		Stage IA -	T1, N0, M0, S0
pTis -	Intratubular tumor, no invasion		Stage IB -	T2-T4, N0, M0, S0
pT1 -	Testis and epididymis only; no vascular invasion or penetration of tunica albuginea		Stage IS -	any T, N0, M0, S1-S3
			Stage IIA -	any T, N1, M0, S0-S1
pT2 -	Testis and epididymis with vascular invasion or through tunica albuginea to involve tunica vaginalis		Stage IIB -	any T, N2, M0, S0-S1
			Stage IIC -	any T, N3, M0, S0-S1
pT3 -	Spermatic cord		Stage IIIA-	any T, any N, M1a, S0-S1
pT4 -	Scrotum		Stage IIIB-	any T, any N, M0-M1a, S2
pNx -	Unknown nodal status		Stage IIIC-	any T, any N, M0-M1a, S3, any T, any N, M1b, any S
pN0 -	No regional node involvement			
pN1 -	Node mass or single nodes ≤2 cm; ≤5 nodes involved (no node >2 cm)			
pN2 -	Node mass >2 but <5 cm; or >5 nodes involved, none >5 cm; or extranodal tumor			
pN3 -	Node mass >5 cm			
Mx -	Unknown status of distant metastases			
M0 -	No distant metastases			
M1a -	Nonregional nodal or lung metastases			
M1b -	Distant metastasis other than nonregional nodal or lung			
SX -	No marker studies available			
S0 -	All marker levels normal			
	LDH**	hCG (mIU/ml)	AFP(ng/ml)	
S1 -	<1.5 X N	+ <5,000	+ <1,000	
S2 -	1.5-10 X N	or 5,000-50,000	or 1,000-10,000	
S3 -	>10 X N	or >50,000	or >10,000	
N = normal value for assay				

Boden/Gibb (64)	Mem. Sloan Kettering Cancer Center	Mass. General (73)
A - Testis only	A - Testis and adnexa	I - Testis only
B - Regional nodal involvement	B - Infradiaphragmatic nodal metastases	II - Retroperipeptoneal involvement
C - Spread beyond retro-peritoneal nodes	B1 - <5 cm	IIA - <2cm
	B2 - 5 - 10 cm	IIB - ≥2 cm
	B3 - >10 cm	IIIB - Supraclavicular and mediastinal
	C - Spread beyond retroperitoneal nodes	involvement

Skinner (74)	M.D. Anderson (67)	Royal Marsden (66, 69)
A - Testis only	I - Testis only	I - Testis only; IM cont. positive serologic evidence of tumor after orchiectomy
B - Infradiaphragmatic involvement	IIA - negative lymphangiogram but pathology positive retroperit. nodes	II - Infradiaphragmatic nodal involvement
B1 - <6 nodes, no extranodal	IIB - Positive lymphangiogram	IIA - <2 cm
B2 - > 6 nodes or any node > 2 cm	IIIA - Supraclavicular nodes	IIB - 2 - 5 cm
B3 - Bulky disease (>5 cm)	IIIB1 - Gynecomastia lacking gross tumor	IIC - >5 cm
C - Supradiaphragmatic involvement	IIIB2 - Lung metastasis (no more than 5 nodules per lung and not >2 cm)	III - Supraclavicular or mediastinal involvement
	IIIB3 - Advanced lung	IV - Extranodal metastases
	IIIB4 - Advanced abdominal or obstructive uropathy	IVL - Lung metastases
	IIIB5 - Visceral disease, excluding lung	IVH - Liver metastases

*Abbreviations: TNM - tumor, nodes, metastases; AFP - alpha-fetoprotein; AJCC - American Joint Committee on Cancer; UICC - International Union Against Cancer; hCG - human chorionic gonadotropin; LDH - lactate dehydrogenase.
**LDH levels expressed as elevations above upper limit of normal (N).
[†]Adapted from references 63a and 65.

the confusion of seminoma with embryonal carcinoma) can be attributed to delayed or incomplete fixation. If the testis is placed intact in fixative and sent to the pathology laboratory, a several-hour delay in dissection may result in suboptimal morphology, since the testicular tunics do not permit ready access of fixative to the neoplasm. If for some reason it is not possible for a specimen to be evaluated promptly by a pathologist, it is preferable for the surgeon to bisect the specimen with a single sagittal cut before placing it in fixative and sending it to the laboratory. This approach is also suboptimal because it prevents the gross inspection of the intact, unfixed specimen by the pathologist and does not allow the harvesting of fresh tissue for ancillary studies. It may also cause difficulty in judging whether the neoplasm has grown through the tunica albuginea, since the tumor may bulge beyond the incision and protrude onto the surface of the tunica albuginea, although close inspection can usually resolve this problem.

A radical orchiectomy is performed for virtually all suspected testicular neoplasms because of the high probability that a testicular mass represents a malignant tumor. The specimen therefore consists of the testis and the surrounding tunica vaginalis, the paratesticular structures (epididymis and soft tissues), and a length of spermatic cord. External inspection of the tunica vaginalis should be performed for possible tumor penetration, followed by opening of the parietal layer of the tunica vaginalis testis. Any fluid present should be measured and described. The length of spermatic cord should be measured, serially cut at regular intervals, and inspected for gross evidence of neoplasm. The proximal cord margin should be separately submitted as one block, any abnormal-appearing areas submitted as additional blocks, or, if no grossly abnormal areas are apparent, a slice from the middle and distal cord submitted. It is best to take sections of the cord before incising the testis in order to avoid the common artifactual contamination of the cord (88). The parietal layer of the tunica vaginalis should then be removed, and the external aspect of the testis inspected and gently palpated, with any abnormalities noted.

The testis should be measured in three dimensions, weighed, and bisected in a sagittal plane from anterior to posterior toward the epididymal head. The cut surface of the neoplasm should be described, its relationship to the tunica albuginea noted, and its size recorded. Foci of hemorrhage and necrosis, translucent cartilage, cysts, fleshy encephaloid areas, and evidence of multifocality should be noted. Special attention should be directed to see if there is paratesticular extension at the mediastinum or invasion of the tunica albuginea. Photographs and samples for electron microscopy, flow cytometry, molecular biologic analyses, and karyotyping studies may be obtained at this point, although these techniques are not required for diagnosis of most cases and are primarily for research purposes. Additional parallel cuts, perpendicular to the original cut, should then be performed at regular intervals, leaving the tunica albuginea intact to hold the specimen together.

The specimen should then be placed in an adequate volume of fixative and allowed to fix thoroughly before the submission of additional blocks; overnight fixation is required for formalin. Ten percent neutral-buffered formalin is a satisfactory fixative but others may be used depending on individual preference. One study noted improved cytologic detail with more acidic fixatives (84a). Adequate fixation is crucial since the distinction of seminoma from nonseminomatous germ cell tumors may primarily depend on cytologic features that may be obscured by poor tissue preservation.

Following fixation, any observations additional to those already made should be noted. Representative blocks of all the different-appearing areas should be submitted, with a minimum number of one block for each centimeter of maximum tumor dimension. Foci with hemorrhage and necrosis should be represented in the sampling, as well as blocks to include the tunica albuginea and subjacent parenchyma. For tumors with the gross appearance of seminoma, we recommend submission of at least 10 blocks of the neoplasm, even if it appears homogeneous, because of the possibility of detecting small foci of nonseminomatous elements that may alter the therapy. Small tumors should be entirely submitted. A representative section of the non-neoplastic testis and the hilum should be submitted, as well as a representative section of any area of testicular scarring.

It should be emphasized that these are general guidelines, and tumors with an extremely variegated gross appearance may require more sections. In addition, in some situations more sections may be required, such as in a patient who appears to have, on initial examination, a pure seminoma but has an elevated alphafetoprotein (AFP) level (87). After the tumor is sampled, the epididymis should be incised by multiple cuts perpendicular to its long axis, any abnormalities noted, and an appropriate block submitted. Germ cell tumors, particularly seminoma and embryonal carcinoma, are friable, making knife implantation on tissue surfaces and into vascular spaces common (88); care during specimen sampling, with the utilization of clean instruments, reduces the frequency of this artifact, which may result in an erroneous diagnosis of extratesticular extension or vascular invasion.

The final pathology report should provide a histologic classification of the neoplasm, an assessment of the presence or absence of lymphatic or blood vessel invasion, information regarding the local extent of the tumor (including the status of the spermatic cord margin) and, for mixed germ cell tumors, an estimate of the percentage of each tumor component (88a).

FROZEN SECTION EXAMINATION

Frozen sections are not routinely required for the management of patients with testicular tumors since the neoplastic nature of the tumor is often evident preoperatively by virtue of serum marker studies and testicular ultrasound, and orchiectomy is required for treatment. If there is clinical ambiguity concerning the neoplastic nature of a testicular mass, frozen section evaluation of a biopsy obtained by an inguinal approach may permit testicular conservation if a clearly benign lesion can be identified (84,85,89). This approach has been applied most frequently to epidermoid cysts (77,83,84), although biopsies for permanent sections of the surrounding testis should also be obtained to exclude intratubular germ cell neoplasia and ensure the diagnosis (79, 80,86). A neoplasm that abuts the tunica albuginea or is entirely paratesticular is more likely to be benign (for example, an adenomatoid tumor) than an intraparenchymal mass, and enucleation of such a neoplasm on the basis of well-prepared frozen sections is justified. Frozen section is particularly likely to be beneficial in allowing con-servative surgical management in cases in which the location and gross appearance of a mass are suggestive of a non-neoplastic process, such as fibromatous periorchitis (see chapter 8). It may also be employed when the patient's age, preoperative evaluation, or both, suggest the likelihood of an unusual, possibly benign, neoplasm as illustrated by a recent case of hemangioma treated conservatively (88b).

Hermanek (81) reviewed the experience with 70 testicular tumors diagnosed by biopsy and frozen section evaluation. This established the correct diagnosis in 81 percent of the cases, and a second biopsy established the correct diagnosis in an additional 11 percent. In four patients no definite diagnosis was established at frozen section, and in one patient a mature teratoma was misinterpreted as an epidermoid cyst, necessitating reoperation with orchiectomy. In our experience with frozen sections on orchiectomy specimens, it is often difficult to subcategorize germ cell tumors with total confidence, but subtyping does not affect surgical management.

CYTOLOGIC EXAMINATION

Cytology does not play a significant role in the diagnosis of primary testicular neoplasms, but aspiration cytology of enlarged lymph nodes or visceral masses is useful in confirming metastases (82). It should be emphasized that a negative result in this context does not exclude a metastasis because of the frequently focal nature of viable metastatic tumor. The distinction of seminoma from nonseminomatous germ cell tumors can generally be made in a reliable fashion (76,78,82), but it may not be possible to distinguish among the various nonseminomatous germ cell tumors (82). Furthermore, at metastatic sites it may not be possible, with cytologic examination alone, to distinguish embryonal carcinoma or yolk sac tumor from undifferentiated carcinoma or poorly differentiated adenocarcinoma of somatic origin (82).

EPIDEMIOLOGY

Most epidemiologic studies utilize medical records or death certificates as diagnostic sources and discuss "testicular cancer" in a generic sense. Because about 95 percent of primary malignant tumors of the testis are germ cell tumors, the

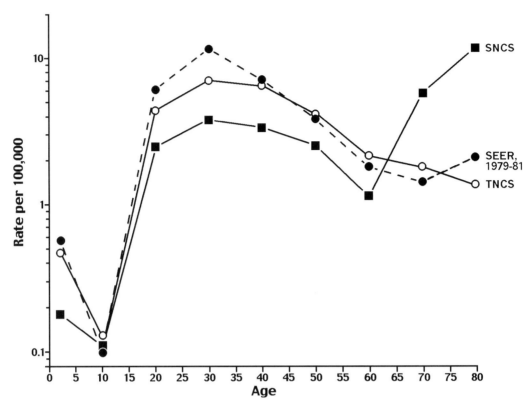

Figure 1-23
INCIDENCE OF TESTICULAR CANCER VERSUS AGE

Three separate studies examining the incidence of testicular cancer with age demonstrate a small peak in infancy, a nadir at 10 years, an increasing incidence following puberty, and a second peak at roughly age 30 years, with a slow decline thereafter. Another peak occurring in some studies in the elderly is not due to germ cell tumors but lymphomas and secondary malignancies. Abbreviations: SNCS - Second National Cancer Survey; TNCS - Third National Cancer Survey; SEER - Surveillance, Epidemiology, and End Results Program. (Fig. 1 from Brown LM, Pottern LM, Hoover RN, Devesa SS, Aselton P, Flannery JT. Testicular cancer in the United States: trends in incidence and mortality. Int J Epidemiol 1986;15:164–70.)

results of these studies generally apply only to germ cell tumors and cannot be extrapolated to other primary malignant testicular tumors. When the patients are restricted to those under 50 years, a relatively pure germ cell tumor population can be expected. However, many of the tumors that occur in older patients and that account for the second peak of the bimodal distribution of testicular cancer (fig. 1-23) are not only not of germ cell origin but are of secondary nature, i.e., lymphomas in patients with extratesticular lymphomas or metastatic carcinomas. For instance, in one study 67 percent of malignant testicular tumors in patients over 70 years old were lymphomas (141). The sex cord-stromal tumors also represent a higher proportion of primary neoplasms in older patients. Epidemiologic studies of testicular germ cell tumors are therefore necessarily flawed if they include the older group of

patients without pathologic verification of the nature of their neoplasms. It seems likely that testicular cancers in childhood, although also predominantly of germ cell origin, are fundamentally different from postpubertal germ cell tumors as they are not generally associated with intratubular germ cell neoplasia of the unclassified type (see chapter 2), are almost always of a pure histologic type, and tend to have a more indolent course. The standard epidemiologic observations on testicular cancer, therefore, do not apply to prepubertal patients.

Testicular cancer is relatively rare, accounting for about 1 percent of malignant neoplasms in males, but is the most common malignancy of young men from 15 to 44 years of age (101). The incidence of testicular cancer rises dramatically around puberty, peaks between 25 and 35 years of age, and slowly declines to a relative nadir near age 60, after which a second peak occurs in some studies in the eighth and ninth decades due to secondary neoplasms involving the testis (fig. 1-23). The current incidence of testicular cancer in the United States is approximately 6 cases per 100,000 of the white male population (133).

Specific subtypes of testicular germ cell tumors tend to occur at different ages. Seminomas characteristically are seen in patients who are roughly 10 years older than those with nonseminomatous germ cell tumors (40.5 years and 31.7 years, respectively [120]). Spermatocytic seminomas occur in a significantly older population (average, 58.8 years [120]). Most epidemiologic studies, however, do not separately analyze the various subtypes.

The incidence of testicular cancer in the United States has increased, for unclear reasons (166), from 46 to 100 percent over the time period from 1936 to 1976 (150); this upward trend is reflected in incidences observed in Denmark (128,139), Norway (119), England (141), Scotland (97), Australia (154), and New Zealand (140). In several northern European countries the incidence has increased at 2 to 5 percent per year throughout various intervals during the last half of the 20th century, leading to a doubling of the age-standardized incidence every 15 to 25 years (90). Some studies noted a leveling of this upward trend in European countries for those born during World War II, only to have the trend continue after the war (96,119). In the Scottish study, the increase was mainly in the nonseminomatous group of tumors (97), but the rates for all types of germ cell tumors increased in Connecticut (166). Another analysis demonstrated a worldwide increase in incidence in both low risk and high risk populations and in age groups characteristically affected by seminomas and nonseminomatous germ cell tumors (113). It is of interest to note that this increase does not appear to apply to pediatric cases but becomes manifest in adolescents (129).

There are wide variations in the incidence of testicular cancer in different countries. The overall annual incidence in the United States is 3.6 (Connecticut) to 4.3 (Seattle) cases per 100,000 male population whereas in Switzerland the annual incidence is as high as 9.3 cases per 100,000 male population, in Denmark 8.5 (139), in Japan (Nagasaki) 1.1, and in Cuba 0.3 (129). White

males in the United States have a higher incidence, 4.7 to 6.3 cases per 100,000 male population (133), than the nonwhite population. Further racial variations are apparent in the United States, with the highest rates in the white population, followed by Hispanics (3.1 per 100,000), Japanese (1.7), blacks (0.9), and Chinese (0.4) (122). There is some evidence for the operation of environmental factors since Hispanics, Japanese, and Chinese who migrate to the United States have incidences intermediate between their country of origin and their country of adoption, although no effect of migration could be demonstrated in the black population (151). The only nonwhite race with a comparably high incidence of testicular cancer is the Maoris of New Zealand (112,163), although native Hawaiians, native Alaskans, and native Americans have higher rates than do other "nonwhite" populations (155). A compilation of testicular cancer incidences for different countries, and in some instances, for racial or ethnic groups within a country, is provided in Table 1-5.

Numerous studies have attempted to identify possible environmental or other etiologic agents in the development of testicular cancers. Several studies have documented an increased risk of testicular cancer in higher socioeconomic classes and in professional workers relative to manual workers (91,103,115,127,131,140,148,155,159). To what extent these data concerning socioeconomic class are skewed by the simultaneous operation of racial (genetic) factors is not clear. Such differences are nonetheless identifiable in cohorts from the early 20th century in England and Wales (103), among populations that would be expected to be relatively homogeneous. At least one study has related the increased frequency of testicular cancer in the higher socioeconomic classes to a higher prevalence of detectable titers of Epstein-Barr virus in this population and hypothesized a possible role for the Epstein-Barr virus in the pathogenesis of testicular germ cell tumors (92). In keeping with this observation, an increased frequency of testicular germ cell tumors, characteristically occurring at a somewhat younger average age, is described in patients with the acquired immunodeficiency syndrome (123,164), as well as in patients with other forms of immunosuppression (123). However, Epstein-Barr virus proteins and nucleic acids are not detected in tumor cells by

Table 1-5

ANNUAL INCIDENCE OF TESTICULAR CANCER IN VARIOUS LOCATIONS PER 100,000 MALE POPULATION*

Switzerland (Basel)	9.3
Switzerland (Zurich)	9.0
Switzerland (Vand)	8.9
Denmark	8.5
Switzerland (Geneva)	7.6
New Zealand, Maori	7.1
Germany (Hamburg)	6.7
USA (California, Alameda County), whites	6.3
USA (Hawaii), whites	6.2
Germany	6.1
Norway	6.1
USA (San Francisco Bay area), whites	5.9
Switzerland (Neuchatel)	5.6
New Zealand, non-Maori	5.6
France (Bas-Rhin)	5.1
USA (Connecticut), whites	4.7
UK (Scotland)	4.6
Israel, Jews born in Europe or America	4.2
France (Doubs)	3.9
Canada (Ontario)	3.8
Australia (New South Wales)	3.8
Sweden	3.6
UK (England and Wales)	3.5
Italy (Lombardy Region, Varese Province)	3.5
Netherlands (Eindhoven)	3.4
Hungary	3.4
Canada	3.3
Iceland	3.2
USA (Hawaii), Hawaiian	3.2
Yugoslavia (Slovenia)	3.2
Ireland (Southern)	3.1
Poland (Cracow)	2.9
Czechoslovakia (Slovakia)	2.9
France (Clavados)	2.7
Poland (Warsaw)	2.3
Brazil (Sao Paulo)	2.2
Canada (Quebec)	2.2
Israel, all Jews	.2.2
Costa Rica	2.0
USA (San Francisco Bay area) Chinese	2.0
New Zealand, Pacific Polynesian Islanders	1.8
Finland	1.7
Israel, Jews born in Israel	1.6
Israel, Jews born in Africa or Asia	1.5
USA (Hawaii), Japanese	1.5
USA (Hawaii), Chinese	1.4
Hong Kong	1.2
Spain (Navarra)	1.2
USA (San Francisco Bay area), blacks.	1.2
USA (San Francisco Bay area, Filipinos	1.2
Columbia (Cali)	1.1
USA (San Francisco Bay area), Japanese	1.1
Singapore, Chinese	1.0
Pureto Rico	1.0
USA (California, Almeda County), blacks	1.0
India (Mumbai)	0.9
Israel, non-Jews	0.5
Antilles	0.4
USA (Hawaii), Filipinos	0.3
USA (Connecticut), blacks	0.2
Martinique	0.0

*Data from reference 133.

immunohistochemical and in situ hybridization techniques, respectively (144).

A higher incidence of testicular cancers is seen in individuals involved in food manufacture and preparation, farming, and among draftsmen (127); in sales and service workers, physicians, production supervisors, and motor vehicle mechanics (140); in professions with an exposure to heat, fertilizers, phenols, fumes, or smoke (116); in workers exposed to temperature extremes (165); in fire fighters (94); in electrical workers, foresters, fishermen, and paper and printing workers (159); in leather workers (93,126); in aircraft repairmen (110,111); in metal workers (146); and in police officers exposed to hand-held radar (104). Most such associations, however, remain weak and some are disputed (140), which has led to the conclusion that occupational status is not of major etiologic importance in testicular cancer (112,162).

Other factors that have been linked to possible increased risk for testis cancer include: a single marital status (increasing the risk for nonseminomatous but not seminomatous tumors [135]), a history of an inguinal hernia (114,143,158,161), although some believe that the association with inguinal hernia represents a false-positive association due to the confusion of cryptorchidism with hernia (151), past mumps orchitis (100, 158), a prior history of a sexually transmitted disease (160), exposure to estrogenic compounds in utero (99,105,156), a dizygotic twin (99), a maternal history of hyperemesis during gestation (117), neonatal jaundice (91), low or high birth weight (91), testicular atrophy with oligospermia and hypofertility (116), Down's syndrome (95,98,107,108a,149a), Klinefelter's syndrome (153), Marfan's syndrome (107), dysplastic nevus syndrome (152), certain human leukocyte antigen (HLA) haplotypes (A-10, Bw35 [125]; Aw24 [for metastatic tumors] [102]; A3, Aw32, Aw33, B5, B7 [142]; B13, Bw-41 [108,109]; DR5 [121,138,142], and Dw7 [106]), ichthyosis (124), testicular trauma (100,160), a maternal history of breast cancer (132), early puberty (131,132,161), a tall stature (114,157), and exogenous hormone administration (134,145). There is an increased frequency of sarcoidosis in patients with testicular cancer, but the tumor usually occurs first (144a). (Sometimes, however, noncaseating granulomas reflect a reaction to tumor [usually seminoma] that may not be apparent at first inspection [159a].) An increased frequency of rare alleles of the variable number of the tandem repeat region flanking the Ha-ras1 oncogene has been demonstrated in testicular cancer patients, supporting a genetic factor (149). The association of testicular germ cell tumors with Klinefelter's syndrome was not confirmed in a recent study, but there was a significant association of Klinefelter's syndrome with mediastinal germ cell tumors (107), a finding supported in other studies (136). A protective effect has been associated with exercise (114,160,161), a prior history of infectious mononucleosis (132) (in apparent contradiction of the previously described positive association with elevated titers to the Epstein-Barr virus [92]), a history of acne (105), and antenatal life during World War II (96,119, 128). Four factors that have not been convincingly associated with testicular cancer include: 1) tobacco use, 2) alcohol use, 3) radiation exposure, and 4) prior vasectomy (112,118,130,137,147, 160). In summary, it is apparent that numerous associations with testicular cancer are described, but most associations are not confirmed. There are, however, five well-established, positive associations with testicular cancer that are now considered in greater detail: 1) cryptorchidism, 2) a prior testicular germ cell tumor, 3) a family history of testicular germ cell tumor, 4) certain intersex syndromes, and 5) infertility.

Cryptorchidism

Cryptorchidism has one of the strongest positive associations with testicular cancer (207). The frequency of past (corrected) or current cryptorchidism in patients with testicular germ cell tumors is between 3.5 and 14.5 percent of cases in various series (171,171a,179,181,184,188,196,197, 200), despite a low overall prevalence of cryptorchidism in the general population (in one study as low as 0.25 percent [192] and 2.7 percent in a case-control study [206]). The calculated increased risk for testicular cancer in patients with cryptorchidism has varied, predominantly because of the variable estimates of this condition in the control population, from 2.5 to 35 times that for the noncryptorchid male population (169,173,176,181,184,188,190,192,197,198,201, 204,207,208). The most frequently cited figure is 10 to 14 times the risk of the control population, although several recent studies have suggested a lower figure, on the order of a 3.5 to 5 times elevated risk (176,197,198). Giwercman and colleagues (176) found that the increased risk did not become manifest before age 20 years, so that screening procedures need not begin until then.

The mechanism by which cryptorchidism predisposes to the development of germ cell tumors is not clear. Several studies have documented that the increased risk is not limited to the cryptorchid testis, and the contralateral testis is also at increased risk (174,185,198,201,204) although at a lower rate (198,203,204). One study, however, failed to find an elevated risk for the noncryptorchid testis (200). The presence of oligospermia in 15 to 25 percent of patients with unilateral cryptorchidism (167) and an increased frequency of genitourinary anomalies other than cryptorchidism in patients with testicular cancer (including ureteral duplication and ectopy, hypospadias, and ectopic kidneys [189,198,199,205]) have led to the conclusion that patients with cryptorchidism may have a generalized defect in genitourinary embryogenesis with bilaterally dysgenetic gonads predisposing to neoplasia (172). Furthermore, cryptorchidism and other genitourinary anomalies may mark patients in whom testicular cancers develop on a familial basis since such anomalies occur with increased frequency in cases with an apparent familial basis compared to apparently sporadic cases (206). The absence of a demonstrable effect of orchidopexy in reducing the rate of testicular cancer in previously cryptorchid gonads (168,171a,196,198,201), a conclusion contradicted in other studies (207), is another feature that favors a developmental basis for the increased risk associated with cryptorchidism. The fact that there is a gradient of increased risk associated with the degree of ectopy, with abdominal testes showing the greatest increased risk and inguinal testes the least (174,185), does not contradict this hypothesis if it is assumed that the greatest degree of ectopy reflects the greatest perturbation in embryogenesis. Similar arguments may apply for the greater risk associated with an undescended testis in patients with unilateral cryptorchidism compared to a descended testis (204). The increased risk previously mentioned in association with testicular atrophy, hypofertility, and oligospermia in the absence of cryptorchidism (180) may also reflect dysembryogenesis.

A higher proportion of seminomas are associated with cryptorchidism than other germ cell tumors (170,190,191), and the proportion of seminomas is greater for abdominal cryptorchid testes (89 percent) than for inguinal testes (78 percent) (179). These figures contrast with the 50 percent frequency of seminoma amongst testicular germ cell tumors in general (183). Because of the greatly increased risk of testicular cancer in patients with a history of cryptorchidism, testicular biopsies have been recommended as a method of identifying these at-risk patients (177). The identification of intratubular germ cell neoplasia of the unclassified type (IGCNU; "carcinoma in situ") in the testes of patients with cryptorchidism appears to be a reliable method of identifying patients at risk, as only one testicular cancer developed in over 1,500 cryptorchid patients with negative testicular

biopsies followed for 8 years (177). On the other hand, invasive testicular germ cell tumors are estimated to occur in at least 50 percent of patients with a positive biopsy for IGCNU (202). The frequency of IGCNU in patients with cryptorchidism varied from 2 to 8 percent in different studies (177,178,187,195) and represents an approximate four-fold increase over the general male population (178). A single-time postpubertal testicular biopsy appears to be sufficient for the identification of cryptorchid patients with IGCNU, but each testis should be biopsied (175). The currently suggested age for these biopsies is 18 to 20 years (175). It does not appear that at-risk patients can be reliably identified by testicular biopsy in the prepubertal period, for instance at orchidopexy (193a). Nistal et al. (193) suggested that the usual anterosuperior location of testicular biopsies may miss some cases of IGCNU in patients with cryptorchidism and severe atrophy of the seminiferous tubules. These authors reported two patients in whom IGCNU was visualized only in intact tubules near the rete testis, and in whom a conventional biopsy would not have sampled the lesion. Accordingly, they suggest a posterior biopsy in cryptorchid patients who have an initial biopsy showing severe germ cell hypoplasia (193). Not all authorities agree that cryptorchid testes should be biopsied for the investigation of IGCNU (194). Immunostains directed against placental alkaline phosphatase (PLAP) highlight the cytoplasmic membranes of IGCNU and can assist in its recognition (see chapter 2).

Orchidopexy, even at an early age, has not generally been shown to reduce the subsequent development of germ cell tumors in originally cryptorchid testes (168,196,198,201), although it has been argued that the data are insufficient to reach a firm conclusion (203). Some urologists, however, feel that early orchidopexy may reduce the likelihood of subsequent infertility (182). Furthermore, the placement of the cryptorchid testis in the scrotum may permit better clinical assessment of the gonad if biopsy and prophylactic orchiectomy are not performed. A recent study, however, failed to show any differences in clinical stages of patients with corrected and uncorrected cryptorchidism in whom germ cell tumors developed (186).

Bilateral Testicular Germ Cell Tumors

Patients with a past or current testicular germ cell tumor are at definite increased risk for a contralateral testicular germ cell tumor (209–211,213,221). In two large series the frequency of simultaneous or subsequent testicular cancer was 1.9 percent and 2.7 percent (218,220), but has ranged from 4 to 5 percent in other studies (211,212,222). Such frequencies correspond to an elevated risk calculated to be more than 20 times higher than that of the general population (210,220). This risk is even greater if the second testis is cryptorchid or atrophic (215,225). In biopsies of the contralateral testis of patients with a history of testicular cancer, 4.5 to 5.7 percent were found to have IGCNU (214,215, 219), but this frequency increased significantly (to 23 percent in one study [215]) when the opposite testis was either cryptorchid or atrophic (215,216,219). The interval between the two cancers is variable but can be lengthy. Kristianslund et al. (218) and Zingg (225) reported that 50 percent of second germ cell tumors occurred within 3 years and 5 years of the initial diagnosis, respectively. Because some second tumors may not be diagnosed for more than a decade after the first, the average interval in one report was 8.8 years (224). One study claimed the risk of a second primary tumor was greater if the initial neoplasm was a nonseminomatous germ cell tumor rather than a seminoma (220). Although the histologic types of the two tumors in a given patient are often discordant (225), there is a tendency for patients with seminoma to have a second seminoma rather than a nonseminomatous tumor (218); a similar tendency is not apparent for nonseminomatous tumors (218). A family history of testicular cancer in a patient with this disease increases the risk of bilaterality four-fold (211,217). There is also an increased frequency of bilateral tumors in patients with bilateral cryptorchidism and occurrence of the first tumor at a young age (214). If the patient receives chemotherapy for the first tumor, the risk of a second tumor is decreased (209).

One means of identifying patients with testicular cancer at risk for a second primary tumor is the examination of testicular biopsies for IGCNU. Von der Maase and co-workers (223) found a 5.4 percent frequency of IGCNU in the contralateral testis of patients with testicular germ cell tumors; 30 percent of these patients already had a second tumor at the time of diagnosis of IGCNU, and 50 percent of the remainder had a second primary germ cell tumor within 5 years of the diagnosis of IGCNU. None of 473 patients with testicular cancer who did not have IGCNU in a biopsy of the opposite testis had a second testicular cancer at follow-up of 12 to 96 months.

Familial Testicular Cancer

Tollerud et al. (241), in a case-control study, found a 2.2 percent frequency of testicular cancer in first-degree male relatives of patients with testicular cancer, with the control population having a frequency of 0.4 percent, a six-fold increased risk for this population (230,241); the risk for brothers appears greater than the risk for fathers (233,243) or sons (233). Other studies confirmed this excess risk (227,227a,229,236). Additionally, with familial testis cancer there is an excessive risk of bilaterality that occurs in 8.1 to 14.2 percent of patients (227,230,233) and a tendency for earlier age of onset compared to "sporadic" cases (233). Other observations include greater differences in the age of onset and less tendency for concordant histology as the genetic differences between the relatives become greater (i.e., from twins, to brothers, to fathers and sons) (227). An increased frequency of cryptorchidism as well as inguinal hernia and hydrocele in first-degree male relatives of patients with testis cancer supports an inherited tendency for urogenital dysembryogenesis as a possible etiology (241), although this observation has not been demonstrated in all studies (233). A genetic factor is also supported by the demonstration of an increased frequency of certain rare alleles associated with the Ha-*ras*1 proto-oncogene in patients with testicular germ cell tumors, especially those with bilateral occurrence or early age of onset (239). There is also a recent report of five testicular germ cell tumors occurring in the relatives of children with bone and soft tissue sarcomas, leading to the speculation that testicular germ cell tumors may represent part of the spectrum of the Li-Fraumeni cancer syndrome (231). Discrepant results, however, have been obtained concerning the occurrence of p53 abnormalities in the tumors, with the preponderance of evidence being that p53 mutations are not a significant factor in testicular germ cell tumors, despite the common occurrence of p53 overexpression, as detected by immunohistochemistry (226,228,232,235,237,238,240, 242,244,245); germ line p53 mutations therefore do not appear to be associated with testicular germ cell tumors that commonly overexpress wild-type p53 protein (238). Another study failed to find any increase in nontesticular cancers in the families of patients with testicular cancer, supporting a lack of a generalized genetic cancer risk (234). Recent genetic linkage studies in cases of familial testicular cancer have found the strongest evidence for "susceptibility genes" on chromosomes 3, 5, 12, and 18 (234a).

Intersex Syndromes

There are several intersex syndromes associated with an increased risk for a germ cell tumor: certain forms of gonadal dysgenesis, true hermaphroditism, and male pseudohermaphroditism due to androgen insensitivity syndrome (254,255).

The term gonadal dysgenesis is somewhat ambiguous but when applied to the testes implies that they are not only abnormal morphologically (often showing severe regressive changes or "streak" morphology, possibly in conjunction with ovarian-type stroma) but also have failed to induce full masculinization of target organs and regression of mullerian structures. Substantial risks of germ cell tumors are associated with gonadal dysgenesis in patients who have a Y chromosome. These disorders include: 46,XY pure gonadal dysgenesis (Swyer's syndrome), in which bilateral streak gonads composed of ovarian-type stroma are present in a phenotypic female with infantile internal genitalia; mixed gonadal dysgenesis in which the patients have combinations of a streak gonad and testis, female internal genitalia, and ambiguous external genitalia; and dysgenetic male pseudohermaphroditism in which bilaterally dysembryogenetic cryptorchid testes with hypoplastic tubules, sometimes with ovarian-type stroma, occur in patients with incompletely masculinized external genitalia and both mullerian and wolffian structures in the internal genitalia (255). Tumors are estimated to occur in at least 25 to 30 percent of patients with these syndromes, the most common of which is gonado-

blastoma (247,255). Since neoplasms may develop during childhood, early gonadectomy is indicated. Gonadal biopsy may successfully identify patients with gonadal dysgenesis who are at risk; four phenotypic male children with 45,X/46,XY mixed gonadal dysgenesis had IGCNU identified on biopsy, leading to prophylactic orchiectomy (251). About 8 percent of children and adolescents with gonadal dysgenesis have IGCNU independent of a gonadoblastoma (253). An increased risk of germ cell tumor is also associated with true hermaphroditism, with IGCNU being reported in a rare case (253) and malignant tumors in 2.6 percent of the reported cases (255).

Male pseudohermaphrodites with androgen insensitivity syndrome lack fully functional androgen-binding receptor; they have maldescended testes with solid immature tubules, markedly decreased or absent germ cells, ovarian-type stroma, Leydig cell hyperplasia, and, frequently, hamartomatous nodules and Sertoli cell adenomas (246,254–256). These patients also have a substantially increased frequency of malignant germ cell tumors, which occur in 5 to 10 percent of the patients (248,249,254,256). Most such tumors occur following pubescence, with the risk increasing substantially with age (248). A 22 percent frequency of malignant tumors is reported in patients older than 30 years (250). IGCNU may also be identified on gonadal biopsy (252).

Infertility

When analyzing patients with infertility, it is difficult to separate those who are infertile because of either cryptorchidism or gonadal dysgenesis from those who are not. An association of male infertility with an increased risk of germ cell tumors is therefore expected, given the association of infertility with cryptorchidism and gonadal dysgenesis and the already discussed proclivity of patients with these disorders to develop testicular germ cell tumors. In support of this, one study found a 22 percent frequency of cryptorchidism in infertile patients with IGCNU (261). Swerdlow et al. (262) did not feel there was any clear evidence that infertility in the absence of cryptorchidism was significantly associated with an increased risk of testicular cancer. Giwercman et al. (257) noted a frequency of

IGCNU in subfertile men of 0.4 to 1.1 percent, and Gondos and Migliozzi (258) cited a similar figure of 0.5 to 1 percent. Comparable figures appear in other studies (259,260,263). It is therefore apparent that patients with infertility as a whole are at increased risk for testicular germ cell tumors, especially if there is a history of cryptorchidism or testicular atrophy. Such patients are likely to have severe oligospermia or azoospermia.

GENERAL CLINICAL ASPECTS

The clinical aspects of specific tumors are addressed in detail in the pertinent sections, however some general remarks are made here. Most patients with testicular tumors present with self-identified palpable masses (generalized enlargement or distinct nodules) and less commonly with local pain (269), which was present in only 11 percent of the cases in one large series (266a). It is not generally appreciated, however, that a substantial number of patients with tumors (11 percent for those with seminomas) (278) may have normal-sized or even smaller testes, perhaps because of the tendency for germ cell tumors to occur in atrophic testes or to undergo necrosis with scarring ("burnt-out" germ cell tumors; see chapter 5) (275). In one series (266a), 6 percent of patients had no self-identified mass but one was detected on careful clinical palpation in these cases. The presence of a hydrocele may compromise detection of a mass. The more aggressive tumors, more commonly than the others, may manifest with symptoms secondary to metastases, and this is also true for tumors that develop in cryptorchid testes because of their inaccessibility to palpation. This results in larger tumors in cryptorchid testes than in normally located testes (269). Two percent of patients present with metastases in the absence of a palpable mass (266a). In one unusual case, a seminoma in an undescended testis invaded the appendix and the resultant acute appendicitis was the clinical presentation (273). Torsion of an intra-abdominal testis may also mimic appendicitis, with the neoplasm incidentally discovered at laparotomy (270).

The overwhelming majority of testicular tumors are of germ cell origin (95 percent [269]), typically occur in young adults, and are inherently malignant but are now almost always curable. The right testis is affected more frequently than the left, with an approximate 5 to 4 ratio (269,271). Sex cord–stromal tumors are much less common and tend to occur over a wider age range than the germ cell tumors and, unlike the germ cell tumors, are more often benign. Germ cell tumors and sex cord–stromal tumors may exceptionally occur as apparent primary tumors in the paratesticular structures (265,266,276), although paratesticular involvement is much more often due to direct spread or metastasis from primary testicular neoplasms.

Occasionally patients present with endocrine manifestations, gynecomastia being the most common, which occur in approximately 4 percent of adults with a germ cell tumor (274). This usually reflects human chorionic gonadotropin (hCG) production by a germ cell tumor which causes secondary Leydig cell hyperplasia with increased estrogen production. Because of the association with hCG production, gynecomastia, when due to a germ cell tumor, is seen in patients with tumors having a trophoblastic component (choriocarcinoma or seminoma) or embryonal carcinoma with syncytiotrophoblast cells. Thyrotoxicosis may also occur secondary to hCG production because of its thyroid stimulating hormone (TSH)-like activity. Patients with metastatic choriocarcinoma and hyperthyroidism may have elevated levels of "molar" TSH with normal levels of pituitary TSH, and gynecomastia may accompany hyperthyroidism in some instances (274). Direct production of androgens or estrogens by tumors in the sex cord–stromal group may cause pseudoprecocity and gynecomastia (see chapter 6), respectively. Other manifestations have included exophthalmos (in two patients with seminoma [268,277]), carcinoid syndrome (in five patients with apparently primary carcinoid tumors [279]), hyperandrogenism with polycythemia (a seminoma with syncytiotrophoblast cells and Leydig cell hyperplasia [272]), paraneoplastic hypercalcemia (seven patients with seminoma [264a]), autoimmune hemolytic anemia (a seminoma [267]), Cushing's syndrome (see chapter 7), and limbic encephalopathy (germ cell tumors [264,278a]).

REFERENCES

Introduction

1. Atkin NB, Baker MC. i(12p): specific chromosomal marker in seminoma and malignant teratoma of the testis? Cancer Genet Cytogenet 1983;10:199–204.
2. Berthelsen JG, Skakkebaek NE. Value of testicular biopsy in diagnosing carcinoma in situ testis. Scand J Urol Nephrol 1981;15:165–8.
3. Berthelsen JG, Skakkebaek NE, von der Maase H, Sorensen BL, Mogensen P. Screening for carcinoma in situ of the contralateral testis in patients with germinal testicular cancer. Br Med J 1982;285:1683–6.
4. Bosl GJ, Dmitrovsky E, Reuter VE, et al. Isochromosome of the short arm of chromosome 12: clinically useful markers for male germ cell tumors. JNCI 1989;81:1874–8.
5. de Jong B, Oosterhuis JW, Castedo SM, Vos A, te Meerman GJ. Pathogenesis of adult testicular germ cell tumors. A cytogenetic model. Cancer Genet Cytogenet 1990;48:143–67.
6. El-Naggar AK, Ro JY, McLemore D, Ayala AG, Batsakis JG. DNA ploidy in testicular germ cell neoplasms: histogenetic and clinical implications. Am J Surg Pathol 1992;16:611–8.
7. Gibas Z, Prout GR, Pontes JE, Sandberg AA. Chromosome changes in germ cell tumors of the testis. Cancer Genet Cytogenet 1986;19:245–52.
8. Lachman MF, Ricci A Jr, Kosciol C. DNA ploidy in testicular germ cell tumors: can an atypical seminoma be identified? Conn Med 1995;59:133–6.
9. Mostofi FK, Sesterhenn IA. Histological typing of testis tumours. International histological classification of tumors, World Health Organization, Berlin: Springer, 1998.
10. Muller J, Skakkebaek NE. Abnormal germ cells in maldescended testes: a study of cell density, nuclear size and deoxyribonucleic acid content in testicular biopsies from 50 boys. J Urol 1984;131:730–3.
11. Oosterhuis JW, Castedo SM, de Jong B, et al. Ploidy of primary germ cell tumors of the testis. Pathogenetic and clinical relevance. Lab Invest 1989;60:14–21.
12. Samaniego F, Rodriguez E, Houldsworth J, et al. Cytogenetic and molecular analysis of human male germ cell tumors: chromosome 12 abnormalities and gene amplification. Genes Chrom Cancer 1990;1:289–300.
13. Skakkebaek NE. Abnormal morphology of germ cells in two infertile men. Acta Pathol Microbiol Scand [A] 1972;80:374–8.
14. Skakkebaek NE. Possible carcinoma-in-situ of the undescended testis. Lancet 1972;2:516–7.
15. Skakkebaek NE. Carcinoma in situ of the testis: frequency and relationship to invasive germ cell tumours in infertile men. Histopathology 1978;2:157–70.
16. Skakkebaek NE, Berthelsen JG, Giwercman A, Müller J. Carcinoma-in-situ of the testis: possible origin from gonocytes and precursor of all types of germ cell tumours except spermatocytoma. Int J Androl 1987;10:19–28.
17. Skakkebaek NE, Berthelsen JG, Visfeldt J. Clinical aspects of testicular carcinoma-in-situ. Int J Androl 1981;4(Suppl):153–62.

Embryology, Anatomy, and Histology

18. Carlson BM. Patten's foundations of embryology. 5th ed. New York: McGraw-Hill, 1988:567–80.
19. Clermont Y. The cycle of the seminiferous epithelium in man. Am J Anat 1963;112:35–51.
20. Comrack DH. Ham's histology. 9th ed. Philadelphia: JB Lippincott, 1987:651–77.
21. Gier HT, Marion GB. Development of the mammalian testis. In: Johnson AD, Gomes WR, Vandmard NL, eds. The testis, Vol. 1. New York: Academic Press, 1970:1–42.
22. Giwercman A, Müller J, Skakkebaek NE. Prevalence of carcinoma in situ and other histopathological abnormalities in testes from 399 men who died suddenly and unexpectedly. J Urol 1991;145:77–80.
23. Gruenwald P. The development of the sex cords in the gonads of man and mammals. Am J Anat 1942;70:359–97.
24. Guarch R, Pesce C, Puras A, Lazaro J. A quantitative approach to the classification of hypospermatogenesis in testicular biopsies for infertility. Hum Pathol 1992;23:1032–7.
25. Halley JB. The infiltrative activity of Leydig cells. J Pathol Bacteriol 1961;81:347–53.
26. Hollinshead WH. Textbook of anatomy. 3rd ed. Hagerstown, MD: Harper and Row, 1974:732–6.
27. Lennox B, Ahmad KN, Mack WS. A method for determining the relative total length of the tubules in the testis. J Pathol 1970;102:229–38.
27a. Mai KT. Cytoplasmic eosinophilic granular change of the ductal efferentes: a histological, immunohisto-chemical, and electron microscopic study. J Urol Pathol 1994;2:273–82.
28. McLaren A. Development of the mammalian gonad: the fate of the supporting cell lineage. Bioessays 1991;13:151–6.
29. Neville AM, Grigor KM. Structure, function, and development of the human testis. In: Pugh RC, ed. Pathology of the testis. Oxford: Blackwell Scientific, 1976:1–37.
30. Nochomovitz LE, Orenstein JM. Adenocarcinoma of the rete testis: review and regrouping of reported cases and a consideration of miscellaneous entities. J Urogenit Pathol 1991;1:11–40.
31. Rutgers JL. Advances in the pathology of intersex syndromes. Hum Pathol 1991;22:884–91.
32. Sadler TW. Langman's medical embryology. 5th ed. Baltimore: Williams & Wilkins, 1985:258–80.
32a. Schned AR, Memoli VA. Coarse granular cytoplasmic change of the epididymis. An immunohistochemical and ultrastructural study. J Urol Pathol 1994;2:213–22.
33. Shah VI, Ro JY, Amin MB, Mullick S, Nazeer T, Ayala AG. Histologic variations in the epididymis: findings in 167 orchiectomy specimens. Am J Surg Pathol 1998;22:990–6.
34. Sohval AR, Churg J, Gabrilove JL. Ultrastructure of feminizing testicular Leydig cell tumors. Ultrastruc Pathol 1982;3:335–45.
35. Trainer TD. Histology of the normal testis. Am J Surg Pathol 1987;11:797–809.

36. van Wagenen G, Simpson ME. Embryology of the ovary and testis: Homo sapiens and Macaca mulatta. New Haven: Yale University Press, 1965.

37. Wartenberg H. Differentiation and development of the testes. In: Burger H, de Kretser D, eds. The testis. 2nd ed. New York: Raven Press, 1989:67–118.

38. Wheeler JE. Histology of the fertile and infertile testis. Monogr Pathol 1991;33:56–103.

39. Williams PL, Warwick R. Gray's anatomy. 36th ed. Philadelphia: WB Saunders, 1980:1410–7.

Classification

40. Collins DH, Pugh RC. Classification and frequency of testicular tumours. Br J Urol 1964;36(Suppl):1–11.

41. Dixon FJ, Moore RA. Tumors of the male sex organs. Atlas of Tumor Pathology, 1st series, Fascicles 31b and 32. Washington, D.C.: Armed Forces Institute of Pathology, 1952.

42. Dixon FJ, Moore RA. Testicular tumors: a clinicopathologic study. Cancer 1953;6:427–54.

43. Dunphy CH, Ayala AG, Swanson DA, Ro JY, Logothetis C. Clinical stage I non-seminomatous and mixed germ cell tumors of the testis. A clinicopathologic study of 93 patients on a surveillance protocol after orchiectomy alone. Cancer 1988;62:1202–6.

44. Freedman LS, Parkinson MC, Jones WG, et al. Histopathology in the prediction of relapse of patients with stage I testicular teratoma treated by orchidectomy alone. Lancet 1987;2:294–8.

45. Friedman NB, Moore RA. Tumors of the testis: a report on 922 cases. Milit Surgeon 1946;99:573–93.

46. Melicow MM. Classification of tumors of the testis: a clinical and pathological study based on 105 primary and 13 secondary cases in adults, and 3 primary and 4 secondary cases in children. J Urol 1955;73:547–4.

47. Mostofi FK. Comparison of various clinical and pathological classifications of tumors of testes. Semin Oncol 1979;6:26–30.

48. Mostofi FK, Price EB Jr. Tumors of the male genital system. Atlas of Tumor Pathology, 2nd Series, Fascicle 8. Washington D.C.: Armed Forces Institute of Pathology, 1973.

49. Pugh RC. Testicular tumours–introduction. In: Pugh RC, ed. Pathology of the testis. Oxford: Blackwell Scientific, 1976:139–59.

50. Pugh RC, Parkinson C. The origin and classification of testicular germ cell tumours. Int J Androl 1981;4(Suppl):15–25.

51. Talerman A, Haije WG, Baggerman L. Serum alpha fetoprotein (AFP) in patients with germ cell tumors of the gonads and extragonadal sites: correlation between endodermal sinus (yolk sac) tumor and raised serum AFP. Cancer 1980;46:380–5.

52. Willis RA. Pathology of tumours. 4th ed. London: Butterworth, 1967:959–1003.

Spread and Metastasis

53. Bredael JJ, Vugrin D, Whitmore WF Jr. Autopsy findings in 154 patients with germ cell tumors of the testis. Cancer 1982;50:548–51.

54. de Bruin MJ, Oosterhof GO, Debruyne FM. Nerve-sparing retroperitoneal lymphadenectomy for low stage testicular cancer. Br J Urol 1993;71:336–9.

55. Donohue JP. Metastatic pathways of nonseminomatous germ cell tumors. Semin Urol 1984;2:217–29.

56. Donohue JP, Thornhill JA, Foster RS, Rowland RG, Bihrle R. Primary retroperitoneal lymph node dissection in clinical stage A non-seminomatous germ cell testis cancer. Review of the Indiana University experience 1965-1989. Br J Urol 1993;71:326–35.

57. Grady RW, Ross JH, Kay R. Patterns of metastatic spread in prepubertal yolk sac tumor of the testis. J Urol 1995;153:1259–61.

58. Jacobsen GK. Malignant Sertoli cell tumors of the testis. J Urol Pathol 1993;1:233–55.

59. Morse MJ, Whitmore WF. Neoplasms of the testis. In: Walsh PC, Gittes RF, Perlmutter AD, Stamey TA, eds. Campbell's urology. Philadelphia: WB Saunders, 1986:1535–82.

60. Mostofi FK, Price EB Jr. Tumors of the male genital system. Atlas of Tumor Pathology, 2nd Series, Fascicle 8. Washington D.C.: Armed Forces Institute of Pathology, 1973.

61. Richie JP. Diagnosis and staging of testicular tumors. In: Skinner DG, Lieskovsky G, eds. Diagnosis and management of genitourinary cancer. Philadelphia: WB Saunders, 1988:498–507.

62. Sweetenham JW, Whitehouse JM, Williams CJ, Mead GM. Involvement of the gastrointestinal tract by metastases from germ cell tumors of the testis. Cancer 1988;61:2566–70.

63. Thackray AC, Crane WA. Seminoma. In: Pugh RC, ed. Pathology of the testis. Oxford: Blackwell Scientific, 1976:164–98.

Staging

63a. American Joint Committee on Cancer. Testis. In: Fleming ID, Cooper JS, Henson DE, et al., eds. AJCC cancer staging manual. Philadelphia: Lippincott-Raven, 1997:225–30.

64. Boden G, Gibb R. Radiotherapy and testicular neoplasms. Lancet 1951;2:1195–7.

65. Bosl GJ, Sheinfeld J, Bajorin DF, Motzer RJ. Cancer of the testis. In: DeVita VT Jr, Hellman S, Rosenberg SA, eds. Cancer: principles and practice of oncology. 5th ed. Philadelphia: Lippincott-Raven, 1997:1397–425.

66. Hendry WF, Barrett A, McElwain TJ, Wallace DM, Peckham MJ. The role of surgery in the combined management of metastases from malignant teratomas of testis. Br J Urol 1980;52:38–49.

66a. International Union Against Cancer. TNM classification of malignant tumors. Sobin LH, Wittekind CH, eds. 5th ed. New York: Wiley-Liss, 1997:174–9.

67. Johnson DE. Clinical staging. In: Donohue JP, ed. Testis tumors. Baltimore: Williams & Wilkins, 1983:131–44.

68. Klepp O, Flodgren P, Maartman-Moe H, et al. Early clinical stages (CS1, CS1Mk+ and CS2A) of non-seminomatous testis cancer. Value of pre- and post-orchiectomy serum tumor marker information in prediction of retroperitoneal lymph node metastases. Swedish-Norwegian Testicular Cancer Project (SWENOTECA). Ann Oncol 1990;1:281–8.

69. Morse MJ, Whitmore WF. Neoplasms of the testis. In: Walsh PC, Gittes RF, Perlmutter AD, Stamey TA, eds. Campbell's urology. Philadelphia: WB Saunders, 1986:1535–82.

70. Mostofi FK. Comparison of various clinical and pathological classifications of tumors of testes. Semin Oncol 1979;6:26–30.

71. Richie JP, Garnick MB, Finberg H. Computerized tomography: how accurate for abdominal staging of testis tumors. J Urol 1982;127:715–7.

72. Rowland RG, Weisman D, Williams SD, Einhorn LH, Klatte EC, Donohue JP. Accuracy of preoperative staging in stages A and B nonseminomatous germ cell testis tumors. J Urol 1982;127:718–20.

73. Shipley WU. The role of radiation in the management of adult germinal testis tumors. In: Einhorn LH, ed. Testicular tumors. New York: Masson, 1980:47–67.

74. Skinner DG. Non-seminomatous testis tumors: a plan of management based on 96 patients to improve survival in all stages by combined therapeutic modalities. J Urol 1969;115:65–9.

75. Thomas G, Jones W, VanOosterom A, Kawai T. Consensus statement on the investigation and management of testicular seminoma 1989. Prog Clin Biol Res 1990;357:285–94.

Gross, Frozen Section, and Cytologic Examination

76. Balslev E, Francis D, Jacobsen GK. Testicular germ cell tumors. Classification based on fine needle aspiration biopsy. Acta Cytol 1990;34:690–4.

77. Buckspan M, Skeldon SC, Klotz PG, Pritzker KP. Epidermoid cysts of the testicle. J Urol 1985;134:960–1.

78. Caraway NP, Fanning CV, Amato RJ, Sneige N. Fine-needle aspiration cytology of seminoma: a review of 16 cases. Diagn Cytopathol 1995;12:327–33.

79. Dieckmann KP, Loy V. Epidermoid cyst of the testis: a review of clinical and histogenetic considerations. Br J Urol 1994;73:436–41.

80. Heidenreich A, Zumbe J, Vorreuther R, Klotz T, Vietsch H, Engelmann UH. Testicular epidermoid cyst: orchiectomy or enucleation resection? Urologe A 1996;35:1–5.

81. Hermanek P. Frozen section diagnosis in tumors of the testis. Possibilities, limitations, indications. Pathol Res Pract 1981;173:54–65.

82. Highman WJ, Oliver RT. Diagnosis of metastases from testicular germ cell tumours using fine needle aspiration cytology. J Clin Pathol 1987;40:1324–33.

83. Kressel K, Hartmann M. Nongerminal, benign testicular tumors–report of experiences. Urologe [A] 1988;27:96–8.

84. Kressel K, Schnell D, Thon WF, Heymer B, Hartmann M, Altwein JE. Benign testicular tumors: a case for testis preservation? Eur Urol 1988;15:200–4.

84a. Krivosic I. Comment fixer les séminomes. Ann Pathol 1993;13:45–7.

85. MacLennan GT, Quinonez GE, Cooley M. Testicular juvenile capillary hemangioma: conservative management with frozen-section examination. A case report. Can J Surg 1994;37:493–4.

86. Manivel JC, Reinberg Y, Niehans GA, Fraley EE. Intratubular germ cell neoplasia in testicular teratomas and epidermoid cysts. Correlation with prognosis and possible biologic significance. Cancer 1989;64:715–20.

87. Nazeer T, Ro JY, Amato B, Ordonez NG, Ayala AG. Histologically pure seminoma (HPS) with elevated alpha-fetoprotein (AFP): a clinicopathologic and immunohistochemical study of ten cases [Abstract]. Mod Pathol 1996;9:79A.

88. Nazeer T, Ro JY, Kee KH, Ayala AG. Spermatic cord contamination in testicular cancer. Mod Pathol 1996;9:762–6.

88a. Ro JY, Amato RJ, Ayala AG. What does the pathology report really mean? Semin Urol Oncol 1996;14:2–7.

88b. Slaughenhoupt BL, Cendron M, Al-Hindi HN, Wallace EC, Ucci A. Capillary hemangioma of the testis. J Urol Pathol 1996;4:283–8.

89. Wegner HE, Herbst H, Loy V, Dieckmann KP. Testicular dermoid cyst in a 10-year-old child: case report and discussion of etiopathogenesis, diagnosis, and treatment. Urol Int 1995;54:109–11.

Epidemiology

90. Adami HO, Bergstrom R, Mohner M, et al. Testicular cancer in nine northern European countries. Int J Cancer 1994;59:33–8.

91. Akre O, Ekbom A, Hsieh CC, Trichopoulos D, Adami HO. Testicular nonseminoma and seminoma in relation to perinatal characteristics. JNCI 1996;88:883–9.

92. Algood CB, Newell GR, Johnson DE. Viral etiology of testicular tumors. J Urol 1988;139:308–10.

93. Anonymous. Testicular cancer in leather workers–Fulton County, New York. MMWR 1989;38:105–6.

94. Bates MN, Lane L. Testicular cancer in fire fighters: a cluster investigation. N Z Med J 1995;108:334–7.

95. Benson RC Jr, Beard CM, Kelalis PP, Kurland LT. Malignant potential of the cryptorchid testis. Mayo Clin Proc 1991;66:372–8.

96. Bergstrom R, Adami HO, Mohner M, et al. Increase in testicular cancer incidence in six European countries: a birth cohort phenomenon. JNCI 1996;88:727–33.

97. Boyle P, Kaye SB, Robertson AG. Changes in testicular cancer in Scotland. Eur J Cancer Clin Oncol 1987;23:827–30.

98. Braun DL, Green MD, Rausen AR, et al. Down's syndrome and testicular cancer: a possible association. Am J Pediatr Hematol Oncol 1985;7:208–11.

99. Braun MM, Ahlbom A, Floderus B, Brinton LA, Hoover RN. Effect of twinship on incidence of cancer of the testis, breast, and other sites (Sweden). Cancer Causes Control 1995;6:519–24.

100. Brown LM, Pottern LM, Hoover RN. Testicular cancer in young men: the search for causes of the epidemic increase in the United States. J Epidemiol Comm Health 1987;41:349–54.

101. Brown LM, Pottern LM, Hoover RN, Devesa SS, Aselton P, Flannery JT. Testicular cancer in the United States: trends in incidence and mortality. Int J Epidemiol 1986;15:164–70.

102. Carr BI, Bach FA. Possible association between HLA-Aw24 and metastatic germ-cell tumours. Lancet 1979;1:1346–7.

103. Davies JM. Testicular cancer in England and Wales: some epidemiological aspects. Lancet 1981;1:928–32.

104. Davis RL, Mostofi FK. Cluster of testicular cancer in police officers exposed to hand-held radar. Am J Ind Med 1993;24:231–3.

105. DePue RH, Pike MC, Henderson BE. Estrogen exposure during gestation and risk of testicular cancer. JNCI 1983;71:1151–5.

106. DeWolf WC, Lange PH, Einarson ME, Yunis EJ. HLA and testicular cancer. Nature 1979;277:216–7.

107. Dexeus FH, Logothetis CJ, Chong C, Sella A, Ogden S. Genetic abnormalities in men with germ cell tumors. J Urol 1988;140:80–4.

108. Dieckmann KP, Klan R, Bunte S. HLA antigens, Lewis antigens, and blood groups in patients with testicular germ-cell tumors. Oncology - Basel 1993;50:252–8.

108a. Dieckmann KP, Rübe C, Henke RP. Association of Down's syndrome and testicular cancer. J Urol 1997;157:1701–4.

109. Dieckmann KP, von Keyserlingk HJ. HLA association of testicular seminoma. Klin Wochenschr 1988;66:337–9.

110. Ducatman AM, Conwill DE, Crawl J. Germ cell tumors of the testicle among aircraft repairmen. J Urol 1986;136:834–6.

111. Foley S, Middleton S, Stitson D, Mahoney M. The incidence of testicular cancer in Royal Air Force personnel. Br J Urol 1995;76:495–6.

112. Forman D, Gallagher R, Moller H, Swerdlow TJ. Aetiology and epidemiology of testicular cancer: report of consensus group. Prog Clin Biol Res 1990;357:245–53.

113. Forman D, Moller H. Testicular cancer. Cancer Surv 1994;19–20:323–41.

114. Gallagher RP, Huchcroft S, Phillips N, et al. Physical activity, medical history, and risk of testicular cancer (Alberta and British Columbia, Canada). Cancer Causes Control 1995;6:398–406.

115. Graham S, Gibson R, West D, Swanson M, Burnett W, Dayal H. Epidemiology of cancer of the testis in upstate New York. JNCI 1977;58:1255–61.

116. Haughey BP, Graham S, Brasure J, Zielezny M, Sufrin G, Burnett WS. The epidemiology of testicular cancer in upstate New York. Am J Epidemiol 1989;130:25–36.

117. Henderson BE, Benton B, Jing J, Yu MC, Pike MC. Risk factors for cancer of the testis in young men. Int J Cancer 1979;23:598–602.

118. Hewitt G, Logan CJ, Curry RC. Does vasectomy cause testicular cancer? Br J Urol 1993;71:607–8.

119. Hoff Wanderas E, Tretli S, Fossa SD. Trends in incidence of testicular cancer in Norway 1955-1992. Eur J Cancer 1995;31A:2044–8.

120. Jacobsen GK, Barlebo H, Olsen JK, et al. Testicular germ cell tumours in Denmark 1976-1980: pathology of 1058 consecutive cases. Acta Radiol Oncol 1984;23:239–47.

121. Kratzik C, Aiginger P, Kuzmits R, et al. HLA-antigen distribution in seminoma, HCG-positive seminoma and non-seminomatous tumours of the testis. Urol Res 1989;17:377–80.

122. Lanson Y. Epidemiology of testicular cancers. Prog Clin Biol Res 1985;203:155–9.

123. Leibovitch I, Baniel J, Rowland RG, Smith ER Jr, Ludlow JK, Donohue JP. Malignant testicular neoplasms in immunosuppressed patients. J Urol 1996;155:1938–42.

124. Lykkesfeldt G, Bennett P, Lykkesfeldt AE, et al. Testis cancer. Ichthyosis constitutes a significant risk factor. Cancer 1991;67:730–4.

125. Majsky A, Abrahamova J, Korinkova P, Bek V. HLA system and testicular germinative tumours. Oncology 1979;36:228–31.

126. Marshall EG, Melius JM, London MA, Nasca PC, Burnett WS. Investigation of a testicular cancer cluster using a case-control approach. Int J Epidemiol 1990;19:269–73.

127. McDowall ME, Balarajan R. Testicular cancer mortality in England and Wales 1971-80: variations by occupation. J Epidemiol Comm Health 1986;40:26–9.

128. Moller H. Clues to the aetiology of testicular germ cell tumours from descriptive epidemiology. Eur Urol 1993;23:8–13.

129. Moller H, Jorgensen N, Forman D. Trends in incidence of testicular cancer in boys and adolescent men. Int J Cancer 1995;61:761–4.

130. Moller H, Knudsen LB, Lynge E. Risk of testicular cancer after vasectomy: cohort study of over 73,000 men. BMJ 1994;309:295–9.

131. Moller H, Skakkebaek NE. Risks of testicular cancer and cryptorchidism in relation to socio-economic status and related factors: case-control studies in Denmark. Int J Cancer 1996;66:287–93.

132. Moss AR, Osmond D, Bacchetti P, Torti FM, Gurgin V. Hormonal risk factors in testicular cancer: a case control study. Am J Epidemiol 1986;124:39–52.

133. Muir C, Waterhouse J, Mack T, Powell J, Whelan S. Cancer incidence in five continents, Vol 5. Lyon, France: International Agency for Research on Cancer, 1987.

134. Neoptolemos JP, Locke TJ, Fossard DP. Testicular tumour associated with hormonal treatment for oligospermia [Letter]. Lancet 1981;2:754.

135. Newell GR, Spitz MR, Sider JG, Pollack ES. Incidence of testicular cancer in the United States related to marital status, histology, and ethnicity. JNCI 1987;78:881–5.

136. Nichols CR, Heerema NA, Palmer C, Loehrer PJ Sr, Williams SD, Einhorn LH. Klinefelter's syndrome associated with mediastinal germ cell neoplasms. J Clin Oncol 1987;5:1290–4.

137. Nienhuis H, Goldacre M, Seagroatt V, Gill L, Vessey M. Incidence of disease after vasectomy: a record linkage retrospective cohort study. BMJ 1992;304:743–6.

138. Oliver RT. HLA phenotype and clinicopathological behaviour of germ cell tumours: possible evidence for clonal evolution from seminomas to nonseminomas. Int J Androl 1987;10:85–93.

139. Osterlind A. Diverging trends in incidence and mortality of testicular cancer in Denmark, 1943–1982. Br J Cancer 1986;53:501–5.

140. Pearce N, Sheppard RA, Howard JK, Fraser J, Lilley BM. Time trends and occupational differences in cancer of the testis in New Zealand. Cancer 1987;59:1677–82.

141. Pike MC, Chilvers CE, Bobrow LG. Classification of testicular cancer in incidence and mortality statistics. Br J Cancer 1987;56:83–5.

142. Pollack MS, Vugrin D, Hennessy W, Herr HW, Dupont B, Whitmore WF Jr. HLA antigens in patients with germ cell cancers of the testis. Cancer Res 1982;42:2470–3.

143. Prener A, Engholm G, Jensen OM. Genital anomalies and risk for testicular cancer in Danish men. Epidemiology 1996;7:14–9.

144. Rajpert-De Meyts E, Hording U, Nielsen HW, Skakkebaek NE. Human papillomavirus and Epstein-Barr virus in the etiology of testicular germ cell tumours. APMIS 1994;102:38–42.

144a. Rayson D, Burch PA, Richardson RL. Sarcoidosis and testicular carcinoma. Cancer 1998;83:337–43.

145. Reyes FI, Faiman C. Development of a testicular tumour during cisclomiphene therapy. Can Med Assoc J 1973;109:502–6.

146. Rhomberg W, Schmoll HJ, Schneider B. High frequency of metal workers among patients with seminomatous tumors of the testis: a case-control study. Am J Ind Med 1995;28:79–87.

147. Rosenberg L, Palmer JR, Zauber AG, et al. The relation of vasectomy to the risk of cancer. Am J Epidemiol 1994;140:431–8.

148. Ross RK, McCurtis JW, Henderson BE, Menck HR, Mack TM, Martin SP. Descriptive epidemiology of testicular and prostatic cancer in Los Angeles. Br J Cancer 1979;39:284–92.

149. Ryberg D, Heimdal K, Fossa SD, Borresen AL, Haugen A. Rare Ha-ras1 alleles and predisposition to testicular cancer. Int J Cancer 1993;53:938–40.

149a. Satgé D, Sasco AJ, Curé H, Leduc B, Sommelet D, Vekemans MJ. An excess of testicular germ cell tumors in Down's syndrome: three case reports and a review of the literature. Cancer 1997;80:929–35.

150. Schottenfeld D, Warshauer ME, Sherlock S, Zauber AG, Leder M, Payne R. The epidemiology of testicular cancer in young adults. Am J Epidemiol 1980;112:232–46.

151. Senturia YD. The epidemiology of testicular cancer. Br J Urol 1987;60:285–91.

152. Sigg C, Pelloni F. Dysplastic nevi and germ cell tumors of the testis—a possible further tumor in the spectrum of associated malignancies in dysplastic nevus syndrome. Dermatologica 1988;176:109–10.

153. Sogge MR, McDonald SD, Cofold PB. The malignant potential of the dysgenetic germ cell in Klinefelter's syndrome. Am J Med 1979;66:515–8.

154. Stone JM, Cruickshank DG, Sandeman TF, Matthews JP. Trebling of the incidence of testicular cancer in Victoria, Australia (1950–1985). Cancer 1991;68:211–9.

155. Swerdlow AJ. The epidemiology of testicular cancer. Eur Urol 1993;23(Suppl 2):35–8.

156. Swerdlow AJ, Huttly SR, Smith PG. Prenatal and familial associations of testicular cancer. Br J Cancer 1987;55:571–7.

157. Swerdlow AJ, Huttly SR, Smith PG. Testis cancer: postnatal hormonal factors, sexual behaviour and fertility. Int J Cancer 1989;43:549–53.

158. Swerdlow AJ, Huttly SR, Smith PG. Testicular cancer and antecedent diseases. Br J Cancer 1987;55:97–103.

159. Swerdlow AJ, Skeet RG. Occupational associations of testicular cancer in south east England. Br J Indust Med 1988;45:225–30.

159a. Tjan-Heijnen VC, Vlasveld LT, Pernet FP, Paulwels P, De Mulder PH. Coincidence of seminoma and sarcoidosis: a myth or fact? Ann Oncol 1998;9:321–5.

160. United Kingdom Testicular Cancer Study Group. Social, behavioural and medical factors in the aetiology of testicular cancer: results from the UK study. Br J Cancer 1994;70:513–20.

161. United Kingdom Testicular Cancer Study Group. Aetiology of testicular cancer: association with congenital abnormalities, age at puberty, infertility, and exercise. Br Med J 1994;308:1393–9.

162. Van den Eeden SK, Weiss NS, Strader CH, Daling JR. Occupation and the occurrence of testicular cancer. Am J Indust Med 1991;19:327–37.

163. Wilkinson TJ, Colls BM, Schluter PJ. Increased incidence of germ cell testicular cancer in New Zealand Maoris. Br J Cancer 1992;65:769–71.

164. Wilson WT, Frenkel E, Vuitch F, Sagalowsky AI. Testicular tumors in men with human immunodeficiency virus. J Urol 1992;147:1038–40.

165. Zhang ZF, Vena JE, Zielezny M, et al. Occupational exposure to extreme temperature and risk of testicular cancer. Arch Environ Health 1995;50:13–8.

166. Zheng T, Holford TR, Ma Z, Ward BA, Flannery J, Boyle P. Continuing increase in incidence of germ-cell testis cancer in young adults: experience from Connecticut, USA, 1935-1992. Int J Cancer 1996;65:723–9.

Cryptorchidism

167. Bar-Maor JA, Nissan S, Lernau OZ, Oren M, Levy E. Orchidopexy in cryptorchidism assessed by clinical, histologic and sperm examinations. Surg Gynecol Obstet 1979;118:855–9.

168. Batata MA, Chu FC, Hilaris BS, Whitmore WF, Golbey RB. Testicular cancer in cryptorchids. Cancer 1982;49:1023–30.

169. Brendler H. Cryptorchidism and cancer. Prog Clin Biol Res 1985;203:189–96.

170. Collins DH, Pugh RC. Classification and frequency of testicular tumours. Br J Urol 1964;36(Suppl):1–11.

171. DePue RH, Pike MC, Henderson BE. Estrogen exposure during gestation and risk of testicular cancer. JNCI 1983;71:1151–5.

171a. Dow JA, Mostofi FK. Testicular tumors following orchiopexy. South Med J 1967;60:193–5.

172. Fram RJ, Garnick MB, Retik A. The spectrum of genitourinary abnormalities in patients with cryptorchidism, with emphasis on testicular carcinoma. Cancer 1982;50:2243–5.

173. Gallagher RP, Huchcroft S, Phillips N, et al. Physical activity, medical history, and risk of testicular cancer (Alberta and British Columbia, Canada). Cancer Causes Control 1995;6:398–406.

174. Gilbert JB, Hamilton JB. Studies in malignant testis tumors: III - incidence and nature of tumors in ectopic testes. Surg Gynecol Obstet 1940;71:731–43.

175. Giwercman A, Bruun E, Frimodt-Moller C, Skakkebaek NE. Prevalence of carcinoma-in-situ and other histopathologic abnormalities in testes of men with a history of cryptorchidism. J Urol 1989;142:998–1002.

176. Giwercman A, Grindsted J, Hansen B, Jensen OM, Skakkebaek NE. Testicular cancer risk in boys with maldescended testis: a cohort study. J Urol 1987;138:1214–6.

177. Giwercman A, Muller J, Skakkebaek NE. Carcinoma in situ of the undescended testis. Semin Urol 1988;6:110–9.

178. Giwercman A, von der Maase H, Skakkebaek NE. Epidemiological and clinical aspects of carcinoma in situ of the testis. Eur Urol 1993;23:104–10.

179. Halme A, Kellokumpu-Lehtinen P, Lehtonen T, Teppo L. Morphology of testicular germ cell tumours in treated and untreated cryptorchidism. Br J Urol 1989;64:78–83.

180. Haughey BP, Graham S, Brasure J, Zielezny M, Sufrin G, Burnett WS. The epidemiology of testicular cancer in upstate New York. Am J Epidemiol 1989;130:25–36.

181. Henderson BE, Benton B, Jing J, Yu MC, Pike MC. Risk factors for cancer of the testis in young men. Int J Cancer 1979;23:598–602.

182. Hezmall HP, Lipshultz LI. Cryptorchidism and infertility. Urol Clin North Am 1982;9:361–9.

183. Jacobsen GK, Barlebo H, Olsen J, et al. Testicular germ cell tumours in Denmark 1976–1980: pathology of 1058 consecutive cases. Acta Radiol Oncol 1984;23:239–47.

184. Javadpour N, Bergman S. Recent advances in testicular cancer. Curr Prob Surg 1978;15:1–64.

185. Johnson DE, Woodhead DM, Pohl DR, Robison JR. Cryptorchidism and testicular tumorigenesis. Surgery 1968;63:919–22.

186. Jones BJ, Thornhill JA, O'Donnell B, et al. Influence of prior orchiopexy on stage and prognosis of testicular cancer. Eur Urol 1991;19:201–3.

187. Krabbe S, Skakkebaek NE, Berthelsen JG, et al. High incidence of undetected neoplasia in maldescended testes. Lancet 1979;1:999–1000.

188. Lanson Y. Epidemiology of testicular cancers. Prog Clin Biol Res 1985;203:155–9.

189. Li FP, Fraumeni JF Jr. Testicular cancers in children: epidemiologic characteristics. JNCI 1972;48:1575–82.

190. Miller A, Seljelid R. Histopathologic classification and natural history of malignant testis tumors in Norway, 1959–1963. Cancer 1971;28:1054–62.

191. Morrison AS. Cryptorchidism, hernia, and cancer of the testis. JNCI 1976;56:731–3.

192. Mostofi FK. Testicular tumors: epidemiologic, etiologic, and pathologic features. Cancer 1973;32:1186–201.

193. Nistal M, Codesal J, Paniagua R. Carcinoma in situ of the testis in infertile men. A histological, immunocytochemical, and cytophotometric study of DNA content. J Pathol 1989;159:205–10.

193a. Parkinson MC, Swerdlow AJ, Pike MC. Carcinoma in situ in boys with cryptorchidism: when can it be detected? Br J Urol 1994;73:431–5.

194. Oliver RT. Germ cell cancer of the testes. Curr Opin Oncol 1995;7:292–6.

195. Pedersen KV, Boiesen P, Zetterlund CG. Experience of screening for carcinoma-in-situ of the testis among young men with surgically corrected maldescended testes. Int J Androl 1987;10:181–5.

196. Pike MC, Chilvers C, Peckham MJ. Effects of age at orchidopexy on risk of testicular cancer. Lancet 1986;1:1246–8.

197. Pottern LM, Brown LM, Hoover RN, et al. Testicular cancer risk among young men: role of cryptorchidism and inguinal hernia. JNCI 1985;74:377–81.

198. Prener A, Engholm G, Jensen OM. Genital anomalies and risk for testicular cancer in Danish men. Epidemiology 1996;7:14–9.

199. Sakashita S, Koyanagi T, Tsuji I, Arikado K, Matsuno T. Congenital anomalies in children with testicular germ cell tumor. J Urol 1980;124:889–91.

200. Schottenfeld D, Warshauer ME, Sherlock S, Zauber AG, Leder M, Payne R. The epidemiology of testicular cancer in young adults. Am J Epidemiol 1980;112:232–46.

201. Senturia YD. The epidemiology of testicular cancer. Br J Urol 1987;60:285–91.

202. Skakkebaek NE, Berthelsen JG, Giwercman A, Müller J. Carcinoma-in-situ of the testis: possible origin from gonocytes and precursor of all types of germ cell tumours except spermatocytoma. Int J Androl 1987;10:19–28.

203. Swerdlow AJ. The epidemiology of testicular cancer. Eur Urol 1993;23(Suppl 2):35–8.

204. Swerdlow AJ, Huttly SR, Smith PG. Testicular cancer and antecedent disease. Br J Cancer 1987;55:97–103.

205. Swerdlow AJ, Stiller CA, Wilson LM. Prenatal factors in the aetiology of testicular cancer: an epidemiological study of childhood testicular cancer deaths in Great Britain, 1953–73. J Epidemiol Comm Health 1982;36:96–101.

206. Tollerud DJ, Blattner WA, Fraser MC, et al. Familial testicular cancer and urogenital developmental anomalies. Cancer 1985;55:1849–54.

207. United Kingdom Testicular Cancer Study Group. Aetiology of testicular cancer: association with congenital abnormalities, age at puberty, infertility, and exercise. Br Med J 1994;308:1393–9.

208. Whitaker RH. Neoplasia in cryptorchid men. Semin Urol 1988;6:107–9.

Synchronous/Metachronous Tumors

209. Bokemeyer C, Schmoll HJ, Schoffski P, Harstrick A, Bading M, Poliwoda H. Bilateral testicular tumours: prevalence and clinical implications. Eur J Cancer 1993;29A:874–6.

210. Colls BM, Harvey VJ, Skelton L, Thompson PI, Frampton CM. Bilateral germ cell testicular tumors in New Zealand: experience in Auckland and Christchurch 1978–1994. J Clin Oncol 1996;14:2061–5.

211. Dieckmann KP, Becker T, Jonas D, Bauer HW. Inheritance and testicular cancer. Arguments based on a report of 3 cases and a review of the literature. Oncology 1987;44:367–77.

212. Dieckmann KP, Boeckmann W, Brosig W, Jonas D, Bauer HW. Bilateral testicular germ cell tumors. Report of nine cases and review of the literature. Cancer 1986;57:1254–8.

213. Dieckmann KP, Loy P, Buttner P. Prevalence of bilateral testicular germ cell tumours and early detection based on contralateral testicular intra-epithelial neoplasia. Br J Urol 1993;71:340–5.

214. Dieckmann KP, Loy V. Prevalence of bilateral testicular germ cell tumors and early detection by testicular intraepithelial neoplasia. Eur Urol 1993;23(Suppl 2):22–3.

215. Giwercman A, Berthelsen JG, Muller J, von der Maase H, Skakkebaek NE. Screening for carcinoma-in-situ of the testis. Int J Androl 1987;10:173–80.

216. Harland SJ, Cook PA, Fossa SD, et al. Risk factors for carcinoma in situ of the contralateral testis in patients with testicular cancer. An interim report. Eur Urol 1993;23:115–8.

217. Hayakawa M, Mukai K, Nagakura K, Hata M. A case of simultaneous bilateral germ cell tumors arising from cryptorchid testes. J Urol 1986;136:470–2.

218. Kristianslund S, Fossä SD, Kjellevold K. Bilateral malignant testicular germ cell cancer. Br J Urol 1986;58:60–3.

219. Loy V, Dieckmann KP. Prevalence of contralateral testicular intraepithelial neoplasia (carcinoma in situ) in patients with testicular germ cell tumour. Results of the German multicentre study. Eur Urol 1993;23:120–2.

220. Osterlind A, Berthelsen JG, Abildgaard N, et al. Incidence of bilateral testicular germ cell cancer in Denmark, 1960–84: preliminary findings. Int J Androl 1987;10:203–8.

221. Reinberg Y, Manivel JC, Zhang G, Reddy PK. Synchronous bilateral testicular germ cell tumors of different histologic type. Pathogenetic and practical implications of bilaterality in testicular germ cell tumors. Cancer 1991;68:1082–5.

222. Scheiber K, Ackermann D, Studer UE. Bilateral testicular germ cell tumors: a report of 20 cases. J Urol 1987;138:73–6.

223. von der Maase H, Rorth M, Walbom-Jorgensen S, et al. Carcinoma in situ of contralateral testis in patients with testicular germ cell cancer: study of 27 cases in 500 patients. Br Med J 1986;293:1398–401.

224. Ware SM, Heyman J, Al-Askari S, Morales P. Bilateral testicular germ cell malignancy. Urology 1982;19:366–72.

225. Zingg EJ, Zehntner C. Bilateral testicular germ cell tumors. Prog Clin Biol Res 1985;203:673–80.

Familial Tumors

226. Bartkova J, Bartek J, Lukas J, et al. p53 protein alterations in human testicular cancer including pre-invasive intratubular germ-cell neoplasia. Int J Cancer 1991;49:196–202.

227. Dieckmann KP, Becker T, Jonas D, Bauer HW. Inheritance and testicular cancer. Arguments based on a report of 3 cases and a review of the literature. Oncology 1987;44:367–77.

227a. Dieckmann KP, Pichlmeier U. The prevalence of familial testicular cancer: an analysis of two patient populations and a review of the literature. Cancer 1997;801954–60.

228. Fleischhacker M, Strohmeyer T, Imai Y, Slamon DJ, Koeffler HP. Mutations of the p53 gene are not detectable in human testicular tumors. Mod Pathol 1994;7:435–9.

229. Forman D, Oliver RT, Brett AR, et al. Familial testicular cancer: a report of the UK family register, estimation of risk and an HLA class 1 sib-pair analysis. Br J Cancer 1992;65:255–62.

230. Fuller DB, Plenk HP. Malignant testicular germ cell tumors in a father and two sons. Case report and literature review. Cancer 1986;58:955–8.

231. Hartley AL, Birch JM, Kelsey AM, Marsden HB, Harris M, Teare MD. Are germ cell tumors part of the Li-Fraumeni cancer family syndrome? Cancer Genet Cytogenet 1989;42:221–6.

232. Heimdal K, Lothe RA, Lystad S, Holm R, Fossa SD, Borresen AL. No germline TP53 mutations detected in familial and bilateral testicular cancer. Genes Chrom Cancer 1993;6:92–7.

233. Heimdal K, Olsson H, Tretli S, Flodgren P, Borresen AL, Fossa SD. Familial testicular cancer in Norway and southern Sweden. Br J Cancer 1996;73:964–9.

234. Heimdal K, Olsson H, Tretli S, Flodgren P, Borresen AL, Fossa SD. Risk of cancer in relatives of testicular cancer patients. Br J Cancer 1996;73:970–3.

234a. International Testicular Cancer Linkage Consortium. Candidate regions for testicular cancer susceptibility genes. APMIS 1998;106:64–72.

235. Lewis DJ, Sesterhenn IA, McCarthy WF, Moul JW. Immunohistochemical expression of p53 tumor suppressor gene protein in adult germ cell testis tumors: clinical correlation in stage I disease. J Urol 1994;152:418–23.

236. Patel SR, Kvols LK, Richardson RL. Familial testicular cancer: report of six cases and review of the literature. Mayo Clin Proc 1990;65:804–8.

237. Peng HQ, Hogg D, Malkin D, et al. Mutations of the p53 gene do not occur in testis cancer. Cancer Res 1993;53:3574–8.

238. Riou G, Barrois M, Prost S, Terrier MJ, Theodore C, Levine AJ. The p53 and mdm-2 genes in human testicular germ-cell tumors. Mol Carcinog 1995;12:124–31.

239. Ryberg D, Heimdal K, Fossa SD, Borresen AL, Haugen A. Rare Ha-ras1 alleles and predisposition to testicular cancer. Int J Cancer 1993;53:938–40.

240. Schenkman NS, Sesterhenn IA, Washington L, et al. Increased p53 protein does not correlate to p53 gene mutations in microdissected human testicular germ cell tumors. J Urol 1995;154:617–21.

241. Tollerud DJ, Blattner WA, Fraser MC, et al. Familial testicular cancer and urogenital developmental anomalies. Cancer 1985;55:1849–54.

242. Ulbright TM, Orazi A, de Riese W, et al. The correlation of p53 protein expression with proliferative activity and occult metastases in clinical stage I non-seminomatous germ cell tumors of the testis. Mod Pathol 1994;7:64–8.

243. Westergaard T, Olsen JH, Frisch M, Kroman N, Nielsen JW, Melbye M. Cancer risk in fathers and brothers of testicular cancer patients in Denmark. A population-based study. Int J Cancer 1996;66:627–31.

244. Wu WJ, Kakehi Y, Habuchi T, et al. Allelic frequency of p53 gene codon 72 polymorphism in urologic cancers. Jpn J Cancer Res 1995;86:730–6.

245. Ye DW, Zheng J, Qian SX, et al. p53 gene mutations in Chinese human testicular seminoma. J Urol 1993;150:884–6.

246. Collins GM, Kim DU, Logrono R, Rickert RR, Zablow A, Breen JL. Pure seminoma arising in androgen insensitivity syndrome (testicular feminization syndrome): a case report and review of the literature. Mod Pathol 1993;6:89–93.

247. Hughesdon PE, Kumarasamy T. Mixed germ cell tumours (gonadoblastomas) in normal and dysgenetic gonads: case reports and review. Virchows Arch [A] 1970;349:258–80.

248. Manuel M, Katayama KP, Jones HW. The age of occurrence of gonadal tumors in intersex patients. Am J Obstet Gynecol 1976;124:293–306.

249. Morris JM. The syndrome of testicular feminization in male pseudohermaphrodites. Am J Obstet Gynecol 1953;65:1192–211.

250. Morris JM, Mahesh VB. Further observations on the syndrome, "testicular feminization." Am J Obstet Gynecol 1963;87:731–48.

251. Muller J, Skakkebaek NE, Ritzén M, Plöen L, Petersen KE. Carcinoma in situ of the testis in children with 45,X/46,XY gonadal dysgenesis. J Pediatr 1985;106:431–6.

252. Nogales FF Jr, Toro M, Ortega I, Fulwood HR. Bilateral incipient germ cell tumours of the testis in the incomplete testicular feminization syndrome. Histopathology 1981;5:511–5.

253. Ramani P, Yeung CK, Habeebu SS. Testicular intratubular germ cell neoplasia in children and adolescents with intersex. Am J Surg Pathol 1993;17:1124–33.

254. Rutgers JL. Advances in the pathology of intersex syndromes. Hum Pathol 1991;22:884–91.

255. Rutgers JL, Scully RE. Pathology of the testis in intersex syndromes. Semin Diagn Pathol 1987;4:275–91.

256. Rutgers JL, Scully RE. The androgen insensitivity syndrome (testicular feminization): a clinicopathologic study of 43 cases. Int J Gynecol Pathol 1991;10:126–45.

Infertility

257. Giwercman A, Berthelsen JG, Muller J, von der Maase H, Skakkebaek NE. Screening for carcinoma-in-situ of the testis. Int J Androl 1987;10:173–80.

258. Gondos B, Migliozzi JA. Intratubular germ cell neoplasia. Semin Diagn Pathol 1987;4:292–303.

259. Pryor JP, Cameron KM, Chilton CP, et al. Carcinoma in situ in testicular biopsies in men presenting with infertility. Br J Urol 1983;55:780–4.

260. Skakkebaek NE. Carcinoma in situ of the testis: frequency and relationship to invasive germ cell tumours in infertile men. Histopathology 1978;2:157–70.

261. Skakkebaek NE, Berthelsen JG, Visfeldt J. Clinical aspects of testicular carcinoma-in-situ. Int J Androl 1981;4(Suppl):153–62.

262. Swerdlow AJ, Huttly SR, Smith PG. Testis cancer: postnatal hormonal factors, sexual behaviour and fertility. Int J Cancer 1989;43:549–53.

263. West AB, Butler MR, Fitzpatrick J, O'Brien A. Testicular tumors in subfertile men: report of 4 cases with implications for management of patients presenting with infertility. J Urol 1985;133:107–9.

General Clinical Aspects

264. Burton GV, Bullard DE, Walther PJ, Burger PC. Paraneoplastic encephalopathy with testicular carcinoma: a reversible neurologic syndrome. Cancer 1988;62:2248–51.

264a. da Silva MA, Edmondson JW, Eby C, Loehrer PJ Sr. Humoral hypercalcemia in seminomas. Med Pediatr Oncol 1992;20:38–41.

265. Dichmann O, Engel U, Jensen DB, Bilde T. Juxtatesticular seminoma. Br J Urol 1990;66:324–5.

266. Leaf DN, Tucker GR III, Harrison LH. Embryonal cell carcinoma originating in the spermatic cord: case report. J Urol 1974;112:285–6.

266a. Lewis LG. Testis tumors: report of 250 cases. J Urol 1948;59:763–72.

267. Lundberg WB, Mitchell MS. Transient warm autoimmune hemolytic anemia and cryoglobulinemia associated with seminoma. Yale J Biol Med 1977;50:419–27.

268. Mann AS. Bilateral exophthalmos in seminoma. J Clin Endocrinol Metab 1967;27:1500–2.

269. Melicow M. Classification of tumors of the testis: a clinical and pathological study based on 105 primary and 13 secondary cases in adults, and 3 primary and 4 secondary cases in children. J Urol 1955;73:547–74.

270. O'Riordan WD, Sherman NJ. Cryptorchidism and abdominal pain. J Emerg Med 1977;196–7.

271. Pugh RC. Testicular tumours–introduction. In: Pugh RC, ed. Pathology of the testis. Oxford: Blackwell Scientific, 1976:139–59.

272. Reman O, Reynick Y, Casadevall N, et al. Polycythemia and steroid overproduction in a gonadotropin–secreting seminoma of the testis. Cancer 1991;68:2224–9.

273. Sarma DP, Weilbaecher TG, Hatem AA. Seminoma arising in undescended testis clinically presenting as acute appendicitis. J Surg Oncol 1986;31:44–7.

274. Scully RE. Testicular tumors with endocrine manifestations. In: DeGroot LJ, ed. Endocrinology. Philadelphia: WB Saunders, 1995:2442–8.

275. Simpson AH, Calvert DG, Codling BW. The shrinking seminoma. J Roy Soc Med 1990;83:187.

276. Srigley JR, Hartwick RW. Tumors and cysts of the paratesticular region. Pathol Annu 1990;25(pt. 2):51–108.

277. Taylor JB, Solomon DH, Levine RE, Ehrlich RM. Exophthalmos in seminoma: regression with steroids and orchiectomy. JAMA 1978;240:860–1.

278. Thackray AC, Crane WA. Seminoma. In: Pugh RC, ed. Pathology of the testis. Oxford: Blackwell Scientific, 1976:164–98.

278a. Voltz R, Gultekin SH, Rosenfeld MR, et al. A serologic marker of paraneoplastic limbic and brain-stem encephalitis in patients with testicular cancer. N Engl J Med 1999;340:1831–3.

279. Zavala-Pompa A, Ro JY, El-Naggar A, et al. Primary carcinoid tumor of testis. Immunohistochemical, ultrastructural, and DNA flow cytometric study of three cases with a review of the literature. Cancer 1993;72:1726–32.

2
GERM CELL TUMORS: HISTOGENETIC CONSIDERATIONS AND INTRATUBULAR GERM CELL NEOPLASIA

HISTOGENESIS

The observations of Skakkebaek (see page 45) and the evolution of the concept of intratubular germ cell neoplasia indicate that most, but not all, germ cell tumors of the testis evolve from a common neoplastic precursor lesion, intratubular germ cell neoplasia of the unclassified type (IGCNU). In past schemes, two divergent pathways were theorized, one giving rise to seminoma and the second to embryonal carcinoma (48). While seminoma was considered incapable of further differentiation, embryonal carcinoma was felt capable of giving rise to other forms of germ cell tumor such as yolk sac tumor, teratoma, and choriocarcinoma. Mostofi and Sesterhenn (39), however, questioned the accuracy of these concepts, feeling that a malignant germ cell may give rise directly to various forms of tumor and cited the observation of specific types of germ cell tumor differentiation within the tubules as evidence for this belief. Recently, the "end-stage" concept of seminoma has been seriously questioned, although it should be noted that Friedman and Moore (15) felt that seminomas evolved into embryonal carcinomas in their seminal study in 1946.

The common observation of nonseminomatous metastases at autopsy in patients who died subsequent to an orchiectomy that demonstrated only seminoma (see Table 1-3) is consistent with the concept that seminomas may evolve into other types of germ cell tumor (6,25). The group from M.D. Anderson (61) noted the presence of early carcinomatous differentiation on ultrastructural examination of seminomas that were typical by light microscopy. Czaja and Ulbright (7) presented several cases of seminoma with apparent focal evolution into yolk tumor, based both on light microscopic and immunohistochemical evaluations, and similar cases were described by Raghavan et al. (54). Ultrastructural studies of xenografted tumors have identified cells with features intermediate between those of seminoma and yolk sac tumor (37).

Analysis of ploidy patterns in germ cell tumors has demonstrated a higher mean deoxyribonucleic acid (DNA) content in seminomas than in nonseminomatous germ cell tumors, supporting the theory that embryonal carcinoma may evolve from seminoma as gene loss occurs; the loss may be of cancer suppressor genes, with resultant evolution of a more aggressive neoplasm (11,14,30,42). Karyotypic analyses support this hypothesis (11), and demonstrate the common occurrence of a marker chromosome, isochromosome (12p), in seminomas, nonseminomatous germ cell tumors, and IGCNU (1,5,13,16,17,56,57,60,64,67) that leads to an excessive number of genes derived from the short arm of chromosome 12. Over-representation of these genes occurs even in cases lacking isochromosome (12p) (2,16,45,57,60). Other chromosomes that show a consistent pattern of over-representation include: 7, 8, 21, and X (57). Recently, testicular germ cell tumors were commonly noted to have deletions of the short arm of chromosome 11 or to show loss of heterozygosity at various chromosomal loci (especially chromosomes 13, 18, and Y), perhaps correlating with the location of tumor suppressor genes (31–33,46,59). The occurrence of identical reactions in IGCNU and seminomas with certain monoclonal and polyclonal antibodies supports a close relationship, if not identity, between the cells of IGCNU and those of seminoma (18,19,23,28,29,41). Similar ploidy patterns, cytogenetic findings, lectin-binding patterns, and numbers of nucleolar organizer regions in IGCNU and seminoma provide additional support for this close relationship (10–12,14,34,65), and, because of the totipotential nature of the cells of IGCNU, implicate seminoma cells with a totipotential capacity.

The M.D. Anderson group, recognizing the difficulty in reconciling such observations with the older theories of germ cell tumor histogenesis, proposed a different model for germ cell tumor evolution (61). In this tetrahedron model (fig. 2-1), seminoma is the common precursor lesion and embryonal carcinoma arises from

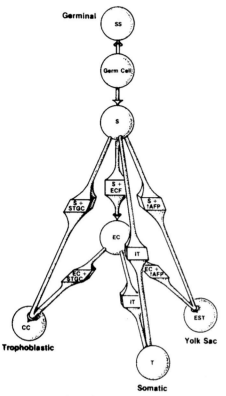

SS – spermatocytic seminoma
S – seminoma
S + ECF – seminoma with early carcinomatous features
EC – embryonal carcinoma
S + STGC – seminoma with syncytiotrophoblastic giant cells
S + ↑AFP – seminoma with elevated alpha–fetoprotein
IT – immature teratoma
EC + STGC – embryonal carcinoma with syncytiotrophoblastic giant cells
EC + AFP – embryonal carcinoma with elevated alpha–fetoprotein
CC – choriocarcinoma
T – mature teratoma
EST – endodermal sinus tumor

Figure 2-1
TETRAHEDRON MODEL OF HISTOGENESIS

In the tetrahedron model of histogenesis, seminoma represents the common precursor for almost all testicular germ cell tumors, with several forms intermediate between seminoma and the nonseminomatous tumors also possible. (Fig. 22 from Srigley JR, Mackay B, Toth P, Ayala A. The ultrastructure and histogenesis of male germ cell neoplasia with emphasis on seminoma with early carcinomatous features. Ultrastruct Pathol 1988;12:67–86.)

seminoma. The other forms of germ cell tumor, representing trophoblastic, somatic (teratomatous), and yolk sac differentiation, may then arise either directly from seminoma or from embryonal carcinoma. This model explains many observations that are difficult to reconcile with the previous concept of two separate pathways, including: the occurrence of seminoma with syncytiotrophoblastic cells and the demonstration of

human chorionic gonadotropin (hCG) within seminoma cells (4,38); the presence of elevated serum alpha-fetoprotein (AFP) levels in some patients with apparently pure testicular seminoma (24, 54); immunohistochemical staining for AFP in embryonal carcinoma (40,41); and the aforementioned common identification of nonseminomatous metastases at autopsy in patients whose orchiectomy showed only seminoma (6,25). Another attribute of this model, given the key role of seminoma as the common precursor, is its reconciliation of the striking similarities of morphology, immunohistochemistry, ultrastructure, DNA content, lectin binding, and numbers of nucleolar organizer regions of IGCNU and seminoma (3,11,12,19,34, 58). Since it is universally acknowledged that IGCNU is the common precursor lesion of the overwhelming majority of germ cell tumors, it is reasonable to hypothesize that seminoma arises as the invasive derivative of IGCNU and that further morphologic diversity usually arises from seminoma. In rare instances, intratubular evolution from IGCNU may occur, perhaps as cancer suppressor genes are lost, to give rise to intratubular differentiated forms of germ cell tumor as described by Mostofi and Sesterhenn (39) and others (62). Similarities in the chromosome composition of IGCNU and adjacent nonseminomatous tumors, which contrast with the chromosome composition of seminoma and its associated IGCNU, confirm that intratubular transformation does occur prior to morphologic change (25,43). This concept has received additional recent support by the demonstration of immunohistochemical differences in IGCNU that correlate with seminomatous or nonseminomatous differentiation (54a). Modification of the tetrahedron model (61) to accommodate the possibility of intratubular differentiation (20), to incorporate the concept of IGCNU, and to provide for a separate pathway for those less common germ cell tumors unassociated with IGCNU, produces a more complete but complicated hypothesis for testicular germ cell tumor histogenesis (fig. 2-2).

Mostofi and Sesterhenn (39) have pointed out that there are problems with the above hypotheses. Most importantly, both seminoma and embryonal carcinoma either do not occur, or are very rare, in infancy when yolk sac tumor and teratoma are essentially the only testicular germ cell tumors encountered. The absence of the purported

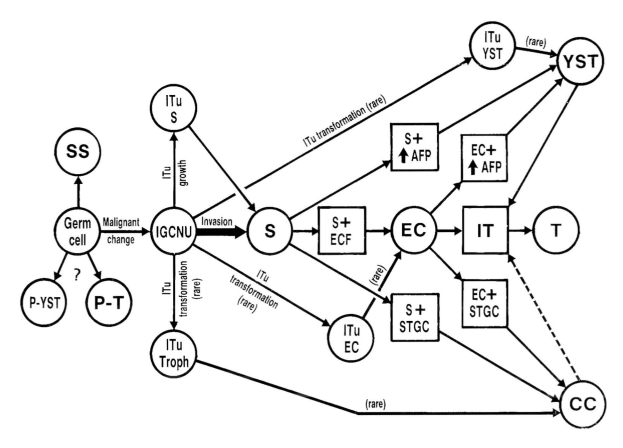

Figure 2-2
REVISED TETRAHEDRON MODEL OF HISTOGENESIS

Seminoma remains the most important precursor, but intratubular differentiation may occur. Also, spermatocytic seminoma and the pediatric germ cell tumors arise from a different pathway. The broken arrow remains a speculative step; smaller print indicates rare lesions. Key: AFP - alpha-fetoprotein; CC - choriocarcinoma; EC - embryonal carcinoma; ECF - early carcinomatous features; IGCNU - intratubular germ cell neoplasia, unclassified; IT - immature teratoma; ITu - intratubular; P-T - pediatric teratoma; P-YST - pediatric yolk sac tumor; S - seminoma; SS - spermatocytic seminoma; STGC - syncytiotrophoblast giant cells; T - teratoma; Troph - trophoblast cells; YST - yolk sac tumor. (Adapted from Ulbright TM, Roth LM. Testicular and paratesticular neoplasms. In: Sternberg SS, Ed. Diagnostic surgical pathology. New York: Raven Press, 1994:1885–947.)

precursor lesion (seminoma) in this age group seems inconsistent with the proposed model of histogenesis. Also, testicular germ cell tumors of infancy are not generally associated with IGCNU (35,36), or at least the association with IGCNU is much less conspicuous than in older patients (21,26,44,55), suggesting that the pathogenesis of germ cell tumors in infancy may be different from that of germ cell tumors in older males. This viewpoint is further supported by an absence of isochromosome (12p) in pediatric germ cell tumors (47). A hitherto undeveloped model of histogenesis may therefore apply to tumors of infancy, but these observations concerning the infantile tumors do not necessarily

invalidate the modified tetrahedron model (61) for most testicular germ cell tumors.

Although the general inability of seminoma to grow in tissue culture or to be reproduced in animal experiments has hindered the laboratory investigation of its precursor role (8), such techniques have proved useful in the evaluation of the precursor role of embryonal carcinoma (9). Pierce et al. (49,51,52) demonstrated that embryonal carcinoma cells from mouse-derived testicular tumors differentiated into teratomatous structures. Cloning experiments have shown that single embryonal carcinoma cells that are transplanted into the peritoneal cavity of mice differentiated into complex "teratocarcinomas" (embryonal carcinoma

Table 2-1

DISTRIBUTION OF TESTICULAR GERM CELL TUMORS IN FOUR SERIES*

	Jacobsen	Von Hochstetter	Pugh	Teppo	Total
Seminoma (48.3 %)	554 (53%)	171 (53%)	1082 (46%)	63 (53%)	1870
classic	515 (49%)	162 (50%)	—‡	---	—
with STGCs§	—	3 (1%)	---	---	—
spermatocytic	13 (1%)	6 (2%)	---	---	—
"anaplastic"	26 (2%)	—	---	---	—
NSGCTs (includes those mixed with S) (51.7%)	499** (47%)	153 (47%)	1291 (54%)	57 (48%)	2000
Pure NSGCTs	145 (14%)	53 (16%)	---	---	—
EC	109 (10%)	35 (11%)	---	---	—
PE	—	0	---	---	—
YST	3 (0.3%)	5 (2%)	53 (2%)	---	—
T	31 (3%)	13 (4%)	---	---	—
mature	—	6 (2%)	---	---	—
immature	—	6 (2%)	---	---	—
"malignant"	—	1 (0.3%)	---	---	—
CC	2 (0.2%)	0	---	---	—
Mixed NSGCTs	352 (33%)	100† (31%)	---	---	—
EC + T	90 (9%)	33 (10%)	---	---	—
S + T	21 (2%)	7 (2%)	---	---	—
S + EC + T	23 (2%)	15 (4%)	---	---	—
S + EC	58 (6%)	24 (7%)	---	---	—
CC + T	3 (0.3%)	1 (0.3%)	---	---	—
CC + EC + T	26 (2%)	13 (4)	---	---	—
CC + EC + T + S	3 (0.3%)	2 (0.6%)	---	---	—
CC + EC	13 (1%)	5 (2%)	---	---	—
Others (including those not assessable)	115 (11%)	0	1238 (52%)	---	—
Total	1053	324	2373	120	3870

*Adapted from references 22,53,63,66.
**Two NSGCTs were not further classified due to extensive necrosis.
†YST was not separately categorized as a component of mixed germ cell tumors.
‡– Indicates not specifically assessed.
§Abbreviations: CC=choriocarcinoma; EC=embryonal carcinoma; NSGCT=nonseminomatous germ cell tumor; PE=polyembryoma; S=seminoma; STGCs=syncytiotrophoblastic giant cells; T=teratoma; YST=yolk sac tumor.

plus teratoma) (27). Furthermore, the overgrowth of "teratocarcinomas" maintained in vitro or in ascites by yolk sac tumor elements supports the differentiation of embryonal carcinoma into yolk sac tumor elements as well as teratomatous elements (52). The ability to form trophoblastic tissue from embryonal carcinoma was suggested by the development of uterine hyperplasia after heterotransplantation of a morphologically typical embryonal carcinoma into cortisone-treated hamsters (50). This work provides convincing evidence for the precursor role of embryonal carcinoma in the formation of other germ cell tumor elements.

Table 2-1 provides a breakdown of the relative frequencies of different types of testicular germ cell tumors in four relatively large studies. Because of differences in nomenclature, it is not possible to provide information regarding some categories. It is apparent that seminomas and nonseminomatous tumors are of approximately equal frequency, with the heterogeneous mixed germ cell tumors constituting the great majority of nonseminomatous neoplasms.

Table 2-2

CLASSIFICATION OF INTRATUBULAR GERM CELL NEOPLASIA*

Intratubular germ cell neoplasia, unclassified

Intratubular germ cell neoplasia, unclassified, with extratubular extension (early seminoma)

Intratubular seminoma
    Classic
    Spermatocytic

Intratubular embryonal carcinoma

Intratubular yolk sac tumor

Intratubular germ cell neoplasia, other forms

---

*Modified from: Scully RE. Testis. In: Henson DE, Albores-Saavedra J, eds. The pathology of incipient neoplasia. Philadelphia, WB Saunders, 1993:384–400.

INTRATUBULAR GERM CELL NEOPLASIA

Intratubular germ cell neoplasia is characterized by the presence of malignant germ cells within the seminiferous tubules. In its most common form, the unclassified type (IGCNU), there is an initial, basal proliferation of undifferentiated, atypical, enlarged germ cells with generally clear cytoplasm that resemble the neoplastic cells of seminoma. IGCNU is considered the common precursor of most germ cell tumors. A classification of intratubular germ cell neoplasia is provided in Table 2-2.

Intratubular Germ Cell Neoplasia, Unclassified Type

General Features. Skakkebaek (136,137) first drew attention to the presence of atypical germ cells in the testes of two infertile men and speculated that these cells represented the preinvasive phase of testicular cancer. The pioneering work of Skakkebaek and his associates in subsequent years verified the accuracy of these observations. Currently, the most controversial aspect of this topic does not involve the morphology or clinical significance of this lesion, but rather the most appropriate terminology for it. Skakkebaek and his co-workers have consistently used the term "carcinoma-in-situ" when describing this lesion; this expression has the merit of conveying the essential information regarding the significance of this finding in familiar terms. Unfortunately, it is histogenetically inaccurate. The intratubular malignant germ cells that Skakkebaek described do not have epithelial features. They do not consistently express cytokeratin (115), and they do not have epithelial junctions on ultrastructural examination (97,135). Furthermore, the invasive neoplasm that they resemble, seminoma, is not a carcinoma. For these reasons the term carcinoma-in-situ is inappropriate. "Seminoma-in-situ" is also not recommended because this lesion may be associated, synchronously or metachronously, with all other invasive germ cell tumors except spermatocytic seminoma. More recently, Skakkebaek and his group have advocated the term "gonocytoma-in-situ" for this lesion (89,140) based on the belief that the malignant cells have features, including their ultrastructure (92) and the results of special stains and immunohistochemistry (140), of prespermatogenic cells. They also consider seminoma, having a similar morphology and ultrastructure to the intratubular lesion and therefore resembling prespermatogenic gonocytes, to be appropriately termed gonocytoma. Koide et al. (104) support this position by suggesting that this intratubular lesion represents a neoplastic reproduction of the germ cells of the fetal testis that, like the atypical germ cells, contain glycogen and a placental-like alkaline phosphatase but which lose these markers shortly after birth. Other studies also support the resemblance of IGCNU to fetal gonocytes (83,101,104). It is furthermore speculated that failure of gonocytes to transform into spermatogonia may be the basis for the tumor development (141a). But gonocytoma-in-situ is still a suboptimal term because the invasive tumor identified on follow-up may not be a seminoma (gonocytoma). The term most widely applied now and utilized here is intratubular germ cell neoplasia, unclassified type (IGCNU); it was agreed upon at an international symposium in 1980 (133). In addition to IGCNU, there are other types of intratubular germ cell neoplasia that show specific forms of differentiation (Table 2-2): intratubular seminoma, intratubular spermatocytic seminoma, intratubular embryonal carcinoma, and, rarely, intratubular yolk sac tumor. Many authors substitute the more inclusive term "intratubular germ cell neoplasia" as a synonym for IGCNU.

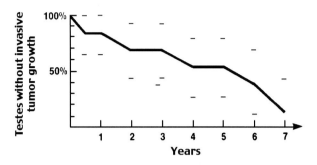

Figure 2-3

THE PROPORTION OF TUMOR-FREE TESTES
AFTER A BIOPSY SHOWING INTRATUBULAR
GERM CELL NEOPLASIA, UNCLASSIFIED

This diagram depicts the percentage of testes that remain free of invasive tumor after a testicular biopsy positive
for intratubular germ cell neoplasia, unclassified type. At 5
years about 50 percent of the patients have developed invasive germ cell tumors, and only a small fraction remain free
of invasive tumors by 7 years. (Fig. 4 from Skakkebaek NE,
Berthelsen JG, Visfeldt J. Clinical aspects of testicular
carcinoma-in-situ. Int J Androl 1981;4(Suppl):153–62.)

The evidence that IGCNU is a form of in situ
neoplasia comes from several sources. In the
original studies of Skakkebaek and colleagues
(141), 50 percent of patients with IGCNU developed invasive germ cell tumors by 5 years of
follow-up, and relatively few patients were free
of invasive tumor at 8 years (fig. 2-3). Rare
patients, however, may not develop a tumor until
15 years after a biopsy showing IGCNU (90).
Furthermore, IGCNU is found at a greater than
expected frequency in populations that are
known to be at increased risk for invasive germ
cell tumors and is not identified in control populations (88). The frequency of IGCNU in patients
with a history of cryptorchidism is 2 to 8 percent
(84,87,92,105,127); patients with a prior germ
cell tumor have a frequency of about 5 percent in
the contralateral testis (73,123,148); the frequency is from 0.4 to 1 percent in patients with
infertility (129,139,150); and 4 of 4 patients with
gonadal dysgenesis in one series had IGCNU
(121) as did 3 of 12 patients with androgen
insensitivity (testicular feminization) syndrome
in another (117). IGCNU is demonstrable in 8
percent of children and adolescents with gonadal
dysgenesis but not in young patients with the
androgen insensitivity syndrome (130). Ploidy
studies have demonstrated that IGCNU is aneuploid, adding further support to its neoplastic

nature (119,138). There is also a remarkably
high frequency of IGCNU in the seminiferous
tubules adjacent to invasive germ cell tumors
(78,97,138). Coffin et al. (78) reported that 98
percent of cases of invasive germ cell tumor had
associated IGCNU when residual seminiferous
tubules were present, an observation that supports the precursor role of IGCNU. Similarities
between the cytogenetic abnormalities in
IGCNU and the adjacent invasive germ cell
tumor support the view that the invasive tumor
is a derivative of IGCNU and provide additional
support for its precursor role (82,145). The frequent association of IGCNU with invasive germ
cell tumors applies to both seminomas and nonseminomatous types, although IGCNU is seen
somewhat more often in nonseminomatous tumors (134). IGCNU, however, has not been associated with spermatocytic seminoma (81,140) and is
infrequent in pediatric cases of yolk sac tumor
and teratoma (96,102,110,111,126,143,144).

IGCNU, in the absence of an invasive tumor,
is asymptomatic and is usually a microscopic
finding in a testicular biopsy performed for other
indications or for screening purposes. As discussed above, there are certain groups of patients who are much more likely to have IGCNU
than the general population. The testis involved
by IGCNU is often smaller than normal (measuring 10 to 12 mL in volume), and there is
usually oligospermia (89). In screening studies
for IGCNU there is a much greater likelihood of
a positive testicular biopsy in the presence of
testicular atrophy (94,108).

Testicular biopsies detect IGCNU with a high
rate of sensitivity. It has been estimated that if
IGCNU involves greater than 2 percent of the
testicular volume, a single biopsy will detect
more than 50 percent of the cases, and if IGCNU
involves more that 10 percent of the testis, a
single biopsy will detect all the cases (72).
Berthelsen and Skakkebaek (72) felt that one or
two biopsy specimens 3 mm in diameter would
detect virtually all cases. In support of this high
sensitivity of testicular biopsy in detecting
IGCNU, only 1 patient among more than 1,500
with infertility or testicular maldescent and negative testicular biopsies developed testicular
cancer on follow-up extending to 8 years (89). In
a second study, 2 of 1858 patients with negative
testicular biopsies contralateral to a germ cell

tumor developed an invasive tumor (80a). In the face of severe atrophy, posterior biopsies near the rete testis may be more productive (125). Because of the high rate of bilaterality of IGCNU (about 40 percent in cases associated with infertility [139]), bilateral biopsy is advocated (129).

The population that requires screening for IGCNU remains somewhat controversial. Giwercman and Skakkebaek (89,90) recommend screening all patients with a history of testicular cancer, all patients with somatosexual ambiguity and a Y chromosome, patients with presumed extragonadal germ cell tumors, and, less strongly, patients with a history of cryptorchidism. Whether patients with oligospermic infertility need biopsy is unclear (89). Biopsy in cryptorchid patients should be delayed until age 18 to 20 years since there is no significant risk of invasive testicular cancer in this group prior to that age (89), and the efficacy of screening at an earlier age appears poor. There is evidence that IGCNU is not easily detectable in at-risk, cryptorchid boys who are prepubertal; the majority of such patients have some abnormal-appearing germ cells with an increased nuclear DNA content (118). No patient among 22 who had a prepubertal biopsy that showed germ cells staining for placental alkaline phosphatase developed a tumor on long-term (mean, 25 years) follow-up (93a). It should be noted that many urologists take issue with the recommendation for biopsy of the contralateral testis in patients with a testicular germ cell tumor; they argue that the yield is low, the procedure is associated with morbidity, and the result, whether positive or negative, does not alter their plan for continued follow-up.

Many male patients with retroperitoneal germ cell tumors who lack clinical evidence of a primary testicular tumor have IGCNU on testicular biopsies (77,79). This is not the case in patients with mediastinal germ cell tumors (79), with rare exceptions (93). This suggests that some of these cases represent metastasis from a regressed, invasive testicular primary tumor (132), although conceivably there may be a "field effect" causing independent neoplasia at both sites. This latter explanation, however, seems unlikely given the high rate of detection of IGCNU in this situation (53 percent in Daugaard's series of 15 patients with retroperitoneal germ cell tumors [79]) and the relatively low rate

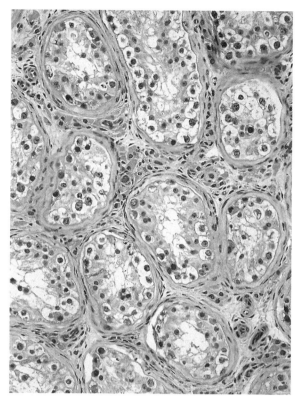

Figure 2-4
INTRATUBULAR GERM CELL NEOPLASIA,
UNCLASSIFIED TYPE
Cells with enlarged nuclei and clear cytoplasm are aligned along the basal aspect of seminiferous tubules lacking spermatogenesis. Sertoli cells are present on the luminal aspect. Note also clusters of Leydig cells in the interstitium.

of IGCNU in the contralateral testis of patients with testicular germ cell tumors (approximately 5 percent). It also fails to explain why a comparable rate of IGCNU is not associated with mediastinal germ cell tumors. For these reasons, it has been suggested that patients with apparent primary retroperitoneal germ cell tumors have testicular biopsies (90).

Gross Findings. A testis harboring IGCNU may appear normal or atrophic. A firmer than usual character may be present secondary to tubular shrinkage and intertubular fibrosis, particularly in cases of "burnt-out germ cell tumors" (see chapter 5). If there is an associated germ cell tumor, the findings characteristic of that lesion are present.

Microscopic Findings. IGCNU consists of enlarged cells with clear cytoplasm that are aligned along the basal portion of seminiferous tubules

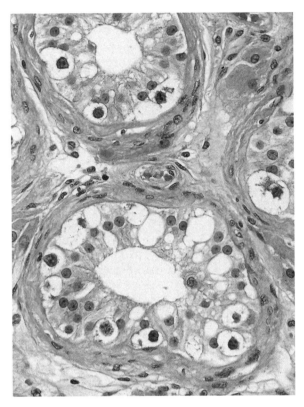

Figure 2-5
INTRATUBULAR GERM CELL NEOPLASIA,
UNCLASSIFIED TYPE
The malignant cells have clear or retracted cytoplasm and enlarged nuclei with one or more nucleoli. Spermatogenesis is absent. Sertoli cells are displaced toward the lumen, and the tubular basement membrane is thickened.

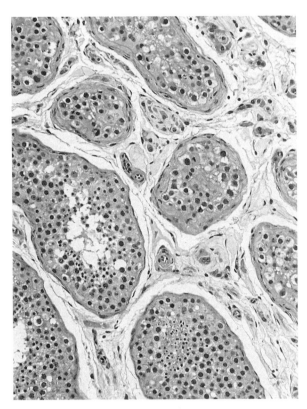

Figure 2-6
INTRATUBULAR GERM CELL
NEOPLASIA, UNCLASSIFIED TYPE
Patchy distribution of intratubular germ cell neoplasia, unclassified type (top), with adjacent normal tubules with active spermatogenesis.

(fig. 2-4). The nuclei are round, significantly larger than those of spermatogonia (median diameter, 9.7 µm versus 6.5 µm, respectively [89]), and are hyperchromatic with one or more prominent nucleoli (fig. 2-5). The nuclear membranes are thickened and irregular. Mitoses may be frequent and can be atypical but are often not conspicuous. The seminiferous tubules involved by IGCNU are usually abnormal, often showing a decreased tubular diameter, thickened peritubular basement membrane and, except in the very early cases, an absence of normal spermatogenic cells (fig. 2-5). Sertoli cells, but not spermatogonia or more mature spermatogenic cells, are characteristically intermingled with IGCNU but show luminal displacement (figs. 2-4, 2-5). If IGCNU is extensive, however, the Sertoli cells can be replaced. In some cases there is a peritubular lymphoid infiltrate and, infrequently, an in-

tratubular granulomatous reaction. Intratubular calcifications occur with increased frequency (39 percent) (102a). Adjacent seminiferous tubules may be completely normal and show intact spermatogenesis (fig. 2-6). The Leydig cells appear normal but may be increased in number (fig. 2-4). In the rare cases described in prepubertal patients, the neoplastic cells, rather than being basally located, were dispersed at various levels throughout the seminiferous tubules (140). The typical adult pattern evolved as the patient aged (120). It is not uncommon for IGCNU to extend into the ductal system of the testis, spreading in a pagetoid pattern into the rete testis and occasionally into the epididymis (107,128). Such spread may produce a confusing histologic picture, similar to that seen in cases of seminoma extending into the rete testis (see page 73 and figs. 3-24, 3-25) (113).

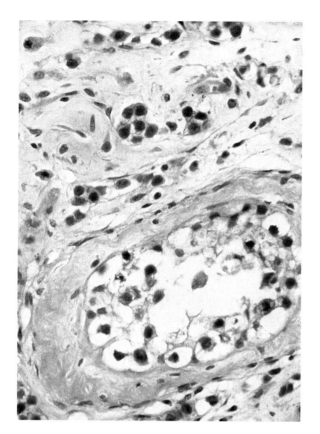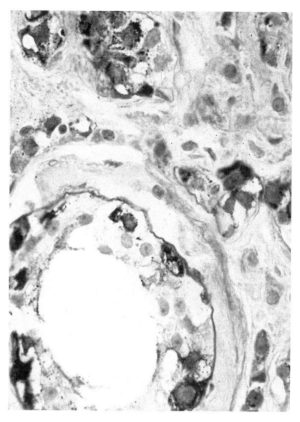

Figure 2-7
INTRATUBULAR GERM CELL NEOPLASIA, UNCLASSIFIED TYPE (IGCNU), WITH EXTRATUBULAR EXTENSION
Left: Small clusters of cells with the morphologic features of seminoma cells are seen in the stroma around a tubule showing IGCNU.
Right: A periodic acid–Schiff (PAS) stain highlights the cells in the stroma. (Fig. 4.10 from Young RH, Scully RE. Testicular tumors. Chicago: ASCP Press, 1990:98.)

In occasional cases of what is predominantly IGCNU, small foci of infiltrating germ cells are seen beyond the basement membranes of the tubules (fig. 2-7). In such cases the descriptive diagnosis, "intratubular germ cell neoplasia unclassified, with extratubular extension," is appropriate. The tumor cells in such cases have the features of seminoma cells (fig. 2-7).

Glycogen is readily demonstrated in the overwhelming majority of cases of IGCNU (fig. 2-8). Coffin et al. (78) found that 46 of 47 (98 percent) cases were periodic acid–Schiff (PAS) positive. Although non-neoplastic spermatogonia and Sertoli cells may also contain glycogen (109), it is typically only in small amounts, making PAS stains quite helpful in the detection of IGCNU. The silver staining technique for the demonstration of nucleolar organizer regions (AgNOR) may also be efficacious for identifying IGCNU; in one

study the AgNOR counts per cell for IGCNU ranged from 19 to 52, with no overlap in AgNOR values for either Sertoli cells or spermatogonia (range, 5 to 18) (122).

Immunohistochemical Findings. Immunostaining discloses placental-like alkaline phosphatase (PLAP) in a high percentage of cases of IGCNU. It appears as membranous (predominantly) and cytoplasmic positivity (fig. 2-9). PLAP positivity was reported in 20 of 24 cases (83 percent) by Jacobsen and Norgaard-Pedersen, 5 of 5 cases by Beckstead, 154 of 155 (99 percent) by Burke and Mostofi, and 52 of 53 cases (98 percent) by Manivel et al. (71,76,100,109). Non-neoplastic spermatogenic cells are almost always PLAP negative. Burke and Mostofi (75) showed an absence of PLAP positivity in the spermatogonia of 469 testicular biopsies lacking IGCNU, although there were four cases with

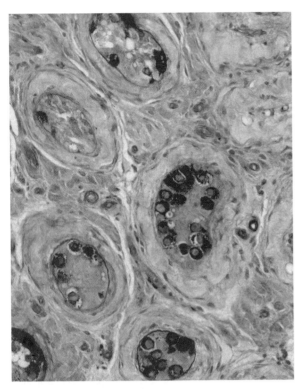

Figure 2-8
INTRATUBULAR GERM CELL NEOPLASIA,
UNCLASSIFIED TYPE
Intense PAS positivity in the neoplastic germ cells.

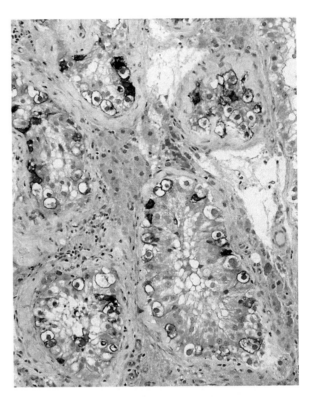

Figure 2-9
INTRATUBULAR GERM CELL NEOPLASIA,
UNCLASSIFIED TYPE
Staining with an antibody directed against placental alkaline phosphatase shows an intense, predominantly membrane-associated positivity in the neoplastic germ cells (anti-placental alkaline phosphatase immunostain).

rare, isolated PLAP positive spermatocytes. PLAP positivity is therefore very useful in confirming IGCNU if the light microscopic findings alone are not entirely diagnostic.

Immunostaining for ferritin has also been proposed as a useful marker for IGCNU. Jacobsen and co-workers (98,99) identified ferritin in 83 percent of cases. Coffin and co-workers (78), however, found only a 2.3 percent frequency of positivity. The reason for this discrepancy is unclear. Several monoclonal antibodies (M2A, 43-9F, TRA-1-60, HB5, HF2, HE11) and antibodies directed against the c-kit proto-oncogene, glutathione-S-transferase π and glycolipid globotriaosylceramide (Gb3) have been used to identify IGCNU with very high sensitivities (69,83,85,86,94a,102b,103). p53 is identifiable in a majority of cases of IGCNU (70), and one study identified DNA mutations by sequence analysis in 39 percent of cases (106), further supporting its malignant nature.

Ultrastructural Findings. On ultrastructural examination the cells of IGCNU have evenly dispersed nuclear chromatin lacking peripheral margination, complex central nucleoli, mitochondria with eccentric cristae, granular intermitochondrial matrix (so-called nuage), annulate lamellae, sparse cisternae of rough endoplasmic reticulum, a high density of free ribosomes, generally abundant glycogen, and only loose, intercellular attachment plaques (68,91,92,124,135). These features are felt to be similar to those of prespermatogenic germ cells, including gonocytes. There is an absence of the synaptinemal complexes that characterize spermatocytic differentiation (92). The ultrastructural features are essentially identical to those of seminoma (95,142).

Special Diagnostic Techniques. Microspectrophotometric methods have demonstrated that the neoplastic cells of IGCNU are aneuploid (119,138). Furthermore, isochromosome (12p), a common cytogenetic anomaly in a variety of testicular germ cell tumors, was identified on karyotypic

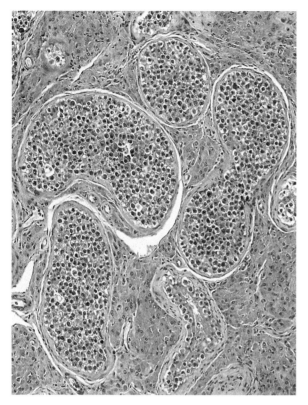

Figure 2-10
INTRATUBULAR SEMINOMA

The tumor cells distend the tubules. Intratubular germ cell neoplasia, unclassified type is also present in a tubule at bottom right of center where neoplastic cells have not proliferated beyond the basal aspect of the tubule.

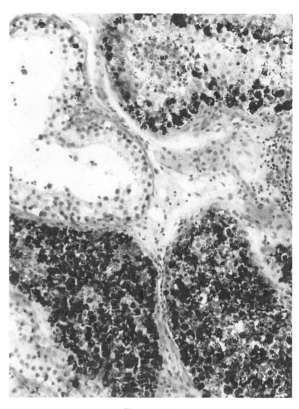

Figure 2-11
INTRATUBULAR SEMINOMA

Intensely PAS-positive cells fill two tubules (bottom). Tubule at top right shows intratubular germ cell neoplasia, unclassified type.

analysis of IGCNU (149). Delahunt et al. (80) noted that IGCNU and seminoma have a similar distribution of nucleolar organizing regions. Hu et al. (96) demonstrated a triploid DNA content within IGCNU associated with an infantile yolk sac tumor by in situ hybridization using a probe specific for a tandem repeat of chromosome 1. A unique transcript of the platelet-derived growth factor alpha-receptor has been identified in IGCNU (as well as in invasive germ cell tumors), but is absent in the non-neoplastic testis; the identification of this transcript by polymerase chain reaction methods may provide a sensitive method for the detection of IGCNU (112).

Differential Diagnosis. Some specific forms of intratubular neoplasia should be distinguished from IGCNU. Intratubular seminoma is characterized by total filling of the seminiferous tubules by seminoma cells (fig. 2-10), in contrast to IGCNU. It almost always is associated with an invasive seminoma, and its cells are intensely PAS positive (fig. 2-11), like those of IGCNU. Rarely, there is a striking granulomatous response within the tubules (fig. 2-12). Intratubular spermatocytic seminoma shows the characteristic polymorphous population that characterizes the invasive tumor, partially or totally fills the seminiferous tubules (figs. 2-13, 2-14), and is associated with invasive spermatocytic seminoma. Intratubular embryonal carcinoma has the cytologic features of that neoplasm. It usually fills the seminiferous tubules and often shows extensive necrosis with occasional calcification (fig. 2-15). Other forms of differentiated intratubular germ cell tumor may also, rarely, be identified but lack the cytologic features and basal disposition of cells of IGCNU (114). Two or more forms of intratubular germ cell neoplasia may coexist, usually IGCNU with either intratubular seminoma or intratubular

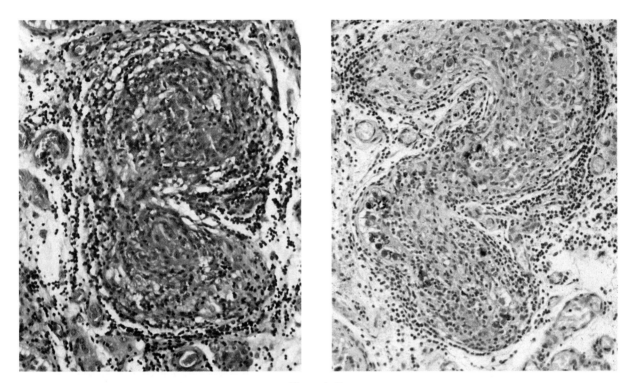

Figure 2-12
INTRATUBULAR SEMINOMA WITH GRANULOMATOUS REACTION
Left: Tubules are filled with epithelioid histiocytes; seminoma cells are inconspicuous.
Right: An immunohistochemical stain for placental alkaline phosphatase highlights the neoplastic germ cells (anti-placental alkaline phosphatase immunostain). (Courtesy of Dr. F. Algaba, Barcelona, Spain.)

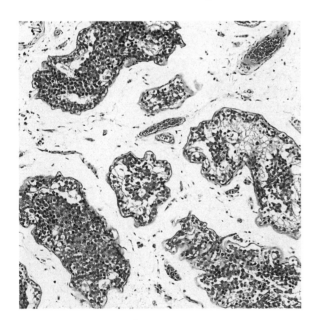

Figure 2-13
INTRATUBULAR SPERMATOCYTIC SEMINOMA
Several tubules are partially involved. The interstitium is edematous.

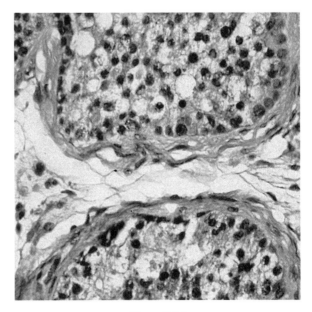

Figure 2-14
INTRATUBULAR SPERMATOCYTIC SEMINOMA
Two tubules contain cells exhibiting the variation in size typical of this neoplasm when seen in invasive form.

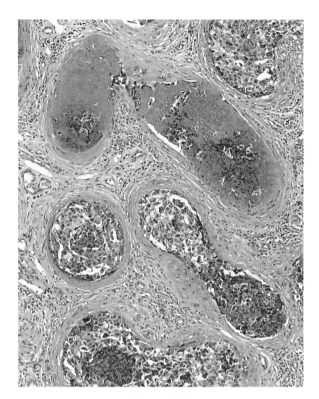

Figure 2-15
INTRATUBULAR EMBRYONAL CARCINOMA
Comedo-type necrosis is present.

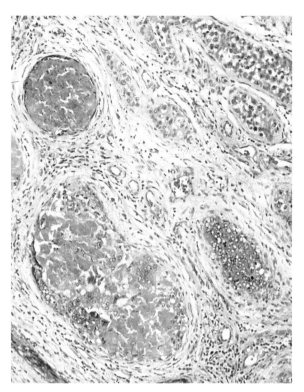

Figure 2-16
INTRATUBULAR EMBRYONAL CARCINOMA
AND INTRATUBULAR SEMINOMA
The intratubular embryonal carcinoma shows the characteristic necrosis, and there is intratubular seminoma in two tubules (top right).

embryonal carcinoma. Less commonly, intratubular seminoma occurs with intratubular embryonal carcinoma (fig. 2-16). In rare prepubertal cases, atypical germ cells with enlarged nuclei and abnormal chromatin may be seen that lack the basal orientation typical of IGCNU and are distributed more randomly in tubules lined by immature Sertoli cells. Whether these rare cases should also be considered IGCNU is not clear, but progression to the usual adult pattern and invasive germ cell tumor has been described (116,120,134). Similar cells have been identified in seminiferous tubules adjacent to pediatric teratomas on rare occasion (131,143), sometimes showing PLAP reactivity (143).

Treatment and Prognosis. The treatment of IGCNU is controversial, with opinions divided between careful follow-up and ablative therapy. Because of the high frequency of progression to an invasive germ cell tumor, there is a growing trend to recommend intervention. Orchiectomy is the treatment of choice in patients with unilat-

eral IGCNU, and low-dose radiation is efficacious in patients with bilateral IGCNU (although sterility is certain). Some patients with invasive testicular cancer who received chemotherapy were shown to have regression of contralateral IGCNU (fig. 2-17), but the reappearance of IGCNU in an occasional patient following chemotherapy casts some doubt on the efficacy of this treatment (74,89,146,147). A recent study demonstrated an estimated risk of recurrent IGCNU following chemotherapy of 21 and 42 percent at 5 and 10 years, respectively (77a)

Other Forms of
Intratubular Germ Cell Neoplasia

In almost all these cases, the intratubular neoplasm occurs simultaneously with an invasive germ cell tumor of the same type, and hence these forms of intratubular germ cell neoplasia are discussed in the sections dealing with the

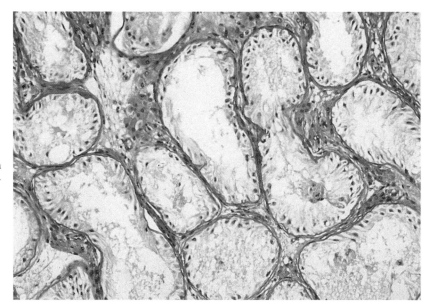

Figure 2-17
TREATMENT EFFECT,
INTRATUBULAR GERM
CELL NEOPLASIA,
UNCLASSIFIED TYPE
The tubules lack neoplastic germ
cells and are lined only by Sertoli cells.

specific form of the invasive lesion. Those that occur commonly are intratubular seminoma, intratubular spermatocytic seminoma, and intratubular embryonal carcinoma. Intratubular forms of yolk sac tumor or trophoblastic neoplasia are rare (114).

REFERENCES

Histogenesis

1. Atkin NB, Baker MC. i(12p): specific chromosomal marker in seminoma and malignant teratoma of the testis? Cancer Genet Cytogenet 1983;10:199–204.
2. Atkin NB, Fox MF, Baker MC, Jackson Z. Chromosome 12-containing markers, including two dicentrics, in three i(12p)-negative testicular germ cell tumors. Genes Chrom Cancer 1993;6:218–21.
3. Bailey D, Baumal R, Law J, et al. Production of monoclonal antibody specific for seminomas and dysgerminomas. Proc Nat Acad Sci USA 1986;83:5291–5.
4. Boseman FT, Giard RW, Kruseman AC, Knijenenburg G, Spaander PJ. Human chorionic gonadothropin and alpha-fetoprotein in testicular germ cell tumors: a retrospective immunohistochemical study. Histopathology 1980;4:673–84.
5. Bosl GJ, Dmitrovsky E, Reuter VE, et al. Isochromosome of the short arm of chromosome 12: clinically useful markers for male germ cell tumors. JNCI 1989;81:1874–8.
6. Bredael JJ, Vugrin D, Whitmore WF Jr. Autopsy findings in 154 patients with germ cell tumors of the testis. Cancer 1982;50:548–51.
7. Czaja JT, Ulbright TM. Evidence for the transformation of seminoma to yolk sac tumor, with histogenetic considerations. Am J Clin Pathol 1992;97:468–77.
8. Damjanov I. Spontaneous and experimental testicular tumors in animals. In: Talerman A, Roth LM, eds. Pathology of the testis and its adnexa. New York: Churchill Livingstone, 1986:193–206.
9. Damjanov I, Solter D. Experimental teratoma. Curr Top Pathol 1974;59:69–130.
10. de Graaff WE, Oosterhuis JW, de Jong B, et al. Ploidy of testicular carcinoma in situ. Lab Invest 1992;66:166–8.
11. de Jong B, Oosterhuis JW, Castedo SM, Vos A, te Meerman GJ. Pathogenesis of adult testicular germ cell tumors. A cytogenetic model. Cancer Genet Cytogenet 1990;48:143–67.
12. Delahunt B, Mostofi FK, Sesterhenn IA, Ribas JL, Avallone FA. Nucleolar organizer regions in seminoma and intratubular malignant germ cells. Mod Pathol 1990;3:141–5.
13. Delozier-Blanchet CD, Walt H, Engel E, Vuagnat P. Cytogenetic studies of human testicular germ cell tumours. Int J Androl 1987;10:69–77.
14. El-Naggar AK, Ro JY, McLemore D, Ayala AG, Batsakis JG. DNA ploidy in testicular germ cell neoplasms. Histogenetic and clinical implications. Am J Surg Pathol 1992;16:611–8.
15. Friedman NB, Moore RA. Tumors of the testis: a report on 922 cases. Milit Surgeon 1946;99:573–93.

16. Geurts van Kessel A, Suijkerbuijk RF, Sinke RJ, Looijenga L, Oosterhuis JW, de Jong B. Molecular cytogenetics of human germ cell tumours: i(12p) and related chromosomal anomalies. Eur Urol 1993;23:23–8.

17. Gibas Z, Prout GR, Pontes JE, Sandberg AA. Chromosome changes in germ cell tumors of the testis. Cancer Genet Cytogenet 1986;19:245–52.

18. Giwercman A, Andrews PW, Jorgensen N, Muller J, Graem N, Skakkebaek NE. Immunohistochemical expression of embryonal marker TRA-1-60 in carcinoma in situ and germ cell tumors of the testis. Cancer 1993;72:1308–14.

19. Giwercman A, Marks A, Bailey D, Baumal R, Skakkebaek NE. M2A–a monoclonal antibody as a marker for carcinoma-in-situ germ cells of the human adult testis. Acta Pathol Microbiol Immunol Scand [A] 1988;96:667–70.

20. Holstein AF. Cellular components of early testicular cancer. Eur Urol 1993;23(suppl 2):9–18.

21. Hu LM, Phillipson J, Barsky SH. Intratubular germ cell neoplasia in infantile yolk sac tumor: verification by tandem repeat sequence in situ hybridization. Diagn Mol Pathol 1992;1:118–28.

22. Jacobsen GK, Barlebo H, Olsen J, et al. Testicular germ cell tumours in Denmark 1976–1980: pathology of 1058 consecutive cases. Acta Radiol Oncol 1984;23:239–47.

23. Jacobsen GK, Norgaard-Pedersen B. Placental alkaline phosphatase in testicular germ cell tumours and carcinoma-in-situ of the testis: an immunohistochemical study. Acta Pathol Microbiol Immunol Scand [A] 1984;92:323–9.

24. Javadpour N. Significance of elevated serum alpha fetoprotein (AFP) in seminoma. Cancer 1980;45:2166–8.

25. Johnson DE, Appelt G, Samuels ML, Luna M. Metastases from testicular carcinoma. Study of 78 autopsied cases. Urology 1976;8:234–9.

26. Jorgensen N, Muller J, Visfeldt J, Giwercman A, Skakkebaek NE. Infantile germ cell tumors associated with carcinoma-in-situ of the testis [Abstract]. Onkologie 1991;14(suppl 4):8.

27. Kleinsmith LJ, Pierce GB. Multipotentiality of single embryonal carcinoma cells. Cancer Res 1964;24:1544–51.

28. Klys HS, Whillis D, Howard G, Harrison DJ. Glutathione S-transferase expression in the human testis and testicular germ cell neoplasia. Br J Cancer 1992;66:589–93.

29. Koide O, Iwai S, Baba K, Iri H. Identification of testicular atypical germ cells by an immunohistochemical technique for placental alkaline phosphatase. Cancer 1987;60:1325–30.

30. Lachman MF, Ricci A Jr, Kosciol C. DNA ploidy in testicular germ cell tumors: can an atypical seminoma be identified? Conn Med 1995;59:133–6.

31. Looijenga LH, Abraham M, Gillis AJ, Saunders GF, Oosterhuis JW. Testicular germ cell tumors of adults show deletions of chromosomal bands 11p13 and 11p15.5, but no abnormalities within the zinc-finger regions and exons 2 and 6 of the Wilms' tumor 1 gene. Genes Chrom Cancer 1994;9:153–60.

32. Lothe RA, Hastie N, Heimdal K, Fossa SD, Stenwig AE, Borresen AL. Frequent loss of 11p13 and 11p15 loci in male germ cell tumours. Genes Chrom Cancer 1993;7:96–101.

33. Lothe RA, Peltomaki P, Tommerup N, et al. Molecular genetic changes in human male germ cell tumors. Lab Invest 1995;73:606–14.

34. Malmi R, Söderström KO. Lectin histochemistry of embryonal carcinoma. APMIS 1991;99:233–43.

35. Manivel JC, Reinberg Y, Niehans GA, Fraley EE. Intratubular germ cell neoplasia in testicular teratomas and epidermoid cysts. Correlation with prognosis and possible biologic significance. Cancer 1989;64:715–20.

36. Manivel JC, Simonton S, Wold LE, Dehner LP. Absence of intratubular germ cell neoplasia in testicular yolk sac tumors in children. Arch Pathol Lab Med 1988;112:641–5.

37. Monaghan P, Raghavan D, Neville M. Ultrastructure of xenografted human germ cell tumors. Cancer 1982;49:683–97.

38. Mostofi FK. Pathology of germ cell tumors of testis: a progress report. Cancer 1980;45:1735–54.

39. Mostofi FK, Sesterhenn IA. Pathology of germ cell tumors of testes. Prog Clin Biol Res 1985;203:1–34.

40. Mostofi FK, Sesterhenn IA, Davis CJ Jr. Immunopathology of germ cell tumors of the testis. Semin Diagn Pathol 1987;4:320–41.

41. Niehans GA, Manivel JC, Copland GT, Scheithauer BW, Wick MR. Immunohistochemistry of germ cell and trophoblastic neoplasms. Cancer 1988;62:1113–23.

42. Oosterhuis JW, Castedo SM, de Jong B, et al. Ploidy of primary germ cell tumors of the testis. Pathogenetic and clinical relevance. Lab Invest 1989;60:14–21.

43. Oosterhuis JW, Gillis AJ, van Putten WJ, de Jong B, Looijenga LH. Interphase cytogenetics of carcinoma in situ of the testis. Numeric analysis of the chromosomes 1, 12 and 15. Eur Urol 1993;23:16–21.

44. Parkinson MC, Ramani P. Intratubular germ cell neoplasia in an infantile testis. Histopathology 1993;23:99–100.

45. Parrington JM, West LF, Heyderman E. Chromosome analysis of parallel short-term cultures from four testicular germ-cell tumors. Cancer Genet Cytogenet 1994;75:90–102.

46. Peng HQ, Bailey D, Bronson D, Goss PE, Hogg D. Loss of heterozygosity of tumor suppressor genes in testis cancer. Cancer Res 1995;55:2871–5.

47. Perlman EJ, Cushing B, Hawkins E, Griffin CA. Cytogenetic analysis of childhood endodermal sinus tumors: a Pediatric Oncology Group study. Pediatr Pathol 1994;14:695–708.

48. Pierce GB Jr, Abell MR. Embryonal carcinoma of the testis. Pathol Annu 1970;4:27–60.

49. Pierce GB Jr, Dixon FJ Jr. Testicular teratomas: I. Demonstration of teratogenesis by metamorphosis of multipotential cells. Cancer 1959;12:573–83.

50. Pierce GB Jr, Dixon FJ Jr, Verney EL. The biology of testicular cancer: II. Endocrinology of transplanted tumors. Cancer Res 1958;18:204–6.

51. Pierce GB Jr, Dixon FJ Jr, Verney EL. Teratocarcinogenic and tissue-forming potentials of cell types comprising neoplastic embryoid bodies. Lab Invest 1960;9:583–602.

52. Pierce GB Jr, Verney EL. An in vitro and in vivo study of differentiation in teratocarcinomas. Cancer 1961;14:1017–29.

53. Pugh RC. Testicular tumours–introduction. In: Pugh RC, ed. Pathology of the testis. Oxford: Blackwell Scientific, 1976:139–59.

54. Raghavan D, Sullivan AL, Peckham MJ, Neville AM. Elevated serum alpha-fetoprotein and seminoma: clinical evidence for a histologic continuum? Cancer 1982;50:982–9.

54a. Rajpert-DeMeyts E, Kvist M, Skakkebaek NE. Heterogeneity of expression of immunohistochemical tumour markers in testicular carcinoma in situ: pathogenetic relevance. Virch Arch 1996;428:133–9.

55. Renedo DE, Trainer TD. Intratubular germ cell neoplasia (ITGCN) with p53 and PCNA expression and adjacent mature teratoma in an infant testis. An immunohistochemical and morphologic study with a review of the literature. Am J Surg Pathol 1994;18:947–52.

56. Samaniego F, Rodriguez E, Houldsworth J. Cytogenetic and molecular analysis of human male germ cell tumors: chromosome 12 abnormalities and gene amplification. Genes Chrom Cancer 1990;1:289–300.

57. Sandberg AA, Meloni AM, Suijkerbuijk RF. Reviews of chromosome studies in urological tumors. III. Cytogenetics and genes in testicular tumors. J Urol 1996;155:1531–56.

58. Schulze C, Holstein AF. On the histology of human seminoma: development of the solid tumor from intratubular seminoma cells. Cancer 1977;39:1090–100.

59. Smith RC, Rukstalis DB. Frequent loss of heterozygosity at 11p loci in testicular cancer. J Urol 1995;153:1684–7.

60. Smolarek TA, Blough RI, Foster RS, Ulbright TM, Palmer CG, Heerema NA. Identification of multiple chromosome 12 abnormalities in human testicular germ cell tumors by two-color fluorescence in situ hybridization (FISH). Genes Chrom Cancer 1995;14:252–8.

61. Srigley JR, Mackay B, Toth P, Ayala A. The ultrastructure and histogenesis of male germ neoplasia with emphasis on seminoma with early carcinomatous features. Ultrastruc Pathol 1988;12:67–86.

62. Stein NA, Jain R. Testicular intratubular origin of choriocarcinoma. Urology 1982;20:296–7.

63. Teppo L. Malignant testicular tumours in Finland. Acta Pathol Microbiol Scand 1969;75:18–26.

64. van Echten J, Oosterhuis JW, Looijenga LH, et al. No recurrent structural abnormalities apart from i(12p) in primary germ cell tumors of the adult testis. Genes Chrom Cancer 1995;14:133–44.

65. van Echten J, van Gurp RJ, Stoepker M, Looijenga LH, de Jong J, Oosterhuis W. Cytogenetic evidence that carcinoma in situ is the precursor lesion for invasive testicular germ cell tumors. Cancer Genet Cytogenet 1995;85:133–7.

66. von Hochstetter AR, Hedinger CE. The differential diagnosis of testicular germ cell tumors in theory and practice: a critical analysis of two major systems of classification and review of 389 cases. Virchows Arch [A] 1982;396:247–77.

67. Vos A, Oosterhuis JW, de Jong B, Buist J, Schraffordt Koops H. Cytogenetics of carcinoma in situ of the testis. Cancer Genet Cytogenet 1990;46:75–81.

Intratubular Germ Cell Neoplasia

68. Albrechtsen R, Nielsen MH, Skakkebaek NE, Wewer U. Carcinoma in situ of the testis. Some ultrastructural characteristics of germ cells. Acta Pathol Microbiol Immunol Scand [A] 1982;90:301–3.

69. Bailey D, Marks A, Stratis M, Baumal R. Immunohistochemical staining of germ cell tumors and intratubular malignant germ cells of the testis using antibody to placental alkaline phosphatase and a monoclonal anti-seminoma antibody. Mod Pathol 1991;4:167–11.

70. Bartkova J, Bartek J, Lukas J, et al. p53 protein alterations in human testicular cancer including pre-invasive intratubular germ-cell neoplasia. Int J Cancer 1991;49:196–202.

71. Beckstead JH. Alkaline phosphatase histochemistry in human germ cell neoplasms. Am J Surg Pathol 1983;7:341–9.

72. Berthelsen JG, Skakkebaek NE. Value of testicular biopsy in diagnosing carcinoma in situ testis. Scand J Urol Nephrol 1981;15:165–8.

73. Berthelsen JG, Skakkebaek NE, von der Maase H, Sorensen BL, Mogensen P. Screening for carcinoma in situ of the contralateral testis in patients with germinal testicular cancer. Br Med J 1982;285:1683–6.

74. Bottomley D, Fisher C, Hendry WF, Horwich A. Persistent carcinoma in situ of the testis after chemotherapy for advanced testicular germ cell tumours. Br J Urol 1990;66:420–4.

75. Burke AP, Mostofi FK. Placental alkaline phosphatase immunohistochemistry of intratubular malignant germ cells and associated testicular germ cell tumors. Hum Pathol 1988;19:663–70.

76. Burke AP, Mostofi FK. Intratubular malignant germ cells in testicular biopsies: clinical course and identification by staining for placental alkaline phosphatase. Mod Pathol 1988;1:475–9.

77. Chen KT, Cheng AC. Retroperitoneal seminoma and intratubular germ cell neoplasia. Hum Pathol 1989;20:493–5.

77a. Christensen TB, Daugaard G, Geertsen PF, von der Maase H. Effect of chemotherapy on carcinoma in situ of the testis. Ann Oncol 1998;9:657–60.

78. Coffin CM, Ewing S, Dehner LP. Frequency of intratubular germ cell neoplasia with invasive testicular germ cell tumors. Histologic and immunocytochemical features. Arch Pathol Lab Med 1985;109:555–9.

79. Daugaard G, von der Maase H, Olsen J, Rorth M, Skakkebaek NE. Carcinoma-in-situ testis in patients with assumed extragonadal germ-cell tumours. Lancet 1987;2:528–30.

80. Delahunt B, Mostofi FK, Sesterhenn IA, Ribas JL, Avallone FA. Nucleolar organizer regions in seminoma and intratubular malignant germ cells. Mod Pathol 1990;3:141–5.

80a. Dieckmann KP, Loy V. The value of the biopsy of the contralateral testis in patients with testicular germ cell cancer: the recent German experience. APMIS 1998;106:13–23.

81. Eble JN. Spermatocytic seminoma. Hum Pathol 1994;25:1035–42.

82. Gillis AJ, Looijenga LH, de Jong B, Oosterhuis JW. Clonality of combined testicular germ cell tumors of adults. Lab Invest 1994;71:874–8.

83. Giwercman A, Andrews PW, Jorgensen N, Muller J, Graem N, Skakkebaek NE. Immunohistochemical expression of embryonal marker TRA-1-60 in carcinoma in situ and germ cell tumors of the testis. Cancer 1993;72:1308–14.

84. Giwercman A, Bruun E, Frimodt-Moller C, Skakkebaek NE. Prevalence of carcinoma-in-situ and other histopathologic abnormalities in testes of men with a history of cryptorchidism. J Urol 1989;142:998–1002.

85. Giwercman A, Lindenberg S, Kimber SJ, Andersson T, Müller J, Skakkebaek NE. Monoclonal antibody 43-9F as a sensitive immunohistochemical marker of carcinoma in situ of human testis. Cancer 1990;65:1135–42.

86. Giwercman A, Marks A, Bailey D, Baumal R, Skakkebaek NE. A monoclonal antibody as a marker for carcinoma-in-situ germ cells of the human adult testis. Acta Pathol Microbiol Immunol Scand [A] 1988;96:667–70.

87. Giwercman A, Muller J, Skakkebaek NE. Carcinoma in situ of the undescended testis. Semin Urol 1988;6:110–9.

88. Giwercman A, Müller J, Skakkebaek NE. Prevalence of carcinoma in situ and other histopathological abnormalities in testes from 399 men who died suddenly and unexpectedly. J Urol 1991;145:77–80.

89. Giwercman A, Skakkebaek NE. Carcinoma-in-situ (gonocytoma-in-situ) of the testis. In: Burger H, de Kretser D, eds. The testis. 2nd ed. New York: Raven Press, 1989:475–91.

90. Giwercman A, von der Maase H, Skakkebaek NE. Epidemiological and clinical aspects of carcinoma in situ of the testis. Eur Urol 1993;23:104–10.

91. Gondos B, Berthelsen JG, Skakkebaek NE. Intratubular germ cell neoplasia (carcinoma in situ): a preinvasive lesion of the testis. Ann Clin Lab Sci 1983;13:185–92.

92. Gondos B, Migliozzi JA. Intratubular germ cell neoplasia. Semin Diagn Pathol 1987;4:292–303.

93. Hailemariam S, Engeler DS, Bannwart F, Amin MB. Primary mediastinal germ cell tumor with intratubular germ cell neoplasia of the testis–further support for germ cell origin of these tumors: a case report. Cancer 1997;79:1031–6.

93a. Hailemariam S, Engeler DS, Bannwart F, et al. Significance of intratubular germ cell neoplasia (ITGCN) in prepubertal testes of patients with cryptorchidism (CO): correlation with clinical reappraisal after two decades [Abstract]. Mod Pathol 1998;11:84A.

94. Harland SJ, Cook PA, Fossa SD, et al. Risk factors for carcinoma in situ of the contralateral testis in patients with testicular cancer. An interim report. Eur Urol 1993;23:115–8.

94a. Hiraoka N, Yamada T, Abe H, Hata J. Establishment of three monoclonal antibodies specific for prespermatogonia and intratubular malignant germ cells in humans. Lab Invest 1997;76:427–38.

95. Holstein AF, Körner F. Light and electron microscopical analysis of cell types in human seminoma. Virchows Arch [A] 1974;363:97–112.

96. Hu LM, Phillipson J, Barsky SH. Intratubular germ cell neoplasia in infantile yolk sac tumor: verification by tandem repeat sequence in situ hybridization. Diagn Mol Pathol 1992;1:118–28.

97. Jacobsen GK, Henriksen OB, von der Maase H. Carcinoma in situ of testicular tissue adjacent to malignant germ-cell tumors: a study of 105 cases. Cancer 1981;47:2660–2.

98. Jacobsen GK, Jacobsen M, Praetorius C. Ferritin as a possible marker protein of carcinoma-in-situ of the testis. Lancet 1980;2:533–4.

99. Jacobsen GK, Jacobsen M, Praetorius C, Strandberg PN. Immunohistochemical demonstration of tumour associated antigens in carcinoma-in-situ of the testis. Int J Androl 1981;4(Suppl):203–10.

100. Jacobsen GK, Norgaard-Pedersen B. Placental alkaline phosphatase in testicular germ cell tumours and carcinoma-in-situ of the testis: an immunohistochemical study. Acta Pathol Microbiol Immunol Scand [A] 1984;92:323–9.

101. Jorgensen N, Giwercman A, Muller J, Skakkebaek NE. Immunohistochemical markers of carcinoma in situ of the testis also expressed in normal infantile germ cells. Histopathology 1993;22:373–8.

102. Jorgensen N, Muller J, Visfeldt J, Giwercmann A, Skakkebaek NE. Infantile germ cell tumors associated with carcinoma-in-situ of the testis [Abstract]. Onkologie 1991;14(suppl 4):8.

102a. Kang JL, Rajpert-De Meyts E, Giwercmann A, Skakkebaek NE. The associaton of testicular carcinoma in situ with intratubular microcalcifications. J Urol Pathol 1996;2:235–42.

102b. Kang JL, Rajpert-De Meyts E, Wiels J, Skakkebaek NE. Expresson of the glycolipid globotriaosylceramide (Gb3) in testicular carcinoma in situ. Virch Arch 1995;426:369–74.

103. Klys HS, Whillis D, Howard G, Harrison DJ. Glutathione S-transferase expression in the human testis and testicular germ cell neoplasia. Br J Cancer 1992;66:589–93.

104. Koide O, Iwai S, Baba K, Iri H. Identification of testicular atypical germ cells by an immunohistochemical technique for placental alkaline phosphatase. Cancer 1987;60:1325–30.

105. Krabbe S, Skakkebaek NE, Berthelsen JG, et al. High incidence of undetected neoplasia in maldescended testes. Lancet 1979;1:999–1000.

106. Kuczyk MA, Serth J, Bokemeyer C, et al. Alterations in the p53 tumor suppressor gene in carcinoma in situ of the testis. Cancer 1996;78:1958–66.

107. Lee AH, Theaker JM. Pagetoid spread into the rete testis by testicular tumours. Histopathology 1994;24:385–9.

108. Loy V, Dieckmann KP. Prevalence of contralateral testicular intraepithelial neoplasia (carcinoma in situ) in patients with testicular germ cell tumour. Results of the German multicentre study. Eur Urol 1993;23:120–2.

109. Manivel JC, Jessurun J, Wick MR, Dehner LP. Placental alkaline phosphatase immunoreactivity in testicular germ cell tumors. Am J Surg Pathol 1987;11:21–9.

110. Manivel JC, Reinberg Y, Niehans GA, Fraley EE. Intratubular germ cell neoplasia in testicular teratomas and epidermoid cysts. Correlation with prognosis and possible biologic significance. Cancer 1989;64:715–20.

111. Manivel JC, Simonton S, Wold SE, Dehner LP. Absence of intratubular germ cell neoplasia in testicular yolk sac tumors in children. A histochemical and immunohistochemical study. Arch Pathol Lab Med 1988;112:641–5.

112. Mosselman S, Looijenga LH, Gillis AJ, et al. Aberrant platelet-derived growth factor alpha-receptor transcript as a diagnostic marker for early human germ cell tumors of the adult testis. Proc Natl Acad Sci U S A 1996;93:2884–8.

113. Mostofi FK, Price EB Jr. Tumors of the male genital system. Atlas of Tumor Pathology, 2nd Series, Fascicle 8. Washington, D.C.: Armed Forces Institute of Pathology, 1973.

114. Mostofi FK, Sesterhenn IA. Pathology of germ cell tumors of testes. Prog Clin Biol Res 1985;203:1–34.

115. Mostofi FK, Sesterhenn IA, Davis CJ Jr. Immunopathology of germ cell tumors of the testis. Semin Diagn Pathol 1987;4:320–41.

116. Muller J. Abnormal infantile germ cells and development of carcinoma-in-situ in maldeveloped testes: a stereological and densitometric study. Int J Androl 1987;10:543–67.

117. Muller J, Skakkebaek NE. Testicular carcinoma in situ in children with the androgen insensitivity (testicular feminisation) syndrome. Br Med J 1984;288:1419–20.

118. Muller J, Skakkebaek NE. Abnormal germ cells in maldescended testes: a study of cell density, nuclear size and deoxyribonucleic acid content in testicular biopsies from 50 boys. J Urol 1984;131:730–3.

119. Muller J, Skakkebaek NE, Lundsteen C. Aneuploidy as a marker for carcinoma-in-situ of the testis. Acta Pathol Microbiol Scand [A] 1981;89:67–8.

120. Muller J, Skakkebaek NE, Nielsen OH, Graem N. Cryptorchidism and testis cancer. Atypical infantile germ cells followed by carcinoma in situ and invasive carcinoma in adulthood. Cancer 1984;54:629–34.

121. Muller J, Skakkebaek NE, Ritzën M, Plöen L, Petersen KE. Carcinoma in situ of the testis in children with 45,X/46,XY gonadal dysgenesis. J Pediatr 1985;106:431–6.

122. Muller M, Lauke H, Hartmann M. The value of the AgNOR staining method in identifying carcinoma in situ testis. Pathol Res Pract 1994;190:429–35.

123. Mumperow E, Lauke H, Holstein AF, Hartmann M. Further practical experiences in the recognition and management of carcinoma in situ of the testis. Urol Int 1992;48:162–6.

124. Nielsen H, Nielsen M, Skakkebaek NE. The fine structure of possible carcinoma-in-situ in the seminiferous tubules in the testis of four infertile men. Acta Pathol Microbiol Scand [A] 1974;82:235–48.

125. Nistal M, Codesal J, Paniagua R. Carcinoma in situ of the testis in infertile men. A histological, immunocytochemical, and cytophotometric study of DNA content. J Pathol 1989;159:205–10.

126. Parkinson MC, Ramani P. Intratubular germ cell neoplasia in an infantile testis. Histopathology 1993;23:99–100.

127. Pedersen KV, Boiesen P, Zetterlund CG. Experience of screening for carcinoma-in-situ of the testis among young men with surgically corrected maldescended testes. Int J Androl 1987;10:181–5.

128. Perry A, Wiley EL, Albores-Saavedra J. Pagetoid spread of intratubular germ cell neoplasia into rete testis: a morphologic and histochemical study of 100 orchiectomy specimens with invasive germ cell tumors. Hum Pathol 1994;25:235–9.

129. Pryor JP, Cameron KM, Chilton CP, et al. Carcinoma in situ in testicular biopsies from men presenting with infertility. Br J Urol 1983;55:780–4.

130. Ramani P, Yeung CK, Habeebu SS. Testicular intratubular germ cell neoplasia in children and adolescents with intersex. Am J Surg Pathol 1993;17:1124–33.

131. Renedo DE, Trainer TD. Intratubular germ cell neoplasia (ITGCN) with p53 and PCNA expression and adjacent mature teratoma in an infant testis. An immunohistochemical and morphologic study with a review of the literature. Am J Surg Pathol 1994;18:947–52.

132. Saltzman B, Pitts WR, Vaughan ED Jr. Extragonadal retroperitoneal germ cell tumors without apparent testicular involvement. A search for the source. Urology 1986;27:504–7.

133. Scully RE. Intratubular germ cell neoplasia (carcinoma in situ). What it is and what should be done about it. Lesson 17, In: Fraley EE, ed. World urology update series, Vol 1. Princeton: Continuing Professional Education Center, 1982:1–8.

134. Scully RE. Testis. In: Henson DE, Albores-Saavedra J, eds. The pathology of incipient neoplasia. 2nd ed. Philadelphia: WB Saunders, 1993:384–400.

135. Sigg C, Hedinger C. Atypical germ cells of the testis. Comparative ultrastructural and immunohistochemical investigations. Virchows Arch [A] 1984;402:439–50.

136. Skakkebaek NE. Possible carcinoma-in-situ of the undescended testis. Lancet 1972;2:516–7.

137. Skakkebaek NE. Abnormal morphology of germ cells in two infertile men. Acta Pathol Microbiol Scand [A] 1972;80:374–8.

138. Skakkebaek NE. Atypical germ cells in the adjacent "normal" tissue of testicular tumours. Acta Pathol Microbiol Scand [A] 1975;83:127–30.

139. Skakkebaek NE. Carcinoma in situ of the testis: frequency and relationship to invasive germ cell tumours in infertile men. Histopathology 1978;2:157–70.

140. Skakkebaek NE, Berthelsen JG, Giwercman A, Müller J. Carcinoma-in-situ of the testis: possible origin from gonocytes and precursor of all types of germ cell tumours except spermatocytoma. Int J Androl 1987;10:19–28.

141. Skakkebaek NE, Berthelsen JG, Muller J. Carcinoma-in-situ of the undescended testis. Urol Clin North Am 1982;9:377–85.

141a. Skakkebaek NE, Rajpert-DeMeyts E, Jørgensen N, et al. Germ cell cancer and disorders of spermatogenesis: an environmental connection? APMIS 1998;106:3–12.

142. Srigley JR, Toth P, Edwards V. Diagnostic electron microscopy of male genital tract tumors. Clin Lab Med 1987;7:91–115.

143. Stamp IM, Barlebo H, Rix M, Jacobsen GK. Intratubular germ cell neoplasia in an infantile testis with immature teratoma. Histopathology 1993;22:69–72.

144. Stamp IM, Jacobsen GK. Infant intratubular germ cell neoplasia [Letter]. Am J Surg Pathol 1995;19:489.

145. van Echten J, van Gurp RJ, Stoepker M, Looijenga LH, de Jong J, Oosterhuis W. Cytogenetic evidence that carcinoma in situ is the precursor lesion for invasive testicular germ cell tumors. Cancer Genet Cytogenet 1995;85:133–7.

146. von der Maase H, Giwercman A, Muller J, Skakkebaek NE. Management of carcinoma-in-situ of the testis. Int J Androl 1987;10:209–20.

147. von der Maase H, Meinecke B, Skakkebaek NE. Residual carcinoma-in-situ of contralateral testis after chemotherapy [Letter]. Lancet 1988;1:477–8.

148. von der Maase H, Rorth M, Walbom-Jorgensen S, et al. Carcinoma in situ of contralateral testis in patients with testicular germ cell cancer: study of 27 cases in 500 patients. Br Med J 1986;293:1398–401.

149. Vos A, Oosterhuis JW, de Jong B, Buist J, Schraffordt Koops H. Cytogenetics of carcinoma in situ of the testis. Cancer Genet Cytogenet 1990;46:75–81.

150. West AB, Butler MR, Fitzpatrick J, O'Brien A. Testicular tumors in subfertile men: report of 4 cases with implications for management of patients presenting with infertility. J Urol 1985;133:107–9.

3
GERM CELL TUMORS: SEMINOMAS

TYPICAL SEMINOMA

Definition. This malignant germ cell tumor is composed of relatively uniform cells, typically with clear cytoplasm, well-defined borders, and nuclei with one or more prominent nucleoli; the cells resemble primitive germ cells. There is almost always an associated lymphoid infiltrate and frequently a granulomatous inflammatory response.

General Features. Chevassu, in 1906, described the essential features of seminoma (1a). Seminoma is now recognized as the most common pure germ cell tumor of the testis and, in some series, is the most common of all germ cell tumors, exceeding in frequency mixed germ cell tumors. In the compilation of Friedman and Moore (6), seminoma constituted 35 percent of all testicular tumors and 36 percent of all testicular germ cell tumors. Dixon and Moore (4) found it constituted 41 percent of testicular germ cell tumors, and in two more recent studies, it accounted for almost 50 percent of such tumors (10,40). The lower frequency in the earlier reports may be due to the patient cohort: they were from military populations which are, on average, younger than the general population of patients with testicular germ cell tumors. Seminomas occur in a somewhat older population than nonseminomatous tumors: the average patient age is 40.5 years (10), 5 to 10 years older than for patients with nonseminomatous tumors (6,10). Seminoma is extremely rare in children under 10 years of age (15,29) and uncommon in adolescents. In a study of 729 seminomas in the series of the British Testicular Tumour Panel, 1 percent occurred in patients 19 years old or younger, 65.4 percent in patients 30 to 49 years, and 1 percent in patients older than 70 years (38). It remains crucial to distinguish seminoma from other forms (nonseminomatous) of germ cell tumor because of different treatments.

The epidemiology and risk factors for seminoma are similar to those of other testicular germ cell tumors. Some patients have shown an increased frequency of human leukocyte antigen (HLA) types DR5 (28) and Bw41 (3). In addition, an increased frequency has been reported among very tall men (36). Some studies report a higher frequency of seminomas associated with cryptorchidism than in the noncryptorchid population with germ cell tumors (8). A higher frequency of testicular germ cell tumors is described in patients with the acquired immunodeficiency syndrome (AIDS), as well as other forms of immunosuppression (19,41), and a disproportionate number of seminomas occur in these cases (19).

Clinical Features. Most patients present with a self-identified mass in the testis, occasionally associated with an ill-defined, aching sensation in the lower abdomen, inguinal area, or scrotum. Acute pain occurs in approximately 10 percent, and may result in delayed diagnosis due to a clinical impression of epididymo-orchitis (23). Seminoma affects the right testis slightly more often (54 percent) than the left (46 percent) (38). About 2.5 percent of patients have initial symptoms secondary to metastatic involvement (27,30), most commonly lumbar pain due to retroperitoneal metastasis, however gastrointestinal bleeding, bone pain, dyspnea and cough, a supraclavicular mass, neurological symptoms, and lower extremity edema may also be presenting symptoms due to spread to other sites (23). About 75 percent of patients present with clinical disease limited to the testis, 20 percent have retroperitoneal involvement, and 5 percent have supradiaphragmatic or organ metastases (35). Such metastases, however, are usually asymptomatic (10). Although 7 to 25 percent of patients with seminomas have a mild elevation of serum human chorionic gonadotropin (hCG) (1b,2,13,14,21,33), the hCG levels are not sufficiently elevated to cause patients to present with clinical gynecomastia, except rarely. Some patients present with infertility and have a small seminoma identified on testicular biopsy. In occasional cases the tumor is an incidental finding on microscopic examination of a cryptorchid testis. Very rarely exophthalmos, apparently due to a paraendocrine abnormality, is a presenting feature (20,37), and paraneoplastic hypercalcemia is also a rare occurrence (1,1c). Current or surgically corrected cryptorchidism is identified in 10 to 30 percent of patients with seminoma (10,38). Seminoma occurs bilaterally in about 2 percent of cases, almost always asynchronously.

Alpha-fetoprotein (AFP) levels are not generally elevated (32,42); if a significantly elevated serum AFP level is identified in a patient with apparently pure seminoma of the testis, it should be interpreted as probably indicating a histologically undetected nonseminomatous element in either the primary tumor or at metastatic sites. Modest AFP elevations may reflect liver disease, including metastatic seminoma to the liver (12). Borderline AFP elevations in histologically pure seminoma did not correlate with a different biologic behavior in one study (26), but this finding warrants further investigation.

Serum hCG levels are elevated in about 10 percent of patients with clinical stage I seminoma and in 25 percent (32) or more (31) of patients with metastatic seminoma; hCG elevations are demonstrable in 80 percent of patients when serum is obtained from the testicular vein (25). In some cases, hCG may be detectable only as an elevated beta subunit (21). An elevated serum hCG is often correlated with the presence of histologically identifiable syncytiotrophoblastic cells in the seminoma (see below). In some studies (5,24), but not others (33,34), elevated serum hCG was associated with a higher rate of relapse and overall poorer prognosis. It may be that modest elevations of hCG are not prognostically important but that higher elevations (greater than 40 IU/L) are (5). It is further suggested that hCG elevations do not indicate greater tumor aggressiveness but correlate with metastatic status (9). The elevations of hCG that occur in seminoma are generally not as great as those that occur in nonseminomatous tumors, particularly those with a choriocarcinomatous component. For example, Javadpour (11) identified 15 of 160 patients with apparently pure seminoma and elevated serum hCG level (2 to 20 ng/mL), with the highest level (without the subsequent identification of a choriocarcinomatous component in a metastasis) being 217 ng/mL (11). This contrasts with the typical elevations of hundreds of thousands of international units per liter in patients with choriocarcinoma (equivalent to more than 900 ng/mL).

Elevated serum levels of the enzyme lactate dehydrogenase (LDH) also occur in patients with seminoma; unfortunately an elevated LDH level is a relatively insensitive tumor marker, occurring in only 82 percent of patients with advanced metastatic seminoma, and is nonspecific in that 7 of 37 patients who were disease free after treatment had elevated LDH levels, and patients with benign testicular lesions may also show such elevations (5).

Most seminomas secrete a placental-like alkaline phosphatase (PLAP) that is apparently biochemically different from placental alkaline phosphatase (22) and somewhat heterogeneous from tumor to tumor (16). Clinical elevation of PLAP is detectable in 33 to 91 percent of stage I seminoma patients and in 40 to 75 percent of patients with metastatic seminoma (32). PLAP levels decline following clinical eradication of the tumor (39). False-positive elevation of PLAP occurs in patients who are heavy smokers, but may be distinguishable from tumor PLAP by the use of different antibodies (17).

Serum levels of neuron-specific enolase (NSE) may be elevated in patients with seminoma; in one study, only 1 of 54 patients with testicular germ cell tumors who were clinically disease free had an elevated NSE level, whereas 8 of 11 patients with metastatic seminoma had high levels (18). The lack of sensitivity and specificity of NSE, however, is described in other studies (7).

Gross Findings. Seminoma usually produces symmetric enlargement of the testis. The tumors average approximately 5 cm (74), with some exceeding 10 cm. In a series of 261 clinical stage I seminomas, 61 percent measured 2 to 6 cm (78a). Many of the largest seminomas occur within an intra-abdominal undescended testis because of its inaccessibility to palpation (114). In some patients with metastatic disease, no testicular enlargement is apparent; the testis is atrophic, and a tiny microscopic tumor or a scarred area ("burnt-out" germ cell tumor, see chapter 5) is identified on histologic examination. In the British Testicular Tumour Panel series, 11 percent of seminomas occurred in normal-sized or, rarely, smaller than normal, testes (123). If gross testicular enlargement is present, prominent, dilated veins may be identified on the surface of the tunica albuginea. The tumor often totally replaces the testis (more than 50 percent of the cases in the series of the British Testicular Tumour Panel) or only leaves a peripheral, compressed crescent of parenchyma. Most seminomas (figs. 3-1–3-4) are solid, well circumscribed, lobulated to multinodular, and bulge above the surrounding parenchyma (figs. 3-1, 3-3), but some are diffuse and smooth (fig. 3-2). Sectioning may disclose more than one nodule (fig. 3-1, top), but such nodules often connect in other planes. Less commonly, truly separate nodules are identified at some distance apart (fig. 3-1, bottom). The tumors are usually soft, fleshy, and encephaloid, but may be firm and fibrous (fig. 3-4C). The cut surface of the tumor is commonly cream-colored (fig. 3-2, above) to tan (fig. 3-1) to pale yellow (fig. 3-2, right) to light pink. Intraparenchymal hemorrhage may occasionally cause a red color (fig. 3-3). Punctate foci of hemorrhage may indicate the presence of trophoblastic elements (fig. 3-4A) (78), but may also be seen in their absence. It is common to identify yellow, granular foci of infarct-type necrosis, sometimes outlined by peripheral hemorrhage (fig. 3-4A,B), and occasional tumors may be extensively necrotic, particularly large ones. About 90 percent of seminomas are grossly confined to the testis; less than 10 percent extend through the tunica albuginea into the epididymis (fig. 3-4C) and beyond (93).

Microscopic Findings. On low-power examination the cells may be arranged in more or less diffuse sheets (fig. 3-5), but closer inspection typically shows delicate, thin fibrous septa (fig. 3-6) or, occasionally, slightly thicker trabeculae coursing through the tumor and in some cases resulting in a solid alveolar pattern (fig. 3-7). The septal framework so characteristic of this tumor is often highlighted by the sprinkling of lymphocytes along the septa (fig. 3-6). Less often, thick, dense fibrous bands subdivide the tumor into discrete, large nodules (fig. 3-8, left), nests, or clusters (fig. 3-9). Occasionally, distinctly separate, sizable tumor nodules are present (fig. 3-8, right), although microscopic multifocality is more often discovered incidentally by examination of grossly unremarkable tissue away from the main tumor. Many seminomas display foci in which the cells grow in cords (fig. 3-10) or, less commonly, trabeculae. In rare cases the tumor cells exhibit a solid tubular pattern (fig. 3-11) (133,134). Miscellaneous patterns that descriptively can be considered as reticular, cystic, hollow tubular, or cribriform are rare (figs. 3-12–3-14); these often appear related to edema that creates pseudoglandular spaces containing lightly staining, eosinophilic, granular fluid (fig. 3-12) (55,61), but

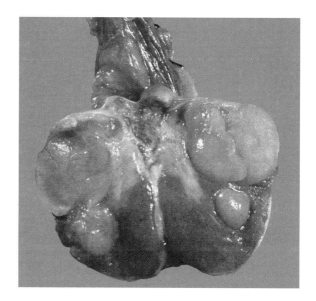

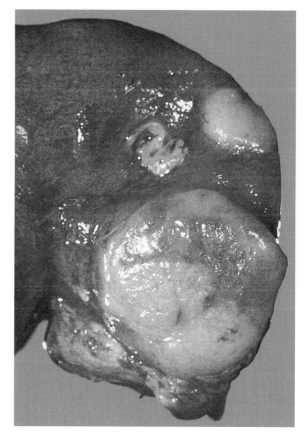

Figure 3-1
SEMINOMA

Top: A lobulated and multinodular, light tan tumor bulges above the cut surface of the surrounding testis. The hemisection on the right shows two separate nodules, but these are seen to be in continuity on the left.

Bottom: Seminoma showing one large mass and a second, separate smaller neoplasm of similar cell type (top right).

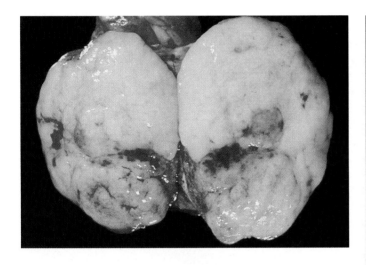

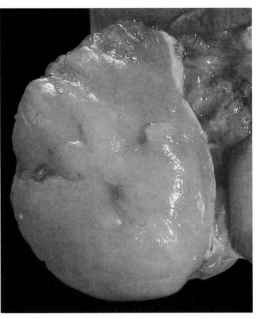

Figure 3-2
SEMINOMA
Fleshy, cream colored tumor with focal hemorrhage (above) and a light yellow tumor (right) replace the testicular parenchyma.

Figure 3-3
SEMINOMA
Hemorrhage into the tumor nodules produces a beefy red appearance. (Fig. 2.4 from Young RH, Scully RE. Testicular tumors. Chicago: ASCP Press, 1990:16.)

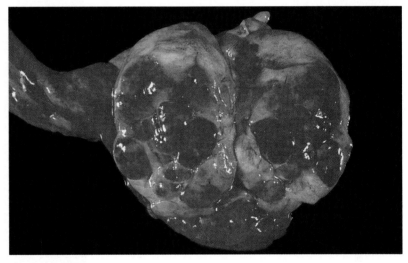

discohesion of seminoma cells may cause somewhat similar patterns (figs. 3-13, 3-14). In almost all seminomas, large, irregular cellular aggregates, small clusters of cells, and single cells are seen to varying extents. Most tumors obliterate the underlying testicular parenchyma, but some small seminomas, and more rarely large tumors, have a predominantly interstitial growth pattern with tubular preservation (fig. 3-15). In rare cases the cells are so widely dispersed in the interstitium that no tumor is grossly apparent (fig. 3-16). This interstitial pattern is more commonly

a focal finding, particularly at the periphery, of otherwise typical tumors. Extensive scarring occurs in some cases (fig. 3-17).

A characteristic feature is an infiltrate of mature lymphocytes; it occurs in almost all cases (63,123) and is marked in 20 to 25 percent (63, 93,123). In a study of 261 clinical stage I seminomas, only 3 tumors (1 percent) lacked lymphocytes (78a). The lymphocytes vary from a delicate sprinkling (fig. 3-7) to thick bands or aggregates (fig. 3-18). They often are most prominent in a perivascular distribution and hence are

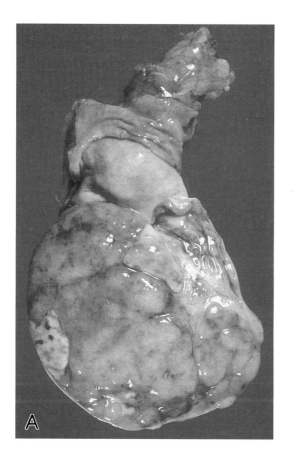

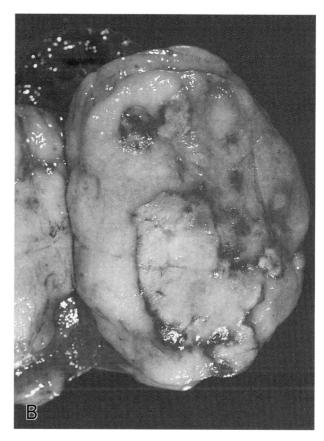

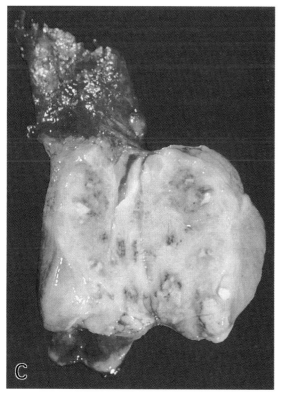

Figure 3-4
SEMINOMA

A: Punctate foci of hemorrhage and foci of necrosis are apparent on the cut surface of this seminoma. Note the prominent lobulation. (Fig. 5 from Ulbright TM, Roth LM. Testicular and paratesticular tumors. In: Sternberg SS, ed. Diagnostic surgical pathology, New York: Raven Press, 1994:1885–947.)

B: Variably sized yellow zones of necrosis focally rimmed by hemorrhage are conspicuous.

C: The white streaks in this case reflected extensive fibrosis in a tumor that prominently involved the epididymis (Fig. 2.2 from Young RH, Scully RE. Testicular tumors. Chicago: ASCP Press, 1990:15.)

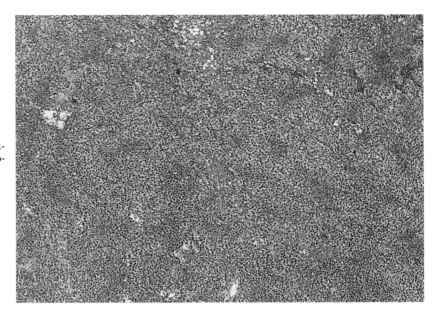

Figure 3-5
SEMINOMA
This tumor has a diffuse, sheet-like pattern. A sprinkling of lymphocytes is seen even at this low power.

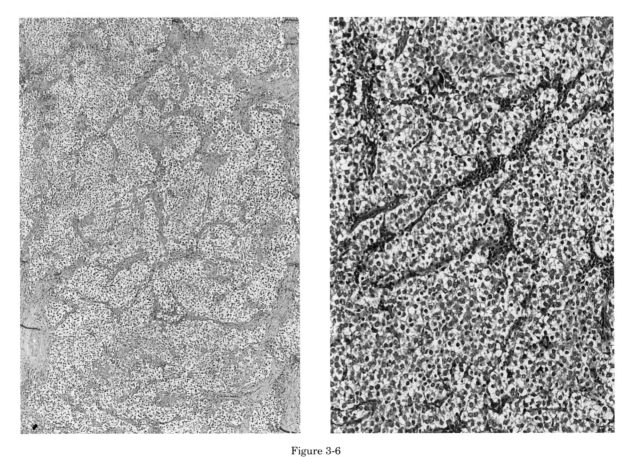

Figure 3-6
SEMINOMA
Typical thin, delicate septa, some of which are barely perceptible, are illustrated on low (left) and high (right) power.

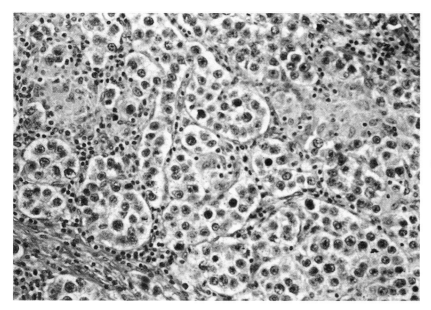

Figure 3-7
SEMINOMA
A solid alveolar pattern is created by thin septa around small nests of cells.

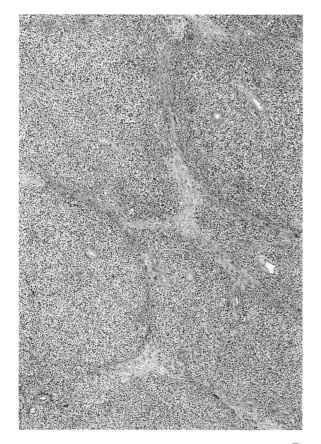
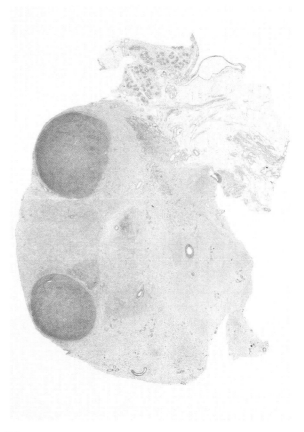

Figure 3-8
SEMINOMA
Left: Multinodular pattern.
Right: Two distinct nodules are present in a scarred parenchyma.

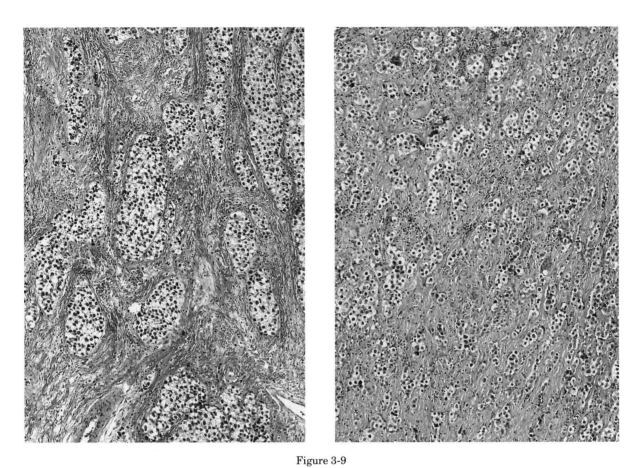

Figure 3-9
SEMINOMA
Left: Prominent fibrous stroma compartmentalizes the tumor into nests and solid pseudotubules.
Right: Extensive fibrous stroma separates small clusters of tumor cells.

Figure 3-10
SEMINOMA
The tumor cells are growing in cords.

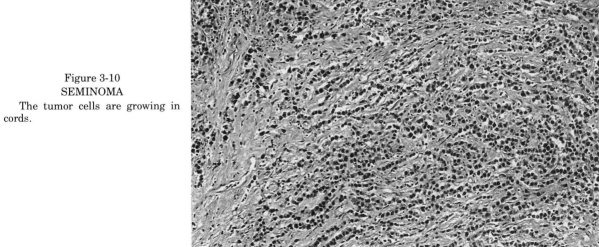

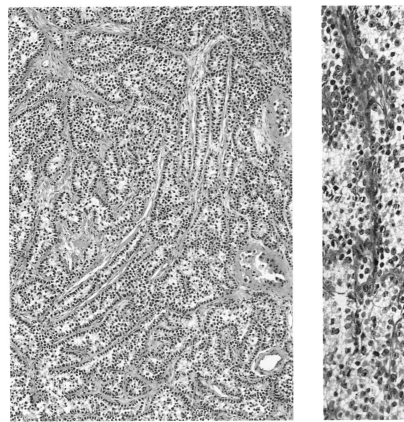
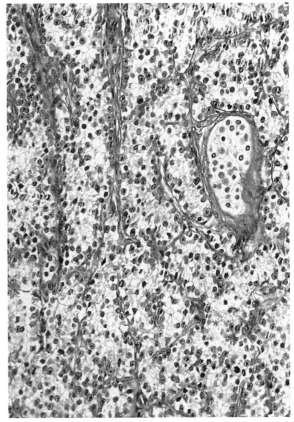

Figure 3-11
SEMINOMA

Left: A tubular pattern is created by central discohesion and a palisade-like arrangement of cells at the periphery of broad, anastomosing cords. Distinction from a Sertoli cell tumor is important in cases of this type.

Right: High-power view of the same case shows the typical cytologic features of seminoma cells.

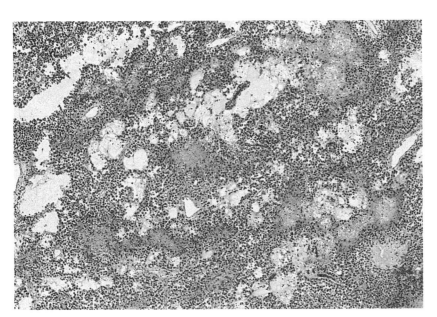

Figure 3-12
SEMINOMA
Edema creates a microcystic pattern.

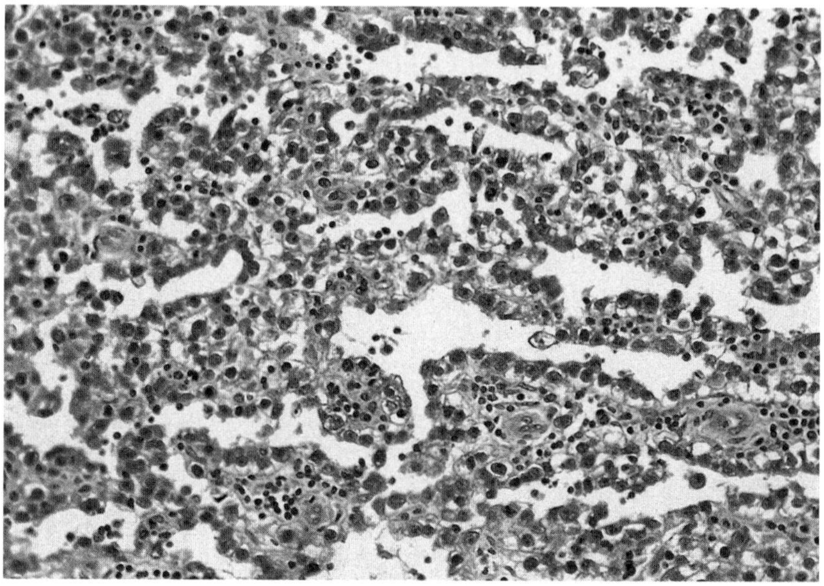

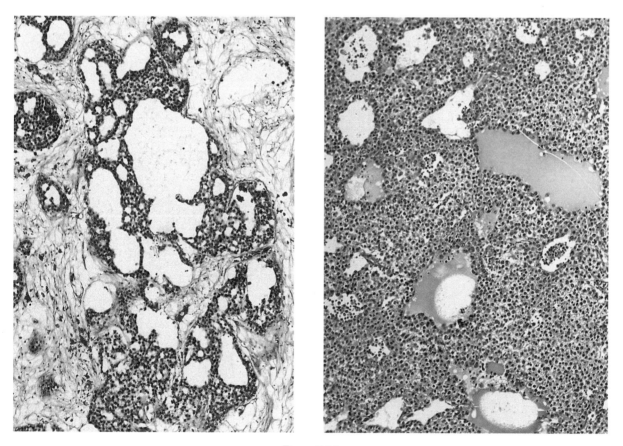

Figure 3-13
SEMINOMA
A pseudoglandular pattern.

Figure 3-14
SEMINOMA
A cribriform pattern with empty spaces (left) and spaces with eosinophilic fluid (right).

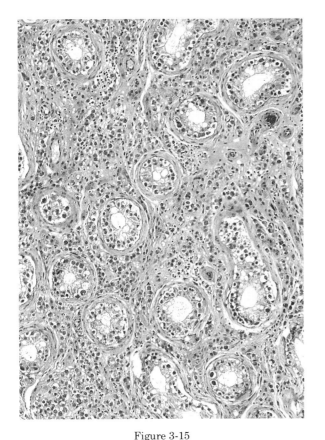

Figure 3-15
SEMINOMA
Interstitial pattern with preservation of preexisting seminiferous tubules.

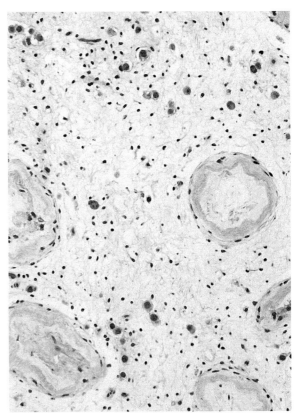

Figure 3-16
SEMINOMA
Widely dispersed tumor cells in the interstitium of an atrophic, cryptorchid testis. This tumor was grossly inapparent. (Courtesy of Drs. T.S. Carlson and D.R. Herbold, Wichita, KS.)

most conspicuous in the fibrous septa of the tumor, but they are also irregularly scattered, usually to a limited extent, among the seminoma cells away from the septa (fig. 3-18). At scanning magnification, local aggregates of lymphocytes may be the first clue to a small focus of seminoma in either the interstitium or the tubules. In up to 18 percent of cases, lymphoid follicles occur (fig. 3-18, right) (123). The majority of the lymphoid elements mark as T cells (43,47,48,121,128,130), and many have gamma/delta receptors and appear to play a role in granuloma formation (135). Occasionally, plasma cells and rarely, eosinophils may be identified in the infiltrate.

A granulomatous reaction occurs in 50 to 60 percent of seminomas (78a,93). This reaction varies from a light, scattered infiltrate of epithelioid histiocytes; to vaguely nodular clusters of such cells (fig. 3-19); to discrete, well-defined granulomas with Langhans-type giant cells. In some in-

stances, the presence of an extensive granulomatous reaction, sometimes with a heavy lymphoid infiltrate, may mask the underlying seminoma cells (fig. 3-20) and cause a misdiagnosis of granulomatous orchitis (see page 306).

Foci of necrosis are common in seminoma (fig. 3-21) and may be extensive; they occur in 46 to 54 percent of cases and are of marked degree in about 12 percent (78a,123). The necrosis generally occurs as discrete foci of the coagulative type, with ghost-like remnants of seminoma cells typically identifiable within the necrotic, eosinophilic zones. Recognition of a necrotic septal framework and small cells consistent with necrotic lymphocytes may help in the diagnosis.

Seminomas often display focal intratubular growth in which the neoplastic cells fill and distend seminiferous tubules (intratubular seminoma) (fig. 3-22). Dixon and Moore (58) identified such

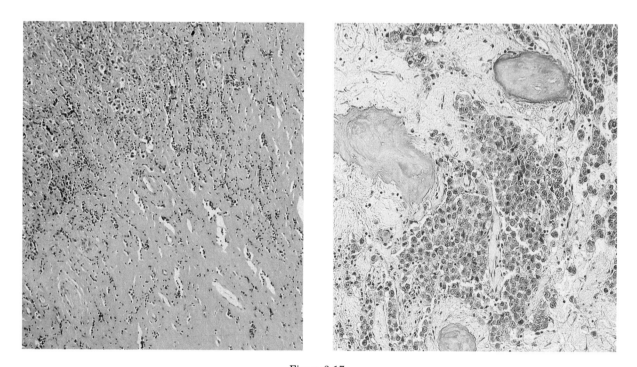

Figure 3-17
SEMINOMA
Left: There is extensive scarring. Note the many lymphocytes and paucity of seminoma cells.
Right: Ossification has occurred in a tumor with extensive stromal sclerosis.

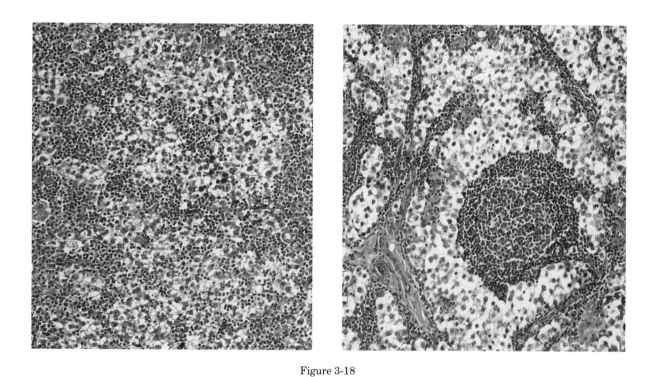

Figure 3-18
SEMINOMA
Left: There is a particularly striking lymphoid infiltrate.
Right: A lymphoid aggregate is seen. (Fig. 2.14 from Young RH, Scully RE. Testicular tumors. Chicago: ASCP Press, 1990:21.)

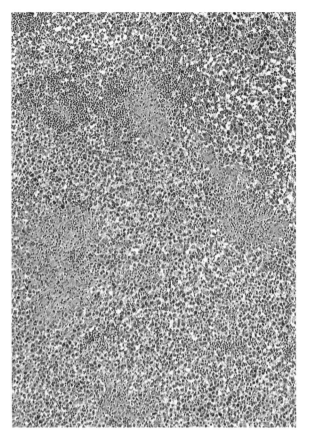

Figure 3-19
SEMINOMA
Granulomatous inflammation characterized by vaguely nodular clusters of epithelioid histiocytes.

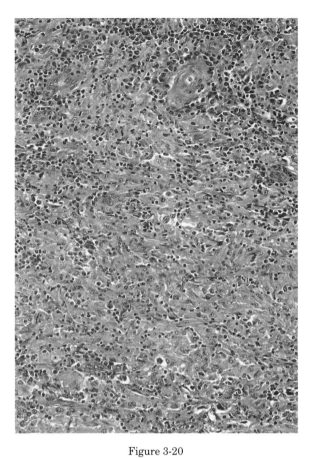

Figure 3-20
SEMINOMA
Extensive granulomatous reaction in a seminoma masking many of the neoplastic cells. Only rare scattered tumor cells are apparent.

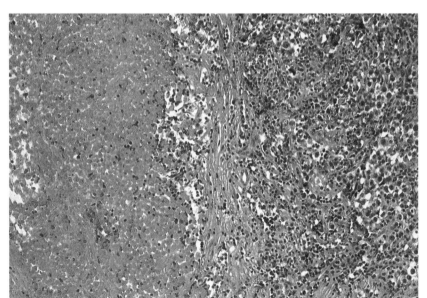

Figure 3-21
SEMINOMA
Necrosis is apparent within the tumor. Ghost outlines of seminoma cells can still be seen in the necrotic region.

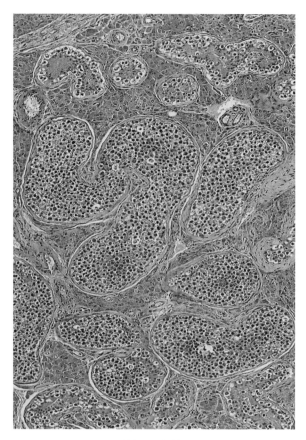

Figure 3-22
SEMINOMA

Intratubular seminoma (adjacent to invasive seminoma not shown) filling and distending the seminiferous tubules. Adjacent tubules show the typical pattern of intratubular germ cell neoplasia of the unclassified type; Leydig cells are hyperplastic.

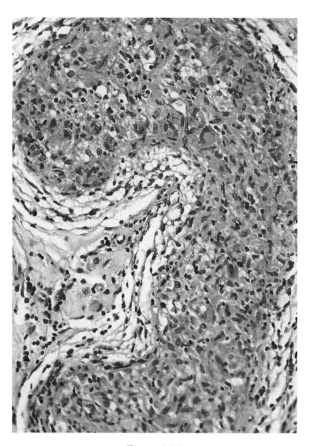

Figure 3-23
SEMINOMA

There is a marked intratubular granulomatous reaction.

growth in 24 percent of their cases. In seminomas that provoke a marked granulomatous reaction, there may also be a prominent intratubular granulomatous response (fig. 3-23). It is also common to see seminoma cells extending into the rete testis, and rarely into the epididymis, in a pagetoid fashion (fig. 3-24), but this phenomenon may also be seen in IGCNU and is not diagnostic of an invasive lesion (104). There are rare seminomas in which the pagetoid intra-rete portion of the tumor predominates (fig. 3-25). Involvement of the rete by invasive seminoma occurs in more than 40 percent of the cases but appears not to have prognostic significance (78a).

Dystrophic calcification may occur within scarred or necrotic foci of seminomas. The presence of calcification, however, should also raise the possibility that the tumor developed from a preexisting gonadoblastoma and that the patient may have gonadal dysgenesis with a consequent higher risk of bilateral germ cell tumors, a more likely possibility if the gonad is cryptorchid (see chapter 5). A careful search is therefore indicated in an attempt to identify gonadoblastoma in this circumstance, although this is an admittedly rare association, despite the common occurrence of calcification (68,87). Rarely ossification occurs within the fibrous septa of seminoma (fig. 3-17, right) (80).

Seminoma cells are round to polygonal and generally have clear to lightly eosinophilic, granular cytoplasm, although in an occasional case a perinuclear rim of dense eosinophilic cytoplasm is present. They measure from 15 to 25 μm in diameter. In adequately fixed specimens a useful diagnostic feature of most seminomas is the distinctly visible cytoplasmic membrane that separates adjacent neoplastic cells (fig. 3-26); this

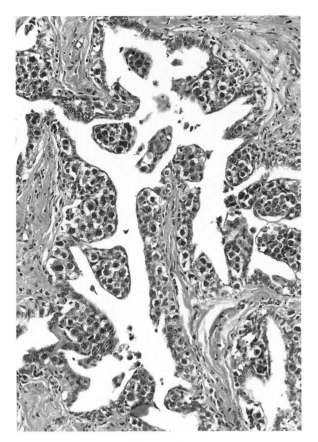

Figure 3-24
SEMINOMA
There is extension of seminoma cells into the rete testis, with intact rete testis epithelium on the luminal aspect.

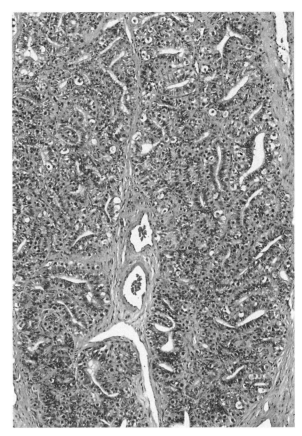

Figure 3-25
SEMINOMA
There is prominent intra-rete extension of seminoma cells with expansion of the rete testis. The enlarged rete caused a palpable mass.

feature contrasts with the syncytial arrangement of embryonal carcinoma in which cytoplasmic borders are indistinct (see page 109, fig. 4-14). The nuclei are large and central or slightly eccentric, with granular chromatin, one, two, or more prominent nucleoli, and an irregularly thickened nuclear membrane (fig. 3-26). The nuclear membrane is typically somewhat flattened rather than perfectly round, causing a "squared-off" appearance (fig. 3-26). Another useful feature is a relatively uniform distribution of nuclei within neoplastic islands such that nuclei are separated from each other by roughly equivalent amounts of cytoplasm (fig. 3-26), in contrast to the overlapping nuclei of embryonal carcinoma. The clear cytoplasm reflects an abundant amount of glycogen that is demonstrable as granular, PAS-positive, diastase-labile deposits (fig. 3-27), with

rare exceptions. Occasionally a seminoma has areas in which the cells have densely eosinophilic to amphophilic cytoplasm, and rarely a tumor consists solely of this cell type. Eccentric positions of the nuclei in such cases result in a plasmacytoid appearance, although a perinuclear hof is lacking (fig. 3-28). Seminoma is very vulnerable to inadequate fixation. The nuclei may be smudgy with loss of detail, sometimes appearing as elongated, densely staining threads (fig. 3-29). A lymphocytic infiltrate and granulomatous reaction are helpful in recognizing these cases. In some tumors there is conspicuous "squeeze" artifact (fig. 3-30) which may be confusing, particularly in a biopsy specimen.

The mitotic activity of seminomas is variable but usually brisk, tending to be greatest at the periphery of lobules where DNA synthesis is

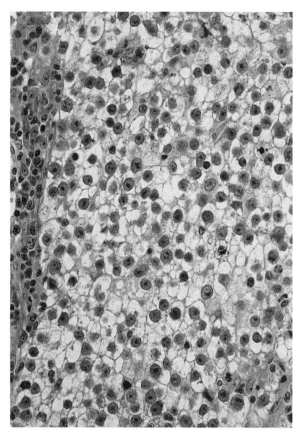

Figure 3-26
SEMINOMA
The tumor cells have abundant clear cytoplasm, well-defined cytoplasmic borders, evenly spaced nuclei (some of which have "squared-off" edges), and prominent central nucleoli.

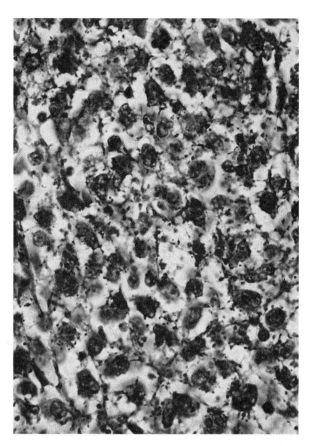

Figure 3-27
SEMINOMA
The tumor cells contain abundant intracytoplasmic glycogen (periodic acid-Schiff stain).

greatest (106). In the past, a high mitotic rate (equal or greater than 3 mitotic figures per high-power field) was employed as a criterion for the recognition of an "anaplastic" subcategory of seminoma (92,93), a subset we, and most others, do not recognize. Recent studies have cast doubt on the value of mitotic activity as a criterion for the recognition of an aggressively behaving seminoma (78a,122,136) and have demonstrated a high mitotic rate (3 or more mitoses per high-power field) in most seminomas (126), a fact that has led some to revise the criteria for anaplastic seminoma to an average of 6 or more mitotic figures per high-power field. The lack of correlation of mitotic activity with prognosis in seminoma, however, argues against even this criterion. Similar findings in classic and "anaplastic" seminomas by ultrastructure, immunohistochemistry, and

lectin-binding analyses provide further evidence against the validity of this category (79,82,122). There remain, nonetheless, occasional seminomas with either focal or more diffuse pleomorphism than is typical (fig. 3-31). In our opinion these are cases that have partially progressed toward embryonal carcinoma in what is likely a multi-step process. Our own approach is not to regard such foci as nonseminomatous differentiation in the absence of clear-cut epithelial features in the form of papillae, glands, or distinct cytokeratin reactivity that contrasts with weaker or absent reactivity in the nonpleomorphic areas of the same tumor. We continue to designate such cases as seminoma, an approach supported by the failure to identify a more aggressive course in the seminomas with ultrastructural evidence of "early carcinomatous features" (117).

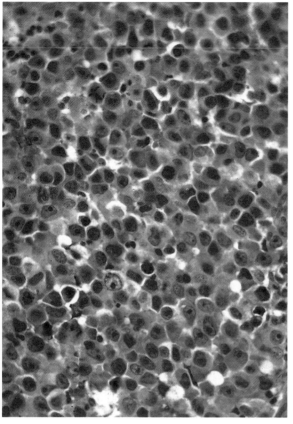

Figure 3-28
SEMINOMA
Dense, amphophilic to eosinophilic cytoplasm and eccentric nuclei cause a plasmacytoid appearance, although perinuclear hofs are absent.

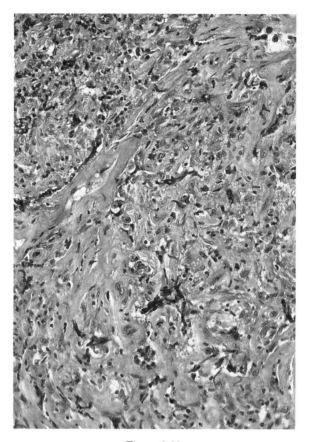

Figure 3-29
SEMINOMA
Many tumor cells have been compressed into darkly staining threadlike forms in a fibrotic stroma. (Fig. 2.22 from Young RH, Scully RE. Testicular tumors. Chicago: ASCP Press, 1990:25.)

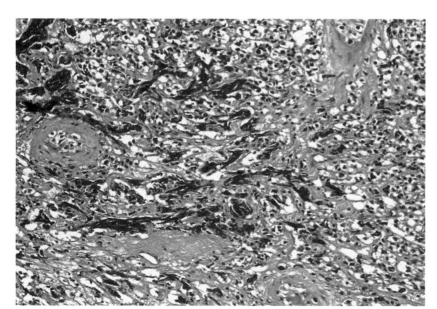

Figure 3-30
SEMINOMA
Prominent "squeeze" artifact is seen.

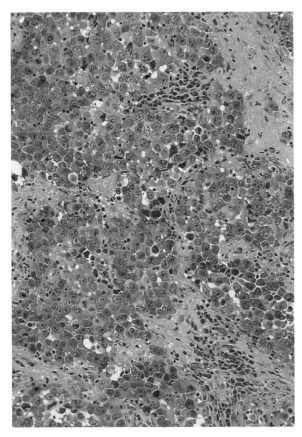

Figure 3-31
SEMINOMA
A pleomorphic area in an otherwise typical neoplasm.

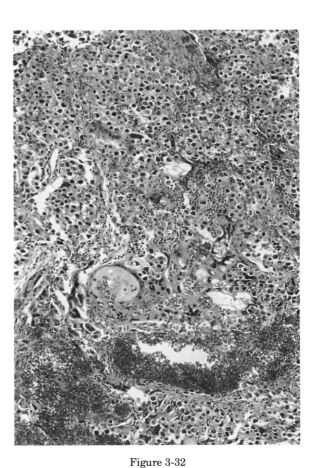

Figure 3-32
SEMINOMA
Prominent syncytiotrophoblastic cells and focal hemorrhage are intermingled with seminoma cells.

Syncytiotrophoblastic cells are seen in 4 to 7 percent of seminomas by routine light microscopy (78a,94), but immunostains directed against hCG highlight cells with syncytiotrophoblastic differentiation in 20 to 25 percent of seminomas (94,127). Sometimes punctate hemorrhagic foci or even blood lakes surrounded by the syncytiotrophoblastic cells are seen (fig. 3-32) and can be a low-power microscopic clue to the diagnosis. In other cases, however, there is no associated hemorrhage (fig. 3-33). The syncytiotrophoblast cells are variable in appearance, sometimes appearing as classic syncytiotrophoblasts with abundant cytoplasm, several or numerous hyperchromatic nuclei, and intracytoplasmic lacunae (fig. 3-34). More commonly they appear as multinucleated giant cells lacking lacunae (figs. 3-32, 3-33). In some instances the cells have relatively scant cytoplasm and contain "mulberry-like" aggre-

gates of nuclei. Some hCG-positive cells are uninucleate and easily blend with the background of seminoma cells (72); some represent intermediate trophoblast cells and are occasionally human placental lactogen (HPL) reactive (86). Most frequently, syncytiotrophoblastic cells are scattered in a multifocal fashion in the tumor, tending to localize in small clusters adjacent to capillaries. An admixture with cytotrophoblasts is lacking. When trophoblastic elements are identified in seminoma, their presence should be recorded as "seminoma with syncytiotrophoblastic cells." The absence of choriocarcinoma should also be explicitly stated.

As mentioned in chapter 1, artifactual implantation of tumor cells into vascular spaces and on tissue surfaces is common in seminoma, and it is important to distinguish this artifact from real invasion of vessels or extratesticular

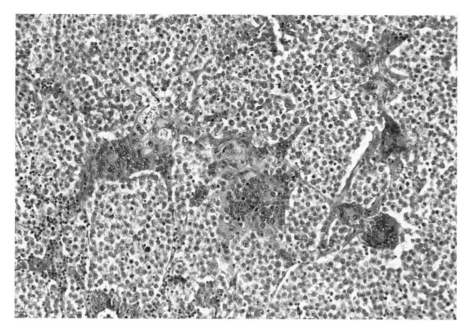

Figure 3-33
SEMINOMA
Scattered syncytiotropho-
blastic cells, some with mulberry-like nuclei.

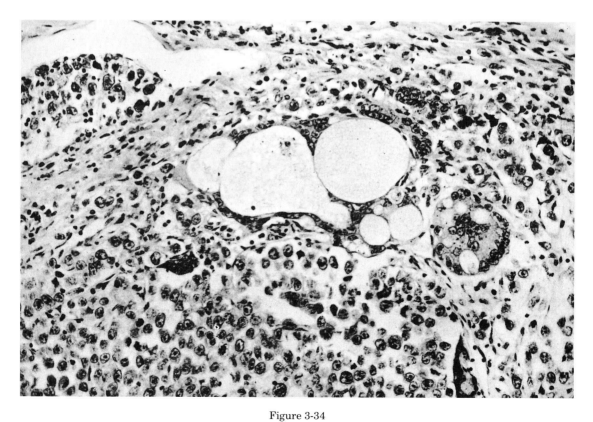

Figure 3-34
SEMINOMA
Syncytiotrophoblastic cells with prominent intracytoplasmic lacunae. (Fig. 41 from Fascicles 31b and 32, First Series.)

Table 3-1

USEFUL IMMUNOSTAINS IN GERM CELL TUMORS

	Pan-keratin	Vimentin	AFP*	Ber-H2	PLAP	hCG
Seminoma	+/−	+	−	−**	+	−[†]
Spermatocytic seminoma	−[‡]	+	−	−	−[§]	−
Embryonal carcinoma	+	−	+/−	+	+	−[†]
Yolk sac tumor	+	+	+	−	+	−[†]
Choriocarcinoma	+	−	−	?	+/−	+
Teratoma	+	+	+/−	−	+/−	−[†]

*Abbreviations: AFP = alpha-fetoprotein; hCG = human chorionic gonadotropin; PLAP = placental-like alkaline phosphatase.
**Rare cells positive.
[†]hCG stains are positive in intermixed syncytiotrophoblastic cells.
[‡]Rare cells may stain for cytokeratin 18.
[§]Immunostains for PLAP may show rare positivity in individual and small groups of tumor cells.

soft tissues. The same guidelines that are discussed in chapter 4 (see page 110) also apply for recognition of this artifact in seminomas.

Immunohistochemical Findings. A summary of immunostains that may be used to aid in the diagnosis of seminoma and other germ cell tumors is provided in Table 3-1. The most useful currently available marker to aid in the recognition of seminoma is anti-placental alkaline phosphatase, which highlights placental-like alkaline phosphatase (PLAP) in a diffuse and membrane-accentuated pattern in 87 to 98 percent of seminomas (fig. 3-35) (73,85,99,124). PLAP positivity, however, is also seen in other germ cell tumors, where it tends to be more focal and cytoplasmic (51), and in some nongerm cell tumors (129). The liver isoenzyme of alkaline phosphatase has also been demonstrated in seminomas but not the intestinal form (50).

As noted previously, 7 to 25 percent of pure seminomas are associated with an elevated serum level of hCG. Immunostaining of such cases usually discloses positivity for hCG in syncytiotrophoblast cells (fig. 3-36), although some hCG positivity occurs in cells that are not recognizable as syncytiotrophoblasts by routine light microscopy (94), suggesting that there is incomplete trophoblastic differentiation or differentiation to intermediate trophoblast (86). hCG reactivity in

seminomas has ranged from 5 to 24 percent (49, 75,94,99,127); typical seminoma cells do not stain for hCG, with rare exceptions (72). Trophoblastic cells are also typically cytokeratin reactive.

Cytokeratin filaments are not abundant in the majority of seminomas, and there are contradictory results concerning the frequency of keratin positivity. Such discrepancies are likely attributable to the specificity of the antibodies and the utilization of different methodologies for antigen retrieval. Reports of cytokeratin positivity range from 0 to 73 percent (46,57,60,61,64,67,88,107a, 114a), with staining usually occurring in isolated cells or small clusters, although some otherwise typical seminomas have, on rare occasions, been diffusely positive (57,61,99). Studies have demonstrated cytokeratins 8 and 18 (molecular weights of 52.5 and 45 kD, respectively) in seminomas (91), with the usual absence of cytokeratin 19 (45,57), which is common in embryonal carcinomas (45). However, Fogel et al. (67), using frozen and paraffin sections, identified scant amounts of cytokeratin 19 in 5 of 26 seminomas, with groups of cells positive in one case. Strong and more than focal positivity for cytokeratin 19 is therefore useful in distinguishing seminoma from embryonal carcinoma, but should not be considered an absolute criterion. Cytokeratins 8, 18, and 19 are readily demonstrated in the syncytiotrophoblast

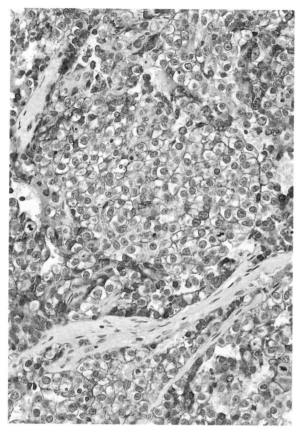

Figure 3-35
SEMINOMA
Positive immunostain for placental-like alkaline phosphatase (PLAP) shows the characteristic membranous pattern.

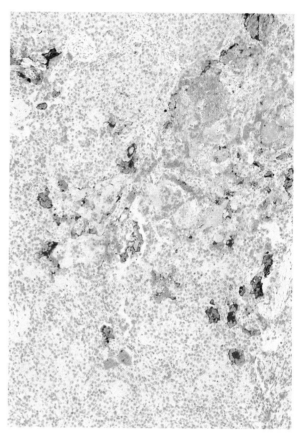

Figure 3-36
SEMINOMA
Prominent syncytiotrophoblastic cells are highlighted by an immunostain for hCG.

cells of seminomas. Cytokeratins 4 and 17, more characteristic of stratified and complex glandular epithelia, can be identified in rare seminomas, as can desmin and neurofilament protein (67). Seminomas associated with borderline serum AFP elevations may disproportionately express cytokeratin 7 (98). The combination of PLAP positivity and cytokeratin negativity (using clones AE1/AE3) appears to be a pattern relatively specific for seminoma in routinely fixed tissues in the absence of antigen retrieval in comparison to other tumors (129). The experience with a cytokeratin cocktail (AE1/AE3 and CAM 5.2) in routinely processed cases showed that seminoma cells are negative to focally reactive, with strong staining of intermixed syncytiotrophoblastic cells (114a).

Seminomas are characteristically positive for vimentin, usually in a small percentage of the tumor cells (57,64,88,107a), although Fogel et al. (67) reported widespread staining in 6 of 26 seminomas and an overall frequency of vimentin positivity of 61 percent. Denk et al. (57) showed patchy positivity for desmosomal-plaque proteins and presented evidence that the poorly developed desmosomes of seminoma are associated with vimentin filaments. Desmoplakins and desmoglein are usually present (67).

LDH, ferritin, and NSE are positive in most seminomas but are nonspecific (76,96,99). Alpha-1-antitrypsin and Leu-7 are positive in 5 percent and 14 percent of cases, respectively (99), whereas angiotensin-converting enzyme was positive in all of 20 germinomas (111).

Unlike yolk sac tumor and some embryonal carcinomas, stains for AFP are negative in seminoma (Table 3-1) (52,77,99). Epithelial membrane antigen (EMA) is also negative in seminoma, as

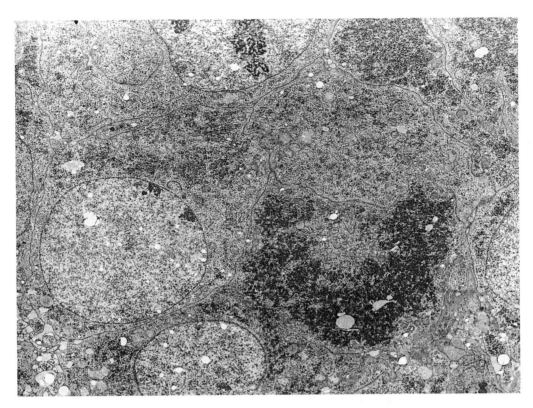

Figure 3-37
SEMINOMA

The seminoma cells have smooth, closely apposed cytoplasmic membranes, abundant glycogen particles, polarization of cytoplasmic organelles, and nuclei with evenly dispersed chromatin. Note "meandering" nucleolus in cell at the top (X8,000).

it is in the great majority of embryonal carcinomas and yolk sac tumors (99,129). Ki-1 (CD30, Ber-H2 antibody) is negative in almost all seminomas and is usually positive in embryonal carcinomas (65,71,102).

The combination of PLAP positivity and EMA negativity, therefore, supports a diagnosis of germ cell tumor (99); if the differential is between seminoma and nonseminomatous germ cell tumor, AFP, Ki-1 (Ber-H2), and selected cytokeratins are useful. Recently, staining for the product of the c-*kit* proto-oncogene has been described in seminomas but not in nonseminomatous germ cell tumors (119). If the differential includes lymphoma and melanoma, stains for leukocyte common antigen and S-100 protein or HMB-45 (which are negative in germ cell tumors, with the exception of S-100 in certain teratomatous elements) are of major value (99).

Ultrastructural Findings. On ultrastructural examination, seminoma cells are closely apposed, with smooth or undulating cell membranes (fig. 3-37). Primitive junctions, most commonly consisting of electron-dense thickenings of the membranes of adjacent cells, are occasionally identified (fig. 3-38) (108a). Such junctions lack well-developed inserting filaments. In some seminomas, more differentiated, epithelial-type junctions and specializations can be found. In these cases, rare, tight junctional complexes are identified, with well-defined desmosomes, as adjacent cells form abortive extracellular lumens with short, projecting microvilli. Complex, interdigitating cell membranes may be identified (105). Such features, suggesting epithelial differentiation, were identified in 4 of 50 cases of seminoma interpreted as showing "early carcinomatous features" (117). Similar features have been noted by some investigators (79,89), but not by others (105). It is likely that seminomas exhibit a spectrum of differentiation, which probably explains the lack of correlation in different studies. Those seminomas with "early carcinomatous features" on ultrastructural examination

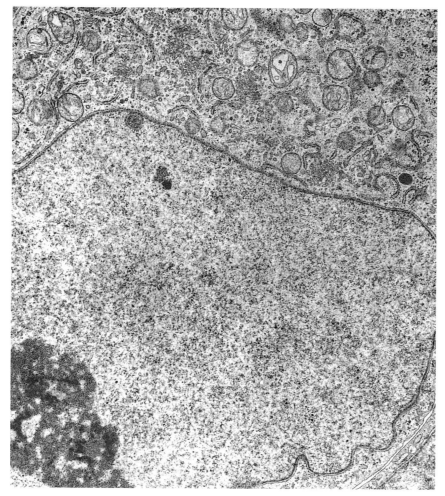

Figure 3-38
SEMINOMA
A portion of a seminoma cell shows polarization of cytoplasmic organelles, which consist of small mitochondria, short stacks of Golgi-like membranes, single strands of rough endoplasmic reticulum, scattered free ribosomes, and a small lysosome. The nucleolus is typically complex, and there is a primitive cell junction at lower right. Note the evenly dispersed chromatin (X16,500).

retained a typical light microscopic morphology and had a typical clinical behavior (117).

The cytoplasm of seminoma cells is primitive. Variable amounts of rosettes of glycogen can be identified, from sparse to superabundant (fig. 3-37) (57a,81,108a). Organelles are usually polarized to one side of the cell (figs. 3-37, 3-38) and consist of mitochondria with tubulovesicular cristae and clear matrices; occasional granular, membrane-bound, lysosome-like bodies; annulate lamellae; and cisternae of rough and smooth endoplasmic reticulum (fig. 3-38). Free ribosomes and polysomes are dispersed in the cytoplasm, and Golgi bodies may be apparent (fig. 3-38). There are occasional droplets of lipid (81).

The nuclei of seminoma cells are round and regular with evenly dispersed, finely granular chromatin. Heterochromatin clumps are distinctly sparse. The nucleoli are large and consist

of complex, "wandering" strands of electron-dense, fibrillar material (figs. 3-37, 3-38) (117).

Special Diagnostic Methods. Analysis of the DNA content of seminomas has shown a mean diploid value 1.6 to 1.8 times the normal, which is significantly higher than in non-seminomatous tumors (mean, 1.4 times the normal) (62,101). The reporting of diploid seminomas is felt to be an incorrect result of flow cytometric analysis caused by extensive lymphoid infiltrates (70). Rukstalis and DeWolf (110) believed that there was a high probability that the loss of cancer suppressor genes contributed to testicular carcinogenesis and implicated a region on chromosome 6 close to the HLA locus (109), although other chromosomes (see below) are more consistently involved in losses. Decreased expression of the retinoblastoma gene has been demonstrated in seminomas (112,120), as well as nonseminomatous germ cell tumors (120), but alterations of the retinoblastoma gene at the DNA level have not been identified (120).

Cytogenetic analysis of seminomas has shown an increased number of chromosomes in the triploid range, leading to the speculation that seminoma may originate from fusion of a postmeiotic haploid cell with a diploid cell or be the result of a meiotic error (54). Certain chromosomes are often over-represented in seminomas (numbers 7, 8, 12, 21, and X) and others may be under-represented (numbers 11, 13, 18, and Y) (54,125). The most common structural cytogenetic abnormality in seminoma is the presence of an isochromosome derived from the short arm of chromosome 12: i(12p), which may be present in multiple copies according to some investigators (54), but not others (56). Copy numbers of i(12p) are fewer in seminomas than in nonseminomatous germ cell tumors (125). Some patients with seminoma lack i(12p), but often have other structural abnormalities involving chromosome 12 (53,54). Isochromosome (12p) is also commonly identified in nonseminomatous germ cell tumors, and cell lines of testicular germ cell tumors commonly contain i(12p) as well as deletions involving the long arm of chromosome 12 (97). The common presence of structural abnormalities in chromosome 12 in seminomas and nonseminomatous tumors has led to the speculation that loss of genetic material from the long arm of chromosome 12 is an important and early step in the malignant transformation of testicular germ cells (97). Some have speculated that such changes may lead to an activation of the K-*ras*-2 protooncogene that maps to this locus (54), but the paucity of N-*ras* and K-*ras* mutations on molecular analysis of testicular germ cell tumors does not support this viewpoint (100).

There are isolated reports concerning the expression of oncogenes in germ cell tumors. Some studies have demonstrated positive immunostaining of seminomas for p62c-myc, the 62-kD protein product of the c-*myc* oncogene (116). N-*myc* expression has been identified in seminomas (90,112,115). The c-*kit* oncogene was expressed in 24 of 30 (80 percent) seminomas, but in only 3 of 40 (7 percent) nonseminomatous germ cell tumors (118), in keeping with the results of a second study (119). Mutations in either the Ki-*ras* or N-*ras* oncogenes at codons 12 or 61

have been reported in 40 percent of seminomas but are present in only some of the seminoma cells, leading to the conclusion that such changes are not an initiating genetic event (95). In another study, five of nine germ cell tumors, including three with seminomatous components, expressed the *hst*-1 oncogene in ribonucleic acid (RNA) blot analyses (132), however a second study indicated that *hst*-1 expression was predominantly found in nonseminomatous tumors rather than in seminomas (118). p53 mutations have also been implicated in seminomas (44, 83,131), but this is disputed by others (66,69, 103,108,113). Immunohistochemical staining for p53 protein correlates with increasing stage in seminomas (84) but probably does not correlate with gene mutation. One study described high levels of c-*mos* expression in seminomas (115)

Analysis of proliferative activity in seminomas, using the monoclonal antibody Ki-67, has demonstrated positive immunostaining in 50 to 80 percent of the cell population, but it did not correlate with the degree of lymphoid reaction or tumor volume (59). Such labeling was relatively homogeneously distributed throughout the tumor. In contrast, thymidine labeling analysis of proliferative activity in seminomas has shown relatively uniform labeling in small tumors but selective peripheral labeling in more advanced seminomas, with a mean labeling index of 11.6 percent (106,107).

Cytologic Findings. Fine needle aspiration cytology of metastases may be helpful in confirming tumor spread or in establishing a diagnosis in patients with occult testicular tumors (161). Seminomas in aspirated smeared preparations consist of loose clusters, occasional sheets, and single cells (fig. 3-39) (159,161–163). The cytoplasm is fragile, and the smearing technique may produce long cytoplasmic tails between groups of cells (162). An important diagnostic feature is a background of cytoplasmic debris that contains glycogen, yielding a striped or "tigroid" staining pattern between the preserved cellular elements in air-dried smears (fig. 3-39) (160,161,163). This tigroid background is not commonly identified in other types of tumors (160), and is probably present in only a minority of seminoma specimens (161). The cells are generally 15 to 20 μm in diameter (in air-dried preparations) (159) and have round to oval nuclei with fine chromatin and one or more prominent nucleoli (159,162). A moderate amount of cytoplasm is present, as well as variably prominent vacuoles, corresponding to cytoplasmic glycogen (159). The cytoplasmic borders are well defined (162). Admixed lymphocytes, plasma cells, and epithelioid cells are common (159,161,162), but these may be less prominent than in tissue sections (161,163).

Differential Diagnosis. Seminoma is confused most often with the solid pattern of embryonal carcinoma. In well-fixed preparations this differential diagnosis should not be problematic. Seminoma, however, is very susceptible to poor fixation, leading to loss of cytoplasm, poorly defined cell borders, and nuclear juxtaposition, all of which are features mimicking embryonal carcinoma (153). For this reason, it is crucial to institute procedures to assure well-fixed material, as discussed in chapter 1. In optimal preparations seminoma has round to "squared off," regular nuclei that are separated from each other by relatively uniform amounts of cytoplasm with well-defined cell borders. Embryonal carcinoma, on the other hand, has more irregularly shaped, vesicular nuclei that appear to overlap in routine sections, and the cell borders are poorly defined. The cytoplasm of embryonal carcinoma cells is more frequently amphophilic to basophilic. A prominent granulomatous and lymphoid reaction favors seminoma, although an occasional embryonal carcinoma has a similar reaction. Embryonal carcinomas lack the characteristic regular septa of seminoma. The presence of true glands and papillae exclude seminoma. In a problematic case, cytokeratin stains are useful: embryonal carcinomas may contain cytokeratin 19, which is either absent or scant in most seminomas (137,141,145). A useful clone is AE1/AE3 which is generally positive in embryonal carcinoma but usually negative in seminoma, at least in routinely processed, paraffin-embedded tissues. Antibodies directed against the Ki-1 antigen (Ber-H2) are essentially negative in seminomas and positive in most embryonal carcinomas (see Table 3-1, page 78) (139,144,149). Recently, a monoclonal antibody, 43-9F, has been reported to stain embryonal carcinomas strongly but seminomas only weakly or not at all (155).

The solid pattern of yolk sac tumor may also mimic seminoma. Usually, however, this pattern is associated with other, more diagnostic patterns

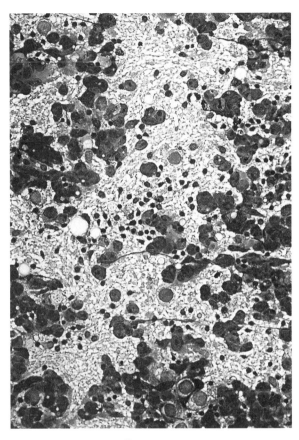

Figure 3-39
SEMINOMA
An air-dried preparation of a needle-aspirated seminoma shows neoplastic cells in loose clusters and as single cells with interspersed lymphocytes. The background shows the characteristic "tigroid" pattern (Diff-Quik).

of yolk sac tumor that permit this distinction with relative ease. Solid foci in yolk sac tumor do not have the typical fibrovascular septa with associated lymphocytes of seminoma. Most of the cells are typically smaller than seminoma cells, do not have their "squared off" nuclear membranes, and typically have less prominent nucleoli. In many cases of solid yolk sac tumor, there are scattered larger cells, unlike seminoma where the cells are more uniform in size, with the exception of syncytiotrophoblasts. Hyaline globules are absent or rare in seminoma and frequent in yolk sac tumors (154), although typically less conspicuous in solid foci. Intercellular basement membrane strongly favors yolk sac tumor. Edema and microcysts or a cribriform pattern in a seminoma may suggest the reticular or cystic pattern of yolk sac tumor, but the cysts are typically more irregular in outline, usually contain exfoliated seminoma cells, and may contain edema fluid, unlike the "clean" microcysts of yolk sac tumor that are lined by spindle-shaped to low cuboidal cells. The lack of other yolk sac tumor-like patterns is also helpful in cases of seminoma. Cytokeratins are demonstrable in most yolk sac tumors using clones AE1/AE3 (and others), but cytokeratins are much more restricted in seminomas (see above). AFP is usually positive in yolk sac tumor and negative in seminoma. The differential with spermatocytic seminoma is discussed in the next section.

Seminomas with syncytiotrophoblastic cells must be distinguished from choriocarcinomas. In typical choriocarcinoma there is an admixture of syncytiotrophoblastic elements with cytotrophoblastic cells, whereas no cytotrophoblastic component occurs in seminoma with syncytiotrophoblasts. Cytotrophoblasts are distinguished from seminoma cells by the absence of the associated lymphocytes and fibrous septa, and greater variation in cell and nuclear size and shape. They, furthermore, usually express hCG, although in a weak and patchy fashion, in contrast to seminoma cells, with rare exceptions.

Malignant lymphoma may be confused with seminoma. Patients with malignant lymphoma are usually older, with the typical mean age being about 60 years (140,142,143,147,148,150, 152). Lymphomas of the testis are more often bilateral (138,140,142,148,150,152), are more frequently associated with extratesticular disease (140), and often have a striking intertubular pattern of growth even in the center of the neoplasm (140,148,151,152), a feature much rarer in seminomas. More definitive, however, are the high-power microscopic features of lymphoma cells, which typically have twisted or angulated nuclei, and a more polymorphous cell population with respect to cell size than in seminoma. The cytoplasm of lymphoma cells is generally less well-defined and not as clear as in seminoma cells. Most seminomas are associated with residual IGCNU. Leukocyte common antigen (LCA; CD45) marks a high percentage of lymphomas but is not identified in seminomas (146), and an opposite pattern is seen with PLAP (156). Other lymphoid markers can be employed if needed (140,146).

Rare "tubular seminomas," composed of closely packed, solid tubules resemble Sertoli cell tumors (157,158). Differentiation depends upon the recognition of the typical cytology of seminoma cells, the presence of abundant cytoplasmic glycogen rather than the large amounts of lipid expected for a Sertoli cell tumor with clear cytoplasm, the association of the seminoma with IGCNU and a lymphoid infiltrate, and, in some cases, the presence of more typical-appearing seminoma with fibrous septa (157,158). PLAP (positive in seminoma, negative in Sertoli cell tumor), inhibin (negative in seminoma, positive in many Sertoli cell tumors), and cytokeratin (often negative in seminoma and frequently positive in Sertoli cell tumor) immunostains can assist with this differential diagnosis.

Rarely, a marked granulomatous reaction in seminoma makes neoplastic cells difficult to identify, and confusion with granulomatous orchitis can occur. Careful, high-power examination identifies seminoma cells; PAS stains and PLAP immunostains highlight them.

Treatment and Prognosis. Most seminomas are extremely sensitive to radiation and chemotherapy. The TNM system has not proved ideal in the stratification of seminoma patients into relevant treatment groups, and a modified Royal Marsden classification (see Table 1-3), with the addition of a stage IID category (maximum diameter, greater than 10 cm), has been advocated for seminoma (190). For seminomas that are clinically confined to the testis, the usual form of treatment following orchiectomy is radiation therapy directed at the ipsilateral inguinal and iliac nodes and the periaortic and pericaval lymph nodes to the level of the diaphragm. Usually about 30 Gy are delivered in fractionated doses over a 3-week interval. Using this treatment a cure rate of 95 percent or better may be expected (164,165,173,177,192). A recent study indicated that patients with clinical stage I or IIA seminoma (Royal Marsden system) can be treated by radiation to a reduced field, omitting the pelvic sites, without increasing the rate of recurrence (167). This would appear to be a reasonable approach for patients without prior inguinal surgery or involvement of the scrotal skin (176). Recurrences are unusual; most develop outside of the radiated field, in the mediastinum (173,188), cervical lymph nodes, or lungs (176). One study, however, demonstrated about equal numbers of relapses in the abdomen or pelvis, mediastinum, and distant sites (191).

In general, surveillance appears to be a less appealing option in early stage seminomas than in nonseminomatous tumors because of the excellent results with radiation with minimal morbidity, the lesser reliability of tumor markers for the detection of recurrence in seminomas compared to nonseminomatous tumors, and a need for a more prolonged period of surveillance due to the slower growth rate of seminomas and the greater frequency of late recurrence (179,183). However, the surveillance approach would save roughly 87 percent of patients with early stage seminoma from radiation and its consequent complications (185). Vascular space invasion in the testicular primary may indicate a subset of seminoma patients who are ineligible for a "surveillance only" approach (181), however, recurrences have also occurred in about 10 percent of patients with no identifiable lymphovascular invasion (as opposed to 20 percent of those with demonstrable lymphovascular invasion) (175). Tumor size of greater than 6 cm also correlates with a significantly increased frequency of relapse (166).

Patients with seminoma metastatic to retroperitoneal sites (stage II or B) are most frequently treated according to the extent of the nodal involvement. For patients with less bulky disease, most authorities continue to advocate radiation therapy, perhaps with additional doses to larger deposits. Survival in this group of patients, when so treated, is 90 to 96 percent (170,191,192). Patients with bulkier retroperitoneal disease (defined by different authors as greater than 5 cm, 6 cm, or 10 cm) are now treated with platinum-based chemotherapy regimens because of high recurrence rates with radiation. In a review of several series, there was an 8 percent recurrence rate with radiation of retroperitoneal tumors between 5 and 10 cm in diameter, and a 35 percent recurrence rate with radiation therapy for retroperitoneal masses exceeding 10 cm in diameter (189). Several studies that included both previously radiated patients as well as previously untreated patients indicate an 80 percent survival for this group, as well as those with stage III (or C) disease. Surgery, beyond the original orchiectomy, does not confer any additional survival benefits (182,185).

Motzer et al. (183), however, advocated the surgical excision of residual masses 3 cm or more in size following the chemotherapy of advanced stage seminoma to determine the presence of persistent neoplasm and therefore the need for additional chemotherapy.

Dixon and Moore (169) found a 4 percent 2-year mortality for seminoma patients having a lymphoid stroma but a 12 percent 2-year mortality for patients whose tumors lacked a lymphoid stroma. Evenson et al. (171) corroborated this, but this correlation was not statistically significant. Vascular invasion was also associated with a worse survival (15.2 versus 5.6 percent 2-year mortality) (169). More recent studies have implicated an elevated level of hCG as a poor prognostic feature of seminoma (168,172, 183), an observation that correlates with the poor prognosis associated with Leydig cell hyperplasia originally identified by Dixon and Moore (169); others, however, have failed to find such a correlation (178,186,187) or to associate a worse prognosis with the presence of syncytiotrophoblastic cells (193). It may be that small elevations of hCG are not associated with a worse prognosis but larger elevations are (172). Elevated hCG levels may correlate with metastatic status rather than indicate a biologically more aggressive tumor (174).

We do not recognize the entity, "anaplastic" seminoma, a purported histologic variant of seminoma with a poorer prognosis (180) (see page 74); a number of subsequent studies agree with us (177a,193,193a).

SPERMATOCYTIC SEMINOMA

Definition. This is a germ cell neoplasm composed of three morphologic varieties of cells. The tumor cells range from 6 to 100 μm in diameter. The tumor lacks cytoplasmic glycogen and is rarely associated with a lymphocytic infiltrate or granulomatous reaction, in contrast to typical seminoma.

General Features. Spermatocytic seminoma, as a distinct entity, was originally described by Masson in 1946 (199) who considered it to mimic spermatogenesis based on the presence of a polymorphous cell population having some resemblance to ordinary spermatogenic cells, including a meiotic-like chromatin pattern

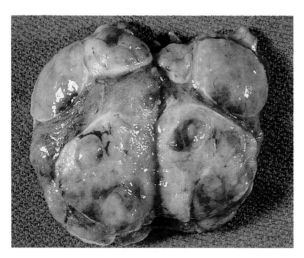

Figure 3-40
SPERMATOCYTIC SEMINOMA
This multinodular gray tumor has a glistening, mucoid quality on the cut surface.

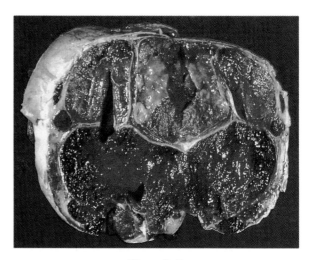

Figure 3-41
SPERMATOCYTIC SEMINOMA
Prominent fibrous septa subdivide a spermatocytic seminoma. There is extensive hemorrhage in the lower portion. (Fig. 2.28 from Young RH, Scully RE. Testicular tumors. Chicago: ASCP Press, 1990:28.)

(see below). Ultrastructural observations supported its differentiation to advanced spermatogenic cells (203). Recent observations, however, have questioned such a relationship since meiotic-specific structures and haploid DNA values are not identified in spermatocytic seminomas (202,205) nor do spermatocytic seminomas bind lectins that are ordinarily reactive for more advanced spermatogenic cells (198).

In two series, spermatocytic seminoma represented 1.2 and 4.5 percent of seminomas (197, 204). It does not occur as a primary tumor in sites other than the testis. The epidemiology is unclear. It is not strongly associated with cryptorchidism (195,204) and does not occur with IGCNU (201) or other forms of germ cell tumor, indicating a different pathogenesis.

Clinical Features. Spermatocytic seminoma tends to occur in older patients than typical seminoma. The average age in three large series was 52, 55, and 58.8 years (194,197,204); it is rare under the age of 30 years (194). Most patients present with painless testicular enlargement (194,204), but occasional patients have pain. Bilaterality, usually asynchronous, occurs in 9 percent of cases (204). Some spermatocytic seminomas undergo sarcomatous transformation (194,196, 200,206). These patients typically have a long history of painless testicular enlargement followed by the recent onset of pain and rapid growth (196,206). Occasionally, they present with metastatic disease (206). Serum marker studies are negative.

Gross Findings. Spermatocytic seminomas exhibit the same range in size as typical seminomas (223). The tumors are well circumscribed and sometimes distinctly multilobulated or multinodular. Occasionally there are separate, multicentric nodules (215b). They typically are soft, friable, and tan-gray, with a mucoid, edematous, or gelatinous cut surface (fig. 3-40) and may show cystic change. Foci of hemorrhage and necrosis may occur, especially in larger tumors (fig. 3-41), but are generally not extensive. Cases with associated sarcoma (see below) are more apt to exhibit hemorrhage or necrosis, with solid, dull gray areas (213,225). Extension beyond the testis is rare in typical cases, but epididymal involvement has been reported (209,220).

Microscopic Findings. A diffuse arrangement of tumor cells is characteristic (fig. 3-42), sometimes with separation of sheets of tumor cells into large nests by a usually scant but occasionally prominent fibrous stroma (fig. 3-43). When the stroma is prominent, it is usually edematous (fig. 3-44). The presence of eosinophilic to basophilic, intercellular edema fluid can lead to a cystic (fig. 3-45) or a pseudoglandular pattern (fig. 3-43), or it may result in trabeculae, small nests, clusters, or single cells (fig. 3-44).

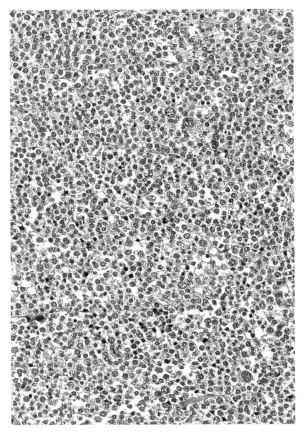

Figure 3-42
SPERMATOCYTIC SEMINOMA
Characteristic diffuse growth.

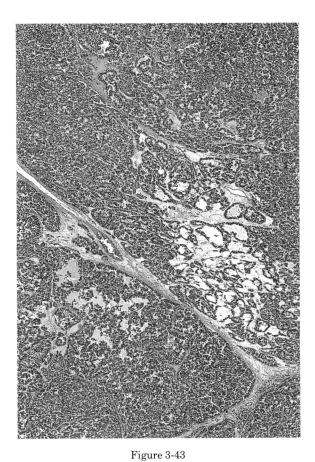

Figure 3-43
SPERMATOCYTIC SEMINOMA
Large nodules within which cells are arranged diffusely
and show a focal pseudoglandular pattern.

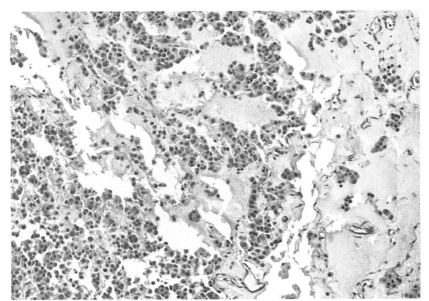

Figure 3-44
SPERMATOCYTIC SEMINOMA
Extensive intercellular edema
causes a pattern of small nests, trabeculae, clusters, and single cells.

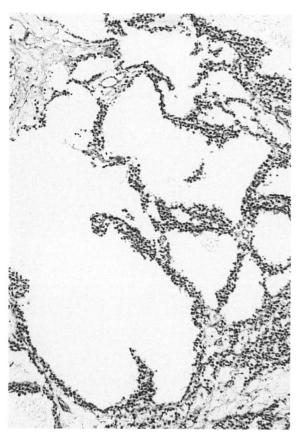

Figure 3-45
SPERMATOCYTIC SEMINOMA
Edema has resulted in a cystic pattern.

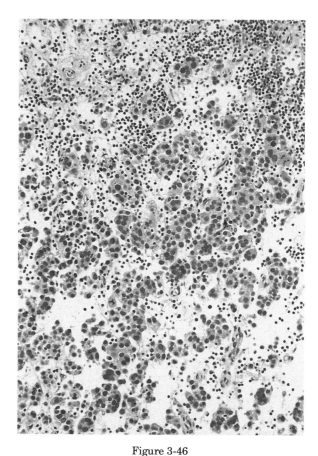

Figure 3-46
SPERMATOCYTIC SEMINOMA
Nests and cords of tumor are intermingled with a moderate lymphoid infiltrate, the latter an unusual feature.

Unlike typical seminoma, spermatocytic seminoma almost always lacks a granulomatous reaction and usually has no or only a scant lymphoid infiltrate; rarely, however, there is a moderate lymphoid infiltrate (fig. 3-46), and we have seen a unique case that closely resembled typical seminoma in that a prominent granulomatous reaction and lymphoid infiltrate were present, although the tumor cells had the usual characteristics of spermatocytic seminoma (fig. 3-47).

A polymorphous cell population is the hallmark of spermatocytic seminoma. There are three types of neoplastic cells: small, averaging 6 to 8 μm in diameter; medium ("intermediate"), averaging 15 to 20 mm in diameter; and giant, averaging 50 to 100 mm in diameter (figs. 3-48, 3-49). The small cells have a densely basophilic nucleus and a scant amount of eosinophilic to basophilic cytoplasm. These cells superficially

resemble lymphocytes, but the homogeneous chromatin pattern and more prominent cytoplasm contrast with lymphocytes. The cells are probably degenerate. The medium-sized (intermediate) cell, the most common, has a round nucleus with finely granular chromatin and a modest amount of cytoplasm. The third cell type, the largest, is the least common. Occasional medium and large cells may have a distinctive filamentous or "spireme" chromatin similar to primary spermatocytes in meiotic prophase (figs. 3-49, 3-50). Nucleoli are variably prominent in these two cell types. Some of the large cells are giant cells that may have two, three, or more nuclei (fig. 3-48). In all cell types, intercellular borders are indistinct.

The mitotic rate of spermatocytic seminomas is often quite brisk and atypical mitoses may occur. Glycogen is usually not demonstrable (209). Prominent intratubular growth is apparent in many

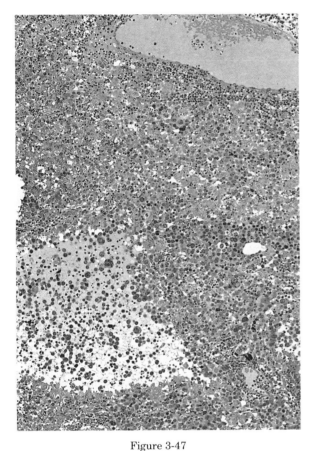

Figure 3-47
SPERMATOCYTIC SEMINOMA
An extremely unusual case with a prominent granulomatous reaction and lymphocytic infiltrate.

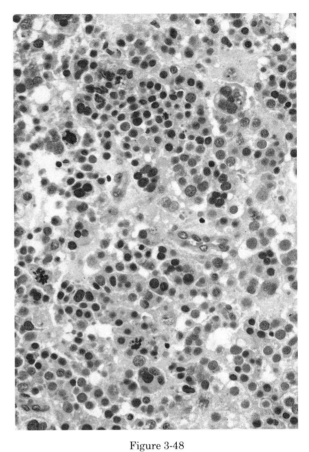

Figure 3-48
SPERMATOCYTIC SEMINOMA
A polymorphic population of neoplastic cells characteristic of spermatocytic seminoma. There are mainly small cells with darkly staining nuclei, and medium-sized cells with paler nuclei; occasional multinucleated giant cells are also present.

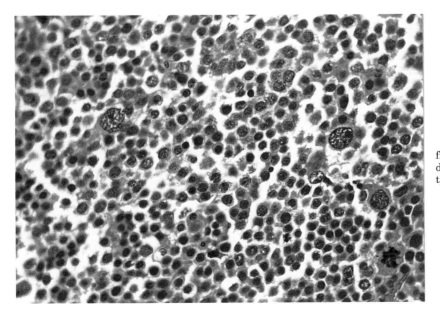

Figure 3-49
SPERMATOCYTIC SEMINOMA
The three cell types, small (superficially resembling lymphocytes), medium-sized, and larger with "spireme" type chromatin, are apparent.

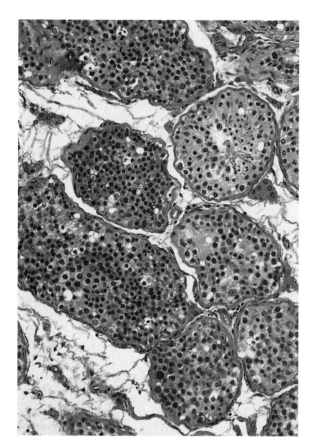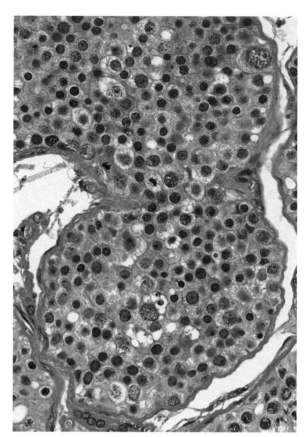

Figure 3-50
INTRATUBULAR SPERMATOCYTIC SEMINOMA
Left: Several tubules are distended by spermatocytic seminoma; one tubule shows normal spermatogenesis.
Right: Note the variable cell size, the round nuclei, and the filamentous ("spireme") chromatin in a few of the larger cells.

cases at the periphery of the tumor (fig. 3-50), but there is an absence of IGCNU (see chapter 2).

An "anaplastic" variant of spermatocytic seminoma has been recently described; this is characterized by a predominance of monomorphous cells with prominent nucleoli, thereby potentially causing confusion with typical seminoma or embryonal carcinoma (fig. 3-51) (208). Typical foci, however, are seen, and the immunohistochemistry, ultrastructure, and clinical course are typical for spermatocytic seminoma (208). In our opinion such cases represent part of the morphologic spectrum of spermatocytic seminoma since nucleoli are of variable prominence in this neoplasm, and there may be areas lacking the typical polymorphism in other cases.

In tumors with associated sarcoma, approximately 6 percent of reported cases (212), the sarcomatous component is often intimately in-termingled with the spermatocytic seminoma (fig. 3-52). The sarcoma is most frequently undifferentiated, consisting of primitive-appearing, oval to spindle-shaped cells arranged in sheets and fascicles (fig. 3-53). Three cases have shown rhabdomyoblastic differentiation (fig. 3-54) (213,216,225). Intratubular spermatocytic seminoma may be adjacent to the sarcoma in some of these cases (fig. 3-53).

Immunohistochemical Findings. Spermatocytic seminomas are nonreactive with a variety of antibodies directed against vimentin, actin, desmin, AFP, hCG, carcinoembryonic antigen, leukocyte common antigen (LCA), and CD30 (209–211). A lack of PLAP reactivity has been reported in some studies (207,215a), although others described positivity in rare cells (209–211). Cytokeratin immunostains are also usually negative, although occasional dot-like positivity

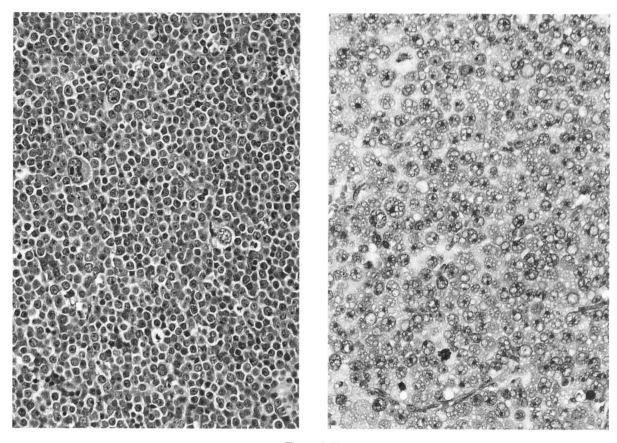

Figure 3-51
"ANAPLASTIC" SPERMATOCYTIC SEMINOMA
There is a predominance of intermediate-sized cells with prominent nucleoli, seen particularly on the right. The three cell types are still appreciable in the figure on the left. (Courtesy of J. Albores-Saavedra, M.D., Dallas, TX.)

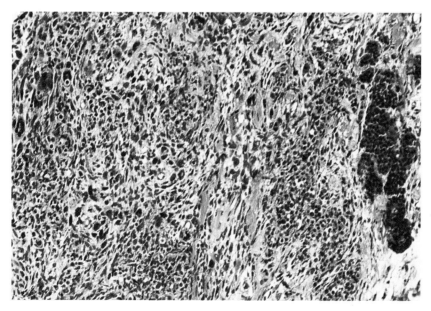

Figure 3-52
SARCOMA WITH
SPERMATOCYTIC SEMINOMA

Residual, poorly preserved spermatocytic seminoma (right) is adjacent to sarcoma. (Fig. 2.33 from Young RH, Scully RE. Testicular tumors. Chicago: ASCP Press, 1990:31.)

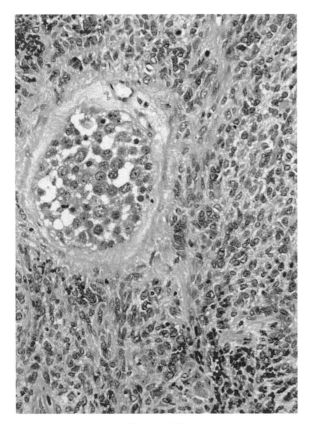

Figure 3-53
SARCOMA WITH SPERMATOCYTIC SEMINOMA
Intratubular spermatocytic seminoma is surrounded by a sarcomatous growth that had the features of embryonal rhabdomyosarcoma.

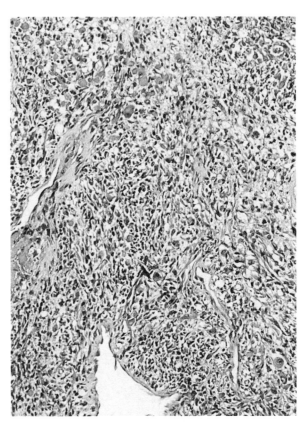

Figure 3-54
RHABDOMYOSARCOMA THAT WAS ASSOCIATED WITH SPERMATOCYTIC SEMINOMA

may be seen with antibodies that react with cytokeratin 18 (210,214).

Ultrastructural Findings. Ultrastructural examination has shown prominent nucleoli with a dispersed nucleolonema and occasional chromosomes having a configuration similar to that of the leptotene stage of meiotic prophase, i.e., filamentous chromosomes with lateral chromatin fibrils (219). Another distinctive feature is the formation of intercellular bridges between adjacent cells, similar to those described in spermatocytic cells (fig. 3-55) (218). One study, however, failed to identify leptotene-type chromosomes or other meiotic-specific features (224); the presence of bridges between neoplastic cells was not considered specific for a meiotic cell (224). Macula adherens–type junctions are present between adjacent cells (fig. 3-56); the Golgi is variably prominent; and there are scanty profiles of rough

endoplasmic reticulum, numerous free ribosomes, scattered mitochondria, scant or absent glycogen, and a thin layer of basal lamina at the periphery of cell nests (fig. 3-56) (219,224). Talerman and co-workers (224) concluded that the ultrastructure of spermatocytic seminoma did not support true spermatocytic differentiation, but that it was a better differentiated form of seminoma that was, perhaps, incompletely differentiating toward spermatocytic cells.

Special Diagnostic Techniques. One study of the DNA content of spermatocytic seminoma showed that most cases were hyperdiploid or peritriploid (224); a second study of 11 tumors showed diploid values in 5 cases, tetraploid values in 3 cases, and aneuploidy in 3 cases (217); a third study of 6 tumors demonstrated diploid values in 2 cases, near diploid values in 2 cases, tetraploidy in 1 case, and aneuploidy (DNA index, 1.35) in 1

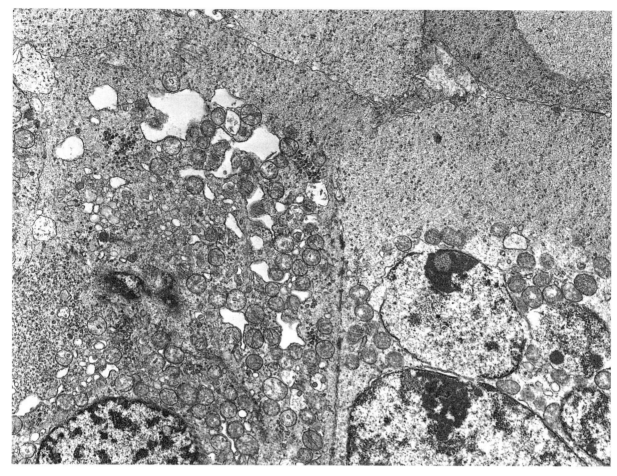

Figure 3-55
SPERMATOCYTIC SEMINOMA
An intercellular bridge links two adjacent cells of a spermatocytic seminoma. Note the intercellular junctions at left and center. Small, round mitochondria are numerous (X13,000).

case (211). A cytophotometric study demonstrated a range of DNA values in the tumor cells: the lymphocyte-like cells had diploid or near diploid values and the giant cells had DNA values ranging up to 42C, while intermediate-sized cells had an intermediate DNA content (221). No haploid values were obtained which argued against a true meiotic-phase neoplasm, a conclusion also supported by morphometric analysis (215). Other studies suggested that the cells of spermatocytic seminoma formed in cycles of polyploidization (215a,222). The ploidy values for spermatocytic seminomas appear to be significantly less than those obtained for typical seminoma (217,224).

Differential Diagnosis. The major entity in the differential diagnosis is typical seminoma. In several series, spermatocytic seminomas had been previously diagnosed as "typical" seminomas (228,229). Table 3-2 lists many of the features useful in this differential (227,229). Immunostains for PLAP can be quite helpful in problematic cases since seminoma is usually diffusely PLAP reactive but spermatocytic seminoma is negative or only focally positive.

The anaplastic variant of spermatocytic seminoma, because of its relatively monomorphic appearance and nucleolar prominence, can be misinterpreted as embryonal carcinoma (226). Many embryonal carcinomas, in addition to having a

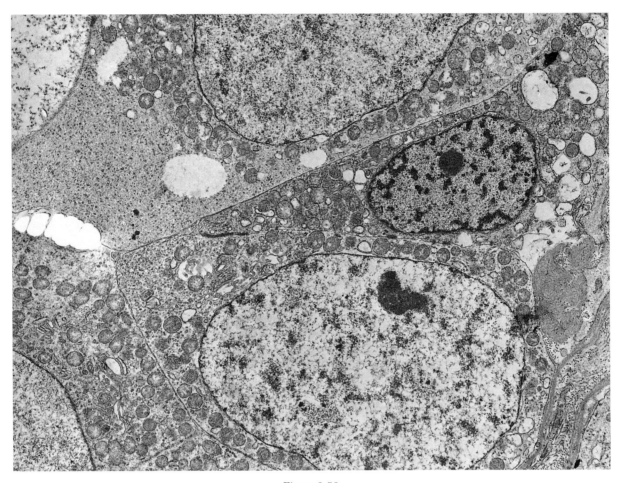

Figure 3-56
SPERMATOCYTIC SEMINOMA
A nest of spermatocytic seminoma is surrounded by a well-defined basement membrane. There are numerous mitochondria, a Golgi apparatus, and round nuclei with dispersed chromatin (X9,750).

solid growth pattern, also form glands and papillae that are not seen in spermatocytic seminoma. Typically, the nuclei of embryonal carcinoma are more irregular than the rounded nuclei of anaplastic spermatocytic seminoma. Furthermore, all of the reported cases of the latter have had foci with the characteristic "tripartite" appearance, a fact that emphasizes the need for thorough sampling and careful examination of any purely solid, putative embryonal carcinoma to exclude an anaplastic spermatocytic seminoma. Absence of IGCNU and lack of more than focal PLAP and cytokeratin reactivity are also supportive of spermatocytic seminoma over embryonal carcinoma.

Lymphoma is another consideration (228). Bilateral involvement is more common in lymphoma, and most lymphomas are associated with extratesticular disease which is virtually never seen in spermatocytic seminoma. Lymphomas typically exhibit an interstitial growth pattern, unlike spermatocytic seminomas. Most crucial are the cytologic differences between the two neoplasms. The cells of lymphoma are usually more uniform in size; the nuclei tend to be less round, with frequent indentations. Immunostains for LCA (CD45) or other lymphoid markers are conclusive in problematic cases.

Treatment and Prognosis. The prognosis of patients with pure spermatocytic seminoma is

Table 3-2

COMPARISON OF THE CLINICAL AND PATHOLOGIC FEATURES OF SPERMATOCYTIC SEMINOMA AND TYPICAL SEMINOMA*

	Spermatocytic Seminoma	Typical Seminoma
Proportion of germ cell tumors	1 - 2%	40 - 50%
Sites	testis only	testis, ovary (dysgerminoma), mediastinum, pineal, retroperitoneum
Association with cryptorchidism	no	yes
Bilaterality	9%	2%
Association with other forms of germ cell tumor	no	yes
Association with IGCNU**	no	yes
Intercellular edema	common	uncommon
Composition	3 cell types,with denser cytoplasm, round nuclei	1 cell type, often clear cytoplasm, less regular nuclei
Stroma	scanty	prominent
Lymphoid reaction	rare to absent	prominent
Granulomas	extremely rare	often prominent
Sarcomatous transformation	occasional	absent
Glycogen	absent to scant	abundant
PLAP staining	absent to scant	prominent
hCG staining	absent	present in 10%
Metastases	extremely rare	common

*Modified from Ulbright TM, Roth LM. Testicular and paratesticular neoplasms. In: Sternberg SS, ed. Diagnostic surgical pathology. New York: Raven Press, 1994:1885–947. Originally adapted from reference 220.
**Abbreviations: IGCNU = intratubular germ cell neoplasia, unclassified; hCG = human chorionic gonadotropin; PLAP = placental-like alkaline phosphatase.

excellent, and there is only one well-documented, pathologically verified case of pure spermatocytic seminoma that metastasized (to para-aortic nodes) (230,232). For this reason, patients with spermatocytic seminoma are managed by orchiectomy, without adjuvant therapy. The patients reported with anaplastic spermatocytic seminoma have also had a good prognosis, a further argument against it representing a distinct clinicopathologic entity.

The excellent prognosis of pure spermatocytic seminoma contrasts with the poor prognosis of spermatocytic seminoma with sarcomatous dedifferentiation. Five of nine patients have died of metastases, most commonly to the lung, which were solely of the sarcomatous component (231,233,234).

REFERENCES

Seminoma: General and Clinical Features

1. Altaffer LF. Paraneoplastic endocrinopathies associated with nonrenal genitourinary tumors. J Urol 1982;127:411–16.

1a. Chevassu M. Tumeurs du testicule. Thèse pour le doctorat en médecine. Paris: Faculté de Médecine de Paris, 1906.

1b. Chisolm GG. Tumour markers in testicular tumours. Prog Clin Biol Res 1985;203:81–91.

1c. da Silva MA, Edmondson JW, Eby C, Loehrer PJ Sr. Humoral hypercalcemia in seminomas. Med Pediatr Oncol 1992;20:38–41.

2. Dieckmann KP, Due W, Bauer HW. Seminoma testis with elevated serum beta-HCG—a category of germ cell cancer between seminoma and nonseminoma. Int Urol Nephrol 1989;21:175–84.

3. Dieckmann KP, von Keyserlingk HJ. HLA association of testicular seminoma. Klin Wochenschr 1988;66:337–9.

4. Dixon FJ, Moore RA. Tumors of the male sex organs. Atlas of Tumor Pathology, 1st series, Fascicles 31b and 32. Washington, D.C.: Armed Forces Institute of Pathology, 1952.

5. Fossa A, Fossa SD. Serum lactate dehydrogenase and human chorionic gonadotropin in seminoma. Br J Urol 1989;63:408–15.

6. Friedman NB, Moore RA. Tumors of the testis: a report on 922 cases. Milit Surgeon 1946;99:573–93.

7. Gross AJ, Dieckmann KP. Neuron-specific enolase: a serum tumor marker in malignant germ-cell tumors? Eur Urol 1993;24:277–8.

8. Halme A, Kellokumpu-Lehtinen P, Lehtonen T, Teppo L. Morphology of testicular germ cell tumours in treated and untreated cryptorchidism. Br J Urol 1989;64:78–83.

9. Hori K, Uematsu K, Yasoshima H, Yamada A, Sakurai K, Ohya M. Testicular seminoma with human chorionic gonadotropin production. Pathol Int 1997;47:592–9.

10. Jacobsen GK, Barlebo H, Olsen J, et al. Testicular germ cell tumours in Denmark 1976–1980. Pathology of 1058 consecutive cases. Acta Radiol Oncol 1984;23:239–47.

11. Javadpour N. Human chorionic gonadotropin in seminoma. J Urol 1984;131:407.

12. Javadpour N. Management of seminoma based on tumor markers. Urol Clin North Am 1980;7:773–81.

13. Javadpour N. The role of biologic tumor markers in testicular cancer. Cancer 1980;45:1755–61.

14. Javadpour N. Tumor markers in testicular cancer—an update. Prog Clin Biol Res 1985;203:141–54.

15. Kay R. Prepubertal testicular tumor registry. J Urol 1993;150:671–4.

16. Koshida K, Stigbrand T, Hisazumi H, Wahren B. Electrophoretic heterogeneity of alkaline phosphatase isozymes in seminoma and normal testis. Tum Biol 1989;10:181–9.

17. Koshida K, Stigbrand T, Munck-Wikland E, Hisazumi H, Wahren B. Analysis of serum placental alkaline phosphatase activity in testicular cancer and cigarette smokers. Urol Res 1990;18:169–73.

18. Kuzmits R, Schernthaner G, Krisch K. Serum neuron-specific enolase: a marker for responses to therapy in seminoma. Cancer 1987;60:1017–21.

19. Leibovitch I, Baniel J, Rowland RG, Smith ER Jr, Ludlow JK, Donohue JP. Malignant testicular neoplasms in immunosuppressed patients. J Urol 1996;155:1938–42.

20. Mann AS. Bilateral exophthalmos in seminoma. J Clin Endocrinol Metab 1967;27:1500–2.

21. Mann K, Siddle K. Evidence for free beta-subunit secretion in so-called human chorionic gonadotropin-positive seminoma. Cancer 1988;62:2378–82.

22. Millan JL, Manes T. Seminoma-derived Nagao isozyme is encoded by a germ-cell alkaline phosphatase gene. Proc Natl Acad Sci U S A 1988;85:3024–8.

23. Morse MJ, Whitmore WF. Neoplasms of the testis. In: Walsh PC, Gittes RF, Perlmutter AD, Stamey TA, eds. Campbell's urology. Philadelphia: WB Saunders, 1986:1535–82.

24. Motzer RJ, Bosl GJ, Geller NL, et al. Advanced seminoma: the role of chemotherapy and adjuvant surgery. Ann Int Med 1988;108:513–8.

25. Mumperow E, Hartmann M. Spermatic cord beta-human chorionic gonadotropin levels in seminoma and their clinical implications. J Urol 1992;147:1041–3.

26. Nazeer T, Ro JY, Amato B, Park YW, Ordonez NG, Ayala AG. Histologically pure seminoma with elevated alpha-fetoprotein: a clinicopathologic study of ten cases. Oncol Rep 1998;5:1425–9.

27. Nilsson S, Anderstrom C, Hedelin H, Unsgaard B. Signs and symptoms of adult testicular tumours. Int J Androl 1981;4(Suppl):146–52.

28. Oliver RT. HLA phenotype and clinicopathological behaviour of germ cell tumours: possible evidence for clonal evolution from seminomas to nonseminomas. Int J Androl 1987;10:85–93.

29. Perry C, Servadio C. Seminoma in childhood. J Urol 1980;124:932–3.

30. Pugh RC. Testicular tumours–introduction. In: Pugh RC, ed. Pathology of the testis. Oxford: Blackwell Scientific, 1976:139–59.

31. Ro JY, Dexeus FH, El-Naggar A, Ayala AG. Testicular germ cell tumors. Clinically relevant pathologic findings. Pathol Annu 1991;26(pt 2):59–87.

32. Rustin GJ, Vogelzang NJ, Sleijfer DT, Nisselbaum JN. Consensus statement on circulating tumour markers and staging patients with germ cell tumours. Prog Clin Biol Res 1990;357:277–84.

33. Scheiber K, Mikuz G, Frommhold H, Bartsch G. Human chorionic gonadotropin positive seminoma: is this a special type of seminoma with a poor prognosis? Prog Clin Biol Res 1985;203:97–104.

34. Schwartz BF, Auman R, Peretsman SJ, et al. Prognostic value of BHCG and local tumor invasion in stage I seminoma of the testis. J Surg Oncol 1996;61:131–3.

35. Smith RH. Testicular seminoma. In: Skinner DG, Lieskovsky G, eds. Diagnosis and management of genitourinary cancer. Philadelphia: WB Saunders, 1988:215–34.

36. Swerdlow AJ, Huttly SR, Smith PG. Testis cancer: postnatal hormonal factors, sexual behaviour and fertility. Int J Cancer 1989;43:549–53.

37. Taylor JB, Solomon DH, Levine RE, Ehrlich RM. Exophthalmos in seminoma: regression with steroids and orchiectomy. JAMA 1978;240:860–2.

38. Thackray AC, Crane WA. Seminoma. In: Pugh RC, ed. Pathology of the testis. Oxford: Blackwell Scientific, 1976:164–98.

39. Tucker DF, Oliver RT, Travers P, Brodmer WF. Serum marker potential of placental alkaline phosphatase-like activity in testicular germ cell tumours evaluated by H17E2 monoclonal antibody assay. Br J Cancer 1985;51:631–9.

40. von Hochstetter AR, Hedinger CE. The differential diagnosis of testicular germ cell tumors in theory and practice: a critical analysis of two major systems of classification and review of 389 cases. Virchows Arch [A] 1982;396:247–77.

41. Wilson WT, Frenkel E, Vuitch F, Sagalowsky AI. Testicular tumors in men with human immunodeficiency virus. J Urol 1992;147:1038–40.

42. Yamamoto H, Ruden U, Stahle E, et al. Pattern of seminoma tissue markers and deletions. Int J Cancer 1987;40:615–9.

Seminoma: Pathologic Findings and Special Studies

43. Akaza H, Kobayashi K, Umeda T, Niijima T. Surface markers of lymphocytes infiltrating seminoma tissue. J Urol 1980;124:827–8.

44. Bartkova J, Bartek J, Lukas J, et al. p53 protein alterations in human testicular cancer including pre-invasive intratubular germ-cell neoplasia. Int J Cancer 1991;49:196–202.

45. Bartkova J, Rejthar A, Bartek J, Kovarik J. Differentiation patterns in testicular germ-cell tumours as revealed by a panel of monoclonal antibodies. Tumor Biol 1987;8:45–56.

46. Battifora H, Sheibani K, Tubbs RR, Kopinski MI, Sun TT. Antikeratin antibodies in tumor diagnosis: distinction between seminoma and embryonal carcinoma. Cancer 1984;54:843–8.

47. Bell DA, Flotte TJ, Bhan AK. Immunohistochemical characterization of seminoma and its inflammatory cell infiltrate. Hum Pathol 1987;18:511–20.

48. Bentley AJ, Parkinson MC, Harding BN, Bains RM, Lantos PL. A comparative morphological and immuno-histochemical study of testicular seminomas and intracranial germinomas. Histopathology 1990;17:443–9.

49. Bosman FT, Giard RW, Kruseman AC, Knijenenburg G, Spaander PJ. Human chorionic gonadothropin and alpha-fetoprotein in testicular germ cell tumors: a retrospective immunohistochemical study. Histopathology 1980;4:673–84.

50. Brehmer-Andersson E, Ljungdahl-Stahle E, Koshida K, Yamamoto H, Stigbrand T, Wahren B. Isoenzymes of alkaline phosphatases in seminomas. An immunohistochemical and biochemical study. APMIS 1990;98:977–82.

51. Burke AP, Mostofi FK. Placental alkaline phosphatase immunohistochemistry of intratubular malignant germ cells and associated testicular germ cell tumors. Hum Pathol 1988;19:663–70.

52. Caillaud JM, Bellet D, Carlu C, Droz JP. Immunohistochemistry of germ cell tumors of the testis: study of hCG and AFP. Prog Clin Biol Res 1985;203:139–40.

53. Castedo SM, de Jong B, Oosterhuis JW, et al. i(12p)-negative testicular germ cell tumors. A different group? Cancer Genet Cytogenet 1988;35:171–8.

54. Castedo SM, de Jong B, Oosterhuis JW, et al. Cytogenetic analysis of ten human seminomas. Cancer Res 1989;49:439–43.

55. Damjanov I, Niejadlik DC, Rabuffo JV, Donadio JA. Cribriform and sclerosing seminoma devoid of lymphoid infiltrates. Arch Pathol Lab Med 1980;104:527–30.

56. Delozier-Blanchet CD, Walt H, Engel E, Vuagnat P. Cytogenetic studies of human testicular germ cell tumours. Int J Androl 1987;10:69–77.

57. Denk H, Moll R, Weybora W, et al. Intermediate filaments and desmosomal plaque proteins in testicular seminomas and non-seminomatous germ cell tumours as revealed by immunohistochemistry. Virchows Arch [A] 1987;410:295–307.

57a. Dickersin GR. Diagnostic electron microscopy: a text/atlas. New York: Igaku-Shoin, 1988.

58. Dixon FJ, Moore RA. Tumors of the male sex organs. Atlas of Tumor Pathology, 1st series, Fascicles 31b and 32. Washington, D.C.: Armed Forces Institute of Pathology, 1952.

59. Düe W, Dieckmann KP, Loy V. Immunohistological determination of proliferative activity in seminomas. J Clin Pathol 1988;41:304–7.

60. Düe W, Loy V. Evidence of interepithelial seminoma spread into the rete testis by immunostaining of paraffin sections with antibodies against cytokeratin and vimentin. Urol Res 1988;16:389–93.

61. Eglen DE, Ulbright TM. The differential diagnosis of yolk sac tumor and seminoma: usefulness of cytokeratin, alpha-fetoprotein, and alpha-1-antitrypsin immunoperoxidase reactions. Am J Clin Pathol 1987;88:328–32.

62. El-Naggar AK, Ro JY, McLemore D, Ayala AG, Batsakis JG. DNA ploidy in testicular germ cell neoplasms. Histogenetic and clinical implications. Am J Surg Pathol 1992;16:611–8.

63. Evensen JF, Fosså SD, Kjellevold K, Lien HH. Testicular seminoma: histological findings and their prognostic significance for stage II disease. J Surg Oncol 1987;36:166–9.

64. Feitz WF, Debruyne FM, Ramaekers FC. Intermediate filament proteins as tissue specific markers in normal and neoplastic testicular tissue. Int J Androl 1987;10:51–6.

65. Ferreiro JA. Ber-H2 expression in testicular germ cell tumors. Hum Pathol 1994;25:522–4.

66. Fleischhacker M, Strohmeyer T, Imai Y, Slamon DJ, Koeffler HP. Mutations of the p53 gene are not detectable in human testicular tumors. Mod Pathol 1994;7:435–9.

67. Fogel M, Lifschitz-Mercer B, Moll R, et al. Heterogeneity of intermediate filament expression in human testicular seminomas. Differentiation 1990;45:242–9.

68. Grantham JG, Charboneau JW, James EM, et al. Testicular neoplasms: 29 tumors studied by high-resolution US. Radiology 1988;157:775–80.

69. Heimdal K, Lothe RA, Lystad S, Holm R, Fossa SD, Borresen AL. No germline TP53 mutations detected in familial and bilateral testicular cancer. Genes Chrom Cancer 1993;6:92–7.

70. Hittmair A, Rogatsch H, Feichtinger H, Hobisch A, Mikuz G. Testicular seminomas are aneuploid tumors. Lab Invest 1995;72:70–4.

71. Hittmair A, Rogatsch H, Hobisch A, Mikuz G, Feichtinger H. CD30 expression in seminoma. Hum Pathol 1996;27:1166–71.

72. Hori K, Uematsu K, Yasoshima H, Yamada A, Sakurai K, Ohya M. Testicular seminoma with human chorionic gonadotropin production. Pathol Int 1997;47:592–9.

73. Hustin J, Collettee J, Franchimont P. Immunohistochemical demonstration of placental alkaline phosphatase in various states of testicular development and in germ cell tumours. Int J Androl 1987;10:29–35.

74. Jacobsen GK, Barlebo H, Olsen J, et al. Testicular germ cell tumours in Denmark 1976–1980. Pathology of 1058 consecutive cases. Acta Radiol Oncol 1984;23:239–47.

75. Jacobsen GK, Jacobsen M. Alpha-fetoprotein (AFP) and human chorionic gonadotropin in testicular germ cell tumours. A prospective immunohistochemical study. Acta Pathol Microbiol Scand [A] 1983;91:165–76.

76. Jacobsen GK, Jacobsen M. Ferritin (FER) in testicular germ cell tumours: an immunohistochemical study. Acta Pathol Microbiol Scand [A] 1983;91:177–81.

77. Jacobsen GK, Jacobsen M, Clausen PP. Distribution of tumor–associated antigens in the various histologic components of germ cell tumors of the testis. Am J Surg Pathol 1981;5:257–66.

78. Jacobsen GK, Talerman A. Atlas of germ cell tumours. Copenhagen: Munksgaard, 1989.

78a. Jacobsen GK, von der Maase H, Specht L, et al. Histopathological features in stage I seminoma treated with orchiectomy only. J Urol Pathol 1995;3:85–94.

79. Janssen M, Johnston WH. Anaplastic seminoma of the testis: ultrastructural analysis of three cases. Cancer 1978;41:538–44.

80. Kahn DG. Ossifying seminoma of the testis. Arch Pathol Lab Med 1993;117:321–2.

81. Koide O, Iwai S. An ultrastructural study on germinoma cells. Acta Pathol Jap 1981;31:755–66.

82. Kosmehl H, Langbein L, Katenkamp D. Lectin histochemistry of human testicular germ cell tumors. Neoplasma 1989;36:29–39.

83. Kuczyk MA, Serth J, Bokemeyer C, et al. Alterations in the p53 tumor suppressor gene in carcinoma in situ of the testis. Cancer 1996;78:1958–66.

84. Lewis DJ, Sesterhenn IA, McCarthy WF, Moul JW. Immunohistochemical expression of P53 tumor suppressor gene protein in adult germ cell testis tumors: clinical correlation in stage I disease. J Urol 1994;152:418–23.

85. Manivel JC, Jessurun J, Wick MR, Dehner LP. Placental alkaline phosphatase immunoreactivity in testicular germ cell tumors. Am J Surg Pathol 1987;11:21–9.

86. Manivel JC, Niehans G, Wick MR, Dehner LP. Intermediate trophoblast in germ cell neoplasms. Am J Surg Pathol 1987;11:693–701.

87. Martin B, Tubiana JM. Significance of scrotal calcifications detected by sonography. J Clin Ultrasound 1988;16:545–2.

88. Miettinen M, Virtanen I, Talerman A. Intermediate filament proteins in human testis and testicular germ-cell tumors. Am J Pathol 1985;120:402–10.

89. Min KW, Scheithauer BW. Pineal germinomas and testicular seminoma: a comparative ultrastructural study with special references to early carcinomatous transformation. Ultrastruc Pathol 1990;14:483–96.

90. Misaki H, Shuin T, Yao M, Kubota Y, Hosaka M. Expression of myc family oncogenes in primary human testicular cancer. Nippon Hinyokika Gakkai Zasshi 1989;80:1509–13.

91. Moll R, Franke WW, Schiller DL, Geiger B, Krepler R. The catalog of human cytokeratins: patterns of expression in normal epithelia, tumors, and cultured cells. Cell 1982;31:11–4.

92. Mostofi FK. Testicular tumors: epidemiologic, etiologic, and pathologic features. Cancer 1973;32:1186–201.

93. Mostofi FK, Price EB Jr. Tumors of the male genital system. Atlas of Tumor Pathology, 2nd Series, Fascicle 8. Washington, D.C.: Armed Forces Institute of Pathology, 1973.

94. Mostofi FK, Sesterhenn IA. Pathology of germ cell tumors of testes. Prog Clin Biol Res 1985;203:1–34.

95. Mulder MP, Keijzer W, Verkerk A, et al. Activated ras genes in human seminoma: evidence for tumor heterogeneity. Oncogene 1989;4:1345–51.

96. Murakami SS, Said JW. Immunohistochemical localization of lactate dehydrogenase isoenzyme 1 in germ cell tumors of the testis. Am J Clin Pathol 1984;81:293–6.

97. Murty VV, Dmitrovsky E, Bosl GJ, Chaganti RS. Nonrandom chromosome abnormalities in testicular and ovarian germ cell tumor cell lines. Cancer Genet Cytogenet 1990;50:67–73.

98. Nazeer T, Ro JY, Amato B, Ordonez NG, Ayala AG. Histologically pure seminoma (HPS) with elevated alpha-fetoprotein (AFP): a clinicopathologic and immunohistochemical study of ten cases [Abstract]. Mod Pathol 1996;9:79A.

99. Niehans GA, Manivel JC, Copland GT, Scheithauer BW, Wick MR. Immunohistochemistry of germ cell and trophoblastic neoplasms. Cancer 1988;62:1113–23.

100. Olie RA, Looijenga LH, Boerrigter L, et al. N- and KRAS mutations in primary testicular germ cell tumors: incidence and possible biological implications. Genes Chrom Cancer 1995;12:110–6.

101. Oosterhuis JW, Castedo SM, de Jong B, et al. Ploidy of primary germ cell tumors of the testis. Pathogenetic and clinical relevance. Lab Invest 1989;60:14–21.

102. Pallesen G, Hamilton-Dutoit SJ. Ki-1 (CD30) antigen is regularly expressed in tumor cells of embryonal carcinoma. Am J Pathol 1988;133:446–50.

103. Peng HQ, Hogg D, Malkin D, et al. Mutations of the p53 gene do not occur in testis cancer. Cancer Res 1993;53:3574–8.

104. Perry A, Wiley EL, Albores-Saavedra J. Pagetoid spread of intratubular germ cell neoplasia into rete testis: a morphologic and immunohistochemical study of 100 orchiectomy specimens with invasive germ cell tumors. Hum Pathol 1994;25:235–9.

105. Pierce GB Jr. Ultrastructure of human testicular tumors. Cancer 1966;19:1963–83.

106. Rabes HM. Proliferation of human testicular tumours. Int J Androl 1987;10:127–37.

107. Rabes HM, Schmeller N, Hartmann A, Rattenhuber U, Carl P, Staehler G. Analysis of proliferative compartments in human tumors. II. Seminoma. Cancer 1985;55:1758–69.

107a. Ramaekers F, Feitz W, Moesker O, et al. Antibodies to cytokeratin and vimentin in testicular tumour diagnosis. Virch Arch [A] 1985;408:127–42.

108. Riou G, Barrois M, Prost S, Terrier MJ, Theodore C, Levine AJ. The p53 and mdm-2 genes in human testicular germ-cell tumors. Mol Carcinog 1995;12:124–31.

108a. Roth LM, Gillespie JJ. Ultrastructure of testicular tumors. In: Talerman A, Roth LM, eds. Pathology of the testis and its adnexa. New York: Churchill-Livingstone, 1986:155–68.

109. Rukstalis DB, Bubley GJ, Donahue JP, Richie JP, Seidman JG, DeWolf WC. Regional loss of chromosome 6 in two urological malignancies. Cancer Res 1989;49:5087–90.

110. Rukstalis DB, DeWolf WC. Molecular biological concepts in the etiology of testicular and other urologic malignancies. Semin Urol 1988;6:161–70.

111. Saint-Andre JP, Alhenc-Gelas F, Rohmer V, Chretien MF, Bigorgne JC, Corvol P. Angiotensin-1-converting enzyme in germinomas. Hum Pathol 1988;19:208–13.

112. Saksela K, Mäkelä TP, Alitalo K. Oncogene expression in small-cell lung cancer cell lines and a testicular germ-cell tumor: activation of the N-myc gene and decreased RB mRNA. Int J Cancer 1989;44:182–5.

113. Schenkman NS, Sesterhenn IA, Washington L, et al. Increased p53 protein does not correlate to p53 gene mutations in microdissected human testicular germ cell tumors. J Urol 1995;154:617–21.

114. Scully RE, Parham AR. Testicular tumors: 1. Seminoma and teratoma. Arch Pathol 1948;45:581–607.

114a. Shah VI, Amin MB, Linden MD, Zarbo RJ. Utility of a selective immunohistochemical (IHC) panel in the detection of components of mixed germ cell tumors (GCT) of testis [Abstract]. Mod Pathol 1998;11:95A.

115. Shuin T, Misaki H, Kubota Y, Yao M, Hosaka M. Differential expression of protooncogenes in human germ cell tumors of the testis. Cancer 1994;73:1721–7.

116. Sikora K, Evan G, Watson J. Oncogenes and germ cell tumours. Int J Androl 1987;10:57–67.

117. Srigley JR, Mackay B, Toth P, Ayala A. The ultrastructure and histogenesis of male germ neoplasia with emphasis on seminoma with early carcinomatous features. Ultrastruc Pathol 1988;12:67–86.

118. Strohmeyer T, Peter S, Hartmann M, et al. Expression of the hst-1 and c-kit protooncogenes in human testicular germ cell tumors. Cancer Res 1991;51:1811–6.

119. Strohmeyer T, Reese D, Press M, Ackermann R, Hartmann M, Slamon D. Expression of the c-kit protooncogene and its ligand stem cell factor (SCF) in normal and malignant human testicular tissue. J Urol 1995;153:511–5.

120. Strohmeyer T, Reissmann P, Cordon-Cardo C, Hartmann M, Ackermann R, Slamon D. Correlation between retinoblastoma gene expression and differentiation in human testicular tumors. Proc Nat Acad Sci USA 1991;88:6662–6.

121. Strutton GM, Gemmell E, Seymour GJ, Walsh MD, Lavin MF, Gardiner RA. An immunohistological examination of inflammatory cell infiltration in primary testicular seminomas. Aust N Z J Surg 1989;59:169–72.

122. Suzuki T, Sasano H, Aoki H, et al. Immunohistochemical comparison between anaplastic seminoma and typical seminoma. Acta Pathol Jap 1993;43:751-7.

123. Thackray AC, Crane WA. Seminoma. In: Pugh RC, ed. Pathology of the testis. Oxford: Blackwell Scientific, 1976:164–98.

124. Uchida T, Shimoda T, Miyata H, et al. Immunoperoxidase study of alkaline phosphatase in testicular tumor. Cancer 1981;48:1455–62.

125. van Echten J, Oosterhuis JW, Looijenga LH, et al. No recurrent structural abnormalities apart from i(12p) in primary germ cell tumors of the adult testis. Genes Chromosomes Cancer 1995;14:133–44.

126. von Hochstetter AR. Mitotic count in seminomas–an unreliable criterion for distinguishing between classical and anaplastic types. Virchows Arch [A] 1981;390:63–9.

127. von Hochstetter AR, Sigg C, Saremaslani P, Hedinger C. The significance of giant cells in human testicular seminomas. A clinicopathological study. Virchows Arch [A] 1985;407:309–22.

128. Wei YQ, Hang ZB, Liu KF. In situ observation of inflammatory cell-tumor cell interaction in human seminomas (germinomas): light, electron microscopic, and immunohistochemical study. Hum Pathol 1992;23:421–8.

129. Wick MR, Swanson PE, Manivel JC. Placental-like alkaline phosphatase reactivity in human tumors: an immunohistochemical study of 520 cases. Hum Pathol 1987;18:946–54.

130. Wilkins BS, Williamson JM, O'Brien CJ. Morphological and immunohistological study of testicular lymphomas. Histopathology 1989;15:147–56.

131. Ye DW, Zheng J, Qian SX, et al. p53 gene mutations in Chinese human testicular seminoma. J Urol 1993;150:884–6.

132. Yoshida T, Tsutsumi M, Sakamoto H, et al. Expression of the HST1 oncogene in human germ cell tumors. Biochem Biophys Res Comm 1988;155:1324–9.

133. Young RH, Finlayson N, Scully RE. Tubular seminoma. Report of a case. Arch Pathol Lab Med 1989;113:414–6.

134. Zavala-Pompa A, Ro JY, El-Naggar AK, et al. Tubular seminoma: an immunohistochemical and DNA flow cytometric study of four cases. Am J Clin Pathol 1994;102:397–401.

135. Zhao X, Wei YQ, Kariya Y, Teshigawara K, Uchida A. Accumulation of gamma/delta T cells in human dysgerminoma and seminoma: roles in autologous tumor killing and granuloma formation. Immunol Invest 1995;24:607–18.

136. Zuckman MH, Williams G, Levin HS. Mitosis counting in seminoma: an exercise of questionable significance. Hum Pathol 1988;19:329–35.

Seminoma: Differential Diagnosis

137. Bartkova J, Rejthar A, Bartek J, Kovarik J. Differentiation patterns in testicular germ-cell tumours as revealed by a panel of monoclonal antibodies. Tumor Biol 1987;8:45–56.

138. Duncan PR, Checa F, Gowing NF, McElwain TJ, Peckham MJ. Extranodal non-Hodgkin's lymphoma presenting in the testicle: a clinical and pathologic study of 24 cases. Cancer 1980;45:1578–84.

139. Ferreiro JA. Ber-H2 expression in testicular germ cell tumors. Hum Pathol 1994;25:522–4.

140. Ferry JA, Harris NL, Young RH, Coen J, Zietman A, Scully RE. Malignant lymphoma of the testis, epididymis, and spermatic cord. A clinicopathologic study of 69 cases with immunophenotypic analysis. Am J Surg Pathol 1994;18:376–90.

141. Fogel M, Lifschitz-Mercer B, Moll R, et al. Heterogeneity of intermediate filament expression in human testicular seminomas. Differentiation 1990;45:242–9.

142. Hamlin JA, Kagan AR, Friedman NB. Lymphomas of the testicle. Cancer 1972;29:1352–6.

143. Hayes MM, Sacks MI, King HS. Testicular lymphoma. A retrospective review of 17 cases. S Afr Med J 1983;64:1014–6.

144. Hittmair A, Rogatsch H, Hobisch A, Mikuz G, Feichtinger H. CD30 expression in seminoma. Hum Pathol 1996;27:1166–71.

145. Lifschitz-Mercer B, Fogel M, Moll R, et al. Intermediate filament protein profiles of human testicular non-seminomatous germ cell tumors: correlation of cytokeratin synthesis to cell differentiation. Differentiation 1991;48:191–8.

146. Niehans GA, Manivel JC, Copland GT, Scheithauer BW, Wick MR. Immunohistochemistry of germ cell and trophoblastic neoplasms. Cancer 1988;62:1113–23.

147. Nonomura N, Aozasa K, Ueda T, et al. Malignant lymphoma of the testis: histological and immunohistological study of 28 cases. J Urol 1989;141:1368–71.

148. Paladugu RR, Bearman RM, Rappaport H. Malignant lymphoma with primary manifestation in the gonad: a clinicopathologic study of 38 patients. Cancer 1980;45:561–71.

149. Pallesen G, Hamilton-Dutoit SJ. Ki-1 (CD30) antigen is regularly expressed in tumor cells of embryonal carcinoma. Am J Pathol 1988;133:446–50.

150. Sussman EB, Hajdu SI, Lieberman PH, Whitmore WF. Malignant lymphoma of the testis: a clinicopathologic study of 37 cases. J Urol 1977;118:1004–7.

151. Talerman A. Primary malignant lymphoma of the testis. J Urol 1977;118:783–6.

152. Turner RR, Colby TV, MacKintosh FR. Testicular lymphomas: a clinicopathologic study of 35 cases. Cancer 1981;48:2095–102.

153. Ulbright TM, Roth LM. Recent developments in the pathology of germ cell tumors. Semin Diagn Pathol 1987;4:304–19.

154. Ulbright TM, Roth LM, Brodhecker CA. Yolk sac differentiation in germ cell tumors: a morphologic study of 50 cases with emphasis on hepatic, enteric and parietal yolk sac features. Am J Surg Pathol 1986;10:151–64.

155. Visfeldt J, Giwercman A, Skakkebaek NE. Monoclonal antibody 43-9F: an immunohistochemical marker of embryonal carcinoma of the testis. APMIS 1992;100:63–70.

156. Wick MR, Swanson PE, Manivel JC. Placental-like alkaline phosphatase reactivity in human tumors: an immunohistochemical study of 520 cases. Hum Pathol 1987;18:946–54.

157. Young RH, Finlayson N, Scully RE. Tubular seminoma. Report of a case. Arch Pathol Lab Med 1989;113:414–6.

158. Zavala-Pompa A, Ro JY, El-Naggar AK, et al. Tubular seminoma. An immunohistochemical and DNA flow cytometric study of four cases. Am J Clin Pathol 1994;102:397–401.

Seminoma: Cytologic Findings

159. Akhtar M, Ali MA, Huq M, Bakry M. Fine needle aspiration biopsy of seminoma and dysgerminoma: cytologic, histologic, and electron microscopic correlations. Diagn Cytopathol 1990;6:99–105.

160. Balslev E, Francis D, Jacobsen GK. Testicular germ cell tumors. Classification based on fine needle aspiration biopsy. Acta Cytol 1990;34:690–4.

161. Caraway NP, Fanning CV, Amato RJ, Sneige N. Fine-needle aspiration cytology of seminoma: a review of 16 cases. Diagn Cytopathol 1995;12:327–33.

162. Highman WJ, Oliver RT. Diagnosis of metastases from testicular germ cell tumours using fine needle aspiration cytology. J Clin Pathol 1987;40:1324–33.

163. Koss LG, Zajicek J. Aspiration biopsy. In: Koss LG, ed. Diagnostic cytology and its histopathologic basis. 4th ed. Philadelphia: JB Lippincott, 1992:1234–402.

Seminoma: Treatment and Prognosis

164. Amichetti M, Fellin G, Bolner A, et al. Stage I seminoma of the testis: long term results and toxicity with adjuvant radiotherapy. Tumori 1994;80:141–5.

165. Babaian RJ, Zagars GK. Testicular seminoma: the M.D. Anderson experience: an analysis of pathological and patient characteristics, and treatment recommendations. J Urol 1988;139:311–4.

166. Banerjee D, Warde PR, Gospodarowicz MK, et al. Stage I testicular seminoma managed by surveillance alone: is flow cytometric DNA analysis of predictive value for relapse [Abstract]. Mod Pathol 1996;9:70A.

167. Brunt AM, Scoble JE. Para-aortic nodal irradiation for early stage testicular seminoma. Clin Oncol 1992;4:165–70.

168. Dieckmann KP, Due W, Bauer HW. Seminoma testis with elevated serum beta-HCG–a category of germ cell cancer between seminoma and nonseminoma. Int Urol Nephrol 1989;21:175–84.

169. Dixon FJ, Moore RA. Tumors of the male sex organs. Atlas of Tumor Pathology, 1st series, Fascicles 31b and 32. Washington, D.C.: Armed Forces Institute of Pathology, 1952.

170. Doornbos JF, Hussey DH, Johnson E. Radiotherapy for pure seminoma of the testis. Radiology 1975;116:401–4.

171. Evensen JF, Fossa SD, Kjellevold K, Lien HH. Testicular seminoma: histological findings and their prognostic significance for stage II disease. J Surg Oncol 1987;36:166–9.

172. Fossa A, Fossa SD. Serum lactate dehydrogenase and human chorionic gonadotropin in seminoma. Br J Urol 1989;63:408–15.

173. Fossa SD, Aass N, Kaalhus O. Radiotherapy for testicular seminoma stage I: treatment results and long-term post irradiation morbidity in 365 patients. Int J Rad Oncol Biol Phys 1989;16:383–8.

174. Hori K, Uematsu K, Yasoshima H, Yamada A, Sakurai K, Ohya M. Testicular seminoma with human chorionic gonadotropin production. Pathol Int 1997;47:592–9.

175. Horwich A, Alsanjari N, A'Hern R, Nicholls J, Dearnaley DP, Fisher C. Surveillance following orchidectomy for stage I testicular seminoma. Br J Cancer 1992;65:775–8.

176. Horwich A, Dearnaley DP. Treatment of seminoma. Semin Oncol 1992;19:171–80.

177. Hunter M, Peschel RE. Testicular seminoma. Results of the Yale University experience, 1964-1984. Cancer 1989;64:1608–11.

177a. Jacobsen GK, von der Maase H, Specht L, et al. Histopathological features in stage I seminoma treated with orchiectomy only. J Urol Pathol 1995;3:85–94.

178. Javadpour N. Human chorionic gonadotropin in seminoma. J Urol 1984;131:407.

179. Kageyama S, Ueda T, Yamauchi T, et al. Mediastinal lymph node metastasis 38 months after surveillance for stage I seminoma: a case report. Hinyokika Kiyo 1994;40:1021–5.

180. Maier JG, Sulak MH, Mittemeyer BT. Seminoma of the testis: analysis of treatment success and failure. Am J Roentgenol Rad Ther Nucl Med 1968;102:596–602.

181. Marks LB, Rutgers JL, Shipley WU, et al. Testicular seminoma: clinical and pathological features that may predict para-aortic lymph node metastases. J Urol 1990;143:524–7.

182. Morse MJ, Whitmore WF. Neoplasms of the testis. In: Walsh PC, Gittes RF, Perlmutter AD, Stamey TA, eds. Campbell's urology. Philadelphia: WB Saunders, 1986:1535–82.

183. Motzer RJ, Bosl GJ, Geller NL, et al. Advanced seminoma: the role of chemotherapy and adjuvant surgery. Ann Int Med 1988;108:513–8.

184. Oliver RT. Limitations to the use of surveillance as an option in the management of stage I seminoma. Int J Androl 1987;10:263–8.

185. Peckham M. Testicular cancer. Acta Oncol 1988;27:439–53.

186. Scheiber K, Mikuz G, Frommhold H, Bartsch G. Human chorionic gonadotropin positive seminoma: is this a special type of seminoma with a poor prognosis? Prog Clin Biol Res 1985;203:97–104.

187. Schwartz BF, Auman R, Peretsman SJ, et al. Prognostic value of BHCG and local tumor invasion in stage I seminoma of the testis. J Surg Oncol 1996;61:131–3.

188. Speer TW, Sombeck MD, Parsons JT, Million RR. Testicular seminoma: a failure analysis and literature review. Int J Radiat Oncol Biol Phys 1995;33:89–97.

189. Thomas G. Management of metastatic seminoma: role of radiotherapy. In: Horwich A, ed. Testicular cancer—clinical investigation and management. New York: Chapman and Hall, 1991:211–31.

190. Thomas G, Jones W, VanOosterom A, Kawai T. Consensus statement on the investigation and management of testicular seminoma 1989. Prog Clin Biol Res 1990;357:285–94.

191. Thomas GM, Rider WD, Dembo AJ, et al. Seminoma of the testis: results of treatment and patterns of failure after radiation therapy. Int J Rad Oncol Biol Phys 1982;8:165–74.

192. Vallis KA, Howard GC, Duncan W, Cornbleet MA, Kerr GR. Radiotherapy for stages I and II testicular seminoma: results and morbidity in 238 patients. Br J Radiol 1995;68:400–5.

193. von Hochstetter AR, Sigg C, Saremaslani P, Hedinger C. The significance of giant cells in human testicular seminomas. A clinicopathological study. Virchows Arch [A] 1985;407:309–22.

193a. Zuckman MH, Williams G, Levin HS. Mitosis counting in seminoma: an exercise of questionable significance. Hum Pathol 1988;19:329–35.

Spermatocytic Seminoma: General and Clinical Features

194. Burke AP, Mostofi FK. Spermatocytic seminoma: a clinicopathologic study of 79 cases. J Urol Pathol 1993;1:21–32.

195. Eble JN. Spermatocytic seminoma. Hum Pathol 1994;25:1035–42.

196. Floyd C, Ayala AG, Logothetis CJ, Silva EG. Spermatocytic seminoma with associated sarcoma of the testis. Cancer 1988;61:409–14.

197. Jacobsen GK, Barlebo H, Olsen JK, et al. Testicular germ cell tumours in Denmark 1976–1980. Pathology of 1058 consecutive cases. Acta Radiol Oncol 1984;23:239–47.

198. Lee MC, Talerman A, Oosterhuis JW, Damjanov I. Lectin histochemistry of classic and spermatocytic seminoma. Arch Pathol Lab Med 1985;109:938–42.

199. Masson P. Étude sur le séminome. Rev Canad Biol 1946;5:361–87.

200. Matoska J, Talerman A. Spermatocytic seminoma associated with rhabdomyosarcoma. Am J Clin Pathol 1990;94:89–95.

201. Muller J, Skakkebaek NE, Parkinson MC. The spermatocytic seminoma: views on pathogenesis. Int J Androl 1987;10:147–56.

202. Romanenko AM, Persidsky YV, Mostofi FK. Ultrastructure and histogenesis of spermatocytic seminoma. J Urol Pathol 1993;1:387–95.

203. Rosai J, Khodadoust K, Silber I. Spermatocytic seminoma. II. Ultrastructural study. Cancer 1969;24:103–16.

204. Talerman A. Spermatocytic seminoma: clinicopathological study of 22 cases. Cancer 1980;45:2169–76.

205. Talerman A, Fu YS, Okagaki T. Spermatocytic seminoma. Ultrastructural and microspectrophotometric observations. Lab Invest 1984;51:343–9.

206. True LD, Otis CN, Delprado W, Scully RE, Rosai J. Spermatocytic seminoma of testis with sarcomatous transformation. A report of five cases. Am J Surg Pathol 1988;12:75–82.

Spermatocytic Seminoma: Pathologic Findings and Special Studies

207. Aguirre P, Scully RE, Dayal Y, DeLellis R. Placental-like alkaline phosphatase reactivity in germ cell tumors of the ovary and testis [Abstract]. Lab Invest 1985;52:2A.

208. Albores-Saavedra J, Huffman H, Alvarado-Cabrero I, Ayala AG. Anaplastic variant of spermatocytic seminoma. Hum Pathol 1996;27:650–5.

209. Burke AP, Mostofi FK. Spermatocytic seminoma: a clinicopathologic study of 79 cases. J Urol Pathol 1993;1:21–32.

210. Cummings OW, Ulbright TM, Eble JN, Roth LM. Spermatocytic seminoma: an immunohistochemical study. Hum Pathol 1994;25:54–9.

211. Dekker I, Rozeboom T, Delemarre J, Dam A, Oosterhuis JW. Placental-like alkaline phosphatase and DNA flow cytometry in spermatocytic seminoma. Cancer 1992;69:993–6.

212. Eble JN. Spermatocytic seminoma. Hum Pathol 1994;25:1035–42.

213. Floyd C, Ayala AG, Logothetis CJ, Silva EG. Spermatocytic seminoma with associated sarcoma of the testis. Cancer 1988;61:409–14.

214. Fogel M, Lifschitz-Mercer B, Moll R, et al. Heterogeneity of intermediate filament expression in human testicular seminomas. Differentiation 1990;45:242–9.

215. Frasik W, Okon K, Sokolowski A. Polymorphism of spermatocytic seminoma. A morphometric study. Anal Cell Pathol 1994;7:195–203.

215a. Kraggerud SM, Berner A, Bryne M, Pettersen EO, Fossa SD. Spermatocytic seminoma as compared to classical seminoma: an immunohistochemical and DNA flow cytometric study. APMIS 1999;107:297–302.

215b. Masson P. Étude sur le séminome. Rev Canad Biol 1946;5:361–87.

216. Matoska J, Talerman A. Spermatocytic seminoma associated with rhabdomyosarcoma. Am J Clin Pathol 1990;94:89–95.

217. Muller J, Skakkebaek NE, Parkinson MC. The spermatocytic seminoma: views on pathogenesis. Int J Androl 1987;10:147–56.

218. Romanenko AM, Persidsky YV, Mostofi FK. Ultrastructure and histogenesis of spermatocytic seminoma. J Urol Pathol 1993;1:387–95.

219. Rosai J, Khodadoust K, Silber I. Spermatocytic seminoma. II. Ultrastructural study. Cancer 1969;24:103–16.

220. Scully RE. Spermatocytic seminoma of the testis: a report of 3 cases and review of the literature. Cancer 1961;14:788–94.

221. Takahashi H. Cytometric analysis of testicular seminoma and spermatocytic seminoma. Acta Pathol Jap 1993;43:121–9.

222. Takahashi H, Aizawa S, Konishi E, Furusato M, Kato H, Ashihara T. Cytofluorometric analysis of spermatocytic seminoma. Cancer 1993;72:549–52.

223. Talerman A. Spermatocytic seminoma: clinicopathological study of 22 cases. Cancer 1980;45:2169–76.

224. Talerman A, Fu YS, Okagaki T. Spermatocytic seminoma. Ultrastructural and microspectrophotometric observations. Lab Invest 1984;51:343–9.

225. True LD, Otis CN, Delprado W, Scully RE, Rosai J. Spermatocytic seminoma of testis with sarcomatous transformation. A report of five cases. Am J Surg Pathol 1988;12:75–82.

Spermatocytic Seminoma: Differential Diagnosis

226. Albores-Saavedra J, Huffman H, Alvarado-Cabrero I, Ayala AG. Anaplastic variant of spermatocytic seminoma. Hum Pathol 1996;27:650–5.

227. Damjanov I. Tumors of the testis and epididymis. In: Murphy WM, ed. Urological pathology. Philadelphia: WB Saunders, 1989:314–79.

228. Rosai J, Silber I, Khodadoust K. Spermatocytic seminoma. I. Clinicopathologic study of six cases and review of the literature. Cancer 1969;24:92–102.

229. Scully RE. Spermatocytic seminoma of the testis: a report of 3 cases and review of the literature. Cancer 1961;14:788–94.

Spermatocytic Seminoma: Treatment and Prognosis

230. Eble JN. Spermatocytic seminoma. Hum Pathol 1994;25:1035–42.

231. Floyd C, Ayala AG, Logothetis CJ, Silva EG. Spermatocytic seminoma with associated sarcoma of the testis. Cancer 1988;61:409–14.

232. Matoska J, Ondrus D, Hornák M. Metastatic spermatocytic seminoma. A case report with light microscopic, ultrastructural, and immunohistochemical findings. Cancer 1988;62:1197–201.

233. Matoska J, Talerman A. Spermatocytic seminoma associated with rhabdomyosarcoma. Am J Clin Pathol 1990;94:89–95.

234. True LD, Otis CN, Delprado W, Scully RE, Rosai J. Spermatocytic seminoma of testis with sarcomatous transformation. A report of five cases. Am J Surg Pathol 1988;12:75–82.

❖❖❖

4

GERM CELL TUMORS: NONSEMINOMATOUS

EMBRYONAL CARCINOMA

Definition. This is a neoplasm composed of primitive-appearing, anaplastic epithelial cells resembling those of early embryonic development arranged in solid, glandular, papillary, or tubular patterns.

General Features. Embryonal carcinoma in pure form accounted for only 2.3 percent of testicular germ cell tumors in one referral series (59); this figure contrasts with that in earlier series showing a frequency of about 20 percent (32,57). This marked difference reflects the current recognition of other tumor types, particularly yolk sac tumor, that were previously grouped with embryonal carcinoma. Approximately 40 percent of all testicular germ cell tumors have an embryonal carcinoma component (41,59), and embryonal carcinoma occurs in 87 percent of nonseminomatous germ cell tumors (41).

An unresolved issue is the point at which differentiation toward teratomatous elements should be recognized and lead to a diagnosis of a mixed germ cell tumor rather than pure embryonal carcinoma. There is a tradition, which we follow, of permitting the inclusion of a minor amount of "primitive mesenchyme" in embryonal carcinomas and not regarding it as a teratomatous component (57,60), despite immunohistochemical evidence that it is a form of early teratomatous differentiation (85). The rationale for this approach derives from the experience of the British Testicular Tumour Panel which identified no difference in survival in patients with embryonal carcinoma regardless of the presence of a stromal component (76). Whether there are important differences, in the current era of chemotherapy, in the courses of patients with embryonal carcinoma with and without a minor component of undifferentiated stroma has not been studied. Ideally, our approach is validated if no such difference is identified.

Embryonal carcinoma most commonly occurs between 25 and 35 years of age, with an average age of 32 years (41), and is extremely rare in prepubertal children and infants (37,56). Patients with human leukocyte antigen (HLA) B-13 may be at increased risk (48). Approximately 80 percent of patients present with a testicular mass that may be associated with pain or discomfort. About 10 percent present with symptoms of metastatic disease, and another 10 percent because of hormonal symptoms, usually gynecomastia. After clinical evaluation only about 40 percent of patients with nonseminomatous tumors have disease limited to the testis at presentation, 40 percent have retroperitoneal involvement, and 20 percent have supradiaphragmatic involvement or visceral organ spread (103). In one study, which staged patients pathologically, 66 percent of patients with a tumor composed predominantly of embryonal carcinoma had metastases (80). There are also rare reports of patients with tumors composed in part of embryonal carcinoma presenting with sudden death due to pulmonary embolism prior to the diagnosis of the testicular tumor (4,83).

Javadpour (45) found alpha-fetoprotein (AFP) elevations in 70 percent of patients with embryonal carcinomas, but it is likely that many of these patients also had a yolk sac tumor component. Although there is the potential for AFP elevation in morphologically pure embryonal carcinoma since an occasional case is immunohistochemically positive (see page 110), Mostofi et al. (59) found no AFP elevation in 24 patients with pure embryonal carcinoma. Elevation of human chorionic gonadotropin (hCG) is reported in 60 percent of patients with embryonal carcinoma (45), reflecting the frequent presence of syncytiotrophoblastic cells in this tumor (59). A similar proportion of patients with advanced stage embryonal carcinoma have elevated serum lactate dehydrogenase (LDH) levels (9), and serum placental-like alkaline phosphatase (PLAP) may also be increased.

Gross Findings. Embryonal carcinoma typically forms a soft, pale gray to pink to tan, granular tumor that tends to bulge from the cut surface; foci of hemorrhage and necrosis may be prominent (figs. 4-1, 4-2). Rarely, the tumor has a firm consistency, at least focally (fig. 4-3). Embryonal carcinomas are usually smaller than seminomas and

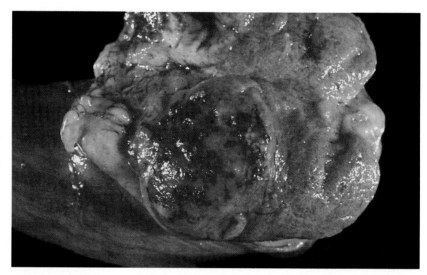

Figure 4-1
EMBRYONAL CARCINOMA
A tan, granular tumor nodule with foci of hemorrhage and necrosis bulges above the cut surface of the testis. The interface of the tumor and adjacent testis is ill-defined in areas.

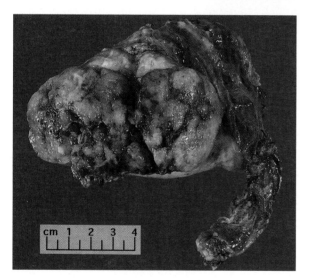

Figure 4-2
EMBRYONAL CARCINOMA
A white to pale pink, solid neoplasm with foci of hemorrhage and cystic degeneration is seen. (Courtesy of Dr. R. Harruff, Seattle, WA.)

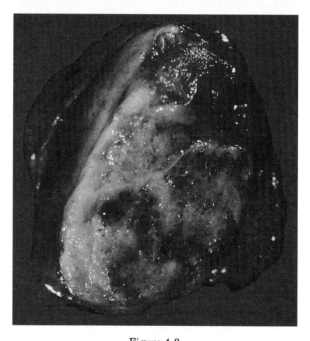

Figure 4-3
EMBRYONAL CARCINOMA
The white areas were firm, and microscopic examination showed prominent fibrosis. (Fig. 3.2 from Young RH, Scully RE. Testicular tumors. Chicago: ASCP Press, 1990:48.)

average about 2.5 cm in diameter (21). Additionally, they tend to blend imperceptibly with the adjacent parenchyma, unlike the more sharply circumscribed seminoma. Local extension into the rete testis, epididymis, or beyond occurs in about 25 percent of the cases (fig. 4-4) (57,80).

Microscopic Findings. Embryonal carcinoma consists of cohesive groups of large cells which can be arranged in several patterns that often coexist (fig. 4-5). Solid sheets of cells, often associated with foci of necrosis both of individual

cells and confluent areas, are common (fig. 4-6), as are glands that may be round or elongated (fig. 4-7). Degenerative spaces may be present and occasionally contain eosinophilic material. There are also frequent papillae, with the tumor cells covering, in a radial fashion, a protruding core of fibrovascular tissue (fig. 4-8). When the

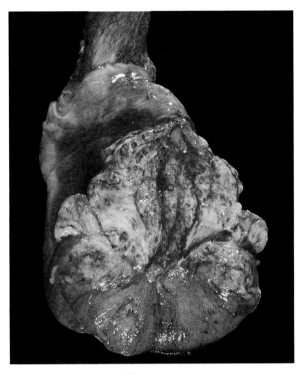

Figure 4-4
EMBRYONAL CARCINOMA
Massive spread of tumor to epididymis and paratesticular soft tissues.

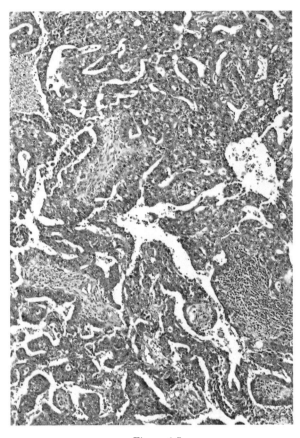

Figure 4-5
EMBRYONAL CARCINOMA
Typical heterogeneous appearance with glandular, papillary, and solid patterns.

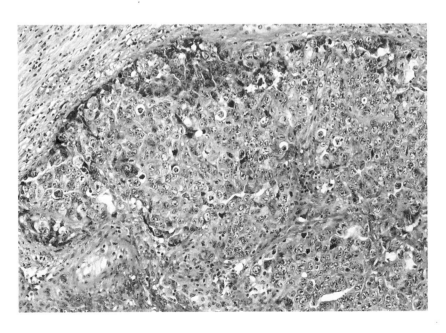

Figure 4-6
EMBRYONAL CARCINOMA:
SOLID PATTERN
A rare gland is also present.

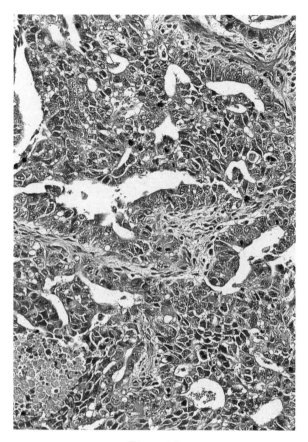

Figure 4-7
EMBRYONAL CARCINOMA
Glands are round and elongated.

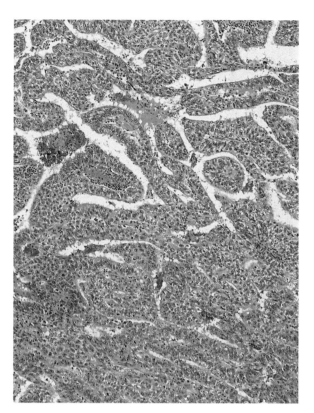

Figure 4-8
EMBRYONAL CARCINOMA: PAPILLARY PATTERN
Neoplastic cells are radially arranged around fibrovascular cores.

vessels are prominent, a "pseudoendodermal sinus" pattern is produced (40), although the tumor cells are larger and more pleomorphic than in yolk sac tumor (see page 122 and figs. 4-30, 4-31). Sometimes papillary processes lack a stromal core and are composed of piled-up, carcinomatous epithelium (fig. 4-9). In Jacobsen's enumeration of patterns of embryonal carcinoma (40), the solid pattern was most common (100 percent), followed by papillary/tubular (78 percent), pseudo-endodermal sinus (15 percent), and double-layered patterns (7 percent). The double-layered pattern, in our opinion, is a diffuse embryoma form of a mixed germ cell tumor composed of embryonal carcinoma and yolk sac tumor (see chapter 5). Jacobsen and Talerman (44) illustrated an unusual variant of embryonal carcinoma in which pleomorphic embryonal carcinoma cells formed blastocyst-like vesicles with a central cavity.

It is common in the solid pattern to find darkly staining, degenerate-appearing, smudged cells. These tend to be particularly prominent at the periphery of cell groups (fig. 4-10) and may be confused with syncytiotrophoblastic cells resulting in a misdiagnosis of choriocarcinoma. Friedman and Moore (32), noting the tendency of the smudged cells to "apply" themselves to adjacent cells, called this the "appliqué" pattern of embryonal carcinoma. A cellular, primitive, undifferentiated stroma of mitotically active, hyperchromatic, oval to spindle cells (fig. 4-11) may constitute a minor component of embryonal carcinoma, as noted earlier (85). The spindle cells are generally located around the epithelial component and do not form a large, expansile sheet. The lymphoid infiltrate and granulomatous reaction associated with seminoma are not prominent features of embryonal carcinoma but are identified in occasional cases (fig. 4-12), as is a prominent fibrous stroma (fig. 4-12), correlating with the occasionally firm gross texture (fig. 4-3).

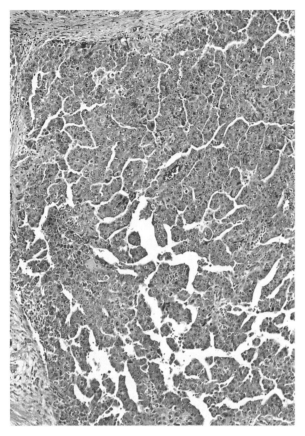

Figure 4-9
EMBRYONAL CARCINOMA
Papillary pattern without fibrovascular cores.

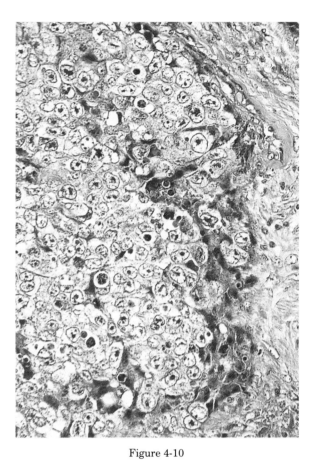

Figure 4-10
EMBRYONAL CARCINOMA
The appliqué pattern results from the degenerate appearance of cells at the periphery of a cellular lobule and imparts a "biphasic" appearance that may mimic choriocarcinoma.

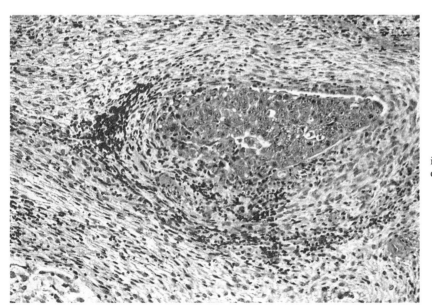

Figure 4-11
EMBRYONAL CARCINOMA
Neoplastic, undifferentiated stroma is associated with typical embryonal carcinoma.

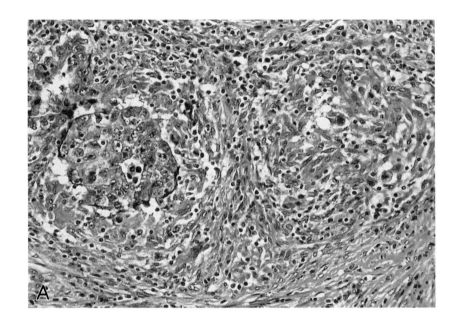

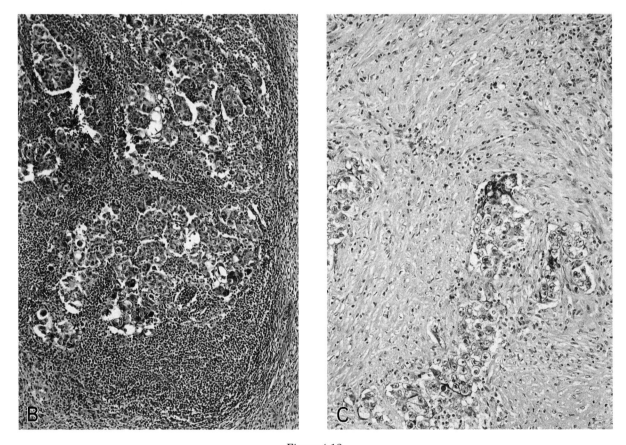

Figure 4-12
EMBRYONAL CARCINOMA
A: A granulomatous reaction surrounds a cluster of embryonal carcinoma cells.
B: A lymphoid infiltrate is striking in another case.
C: Prominent stromal fibrosis is present.

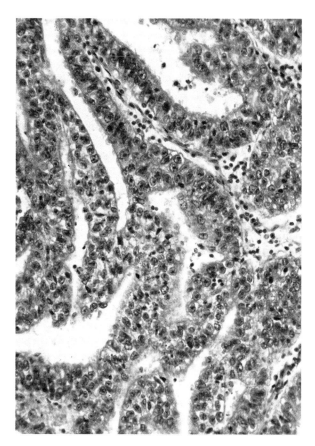

Figure 4-13
EMBRYONAL CARCINOMA
Glandular pattern with columnar cells.

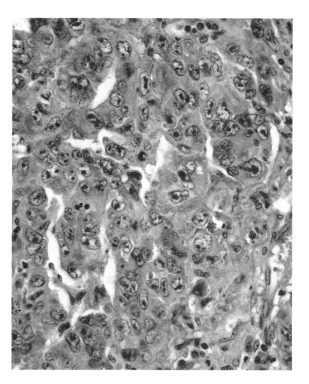

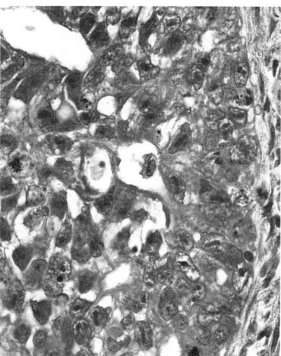

Figure 4-14
EMBRYONAL CARCINOMA

There are pleomorphic, irregularly shaped, vesicular nuclei with large, central nucleoli. The nuclei are crowded, often abut and occasionally overlap. Intercellular borders are often difficult to discern. In top figure, the cytoplasm is eosinophilic to amphophilic; in bottom one it is basophilic.

The tumor cells are usually polygonal, but in glandular foci the lining cells are cuboidal to columnar (fig. 4-13). The usually abundant cytoplasm is slightly granular and varies from basophilic (fig. 4-14, bottom) to amphophilic to eosinophilic (fig 4-14, top) or even clear. Cytoplasmic borders cannot usually be appreciated in light microscopic sections, especially in neoplasms with a solid pattern, causing a syncytial appearance. In semi-thin plastic sections, cell borders are more easily identified, and the nuclei are discrete. The nuclei are large and vesicular, with irregular, coarsely clumped chromatin and prominent parachromatin clearing. The nuclear shape is generally polygonal, but frequently there are deep clefts and irregular contours. One or more very large nucleoli are present (fig. 4-14). Often the crowded nuclei appear to abut or overlap each other (fig. 4-14). The mitotic rate is high. Syncytiotrophoblast cells are common in embryonal

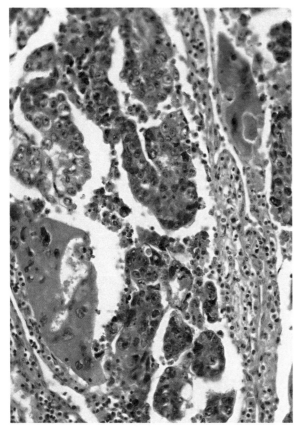

Figure 4-15
EMBRYONAL CARCINOMA
Two syncytiotrophoblast cells are present.

carcinoma (fig 4-15) and, just as with the appliqué pattern, should not lead to the diagnosis of choriocarcinoma.

Toward the periphery, it is common to identify intratubular embryonal carcinoma that is usually extensively necrotic, with darkly staining masses of degenerated, intraluminal neoplastic cells (fig. 4-16). The residual intact nuclei frequently have a smudged appearance, and there is often dystrophic calcification.

Vascular invasion occurs commonly (fig. 4-17) and is an important feature to identify, as it may be used to exclude patients from "surveillance only" protocols. The true frequency of vascular invasion is unclear because most of the studies have assessed mixed germ cell tumors; Moriyama and co-workers (54), for instance, identified vascular invasion in 29 of 45 (64 percent) nonseminomatous germ cell tumors of different stages. In our own experience with nonseminomatous germ cell tumors, the angioinvasive element is disproportionately embryonal carcinoma. Such vascular invasion is often most easily identified at the periphery of the tumor, in the surrounding non-neoplastic testis. Artifactual implantation of tumor into vascular spaces by specimen dissection may mimic vascular invasion but has loosely associated tumor cells dispersed randomly ("floating") in vascular spaces rather than the cohesive groups that conform to the shape of the vessel that are the hallmark of true invasion (fig. 4-17). The association of true vascular invasion with thrombotic material is also helpful (107), as is the usual simultaneous presence of implants on tissue surfaces when artifactual vascular implants occur (67). Retraction artifacts induced by fixation may be misinterpreted as vascular space involvement but lack an endothelial lining. Vascular invasion may also be mimicked by intratubular tumor, but the identification of residual Sertoli cells along the basal aspect of the space or a thickened, peritubular basement membrane confirms an intratubular location in some cases. Extensive necrosis in this circumstance, in our opinion, argues for intratubular rather than intravascular tumor. In addition, seminiferous tubules with intratubular tumor tend to have a more uniform diameter and are nonbranching, whereas vessels with tumor may be less uniform in size and often branch. Immunostaining for endothelial cell markers can resolve this dilemma if routine light microscopy is ambiguous.

Immunohistochemical Findings. Several immunohistochemical stains aid in the differential diagnosis of embryonal carcinoma. Much of the reported AFP positivity probably represents intermixed yolk sac tumor elements, but some typical embryonal carcinomas do stain for AFP (8,90). Niehans et al. (69) identified AFP in 19 of 57 (33 percent) embryonal carcinomas, whereas Mostofi and co-workers (58) found AFP in 2 of 24 (8 percent) pure embryonal carcinomas and in the embryonal carcinoma component of 47 of 377 (12 percent) mixed germ cell tumors. Similarly, Wittekind et al. (105) found no AFP in pure embryonal carcinomas but did report positivity within the embryonal carcinoma component of some mixed germ cell tumors, perhaps indicating early transformation to yolk sac tumor in

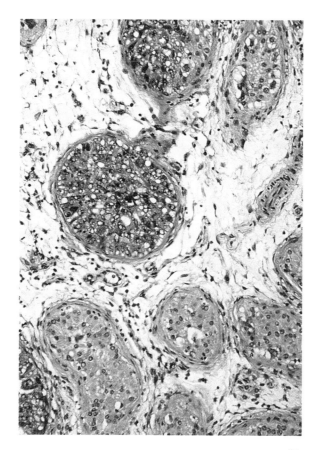
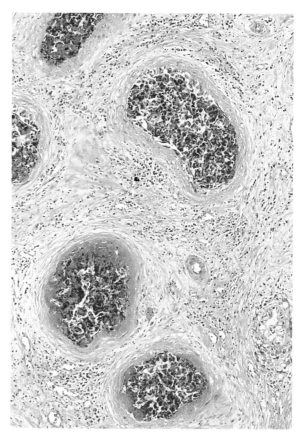

Figure 4-16
EMBRYONAL CARCINOMA
Intratubular embryonal carcinoma consisting of viable epithelium (left) and the more usual darkly staining nuclear debris admixed with partially necrotic cells (right).

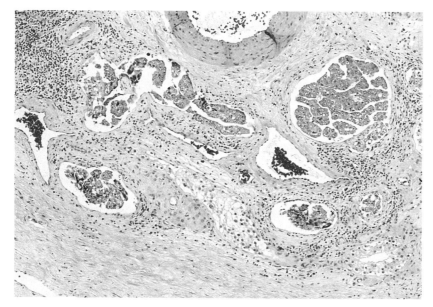

Figure 4-17
EMBRYONAL CARCINOMA:
VASCULAR INVASION
The intravascular tumor conforms to the shape of the vessels.

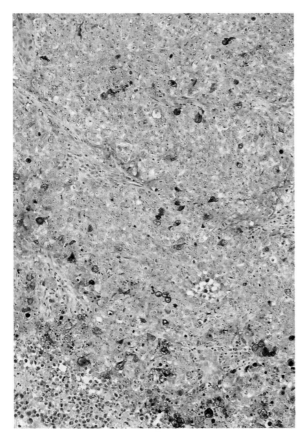

Figure 4-18
EMBRYONAL CARCINOMA
There is focal membranous and cytoplasmic positivity for placental alkaline phosphatase.

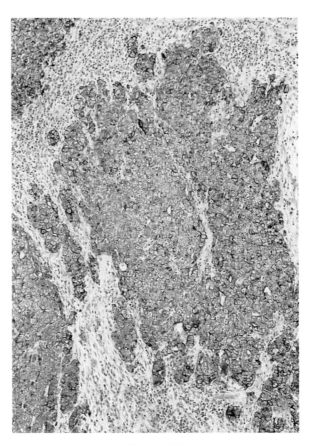

Figure 4-19
EMBRYONAL CARCINOMA
Diffusely positive staining occurs with a broad spectrum anti-cytokeratin "cocktail."

these neoplasms. Such positivity occurs most commonly in scattered cells of the solid pattern.

Recent studies have reported PLAP positivity in 86 to 97 percent of embryonal carcinomas (10,50, 69). Failure to identify PLAP in seven embryonal carcinomas in one study may be related to methodologic differences (95). Burke and Mostofi (10) noted that staining for PLAP was often more intense and focal in embryonal carcinomas than in seminoma, with both cytoplasmic and membrane positivity (fig. 4-18).

Most embryonal carcinomas stain for pancytokeratin (AE1/AE3 and CAM 5.2) as well as cytokeratin classes 8, 18, and 19 (fig. 4-19), with occasional cases also staining for cytokeratins 4 and 17 (7,49,69,84). Most embryonal carcinomas do not react with epithelial membrane antigen (EMA) (69). Positivity with Ber-H2 (Ki-1, CD30) occurs in over 80 percent of cases (fig. 4-20) and

is rarely identified in other forms of germ cell tumor (see Table 3-1) (26,39,71,84). A useful immunohistochemical panel for recognizing a poorly differentiated neoplasm as an embryonal carcinoma is PLAP, pancytokeratin, and CD30 (all typically positive), with EMA (negative).

Several other antigens may be demonstrated in embryonal carcinoma but are diagnostically less useful. LDH-1 is positive in over 50 percent of cases (66), and ferritin in 88 percent (42). Monoclonal antibody 43-9F is strongly reactive in 87 percent of cases, with weak or absent reactivity in seminomas, choriocarcinomas, and most yolk sac tumors (100). Many embryonal carcinomas are strongly positive for p53 in 5 to 50 percent of the cell population, contrasting with weaker and more focal positivity in seminomas (6,97). Alpha-1-antitrypsin, Leu 7, vimentin, and human placental lactogen (HPL) may be demonstrated in a

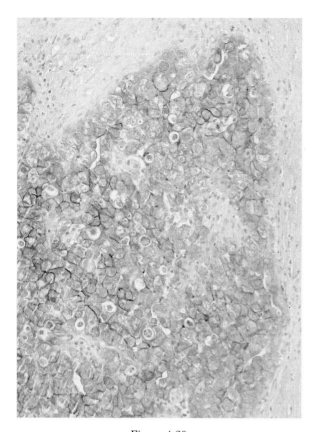

Figure 4-20
EMBRYONAL CARCINOMA
Strong membranous positivity occurs with Ber-H2 (Ki-1, CD30).

small percentage of cases (58,69). Embryonal carcinomas are negative for carcinoembryonic antigen, and beta-hCG is demonstrable only in intermingled syncytiotrophoblastic cells (69); the latter may also stain for inhibin (51a).

Ultrastructural Findings. Ultrastructural examination shows small, extracellular luminal spaces in solid patterns of tumor (fig. 4-21) and larger, more distinctive luminal spaces in overtly glandular patterns (fig. 4-22) (89). Stubby microvilli project into the luminal spaces (fig. 4-21), and tight junctional complexes with well-defined desmosomes are present between cells abutting a lumen (figs. 4-21, 4-22) (80a). The tight junctions of these complexes are frequently quite long; this feature has proved useful in differentiating glandular-pattern embryonal carcinomas from somatic-type adenocarcinomas derived from teratomatous elements (96). The cytoplasm of embryonal carcinoma cells is more

complex than is seen in seminoma, with abundant numbers of ribosomes, frequent arrays of glycogen, and a much more prominent Golgi apparatus and rough endoplasmic reticulum (89). Mitochondria are numerous, and telolysosomes are prominent (fig. 4-21). Scattered lipid droplets are present. Basement membrane often surrounds nests of cells. The nuclei are irregular, with deep indentations, clumps of heterochromatin, and large nucleoli with a "complex meandering appearance" (figs. 4-21, 4-22) (89). Intranuclear cytoplasmic inclusions may be identified.

Special Diagnostic Techniques. Ploidy analysis of embryonal carcinomas has shown a mean deoxyribonucleic acid (DNA) value of 1.43 times the diploid control, a result significantly less than that obtained for seminomas (1.66 times) (70). Nonseminomatous tumors, including embryonal carcinomas, most commonly have single aneuploid stem lines with ploidy values in the triploid range (30). These data have led to the hypothesis that embryonal carcinomas arise from seminomas secondary to the loss of cancer suppressor genes (70). Cytogenetic analysis of embryonal carcinomas has confirmed the presence of isochromosome (i)12p in many cases (20), but some tumors lack this marker chromosome (11). It has been suggested that the formation of i(12p) may alter a proto-oncogene on chromosome 12 (20). There appears to be a general correlation between the number of copies of i(12p) and the aggressiveness of the tumor (20). One study detected a second distinctive chromosomal anomaly involving chromosome 12 that appears to be restricted to nonseminomatous tumors, unlike i(12p) (82). This anomaly is del(12)(q13-q22). An activated form of the N-*ras* gene caused by a point mutation at the codon for amino acid 12 has been identified in cultured "teratocarcinoma" cells, and correlates with the increased aggressiveness of the tumor cells (93). One study identified point mutations at codon 12 of the K-*ras* proto-oncogene in 3 of 25 nonseminomatous tumors (65). Transcripts of the c-*myb* oncogene have also been found in undifferentiated mouse "teratocarcinoma" stem cells but not in their differentiated progeny (33). N-*myc* expression has been identified in embryonal carcinomas but not in non-neoplastic testis (53,86). The proto-oncogenes c-Ki-*ras*, c-Ha-*ras*1, c-*raf*1, N-*myc*, and c-*fos* as well as p53 have

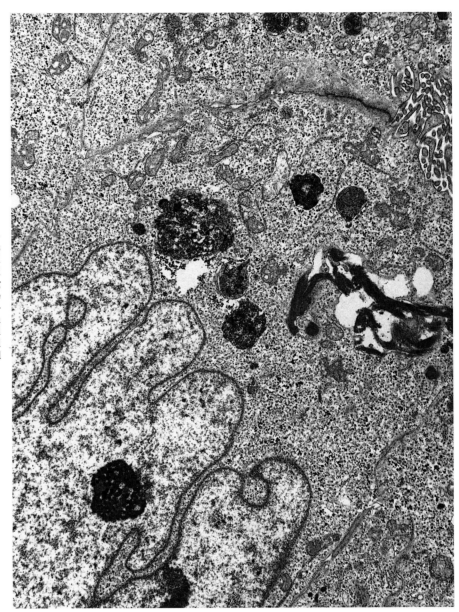

Figure 4-21
EMBRYONAL CARCINOMA
Electron micrograph shows the formation of a luminal space bordered by microvilli (upper right). Note the long tight junction adjacent to the lumen. The nucleus has intricate folds, and the cytoplasm contains granular lysosomal bodies (telolysosomes), small mitochondria, and scattered glycogen granules (X11,000).

been detected in "teratocarcinoma" cell lines, but no mutations of N-*ras* or activation of Ha-*ras* or Ki-*ras* were identified in this study (94). A comprehensive model for these observations, however, has yet to evolve.

Because of the association of germ cell tumors with characteristic cytogenetic anomalies of chromosome 12, genetic analyses may aid in the diagnosis of ambiguous carcinomas at extragenital sites. Four of eight patients with poorly differentiated carcinomas involving midline struc-

tures had abnormalities of chromosome 12, consistent with germ cell tumors (62).

Proliferative activity of embryonal carcinomas, as judged by thymidine uptake, is quite high, with the tumors showing a random pattern of label incorporation (77). This high proliferative index is also reflected by a rapid in vitro tumor doubling time which, in one study, was 17 hours (106).

Human embryonal carcinomas express certain globoseries carbohydrate surface antigens (so-called stage-specific embryonic antigens

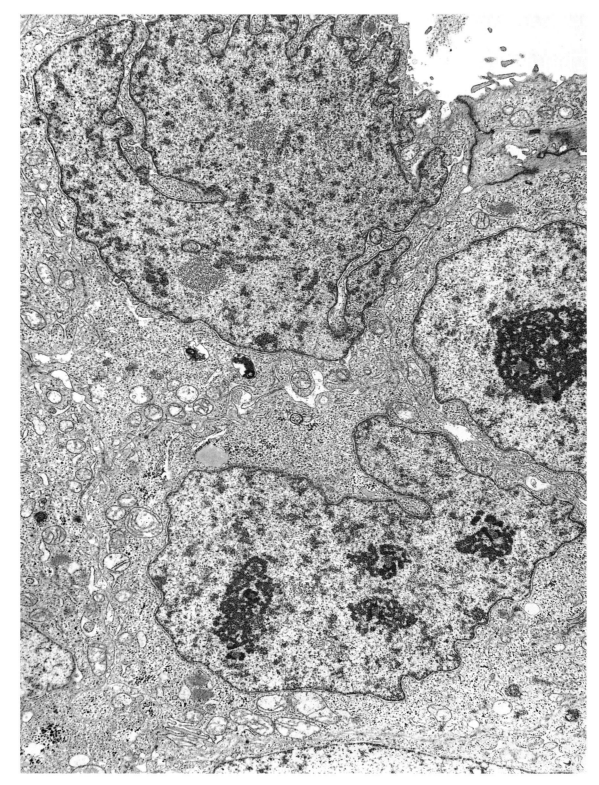

Figure 4-22
EMBRYONAL CARCINOMA

This glandular pattern has a luminal space at upper right, with well-defined junctional complexes. The nuclei are complexly folded and have large, intricate nucleoli. The cytoplasm contains round mitochondria and scattered glycogen granules (X8,300).

[SSEA]) corresponding to primitive embryonic development (SSEA-3) but do not express the more mature phenotype (SSEA-1) (15). Spontaneous differentiation to syncytiotrophoblast cells (13) and, after exposure to retinoic acid, to cells expressing neurofilament proteins is described in tissue culture. Both muscle and neural differentiation were detected immunohistochemically in tumors produced by injecting cultured embryonal carcinoma into mice (14). These data support the capacity of embryonal carcinoma to differentiate into other forms of germ cell tumor. The capacity for such transformation is not predictable by morphology, since certain tissue culture lines are nullipotent, and morphologically similar lines have the capacity to form several different neoplastic types (61,73,74).

Cytologic Findings. In preparations derived from aspirated tumors, embryonal carcinoma appears as tight clusters of pleomorphic epithelium (5) (fig. 4-23). A sheet-like, papillary, or ball-like arrangement may occur (38). Nuclear and cytoplasmic borders may be blurred (5,38). The nuclei are irregularly shaped and pleomorphic, with clumped, unevenly distributed chromatin and one or more prominent nucleoli (38,47). A branching, "right-angle" capillary network may be identified, with the tumor cells forming tight clusters along the branching capillaries (5). A "tigroid" background, as seen in seminomas, is not identified (5). The cohesive nature of embryonal carcinoma aspirates further differentiates it from the more dissociated cellular elements derived from seminomas.

Differential Diagnosis. Most embryonal carcinomas are easily recognized, but occasional confusion with a seminoma or yolk sac tumor occurs. The differentiation of typical and spermatocytic seminoma from embryonal carcinoma has been discussed in chapter 3. A diagnosis of yolk sac tumor is justifiable only when one of the many distinctive patterns of yolk sac tumor is identified (see section on yolk sac tumor). Embryonal carcinomas generally lack these patterns, and although the solid and papillary patterns of the two tumors may be confused, embryonal carcinomas have cells with larger nuclei and greater nuclear pleomorphism than yolk sac tumors. These features, and associated patterns, help distinguish the two tumors, including cases of embryonal carcinoma with the "pseudoendodermal sinus" pattern. The

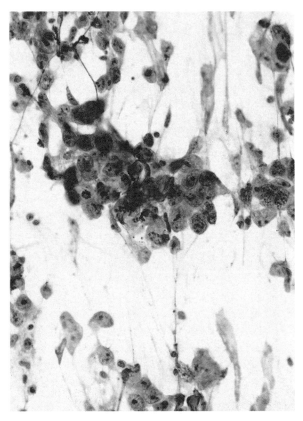

Figure 4-23
EMBRYONAL CARCINOMA

In this preparation from a needle aspirate, cells are arranged in tight clusters, with scattered individual tumor cells. Note the ill-defined cytoplasm, pleomorphic overlapping nuclei, and prominent multiple nucleoli.

common hyaline globules and basement membrane deposits of yolk sac tumor are not seen with any regularity in embryonal carcinomas (99). Staining with Ber-H2 (Ki-1, CD30), positive in most embryonal carcinomas and negative in yolk sac tumor, may also assist with this differential (26), and more than focal AFP positivity favors yolk sac tumor. Solid embryonal carcinomas with degenerate cells (the appliqué pattern; fig. 4-10) may resemble choriocarcinoma but lack the well-defined, biphasic pattern of classic choriocarcinomas. Immunostains for hCG can resolve this differential diagnosis.

A large cell lymphoma, particularly of an immunoblastic phenotype, can be confused with an embryonal carcinoma, and Ki-1–positive, anaplastic large cell lymphoma with a prominent intratubular growth pattern may additionally mimic embryonal carcinoma with an intratubular component (see fig. 7-85) (27). Patients with lymphoma are usually older and may have bilateral testicular involvement. The interstitial growth pattern of many lymphomas is not a feature of embryonal carcinoma, which destroys tubules and usually has distinct epithelial differentiation. Intratubular germ cell neoplasia, unclassified (IGCNU) is often present in the seminiferous tubules adjacent to embryonal carcinomas and is absent in lymphomas. Immunostains for cytokeratins and PLAP are usually positive in embryonal carcinoma and negative in lymphoma (102), although rare Ki-1–positive, anaplastic large cell lymphomas may focally express cytokeratins. Nonetheless, strong and diffuse cytokeratin reactivity and PLAP positivity establish a diagnosis of embryonal carcinoma over Ki-1–positive, anaplastic large cell lymphoma (27). Leukocyte common antigen (LCA), if positive, is also diagnostic, but a high proportion of anaplastic large cell lymphomas are negative for LCA, and some do not express the usual B-cell and T-cell antigens. EMA positivity favors anaplastic large cell lymphoma. CD30 expression (Ki-1, Ber-H2 antibody) is not of diagnostic value since it is commonly positive in both large cell lymphoma and embryonal carcinoma.

Treatment and Prognosis. Embryonal carcinomas are not separated from other nonseminomatous germ cell tumors in current treatment strategies, and the following remarks concerning treatment are applicable to other forms of nonseminomatous germ cell tumor, with the possible exception of pure mature teratoma. The treatment of nonseminomatous tumors clinically limited to the testis is currently controversial. One school of thought advocates retroperitoneal lymph node dissection (RPLND), preferentially nerve sparing (16), to verify lack of extragonadal involvement (75). Patients with negative nodes may then be followed without the need for adjuvant therapy (81). For patients with relapse on follow-up (roughly 10 percent), multiagent, cisplatin-based chemotherapy is instituted. With this approach, a greater than 98 percent cure rate has been demonstrated (81). If positive nodes are identified on RPLND, patients may either be followed or given chemotherapy, depending upon factors such as patient reliability and extent of involvement (79). A 98 to 100 percent survival can be anticipated (81).

Another approach to clinical disease limited to the testis is simple observation following orchiectomy. Before being assigned to a surveillance only category, certain criteria, such as patient reliability for follow-up and absence of marker elevation postorchiectomy, should be met. Approximately 30 percent of patients followed in this manner develop a recurrence (88, 92). It has been suggested that patients with recurrence or those who, although clinical stage I, are found to have occult metastases in the retroperitoneal nodes at RPLND (pathologic stage II), could be placed, prospectively, into a high-risk group if one or more of the following features are identified: 1) the presence of identifiable vascular/lymphatic invasion (12,22,25,29,31,34,36,43,46,54,64,80,88,92,104); 2) advanced local tumor stage (12,34,46,78); 3) the presence of embryonal carcinoma (22,31,36,46,68), particularly if pure (18,43), predominant (63,64,104), or unassociated with teratoma (88); 4) a volume of embryonal carcinoma in excess of 2 mL (1,2); 5) less than a 50 percent teratomatous component (34,104); 6) absence of mature teratoma (36); 7) absence of yolk sac tumor elements (31); 8) the presence of a choriocarcinomatous component (12); 9) high S-phase values as determined by flow cytometry (18,19); 10) high proliferation indices as determined by immunostaining (Ki-67) (1); and 11) tumor DNA indices in the hypertetraploid to hyperpentaploid range (3,17). One study achieved greater success in identifying patients at low risk for metastasis, based on low proliferation values and small volumes of embryonal carcinoma, than identifying those at high risk (2). A preorchiectomy serum AFP of 80 ng/mL or greater (104) and a slower than usual decrease in AFP after orchiectomy (29) also correlate with an increased frequency of recurrence in clinical stage I patients. Such clinical and pathologic findings may be contraindications to management by surveillance only. Sogani and Fair (88) summarized the results of several surveillance only studies and found that 544 of 560 (97 percent) patients were alive without evidence of disease; 405 patients (72 percent) did not require additional treatment beyond orchiectomy.

The generally accepted treatment in the United States for patients with known retroperitoneal involvement of relatively limited extent (6 cm or less of total nodal involvement according to Rowland and Donohue [81]) is RPLND, with either close follow-up (followed by full course chemotherapy if recurrence develops) or limited course, adjuvant therapy. The overall survival in this group of patients is 98 percent with these methods.

For patients with advanced-stage, nonseminomatous germ cell tumors (i.e., bulky retroperitoneal disease or distant metastases), the standard form of treatment is initial cisplatin-based, multidrug chemotherapy followed by surgical resection, if necessary, of residual masses. It has been suggested that patients with residual retroperitoneal masses measuring less than 2 cm in diameter and an embryonal carcinoma in the testis without prechemotherapy marker elevation do not require a RPLND (28). Using this approach survival rates of 70 to 87 percent can be achieved (24,29,55). The nature of the residual mass in postchemotherapy resections has an important bearing on subsequent treatment (98). The presence of viable-appearing, nonteratomatous germ cell tumor in the completely resected residual mass following chemotherapy identifies a subset of patients who are at high risk for relapse (42 percent in one series [35]).

Numerous studies have been performed in order to determine prognosis in patients with advanced-stage, nonseminomatous germ cell tumors. The results of such studies, while showing some inconsistencies, generally agree that the important prognostic factors include estimates of the extent of disseminated disease and the degree of elevation of serum markers. In a study by Einhorn (24), 80 of 81 (99 percent) patients with disseminated, nonseminomatous germ cell tumors identified as "minimal" in extent achieved complete clinical remission, but for patients having "moderate" or "advanced" disease, complete clinical remission was achieved in 89 and 57 percent, respectively. Criteria for advanced extent of disseminated disease included: advanced pulmonary metastases (a mediastinal mass more than 50 percent of the intrathoracic diameter, more than 10 pulmonary metastases per lung field, or multiple pulmonary metastases with the largest metastasis exceeding 3 cm); a palpable abdominal mass with pulmonary metastases; or hepatic, osseous, or central nervous system metastases. A multivariate analysis of 795 patients with metastatic nonseminomatous germ cell tumors identified the following adverse

prognostic features: 1) the presence of liver, bone, or brain metastases; 2) AFP levels exceeding 1,000 IU/L or beta-hCG levels exceeding 10,000 IU/L; 3) a mediastinal mass exceeding 5 cm; 4) 20 or more lung metastases; 5) increasing patient age; and 6) the absence of embryonal carcinoma or a fibrous tissue component in the primary tumor (52). Vogelzang (101) identified levels of serum hCG as the single most important prognostic factor, but also found the volume of the metastases and serum levels of LDH and AFP to be prognostically important. Stoter and colleagues (91) developed a model using multivariate analysis that factored four features into a prognostic equation: 1) the presence of trophoblastic elements in the primary tumor; 2) the serum levels of AFP; 3) the presence of lung metastases; and 4) the size and number of lung metastases. Sledge and co-workers (87) identified serum hCG levels and the proliferative index (as determined by flow cytometry) as important prognostic factors. Using such methods, patients with disseminated nonseminomatous testicular germ cell tumors can often be classified into good prognosis and poor prognosis categories, and treatment may be adjusted accordingly (72).

Obviously, as this discussion indicates, there has been a remarkable turnaround in the prognosis of patients with nonseminomatous testicular germ cell tumors. The combination of effective, multiagent chemotherapy with surgery, as well as the identification of effective agents for "salvage" chemotherapy regimens, have resulted in cures for most patients with testicular germ cell tumors. An analysis of the data presented by Dixon and Moore (21) in the early 1950s shows an overall 5-year survival of 60 percent for patients with testicular germ cell tumors, but a 5-year survival of only 30 percent for those with nonseminomatous tumors; the current survival rate for patients with nonseminomatous germ cell tumors is in excess of 90 percent (23,81). Marrett et al. (51), in a study of death rates from testicular cancer in Ontario from 1964–1982, noted that the reduction in the overall death rate is primarily due to the reduction in the death rate of patients with nonseminomatous tumors.

YOLK SAC TUMOR
(ENDODERMAL SINUS TUMOR)

Definition. This malignant germ cell neoplasm differentiates to form structures typical of the embryonic yolk sac, allantois, and extraembryonic mesenchyme.

General Features. Teilum identified this tumor by noting the resemblance of certain of its structures to the extraembryonic mesoderm and, his most seminal discovery, the close homology between the "glomerulus-like" structures of yolk sac tumor and the endodermal sinuses of the rat placenta (179,180). He also noted its association with other germ cell tumors (177,178), and its differentiation toward structures of the extraembryonic fetal membranes, including the yolk sac and allantois. Additional evidence in support of Teilum's views occurred when AFP was localized both to the embryonic yolk sac as well as to yolk sac tumors (181).

Yolk sac tumor is the most common testicular tumor of children, representing 82 percent of all prepubertal germ cell tumors and occurring more than four times as commonly as testicular teratomas (114). About half (130) to three fourths (112) of childhood cases occur in patients under 2 years of age (167), with a range in one series of from the newborn period to 8.8 years (130). In a tumor registry series of 176 prepubertal boys with testicular yolk sac tumor, the median age was 17 months (139), which is comparable to the mean of 18 months reported by Brosman (112). When yolk sac tumor occurs in a prepubertal child, it is almost always a pure neoplasm, whereas in postpubertal patients it is, with rare exceptions, one component of a mixed germ cell tumor.

The usual age range for adults with either a pure yolk sac tumor or a germ cell tumor with a yolk sac tumor component is 17 to 40 years, but rare cases have been reported in the elderly (166). The reported frequency of yolk sac tumor among adult germ cell tumors depends upon the care with which it is sought. In prospective studies that included multiple sections, yolk sac tumor occurred in 44 percent of nonseminomatous germ cell tumors (174). Our own experience with consultation material is similar to that of Mostofi and co-workers (157): yolk sac tumor is the most commonly overlooked component of testicular germ cell tumors, probably because of its frequently focal nature, as well as continued confusion regarding its distinction from embryonal carcinoma.

There is no association of childhood yolk sac tumor with cryptorchidism, and, whereas the adult forms of germ cell tumor occur four or five times more commonly in the white population than the black population, the incidence of childhood yolk sac tumor is equal in both races (113).

Clinical Features. Children and adults most commonly present with a painless testicular mass (111). From 84 to 94 percent of patients with childhood yolk sac tumor have clinical stage I (or A) disease at presentation (i.e., no clinical/radiologic/ serologic evidence of nodal or distant spread) (129, 139). These data are not available for pure yolk sac tumor in adults. There is evidence that adults with a yolk sac tumor component in a mixed germ cell tumor have a higher frequency of pathologic stage I disease than do patients lacking a yolk sac tumor component (126).

Yolk sac tumor is closely associated with elevated serum levels of AFP. Talerman and co-workers (176) examined the germ cell tumors of 387 patients with known elevated AFP levels. Of the 92 patients with active disease and a demonstrable yolk sac tumor component, all had AFP levels that were substantial: hundreds to thousands of nanograms per milliliter. Significantly less elevated serum AFP levels were identified in some patients with embryonal carcinoma. Jacobsen (132) found elevated serum AFP levels in 36 of 38 (95 percent) patients with a demonstrable yolk sac tumor component. The correlation between elevated serum AFP and yolk sac tumor provides a valuable method for both assisting with the diagnosis as well as monitoring the effects of therapy.

Gross Findings. Most yolk sac tumors are gray-white to tan to yellow, nonencapsulated tumors that often have a somewhat glistening, mucoid quality and frequently show cystic changes on the cut surface (fig. 4-24). Foci of hemorrhage and necrosis may be present and can be extensive, especially in postpubertal patients (fig. 4-25). The texture is usually soft but may be firm. Extratesticular extension may be apparent in a minority of the prepubertal cases (114,166).

Microscopic Findings. Teilum's original descriptions of the various patterns of yolk sac tumor (181) have been further refined by Talerman who recognized nine different patterns (175). We have slightly modified his classification, with the

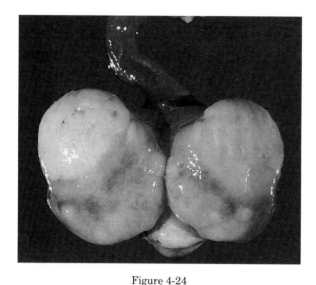

Figure 4-24
YOLK SAC TUMOR
A well-circumscribed tumor with a pale yellow, mucoid cut surface in a 4-month-old.

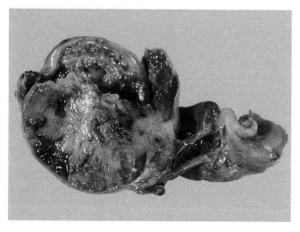

Figure 4-25
YOLK SAC TUMOR
A pure tumor in an adult shows gray tissue, hemorrhagic foci, and cystic degeneration. (Fig. 35 from Ulbright TM, Roth LM. Testicular and paratesticular tumors. In: Sternberg SS, ed. Diagnostic surgical pathology, New York: Raven Press, 1994:1885–947.)

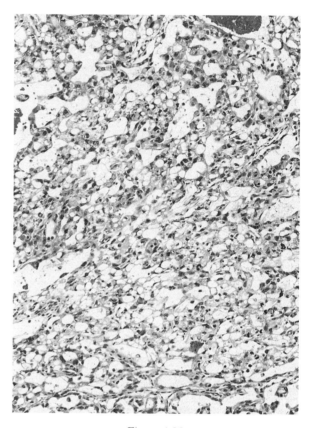

Figure 4-26
YOLK SAC TUMOR
Typical reticular pattern represented by a meshwork of spaces.

etal. These patterns really represent a morphologic continuum, with transitional forms and admixtures of patterns the rule. Similar patterns are observed in both the pediatric and adult forms of the tumor (184).

The reticular pattern of yolk sac tumor is the most common (fig. 4-26). Prominent cytoplasmic vacuoles create a sieve-like appearance while anastomosing, thin cords of neoplastic cells or attenuated cytoplasmic processes create an array of microcysts of varying sizes (figs. 4-26, 4-27). Compression of the nuclei may result in a lipoblastic-like appearance (fig. 4-27). Occasionally the cords of cells disperse as single spindle cells into the surrounding stroma (fig. 4-28). The stroma is often myxoid, and such cases represent hybrids of reticular and myxomatous patterns (see below). It is quite common to see reticular/microcystic patterns of yolk sac tumor intermingled with foci having a more solid appearance. A macrocystic pattern is seen when microcysts coalesce (fig. 4-29).

addition of a few recently described patterns, as follows: 1) reticular (microcystic, vacuolated, honeycomb); 2) macrocystic; 3) endodermal sinus (perivascular, festoon); 4) papillary; 5) solid; 6) glandular-alveolar (including intestinal and endometrioid-like [118,119]); 7) myxomatous; 8) sarcomatoid (spindle cell) (155); 9) polyvesicular vitelline; 10) hepatoid; and 11) pari-

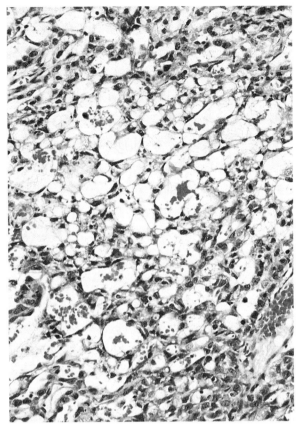

Figure 4-27
YOLK SAC TUMOR
Vacuolated cells resembling lipoblasts and small cysts are present.

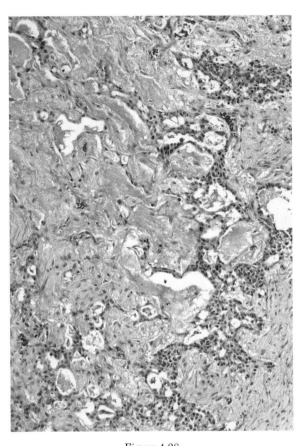

Figure 4-28
YOLK SAC TUMOR
Cords of cells extend from nests with microcysts into a myxoid stroma.

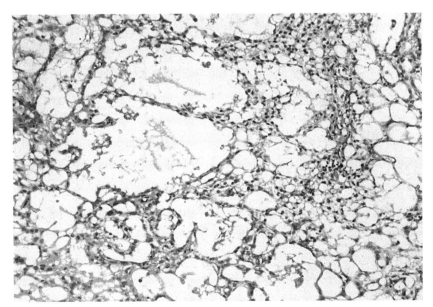

Figure 4-29
YOLK SAC TUMOR
Microcystic and macrocystic patterns are seen.

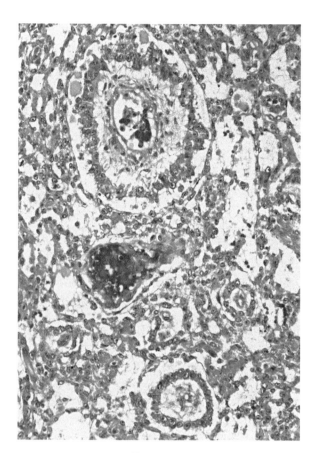

Figure 4-30
YOLK SAC TUMOR
There are anastomosing cords of cells and two endodermal sinus-like structures (Schiller-Duval bodies: the papillary structures lying in spaces and with central blood vessels in their stromal cores). Note also pink-staining basement membrane deposits.

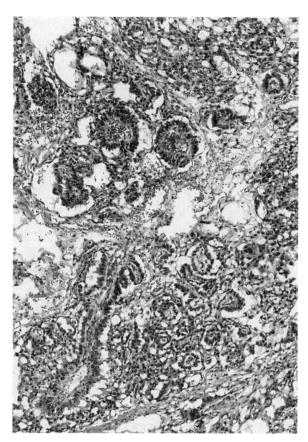

Figure 4-31
YOLK SAC TUMOR
Longitudinally (left bottom) and transversely sectioned endodermal sinus-like structures (Schiller-Duval bodies).

The endodermal sinus pattern of yolk sac tumor is perhaps its most distinctive and is classically characterized by a papillary core of fibrous tissue that, when cut transversely, contains a central small vessel and is ringed on its surface by a layer of malignant-appearing, cuboidal to columnar cells. This total structure is recessed into a small cystic space that is, in turn, lined by flattened tumor cells (fig. 4-30). These "Schiller-Duval bodies" may be cut longitudinally, resulting in an elongated structure (fig. 4-31). Oblique cuts of such structures may result in connective tissue cores that appear to be draped (festooned) by malignant epithelium (fig. 4-32). Abortive endodermal sinus structures that consist of fibrovascular cores of tissue rimmed by malignant cells but that are not recessed into a well-defined cystic

space are common. Jacobsen and Talerman (137) have described such configurations as "atypical perivascular formations." "Labyrinthine" spaces are a frequent feature of neoplasms with endodermal sinus formation (fig. 4-32).

In the papillary pattern, small, irregularly shaped papillae, sometimes with fibrous or hyalinized cores, project into cystic spaces that often contain many detached clusters of tumor cells (fig. 4-33). The tumor cells lining the papillae have a low-columnar to cuboidal profile, and a hobnail configuration of the nuclei may be present. Such papillae may sometimes be superimposed on a festoon (endodermal sinus) type of arrangement (fig. 4-34).

The solid pattern of yolk sac tumor consists of a sheet-like arrangement of polygonal tumor cells, with lightly eosinophilic to clear cytoplasm, well-defined cytoplasmic borders, and non-overlapping,

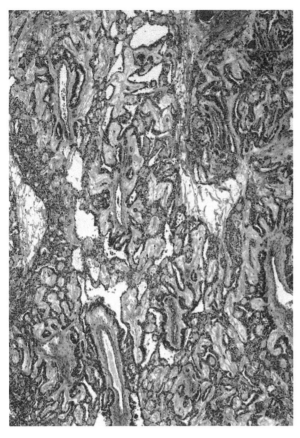

Figure 4-32
YOLK SAC TUMOR
Fibrous and fibrovascular cores are draped or "festooned" by malignant epithelium. Between the cores are interconnecting, irregular, "labyrinthine-like" spaces.

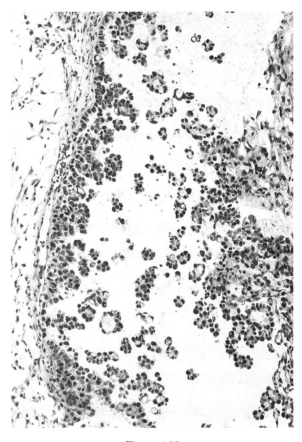

Figure 4-33
YOLK SAC TUMOR:
NONSPECIFIC PAPILLARY PATTERN
Papillae with fibrovascular cores, rimmed by cells with scant cytoplasm and which sometimes have a "hobnail" nuclear arrangement, project into a cystic space. Clusters of exfoliated cells are present in the cyst.

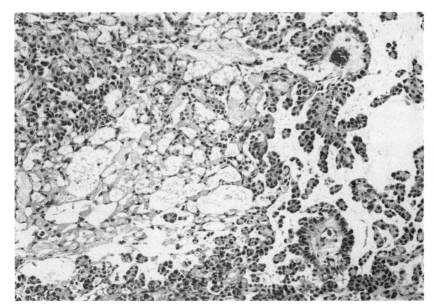

Figure 4-34
YOLK SAC TUMOR
On the right, papillary yolk sac tumor develops from well-defined endodermal sinus-like structures. A microcystic pattern is present in the center.

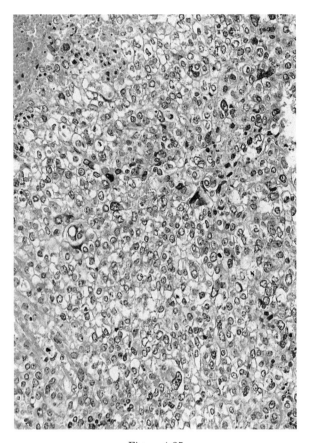

Figure 4-35
YOLK SAC TUMOR: SOLID PATTERN
Note the random pleomorphism and lack of fibrovascular septa (features that contrast with seminoma).

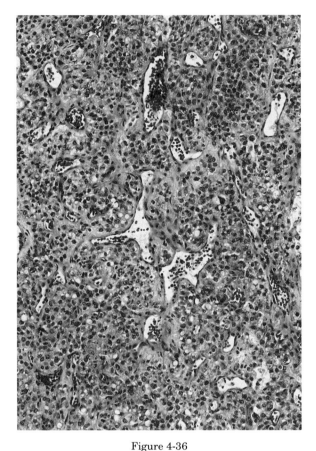

Figure 4-36
YOLK SAC TUMOR
A solid pattern with a prominent vascular network is seen. Foci of this type are nondiagnostic when viewed in isolation.

relatively uniform nuclei with prominent to inconspicuous nucleoli (fig. 4-35). It is common to see occasional, randomly distributed tumor cells with larger nuclei (fig. 4-35). Often there is a prominent vascular network (fig. 4-36), and frequently there are focal microcysts. This pattern shares some histologic features with seminoma, a differential diagnostic problem addressed in chapter 3. In some cases, the cells of solid yolk sac tumor have a blastematous appearance, being small and ovoid with hyperchromatic nuclei (fig. 4-37).

Glandular and alveolar patterns are common in yolk sac tumors, but rarely occur in pure form. Glands often connect with cystic, alveolar-like spaces lined by flattened epithelium, resulting in overlap with the polyvesicular vitelline pattern (fig. 4-38) (see page 128 and figs. 4-46, 4-47). The glands often have enteric features consist-

ing of pseudo-stratified columnar cells with eosinophilic cytoplasm and an apparent apical brush border, but, unlike many teratomatous glands, lack a peripheral smooth muscle layer. A branching and anastomosing pattern is common or more simple, tubular glands may occur (figs. 4-39, 4-40). In some cases the glandular component can be prominent and complex (fig. 4-41). Such enteric-type glands were identified in 34 percent of yolk sac tumors in one series (183). The nuclei of such glandular structures appear less atypical than those of the adjacent nonglandular component. The glands may show basal cytoplasmic vacuolation reminiscent of early secretory phase endometrium (endometrioid-like). Purely glandular yolk sac tumor of intestinal or endometrioid-like type occurs rarely (fig. 4-42), sometimes with elevated serum AFP (119).

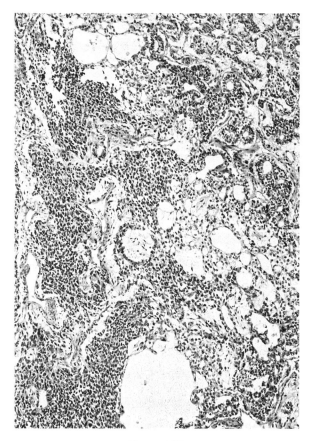

Figure 4-37
YOLK SAC TUMOR
Microcystic and solid patterns, the latter having a blastema-like appearance, are seen.

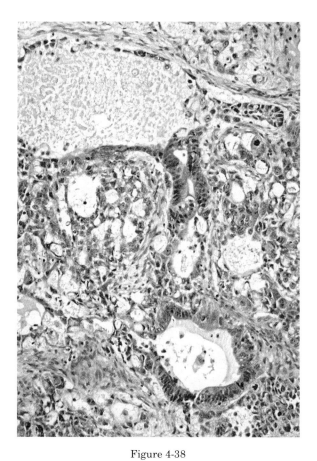

Figure 4-38
YOLK SAC TUMOR
Well-defined foci of columnar, glandular epithelium focally connect to a cystic (vesicle-like) space.

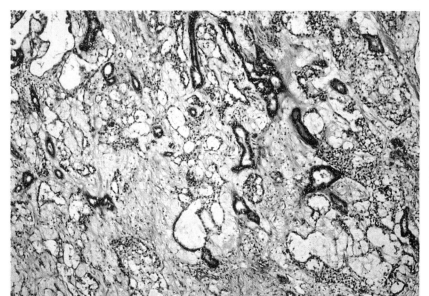

Figure 4-39
YOLK SAC TUMOR
Numerous tubular glands are present in this tumor which also has microcystic and macrocystic patterns.

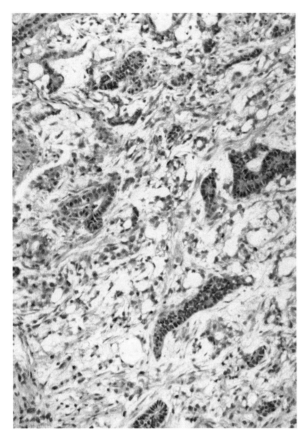

Figure 4-40
YOLK SAC TUMOR: GLANDULAR
AND MICROCYSTIC PATTERNS
The glands in this example are of simple, tubular type.

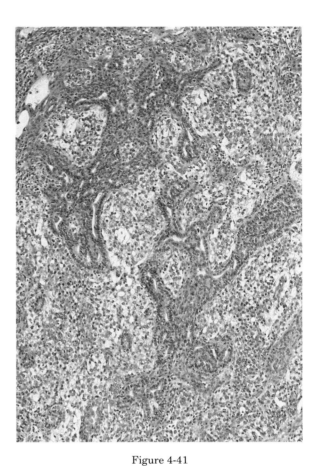

Figure 4-41
YOLK SAC TUMOR
The glandular component in this tumor is prominent, complex, and anastomosing.

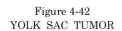

Figure 4-42
YOLK SAC TUMOR
This purely glandular tumor is composed of glands resembling secretory endometrium, with clear supranuclear and subnuclear cytoplasm.

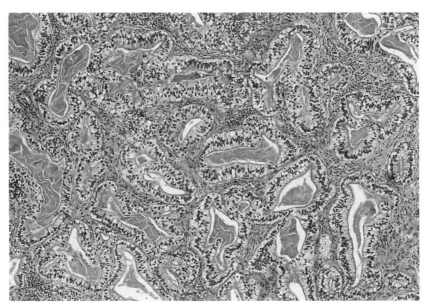

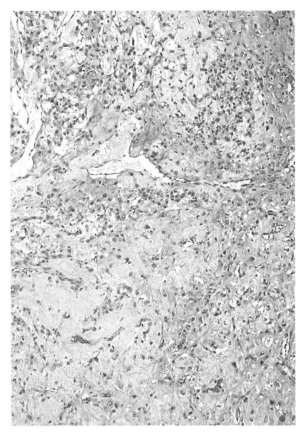

Figure 4-43
YOLK SAC TUMOR
A microcystic pattern (top) blends into a hypocellular, myxoid pattern, with stellate to spindle cells and frequent vessels. This pattern has been described as mesenchyme-like.

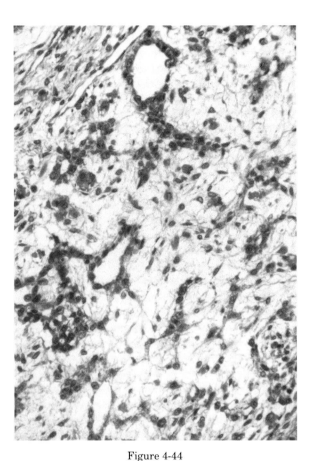

Figure 4-44
YOLK SAC TUMOR
Scattered rhabdomyoblasts are present in a myxoid zone.

A myxoid component is common, particularly in association with a reticular pattern (figs. 4-28, 4-43). The epithelial cells of the reticular pattern gradually disperse into a hyaluronic acid–rich, myxoid stroma and acquire stellate and spindled profiles (fig. 4-43), thereby constituting a myxomatous pattern (168). In addition to the spindled cells in the myxoid background, these foci have a prominent component of blood vessels that led Teilum (181) to describe such areas as "angioblastic mesenchyme." It was his belief that these zones recapitulated the extraembryonic mesenchyme (or the magma reticulare) of the developing gestation. It is noteworthy that such cells, while having a spindled, mesenchymal-like appearance, retain cytokeratin reactivity, supporting their derivation from the epithelial component of reticular yolk sac tumor (152). Michael and

co-workers (152) described the pluripotential nature of the cells of this mesenchyme, noting that they have the capacity to differentiate into skeletal muscle and cartilage (fig. 4-44). The development of such differentiated somatic tissues creates semantic difficulties with respect to the classification of such cases as yolk sac tumor variants or teratomas. Our own approach is to accept scattered foci of such somatic differentiation in an otherwise pure yolk sac tumor as yolk sac tumor, but to regard cohesive nodules of differentiated mesenchyme as teratomatous structures.

Rare yolk sac tumors have a cellular, neoplastic spindle cell component (fig. 4-45). Such foci develop in continuity from classic yolk sac tumor patterns, usually either reticular or myxomatous ones. These sarcomatoid foci retain reactivity for low molecular weight cytokeratins, indicating their derivation from epithelial yolk sac tumor elements and assisting in the distinction

127

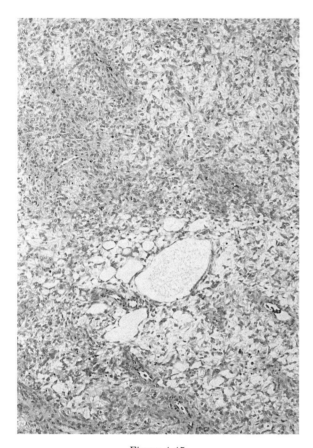

Figure 4-45
YOLK SAC TUMOR
A cellular, focally sarcomatoid pattern composed of oval and spindle cells is adjacent to a microcystic pattern.

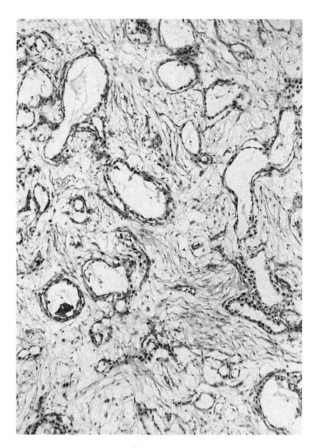

Figure 4-46
YOLK SAC TUMOR:
POLYVESICULAR VITELLINE PATTERN
Vesicles, some with constrictions (upper left), are present in a loose, hypocellular stroma. The vesicles recapitulate the embryonic subdivision of the primary yolk sac (larger) into the secondary yolk sac (smaller). (Fig. 3-19 from Young RH, Scully RE: Testicular tumors. Chicago: ASCP Press, 1990:57.)

from tumors in the sex cord–stromal category that may share some histologic features. Although not well described in the testis, similar cases of mediastinal yolk sac tumor with a prominent spindle cell component are the subject of a recent report (155). Although some may regard these rare tumors as variants of myxomatous or reticular patterns, we prefer to categorize this pattern separately to highlight the need to consider the possibility of yolk sac tumor when confronted with a spindle cell proliferation in limited material.

The polyvesicular vitelline pattern of yolk sac tumor consists of cysts scattered in a variably cellular mesenchyme, which ranges from edematous to fibrous (fig. 4-46). Some of the cysts often show an eccentric constriction, giving rise to a lopsided, figure-eight shape (fig. 4-47). These cysts are lined by a layer of flattened to columnar

epithelium. Often a transition from flattened to a cuboidal or columnar epithelium can be identified within a cyst near the point of constriction (fig. 4-47). The taller epithelial cells may show basal or apical vacuolation of the cytoplasm. Sometimes the lining epithelium has a definite enteric appearance, with apical brush borders. Teilum (180) compared the constricted vesicles of this pattern to the embryonic subdivision of the primary yolk sac into the secondary yolk sac. The polyvesicular vitelline pattern is infrequent in testicular yolk sac tumors (about 8 percent of cases [183]), where it is generally associated with other yolk sac tumor patterns; it occurs more commonly in ovarian neoplasms. It can have a deceptively bland appearance.

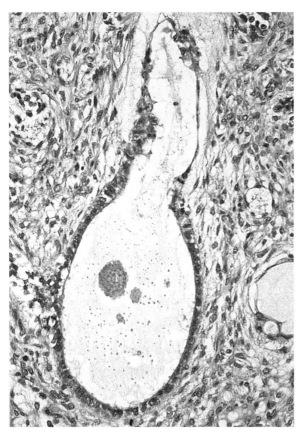

Figure 4-47
YOLK SAC TUMOR
Polyvesicular vitelline pattern shows a single vesicle with epithelium that varies from flat to columnar. Note the eccentric constriction of the vesicle.

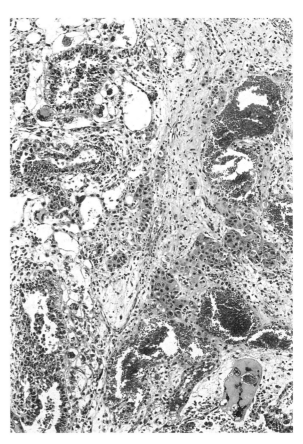

Figure 4-48
YOLK SAC TUMOR
Clusters of hepatoid cells with abundant eosinophilic cytoplasm are at the periphery of a nodule of microcystic yolk sac tumor. Occasional syncytiotrophoblast cells are also present.

Hepatoid patterns occur in approximately 20 percent of yolk sac tumors (135,183), commonly as small clusters of liver-like cells arranged in nests, tubules, or trabeculae (fig. 4-48); the cells are usually intensely immunoreactive for AFP. They are polygonal and have abundant eosinophilic cytoplasm and a large nucleus with a single, prominent nucleolus (fig. 4-49). Bile canaliculi can be identified, but we have not seen bile production. In rare instances, hepatoid foci may compose a large area or even the majority of a yolk sac tumor. Hyaline globules occur commonly in hepatoid foci.

Parietal differentiation refers to the presence of eosinophilic bands of basement membrane material in the extracellular space between neoplastic cells (fig. 4-50). The basement membrane material is felt to represent a recapitulation of the parietal layer of the embryonic yolk sac of the rodent that synthesizes a thick basement membrane (Reichert's membrane) (181,183). It is a common but typically focal finding in yolk sac tumors; 92 percent of cases in a series of 50 yolk sac tumors (of which 36 were testicular in origin) contained such foci (183). Rarely, the basement membrane material may become a predominant element, with neoplastic cells embedded within an eosinophilic matrix (fig. 4-51). Patients with metastatic testicular yolk sac tumors treated by chemotherapy may have recurrences with a pure parietal pattern.

Several series have addressed the frequency of various yolk sac tumor patterns when a four-pattern classification system consisting of reticular, endodermal sinus, solid, and polyvesicular vitelline is used (133,143,183). Most agree that the reticular pattern is most common, followed by solid

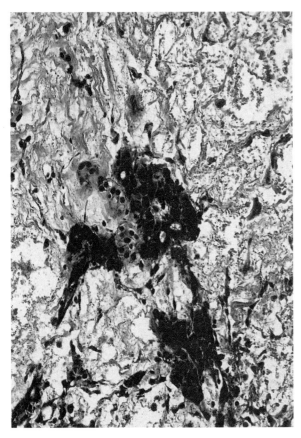

Figure 4-49
YOLK SAC TUMOR
Clusters of hepatoid cells with vesicular nuclei and prominent nucleoli in a myxomatous yolk sac tumor.

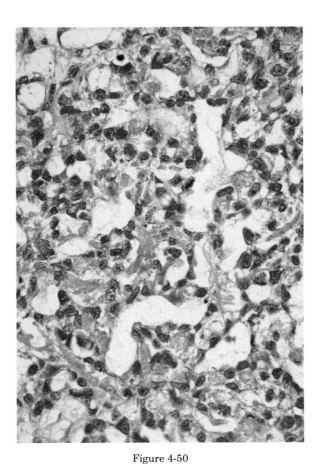

Figure 4-50
YOLK SAC TUMOR
Deposits of eosinophilic, basement membrane material in the extracellular space in a reticular pattern.

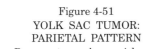

Figure 4-51
YOLK SAC TUMOR:
PARIETAL PATTERN
Basement membrane-rich matrix contains scattered neoplastic cells. Residual microcysts are also apparent.

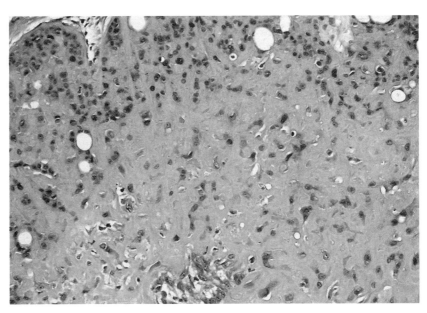

and endodermal sinus patterns; the polyvesicular vitelline pattern is unusual (133,183). Macrocystic, papillary, and endodermal sinus patterns appear to occur more prominently in childhood yolk sac tumors than in the adult form. Jacobsen (133) analyzed the frequency of several yolk sac tumor patterns in a series of 70 cases. She recognized both a "vacuolated network" (91 percent of cases) and a microcystic pattern (67 percent), which we consider to be variants of a reticular pattern. Myxomatous patterns occurred in 51 percent, macrocysts in 44 percent, solid patterns in 27 percent, hepatoid foci in 23 percent, labyrinthine structures in 17 percent, and endodermal sinuses in 9 percent. It is evident that although endodermal sinus structures are a most distinctive feature of yolk sac tumor, one cannot rely on their presence to establish a diagnosis.

Another characteristic finding is the presence of hyaline eosinophilic globules in the cytoplasm of neoplastic cells. These are not specific for yolk sac tumor and can be observed in other malignant neoplasms as well; however they are rarely identified in other forms of testicular germ cell tumor (183). The globules tend to occur in clusters and vary in size from 1 μm or less to more than 50 μm in diameter (fig. 4-52). Sometimes they can be confused with erythrocytes but they are more variable in size and are PAS positive and diastase resistant. Only occasional globules stain for AFP, although other serum proteins may be present. Many observers have felt that they occur both extracellularly and intracellularly; electron micrographs of non-necrotic yolk sac tumor elements, however, verify that the globules are typically intracellular. It is possible that they appear to be extracellular by light microscopy as a consequence of necrosis and cytolysis, with extrusion into the extracellular space, or because the intact cytoplasm that surrounds them is too scant to be seen by light microscopy.

Hematopoietic foci can be identified in an occasional yolk sac tumor, most commonly erythroblasts within the blood vessels or mesenchymal component of the tumor.

An interesting if incompletely understood aspect of yolk sac tumors is the rare association of childhood cases with IGCNU (141,149) whereas adult tumors show IGCNU in most instances. This has led to the hypothesis that childhood yolk sac tumor results from an oligoclonal intratubular

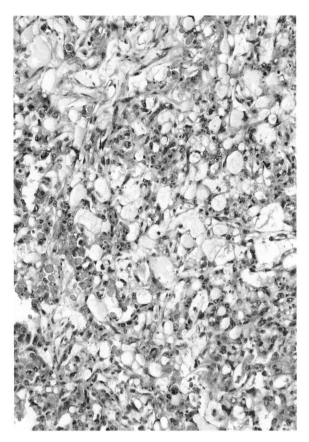

Figure 4-52
YOLK SAC TUMOR
Numerous round, eosinophilic hyaline globules in a microcystic yolk sac tumor.

malignant transformation, in contrast to adult cases (148).

Immunohistochemical Findings. The frequency of AFP positivity in three series of yolk sac tumors varied from 74 to 100 percent (134, 156,160), although childhood cases were more often negative in one study (156), but not in a second (184). Positivity, manifest as a cytoplasmic blush, can be quite focal and patchy (fig. 4-53). Hepatoid foci are often intensely positive. The hyaline globules are usually AFP negative. The AFP staining seen in solid yolk sac tumors is of considerable value in the distinction from seminoma (fig. 4-54) (Table 3-1).

Alpha-1-antitrypsin has been identified in about 50 percent of yolk sac tumors (134,160). Reactivity to carcinoembryonic antigen (CEA) has been reported in occasional cases; 4 of 32 cases (13

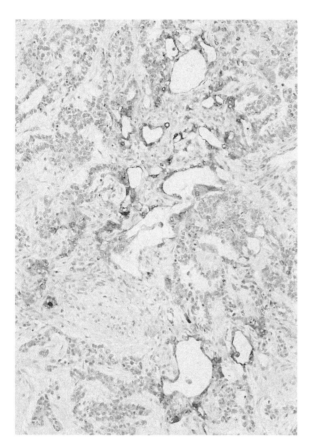

Figure 4-53
YOLK SAC TUMOR
AFP is positive in a microcystic region.

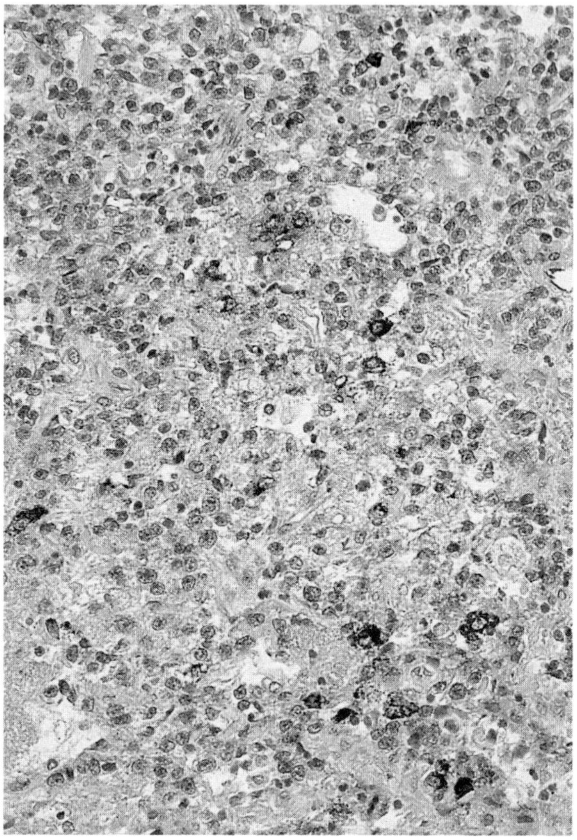

Figure 4-54
YOLK SAC TUMOR
Scattered AFP-positive tumor cells in a solid pattern.

percent) in two series were positive (136,160). The reactivity was apparently localized to enteric glands (136,183). Cytokeratin marks almost all cases and is usually intensely positive (153,160,173); vimentin is routinely seen in the spindle cell component (153). EMA is usually negative (18 out of 19 cases [160]) and therefore useful in helping to distinguish yolk sac tumor from somatic carcinomas in metastatic sites. PLAP reactivity varied from 1 to 85 percent in four studies (115,147,160,172). Laminin is identifiable in the basement membrane component (184), and positivity for albumin, ferritin, neuron-specific enolase, and Leu-7 has been reported in some cases (136,160). p53 is heterogeneously positive in yolk sac tumor (110), and CD34 occurs in a minority of cases, which contrasts with its negativity in seminoma and embryonal carcinoma (172). Also in contrast to embryonal carcinoma, CD30 is absent (122,125,

164,172), and the staining with a cytokeratin cocktail (AE1/AE3 and CAM 5.2) tends to be stronger (172). Two experimental monoclonal antibodies may show some specificity for yolk sac tumor versus other germ cell tumors but have not been employed diagnostically (127).

Different patterns of yolk sac tumor tend to show different immunohistochemical profiles (Amin MB, unpublished observations, 1997). AFP reactivity occurs with greatest frequency in hepatoid, glandular, polyvesicular vitelline, microcystic, and endodermal sinus patterns, whereas myxoid foci are more frequently negative. CD34 reactivity may be seen in glandular, reticular, polyvesicular vitelline, and myxomatous patterns.

Ultrastructural Findings. Electron microscopic examination shows clusters of epithelial cells conjoined by tight junctional complexes and desmosomes (fig. 4-55) and occasionally forming extracellular lumens with apical microvilli.

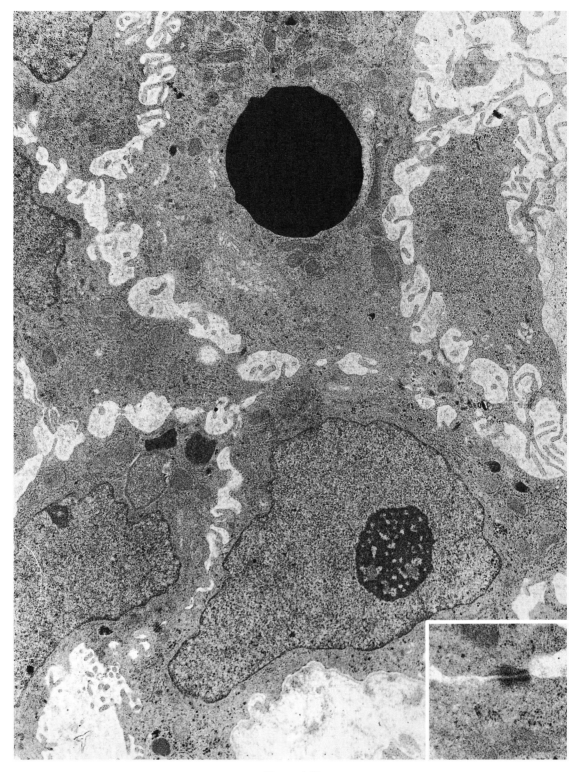

Figure 4-55
YOLK SAC TUMOR

Electron micrograph of a yolk sac tumor with a solid pattern. Note the prominent cytoplasmic processes in the extracellular space, mitochondria often surrounded by rough endoplasmic reticulum, and a densely osmiophilic intracytoplasmic inclusion, representing a hyaline globule. Desmosomes connect adjacent cells (inset) (X8,400; inset X24,000).

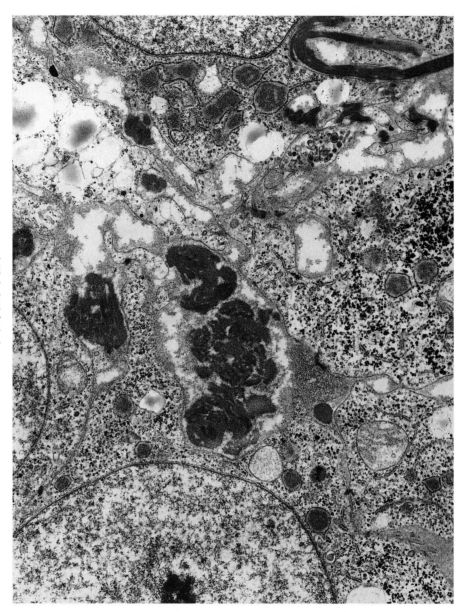

Figure 4-56
YOLK SAC TUMOR
Basement membrane material is present within dilated cisternae of endoplasmic reticulum and also appears as osmiophilic, irregularly shaped deposits in the extracellular space. Note the prominent glycogen particles in the cytoplasm (X15,700).

Abundant extracellular spaces frequently contain bands and irregularly shaped globular deposits of electron-dense basement membrane material (fig. 4-56) (128,161,183), with similar material in the dilated cisternae of the rough endoplastic reticulum of the adjacent cells (174). The deposits within the endoplasmic reticulum often have a central lucent zone, creating a doughnut-like appearance (173). In addition, some cells may show nonmembrane-bound, densely osmiophilic, homogeneous, round cytoplasmic globules corresponding to the hyaline globules (fig. 4-55) (159,183). Glycogen may be conspicuous (128,170). The nuclei are usually irregular in shape and have a thread-like nucleolonema, as seen in seminoma. Enteric glands have microvilli with long anchoring rootlets (fig. 4-57) and glycocalyx with glycocalyceal bodies, as seen in intestinal absorptive cells (183).

Special Diagnostic Techniques. Karyotypic analysis of childhood yolk sac tumors failed to identify the i(12p) marker chromosome that is characteristic of postpubertal testicular germ cell tumors (163,165), but showed frequent

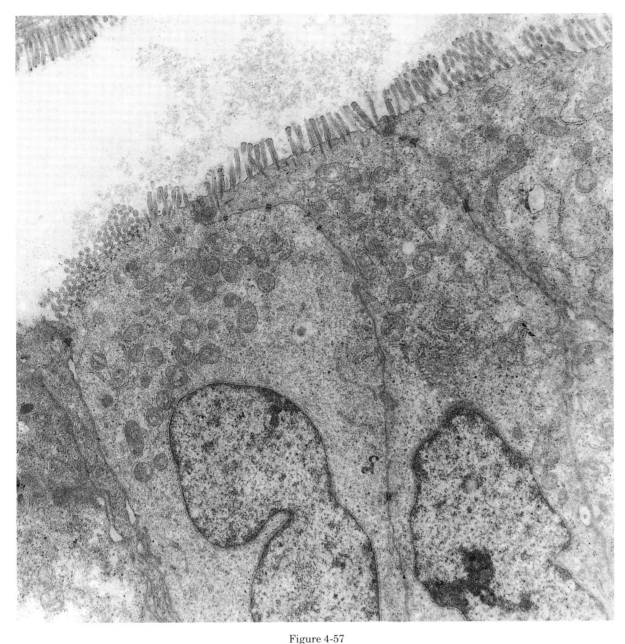

Figure 4-57
YOLK SAC TUMOR
Portion of a glandular pattern in a yolk sac tumor showing prominent apical microvilli with cytoplasmic rootlets (X8,400).

anomalies of chromosomes 1p, 6q, and 3q (165). Furthermore, ploidy analysis of 10 childhood yolk sac tumors demonstrated a diploid DNA value in 3 cases, while the remaining cases showed a peritetraploid value (121). The average DNA index in pediatric cases was 1.91 compared to 1.43 for adult nonseminomatous germ cell tumors, which were rarely diploid (121). These observations, in conjunction with the usual absence of IGCNU in childhood yolk sac tumors (141,149), indicates a different formative pathway. Recent studies using fluorescence in situ hybridization and chromosome-specific probes, however, indicate some numerical chromosomal aberrations in pediatric yolk sac tumors that are also identified in adult cases (138).

Some insight into the formation of yolk sac tumor has been gained by xenograft cultures. Cells from a mixed germ cell tumor that were grown in vitro produced tumors in nude mice that were initially composed of embryonal carcinoma and yolk sac tumor, but which later had the appearance of yolk sac tumor with a peripheral rim of embryonal carcinoma, supporting the differentiation of embryonal carcinoma into yolk sac tumor (185). Additional work using in vitro germ cell lines derived from human tumors showed the potential for differentiation of some but not all embryonal carcinoma cells into yolk sac tumor (158). The xenograft studies of Raghavan and co-workers (154,169) suggest that seminoma may also differentiate to yolk sac tumor, and Czaja and Ulbright (120) supported this concept in their report of several cases of seminoma with peripheral differentiation to yolk sac tumor.

Cytologic Findings. Yolk sac tumor forms tightly arranged, rounded clusters on smears derived from aspirations (108,109). A characteristic pattern is the association of such clusters with a loosely cohesive spindle cell component. The spherical masses may be covered by a layer of flattened tumor cells, but the branching capillary patterns seen in aspirations of embryonal carcinomas are not identified (109). A vague papillary arrangement has been described in several cases (123). The nuclei are ovoid, with irregular nuclear membranes, coarse chromatin, and one or more nucleoli (108). Two cell types have been described, distinguished by their cytoplasmic appearances (108): one has distinct cell borders and a solid cytoplasm with only small vacuoles; the other has indistinct cellular borders, tending to form syncytial clusters of cells, and has a hypervacuolated or bubbly cytoplasm (108,123). The background of yolk sac tumor is often myxoid, with foamy histiocytes (muciphages) (108,123). In addition, intracytoplasmic hyaline globules and intercellular basement membrane material can be identified in some cases (108,123). Seminoma, in contrast to yolk sac tumor, lacks hypervacuolated cells (108).

Differential Diagnosis. The differentiation of solid pattern yolk sac tumor and seminoma is discussed in chapter 3. From a clinical standpoint this distinction is much more crucial than the differentiation of embryonal carcinoma from yolk sac tumor. The latter distinction, however,

may be important in assessing the appropriateness of surveillance-only management, since a yolk sac tumor component has been associated with a decreased frequency of relapse (145). Both embryonal carcinoma and yolk sac tumor may have glandular and papillary patterns, and their distinction is discussed in the section on embryonal carcinoma at the beginning of this chapter. There remain occasional cases in which it is almost arbitrary whether a particular focus represents yolk sac tumor or embryonal carcinoma; our experience with such cases is that the remainder of the neoplasm shows areas of both tumor types and such foci are probably transitional forms. CD30 and AFP stains (Table 3-1) can assist with this differential.

Juvenile granulosa cell tumor is a major consideration in the differential diagnosis of infants with yolk sac tumor (see chapter 6). Juvenile granulosa cell tumors usually occur in infants under 3 months of age, while yolk sac tumor, in our experience and that of others (124a), tends to occur in patients older than 3 months, with rare exceptions (140a). The solid and cystic areas, the latter representing follicle-like structures (117,144), of juvenile granulosa cell tumor may be confused with the solid and reticular-cystic patterns of yolk sac tumor. A high mitotic rate may be seen in each tumor. However, the cells in most juvenile granulosa cell tumors are less primitive in appearance than those of a yolk sac tumor, and the presence of other recognizable yolk sac tumor patterns facilitates proper classification, as does the demonstration of intracellular AFP which does not occur in juvenile granulosa cell tumor. Serum AFP levels in young infants may not be useful in the differential since they do not fall into the "normal" adult range until 8 months of age (186). Stains for inhibin A may be useful in this differential since they are usually positive in juvenile granulosa cell tumor and negative in the limited experience with testicular yolk cell tumor (Kommoss F, unpublished observations, 1998).

Rare purely glandular yolk sac tumors may be confused with immature teratoma (fig. 4-42). The enteric glands of yolk sac tumor lack a circumferential smooth muscle component, unlike most such glands in teratomas (151). In addition, they often branch extensively, unlike the typically more simplified, oval to round glands of teratoma. Additionally teratomatous glands are more evenly distributed with other teratomatous foci, in contrast to yolk sac tumor. In our opinion, strong and more than focal AFP reactivity also favors yolk sac tumor, although staining for AFP may be seen in teratomatous glands.

Sarcomatoid patterns of yolk sac tumor may resemble unclassified forms of sex cord–stromal tumor. The admixture with more distinctive yolk sac tumor patterns, the association with IGCNU, and strong cytokeratin reactivity are features of yolk sac tumor that are useful in this uncommon differential diagnosis.

Invasion of the rete testis by germ cell tumor elements may provoke a hyperplastic reaction of the epithelium, with the development of vacuoles and intracytoplasmic hyaline globules that may be misinterpreted as reticular yolk sac tumor (182). Differentiation depends on the scanning magnification observation of the characteristic branching pattern of the rete testis, and the high-power observation of the bland cytologic features of the hyperplastic rete epithelial cells (182) (see pages 322, 323).

Treatment and Prognosis. The treatment of adults with yolk sac tumor (almost always as a component of a mixed germ cell tumor) does not differ from that outlined for nonseminomatous tumors in the section on embryonal carcinoma.

The approach to pediatric yolk sac tumors remains controversial. The current trend is conservative management of patients who have clinical disease limited to the testis and who lack postorchiectomy elevation of serum AFP. These patients receive close follow-up after radical orchiectomy rather than retroperitoneal lymph node dissection. Chemotherapy may be instituted if relapse occurs (116). The rationale for this approach is based on the more frequent early stage status of pediatric yolk sac tumor compared to adult-type nonseminomatous tumors, with 80 to more than 90 percent of neoplasms confined to the testis at diagnosis (129,139,171). It is also held that pediatric yolk sac tumors behave less aggressively than adult nonseminomatous germ cell tumors (150, 184) and that the frequency of retroperitoneal metastases is low (4 to 14 percent) (129,142), with metastases more commonly developing by hematogenous routes to the lungs (112,124,129). Current chemotherapy is quite effective in treating patients who relapse. Others, however, advocate staging lymph node dissection based on their belief that the nodal metastatic rate is higher than the usual quoted figures and that some yolk sac tumors are not associated with AFP elevation, making early diagnosis of relapse on surveillance-only protocols difficult (140); Kaplan et al. (139) identified AFP elevations in only 84 of 109 (77 percent) prepubertal boys with yolk sac tumor at presentation.

Most recent studies using the latest chemotherapeutic and surgical strategies for treating patients with testicular germ cell tumors do not discriminate between patients having nonseminomatous tumors with and without a yolk sac tumor component. Statistics for patients with nonseminomatous tumors in general are therefore applied to adults having a component of yolk sac tumor in a mixed germ cell tumor. There is, however, evidence that the presence of a yolk sac tumor component in a stage I mixed germ cell tumor of the testis may convey a relatively better prognosis than neoplasms lacking a yolk sac tumor component (126,145). In a study examining surveillance management for postorchiectomy patients with clinical stage I (Royal-Marsden system) nonseminomatous tumors, a multivariate analysis identified a yolk sac tumor component as a significant predictor for the absence of relapse. This finding awaits confirmation in other studies. Of note is the fact that yolk sac tumor elements in patients with metastatic (stage III) testicular cancer have been associated with a poor prognosis (146). This information does not necessarily contradict the prior study but may indicate that yolk sac tumor has both less metastatic potential and less chemosensitivity than does embryonal carcinoma. Hence its prognostic significance varies depending on whether or not it has disseminated. In support of this viewpoint is a study documenting a much higher frequency at autopsy of yolk sac tumor elements during the chemotherapeutic era compared to the prechemotherapeutic era (162).

Childhood yolk sac tumor is currently associated with a good prognosis, although there are some controversial aspects. In a literature review (antedating, for the most part, the revolution in the chemotherapeutic management of testicular germ cell tumors) Brosman (112) identified a significant difference in mortality rates for children with yolk sac tumors who were less than 2 years of age (mortality rate of 11 percent) compared to children older than 2 years (mortality rate of 77 percent). A more recent study from the Pediatric Oncology Group found a 91 percent 5-year survival rate in children with (predominantly) testicular yolk sac tumors and failed to identify a difference in survival with respect to age (131). There was, furthermore, no difference in survival noted for different patterns of yolk sac tumor. These essential points were confirmed in a subsequent larger series (139). It may well be that the natural history of childhood yolk sac tumor in the absence of effective chemotherapy is significantly different according to the age of the patient but that recent advances in treatment have improved survival rates for older children and therefore obscured this difference. Stage remains the single most important prognostic factor in childhood yolk sac tumor, with the great majority (84 to 94 percent) of patients presenting with stage I disease (129,139). In patients with metastatic disease, 50 percent were cured by chemotherapy (139). When relapse occurs in children with yolk sac tumor, the preferred site appears to be the lungs.

CHORIOCARCINOMA AND OTHER RARE FORMS OF TROPHOBLASTIC NEOPLASIA

Definition. Choriocarcinoma is a highly malignant tumor displaying trophoblastic differentiation. It is typically composed of an intimate admixture of syncytiotrophoblast and cytotrophoblast cells.

General Features. Pure choriocarcinoma is rare, representing only 0.3 percent of 6,000 testis tumors in the files of the American Testicular Tumor Registry (205). Focal choriocarcinoma is identified in about 8 percent of testicular germ cell tumors upon careful examination (198), mixed with other forms of germ cell tumor. There are no known distinct epidemiologic features.

Clinical Features. Unlike most other testicular germ cell tumors, patients with pure choriocarcinoma tend to present with symptoms related to metastatic disease rather than a testicular mass. This is due to its frequent early and widespread dissemination prior to the development of a palpable lesion. Indeed, a significant number of patients, even after the establishment of a diagnosis of metastatic choriocarcinoma, do

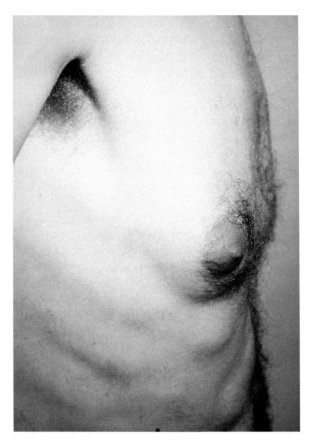

Figure 4-58
GYNECOMASTIA IN A PATIENT
WITH CHORIOCARCINOMA
(Courtesy of Dr. D. Gersell, St. Louis, MO.)

not have palpable abnormalities in the testes. Typical presenting symptoms are hemoptysis, secondary to pulmonary metastases; back pain due to retroperitoneal spread; gastrointestinal bleeding; or neurologic symptoms, secondary to central nervous system involvement. Patients may rarely present with skin metastases (192). The majority of patients are in their second or third decades. No cases have been reported in prepubertal boys. Pure tumors are often associated with marked elevations in serum levels of hCG, with values commonly greater than 100,000 IU/L. As a reflection of hormonal abnormalities associated with hCG elevations, about 10 percent of patients have clinical gynecomastia (215), which may be a presenting complaint (fig. 4-58). Logothetis and co-workers (202) have described a "choriocarcinoma syndrome" dominated by visceral hemorrhage due

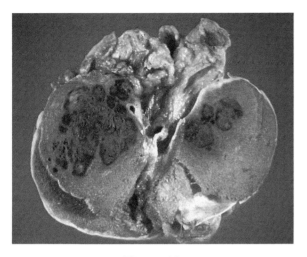

Figure 4-59
CHORIOCARCINOMA
An irregularly shaped, hemorrhagic area in the testis, the typical gross appearance. (Plate IB from Fascicle 8, Second Series.)

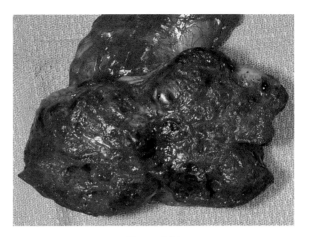

Figure 4-60
CHORIOCARCINOMA
Diffusely hemorrhagic tumor with cystic change and distinct nodules of clotted blood and tumor.

to metastatic choriocarcinoma. Thyrotoxicosis may also occur in these patients secondary to the extreme hCG elevations and the similarity of hCG to thyroid-stimulating hormone (197,202).

Gross Findings. The external appearance of a testis harboring a pure choriocarcinoma is often not distorted, reflecting the typically small size of these tumors. On cut section a centrally necrotic and hemorrhagic nodule is often identified (fig. 4-59), sometimes with ill-defined, gray to tan tissue at the periphery. In other cases, the entire testis may be hemorrhagic, often with some cystic change and separate nodules of clotted blood and tumor (fig. 4-60). Occasionally, only a hemosiderin-containing scar is identified in the testis, despite metastases (see pages 183, 184).

Microscopic Findings. Most choriocarcinomas are extensively hemorrhagic and necrotic (fig. 4-61), often with little viable tumor. Diagnostic foci are typically identified at the periphery of the hemorrhagic/necrotic lesion, where there is usually an admixture of syncytiotrophoblast cells with mononuclear cytotrophoblast cells (fig. 4-62). Identifiable syncytiotrophoblast cells may be found within the hemorrhagic/necrotic area, and such cells may be highlighted by immunostains for hCG (see below). A distinctive feature is prominent blood vessel invasion; clumps of cohesive syncytiotrophoblasts and cytotrophoblasts are often easily identified within vessel lumens. It is

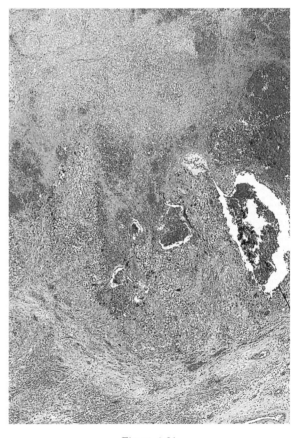

Figure 4-61
CHORIOCARCINOMA
Large areas of hemorrhage and necrosis with a peripheral rim of viable tumor.

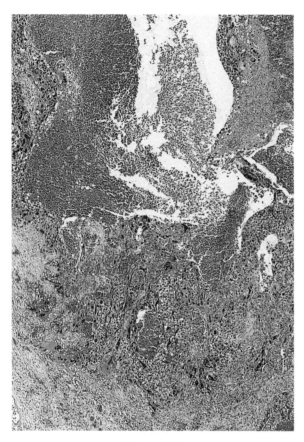

Figure 4-62
CHORIOCARCINOMA
Diagnostic admixture of syncytiotrophoblast and cyto-trophoblast cells at the periphery of a zone of hemorrhage and necrosis.

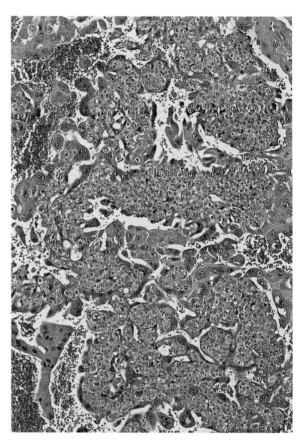

Figure 4-63
CHORIOCARCINOMA
The cytotrophoblast component consists of sheet-like collections of cells with pale cytoplasm and distinct borders that are "capped" by multinucleated cells (syncytiotrophoblasts) with dark, eosinophilic cytoplasm.

necessary to have stringent criteria for the diagnosis of choriocarcinoma since it is common to see syncytiotrophoblast cells without associated cytotrophoblasts in other germ cell tumors.

In the best differentiated examples, the cellular areas show well-defined syncytiotrophoblast cells that "cap" masses of proliferating cytotrophoblast cells by wrapping around their periphery in a pattern often described as villus-like, although stromal cores similar to placental villi are absent (figs. 4-63, 4-64). There is, however, one unique report of a metastatic testicular choriocarcinoma that reproduced villus-like structures with evident stromal cores (212). In other examples, the mixture of syncytiotrophoblasts and cytotrophoblasts appears random (fig. 4-65). In some cases, the cytotrophoblast component predominates, with the syncytiotrophoblast cells being rela-

tively inconspicuous (fig. 4-66). Uncommonly, syncytiotrophoblast cells are rare, creating a "monophasic" appearance (fig. 4-67). Occasionally, areas of distinct separation of syncytiotrophoblast cells are seen; at other times the separation of syncytiotrophoblast from cytotrophoblast is indistinct, but there is a nodular proliferation of trophoblastic cells that range from relatively small to large mononucleated and occasional multinucleated forms (fig. 4-68). Many of the cells in these cases resemble the "intermediate trophoblasts" of gestational tissues (203), having large, single, or occasionally double nuclei and abundant, well-defined, eosinophilic cytoplasm.

Syncytiotrophoblast cells in choriocarcinoma have a variable morphology. They are most easily recognized when they occur as large cells with eosinophilic to amphophilic cytoplasm containing

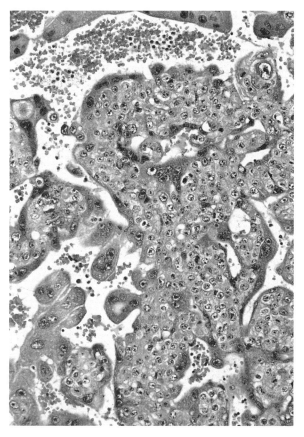

Figure 4-64
CHORIOCARCINOMA
A central collection of pale cytotrophoblast cells is surrounded by multinucleated syncytiotrophoblasts with eosinophilic cytoplasm and vesicular nuclei.

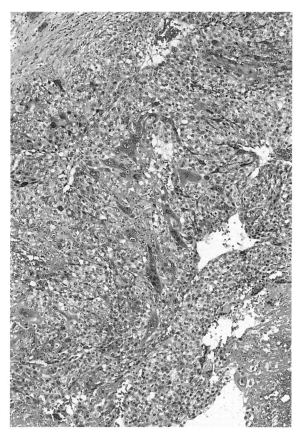

Figure 4-65
CHORIOCARCINOMA
A more or less random admixture of cytotrophoblast cells and larger, syncytiotrophoblast cells, with a subtle impression of the more "classic" mantling of cytotrophoblast by syncytiotrophoblast.

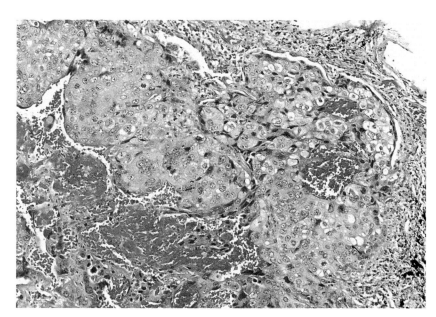

Figure 4-66
CHORIOCARCINOMA
The syncytiotrophoblast cells are less conspicuous and have a focal spindle cell configuration with darkly staining, smudged nuclei.

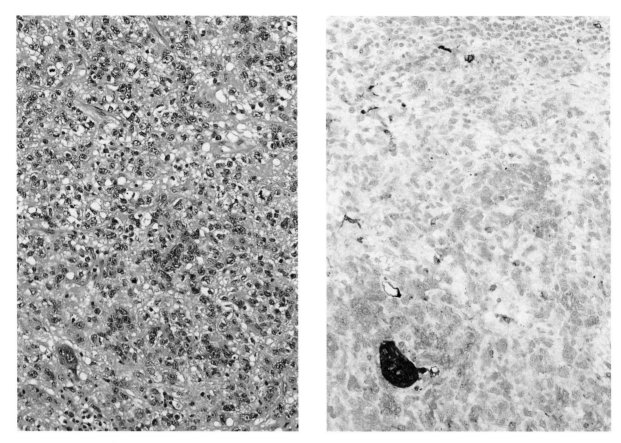

Figure 4-67
"MONOPHASIC" CHORIOCARCINOMA

Left: A sheet-like array of cytotrophoblasts with only a rare syncytiotrophoblast in a "monophasic" choriocarcinoma.

Right: Weak but diffuse positivity for hCG in the predominant cytotrophoblasts, with strong reactivity in the rare syncytiotrophoblasts.

Figure 4-68
CHORIOCARCINOMA

In this case, there is a spectrum of malignant trophoblastic cells from relatively small to large mono-nucleated forms.

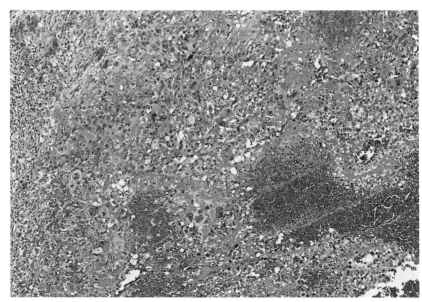

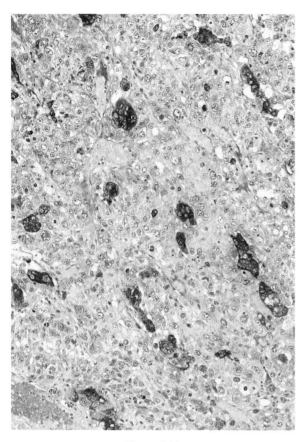

Figure 4-69
CHORIOCARCINOMA
The multinucleated syncytiotrophoblast cells stain intensely with anti-hCG (anti-hCG immunostain).

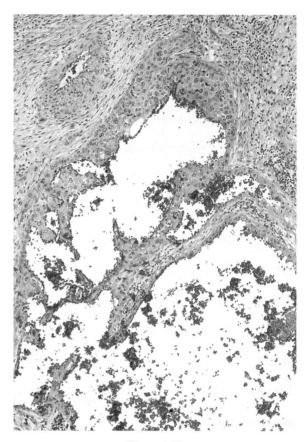

Figure 4-70
LOW-GRADE TROPHOBLASTIC TUMOR
This cystic space contains blood and is lined by squamoid-appearing, non-necrotic trophoblastic cells.

several vesicular to deeply chromatic, irregular, sometimes smudged nuclei (figs. 4-64, 4-65), and having distinct cytoplasmic vacuoles or lacunae (see fig. 3-34). Such vacuoles or lacunae may contain erythrocytes or an eosinophilic precipitate. Nucleoli may be prominent in cells with less dense nuclei. Less distinctive variants of syncytiotrophoblasts occur. In some instances multinucleation is not prominent, but giant nuclei are seen (fig. 4-68). Cytoplasmic vacuoles are often not identified, and in some instances the syncytiotrophoblasts are small and mainly distinguished from their associated cytotrophoblasts by their more deeply staining cytoplasm and somewhat smudged nuclei (fig. 4-66) (200). Syncytiotrophoblasts are mitotically inactive and do not incorporate ^{3}H-thymidine (210), but the mitotic rate in the associated cytotrophoblasts may be high. Often the syncytiotrophoblasts abut thin-walled capillaries that appear to be the source of the hemorrhage in choriocarcinoma.

Cytotrophoblast cells are typically relatively uniform mononucleated cells having clear to amphophilic cytoplasm with well-defined borders and vesicular nuclei (fig. 4-64). They often resemble the cells seen in the solid pattern of yolk sac tumor. In some choriocarcinomas, pleomorphism of the cytotrophoblast component occurs. Immunostains of choriocarcinoma show intense positivity for hCG (fig. 4-69) (see below).

We have seen occasional untreated testicular cases in which mononucleated, squamoid-appearing trophoblastic cells (focally positive for hCG) showed only rare mitoses and lined cystic spaces filled with hemorrhage (fig. 4-70). Lesions with a similar morphology are more frequently identified in metastatic sites following chemotherapy (216), and variants were initially reported in chemotherapy-treated gestational choriocarcinomas (204). Such cases lack the biphasic histology or spectrum of trophoblastic cells associated with choriocarcinoma. It is difficult to believe that such relatively innocuous-appearing lesions portend the more aggressive course generally associated with ordinary choriocarcinoma (see page 146), and future studies may justify the classification of such lesions in a separate subcategory.

A rare form of testicular trophoblastic neoplasia resembles the placental site trophoblastic tumor of the uterus (217,219). The one documented case occurred in a 16-month-old boy and consisted of mostly mononucleate intermediate trophoblast cells in a fibrous to edematous stroma. The cells had a moderate amount of dense, eosinophilic to amphophilic cytoplasm and hyperchromatic, smudged nuclei and occasional binucleate forms (fig. 4-71). Distinct populations of syncytiotrophoblasts and cytotrophoblasts were absent. Small zones of hemorrhage occurred, and the tumor cells invaded vessel walls (217).

Immunohistochemical Findings. Stains for hCG are the most valuable marker for choriocarcinoma and are positive within the syncytiotrophoblast component in essentially all cases (fig. 4-69). They are also positive within occasional, large, mononuclear cells that may represent transitional forms between syncytiotrophoblasts and cytotrophoblasts (199,203,207). The cytotrophoblast cells are generally weakly positive or negative for hCG (figs. 4-67, right, 4-69). Pregnancy-specific beta-1-glycoprotein (SP1) and human placental lactogen (HPL) are also positive within the syncytiotrophoblast cells and within trophoblastic cells of intermediate size (203). Unlike hCG, SP1 and HPL are not identified within the cytotrophoblast cells (203). HPL was strongly and diffusely positive in the above-mentioned placental site trophoblastic tumor of the testis (fig. 4-72), whereas hCG was only focally positive, as expected for intermediate trophoblast cells (217).

Patchy PLAP positivity occurs in 54 percent of choriocarcinomas (207); CEA is demonstrable in 25 percent of cases in both syncytiotrophoblast (201) as well as cytotrophoblast cells (207). Cytokeratins, usually cytokeratins 7, 8, 18, and 19 (193), occur in all cell types (200,207). Unlike seminoma, embryonal carcinoma, and yolk sac tumor, a significant percentage of choriocarcinomas (46

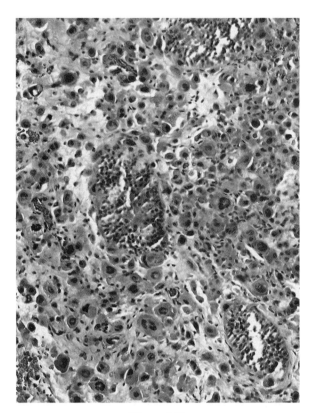

Figure 4-71
PLACENTAL SITE TROPHOBLASTIC TUMOR
Atypical, mostly mononucleate intermediate trophoblast cells in the interstitium. Residual seminiferous tubules are visible.

percent) react with antibodies directed against EMA, mainly in syncytiotrophoblast cells (207). Inhibin is often strongly positive in syncytiotrophoblast cells (Kommoss F, unpublished observations, 1999). A heterogeneous pattern of positivity for p53 has also been identified in choriocarcinomas, but we are unaware that this has any clinical or diagnostic significance (188).

Ultrastructural Findings. On ultrastructural examination, syncytiotrophoblast cells demonstrate several nuclei in a common cytoplasm; there is also a strikingly prominent rough endoplasmic reticulum, with dilated cisternae frequently producing a honeycomb-like pattern (fig. 4-73) (208). The cisternae contain electron-dense, protein-like material that is also identifiable in the surrounding extracellular space (213). Desmosome-like attachments join adjacent cells, both syncytiotrophoblast and cytotrophoblast, and prominent interdigitating microvilli are present on the cell membranes of the syncytiotrophoblasts. In contrast, the cytoplasm of cytotrophoblast cells contains only short profiles of tubular endoplasmic reticulum with numerous free cytoplasmic ribosomes (fig. 4-74). The nuclei of cytotrophoblast cells are more regular and round than those of embryonal carcinoma cells, although heterochromatin clumps and nucleoli remain prominent (213). There also occur cells having features intermediate between syncytiotrophoblasts and cytotrophoblasts (208). The similarity of the nuclei of the syncytiotrophoblast and cytotrophoblast cells supports derivation of the former from the latter (213).

Differential Diagnosis. Choriocarcinoma with extensive hemorrhagic necrosis and scant residual cells must be distinguished from hemorrhagic testicular infarction due to torsion, trauma, thromboembolic disease, or hypercoagulable states. Most patients with testicular infarction have painful, diffuse testicular enlargement, in contrast to most patients with choriocarcinoma. Furthermore, the testis, at least in the earlier stages of hemorrhagic infarction, is edematous, and residual outlines of seminiferous tubules can usually be identified within the infarcted area; such outlines are not identified within the cystic/hemorrhagic portions of extensively necrotic choriocarcinomas. Additional help may be obtained by generous sampling in an attempt to

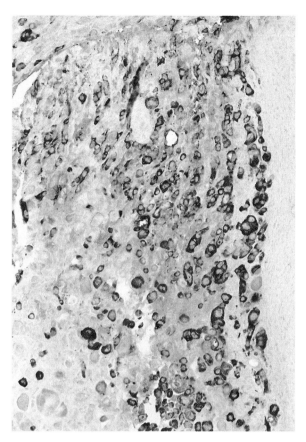

Figure 4-72
PLACENTAL SITE TROPHOBLASTIC TUMOR
Strong positivity for HPL (anti-HPL immunostain).

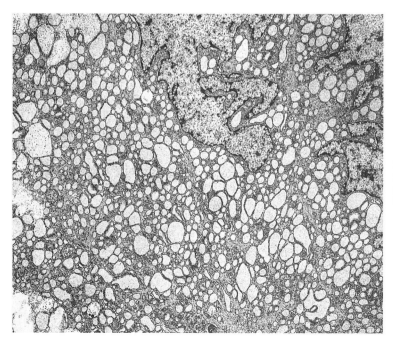

Figure 4-73
CHORIOCARCINOMA

An electron micrograph shows a syncytiotrophoblast cell with very irregularly shaped nuclei in a common cytoplasm. There are numerous dilated cisternae of rough endoplasmic reticulum producing a honeycomb-like pattern.

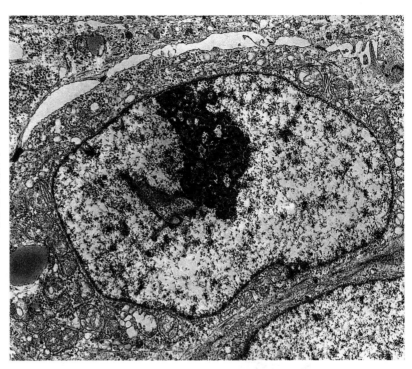

Figure 4-74
CHORIOCARCINOMA

An electron micrograph shows a cytotrophoblast cell with a simple-appearing
cytoplasm contains scattered cisternae of
rough endoplasmic reticulum, mitochondria, and a lipid droplet. The nucleus is
round with a prominent nucleolus. Note
the well-developed desmosomes at upper
left joining it to an adjacent cell.

identify tumor cells. Sections at the periphery of
the lesion and away from it may permit detection
of IGCNU. Immunostains for hCG may identify
residual trophoblastic cells, but the necrosis is
associated with nonspecific staining and a high
background, making interpretation difficult.

Choriocarcinoma must be distinguished from
other testicular germ cell tumors with intermingled syncytiotrophoblast cells. The syncytiotrophoblast cells that occur in seminoma are dispersed as individual cells and small clusters, with
the surrounding neoplasm having the typical
morphology of seminoma including the lymphoid
infiltrate and fibrous septa. In choriocarcinoma,
the cells associated with the syncytiotrophoblasts
are cytotrophoblasts, the tumor usually has a
greater hemorrhagic and necrotic background,
and there is an absence of stromal (fibrous septa)
and lymphoid components.

Most embryonal carcinomas with syncytiotrophoblasts are readily distinguished from
choriocarcinoma. A problem arises in embryonal
carcinomas with the appliqué pattern (see page
106) wherein dark, smudged cells resembling
syncytiotrophoblasts intermix with embryonal
carcinoma cells, creating a biphasic pattern mimicking choriocarcinoma. A lack of hemorrhage in

such a case favors an appliqué pattern of embryonal carcinoma. In difficult cases the differential
is best made with hCG immunostains. We have
seen some cases that have hybrid features of these
two tumors and may represent transitional forms,
as illustrated by Friedman and Moore (196) and
Dixon and Moore (195).

Spread and Metastasis. Choriocarcinoma
may metastasize hematogenously without
lymph node involvement (187). In autopsy studies there is not only involvement of the usual
metastatic sites of testicular germ cell tumors,
but also the lungs (100 percent), liver (86 percent), gastrointestinal tract (71 percent), and
spleen, brain, and adrenal gland (56 percent)
(205). Bredael et al. (190) noted that a disproportionate number of brain metastases at autopsy
in patients with metastatic testicular germ cell
tumors were choriocarcinomas.

Treatment and Prognosis. Because of its
tendency to disseminate widely by hematogenous routes prior to diagnosis, pure choriocarcinoma carries a worse prognosis than other testicular germ cell tumors. Also, a greater amount of
a choriocarcinoma component in mixed germ cell
tumors has an adverse effect on survival (194,195,
206,209). It remains unclear if there is a certain

threshold amount of choriocarcinoma below which a deterioration in prognosis does not occur. Multivariate analyses of clinical prognostic factors in patients with metastatic nonseminomatous germ cell tumors have shown a poor prognosis associated with increased levels of serum hCG (189, 202, 218) and with the identification of choriocarcinomatous or trophoblastic elements in the primary tumor (202,211,214,218). Logothetis et al. (202) described a poor outcome in patients with a "choriocarcinoma syndrome" in whom hemorrhagic visceral metastases, including to the brain, are associated with a high mortality. Despite these findings, some patients with metastatic testicular choriocarcinoma are cured by chemotherapy (191,202). Four of seven patients (57 percent) with metastatic choriocarcinoma, with or without embryonal carcinoma, treated by Logothetis et al. were disease-free on follow-up (202).

The patient with the placental site trophoblastic tumor of the testis was treated by orchiectomy alone and was alive and well 8 years later (217).

TERATOMA

Definition. This is a neoplasm of germ cell origin that differentiates to form somatic-type tissues typical of either adult or embryonic development. Dermoid cyst is recognized as a specific subcategory of teratoma; epidermoid cyst is classified separately (see page 323).

General Features. Teratomas account for about 7 percent of testicular germ cell tumors, although this figure also includes epidermoid cysts (238). Testicular teratomas occur in two distinct age groups, and the prognosis of the lesion differs significantly accordingly (see page 160). They are the second most common germ cell tumor of infancy and childhood, representing 14 to 20 percent of cases (225,241a,250); the mean age at diagnosis is 20 months, and 57 percent occur by 24 months of age. Occurrence beyond 4 years of age is unusual. Teratoma also occurs in postpubertal patients, usually as a component of a mixed germ cell tumor and uncommonly as a pure tumor, in a typical age distribution for a germ cell tumor, most commonly in patients in the second to fourth decades but sporadically in older patients. Teratomatous elements occur in 50 percent of mixed germ cell tumors (222,284).

Associated congenital anomalies have been described in patients with childhood germ cell tumors, including teratomas: inguinal hernia (7 percent), testicular malformation or maldescent (5 percent), other genitourinary tract anomalies (2.5 percent), Down's syndrome (2 percent), Klinefelter's syndrome (1.5 percent), xeroderma pigmentosa (0.5 percent), ataxia (0.5 percent), hemihypertrophy (0.5 percent), spina bifida (0.5 percent), hemophilia (0.5 percent), umbilical hernia (0.5 percent), and retrocaval ureter (0.5 percent) (241). In postpubertal patients, the general epidemiologic features for germ cell tumors appear to apply for teratomas, as detailed in chapter 1.

Manivel et al. (258) noted an absence of IGCNU in the prepubertal testes of patients with teratomas and its frequent presence in postpubertal cases. It was speculated that this reflected a later neoplastic event in the spermatogenic cell line. "Atypical germ cells" adjacent to prepubertal mature teratoma may represent a precursor other than IGCNU, given their usual lack of immunoreactivity with IGCNU markers (PLAP, c-kit) and their different DNA content (243,248,249,271).

It is not unusual for postpubertal patients with pure testicular teratomas to develop metastases that contain nonteratomatous germ cell tumor elements (254,269,274,275). The most likely basis for such a finding, in our opinion, is the development of a precursor element in the testis (usually embryonal carcinoma) that metastasizes but later differentiates in the testis to form teratoma. At the metastatic site, the precursor elements may remain unchanged (or evolve to a different nonteratomatous form) to yield discrepant histologic findings with the testis. Evolution to teratoma may also occur in the metastasis. Evolution to teratoma in both the testis and metastatic site could explain reports of "mature teratoma metastasizing as mature teratoma" (228,251,253,287), although this may also represent direct metastasis of mature teratoma, since vascular invasion by mature teratomatous elements has been identified (263). Alternatively, teratoma in vascular spaces may also represent intravascular "maturation." Regardless, it is important to emphasize that mature teratoma of the adult testis has a definite malignant potential, and maturity should not be equated with benignity (254).

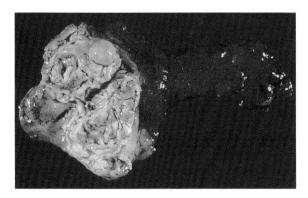

Figure 4-75
TERATOMA
The typical cut surface of a mature teratoma shows multiple cysts that contained serous to mucoid fluid.

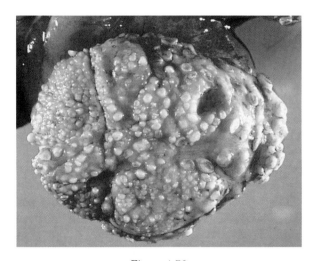

Figure 4-76
TERATOMA
Mainly mature teratoma with nodular excrescences of keratin protruding from small, squamous epithelial-lined cysts. (Fig. 3.38 from Young RH, Scully RE. Testicular tumors. Chicago: ASCP Press, 1990:66.)

Clinical Features. Most patients present because of testicular enlargement. Postpubertal patients, in addition, may have symptoms attributable to metastatic disease. Dixon and Moore (232) identified metastases in 25 percent of patients with teratoma with or without seminoma at presentation; 63 percent of adults with pure teratoma at Indiana University had metastases, but this high proportion possibly reflects selection bias (254). In patients with pure teratoma, the usual serum marker studies are negative, although some adult patients may have marker elevations due to discordant histologies in the testis versus metastases. In addition, several authors have noted that endodermal derivatives in teratomas immunostain for AFP (244,245,263), so some degree of serum AFP elevation is theoretically compatible with a diagnosis of pure teratoma, although we are not aware of any such cases. Children under 8 months may have physiologic AFP "elevation" unrelated to the tumor (241a).

Gross Findings. Pure teratomas are usually nodular and distort the tunica albuginea. Extratesticular extension is rare (231). The cut surface is variably cystic and solid, with the cysts filled with mucoid, keratinous, or serous-type fluid (fig. 4-75). The solid areas may contain translucent, gray-white nodules of cartilage. Small, white to yellow nodular excrescences may represent keratin protruding from the center of squamous epithelial-lined nests (fig. 4-76). Hair is rarely identified except in pure dermoid cysts. Small patches of black pigment often represent melanin-containing choroidal epithelium. Imma-

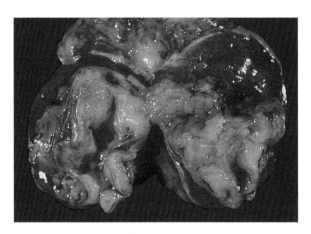

Figure 4-77
IMMATURE TERATOMA
Predominantly solid, encephaloid tissue.

ture tissues are most frequently solid and have an encephaloid, hemorrhagic, or necrotic appearance (fig. 4-77). Dermoid cysts are rare and have a similar appearance to their much more common ovarian counterpart; they are usually unilocular and filled with grumous, keratinous material and hair, with protruding nodules in the cyst wall (fig. 4-78). Particularly large teratomas may be seen in intra-abdominal testes (fig. 4-79) because they do not come to clinical attention as quickly as those in the scrotal sac. Enigmatically, small mature teratomas in adult

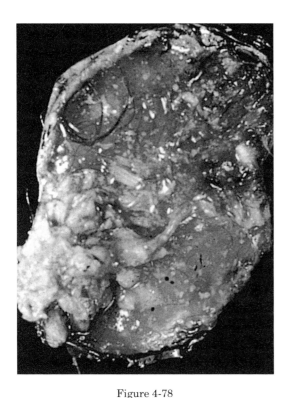

Figure 4-78
DERMOID CYST
A hair-containing cyst with central, keratinous material.
(Fig. 57 from Fascicle 8, 2nd Series.)

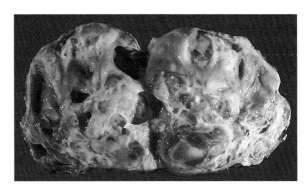

Figure 4-79
MATURE TERATOMA
This large neoplasm replaced an intra-abdominal testis.

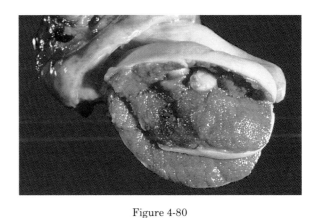

Figure 4-80
MATURE TERATOMA
The patient with this small tumor presented with a retroperitoneal metastasis that contained yolk sac tumor.

testes may be associated with massive retroperitoneal metastases of a different type (fig. 4-80).

Microscopic Findings. *Mature Teratoma.* Mature teratomas contain elements closely resembling normal postnatal tissues; they typically, but not invariably, include structures derived from the three germ layers (figs. 4-81–4-86). Nests of squamous epithelium within a fibrous stroma, some centrally cystic and containing keratin (fig. 4-81), are common. Many cysts are lined by glandular epithelium of enteric type, showing both absorptive and goblet cells (fig. 4-84); some contain only mucinous cells. Other glands are lined by ciliated respiratory-type epithelium. Some glands may be architecturally complex, with frequent outpouchings or a cribriform pattern (fig. 4-83).

Attempts at organ formation are frequently identified, with smooth muscle cells encircling enteric and respiratory epithelial-lined glands, and mimicking intestine and bronchus, respectively (fig. 4-84). Nests of transitional epithelium may also be seen. The stromal tissues often consist of hypocellular fibrous tissue and smooth muscle

and, less commonly, adipose tissue. Foci of neuroglia, sometimes with ependymal differentiation, are common, as are islands of hyaline cartilage which often appear cellular (fig. 4-82, right). Bone is less commonly present but may contain hematopoietic marrow. Pigmented, retinal-type epithelium can be identified in occasional cases (fig. 4-85). Kidney, liver, prostate (302a), pancreas, thyroid (fig. 4-87, left), and choroid plexus are unusual. Although there are rare reports of "struma testis," they have not been confirmed immunohistochemically. A focal surface covering of meninges may rarely be seen with neuroglia (238), and we have seen one case in which meninges were prominent (fig. 4-87, right). Foci resembling mixed tumor of the salivary glands are rarely described (238). Silver stains are positive within the endocrine cells of enteric glandular structures.

149

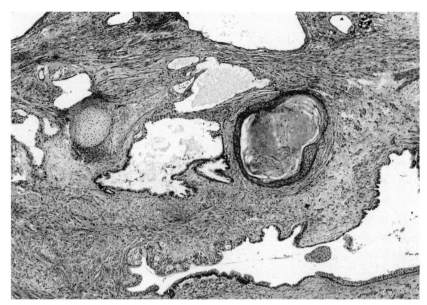

Figure 4-81
TERATOMA
Mature teratoma with a squamous epithelial-lined cyst, a nodule of cartilage, and cysts lined by simple, columnar and cuboidal epithelium. At lower right, the large cyst is partially lined by transitional epithelium.

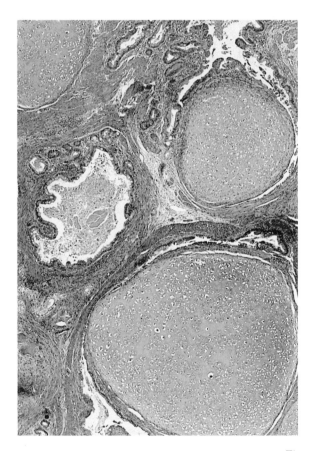

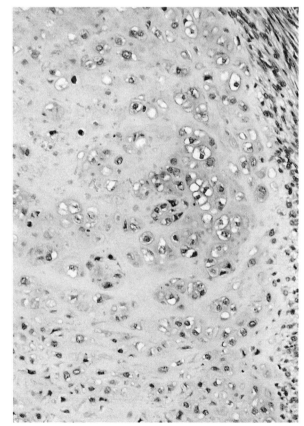

Figure 4-82
TERATOMA
Left: A mature teratoma composed of nodules of cartilage, glandular structures lined by enteric-type epithelium, and fibromuscular stroma.
Right: A cellular cartilaginous component with cytologic atypia.

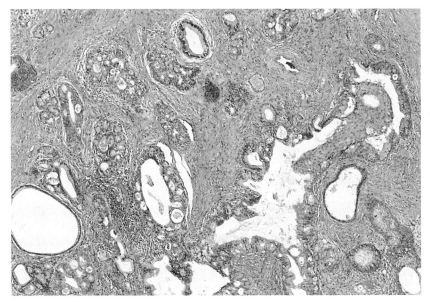

Figure 4-83
TERATOMA
Mature teratoma with complex glands, some with a cribriform pattern.

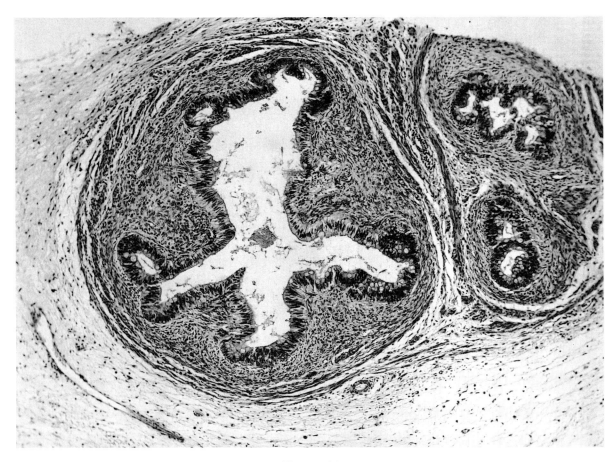

Figure 4-84
TERATOMA
Mature teratoma composed of gut-like structures lined by enteric epithelium with absorptive and goblet cells and encircled by smooth muscle. (Fig. 65 from Fascicles 31b and 32, 1st Series.)

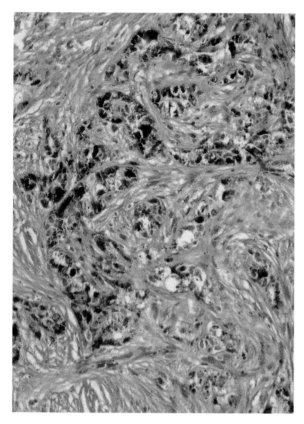

Figure 4-85
TERATOMA
Retinal-type epithelium.

Granulomas may develop in reaction to keratin leakage into the stroma.

Although the microscopic appearance of the elements in mature teratoma generally resembles those normally found in adult tissues, there is often increased cellularity, mild to moderate cytologic atypia, and occasional mitotic activity of both mesenchymal and epithelial tissues (figs. 4-82, 4-86). Such changes are not justification for categorization as immature which is reserved for tumors that resemble embryonic tissues (see below).

In childhood cases, testicular teratomas are usually pure, unassociated with other germ cell tumor types, and many have completely mature histologic features. In contrast to childhood cases, teratomas in postpubertal patients almost always have some immature elements and are usually associated with other forms of germ cell tumor.

Dermoid Cyst. Dermoid cysts are rare, specialized forms of mature teratoma analogous to the common ovarian lesions; they consist of cen-

tral keratinous material, often containing hairs (fig. 4-78), surrounded by a cyst wall composed of keratinizing squamous epithelium with skin appendages, including hair follicles and sebaceous glands (fig. 4-88) (221,223a,224,227,233, 242,285,286). Cartilage, fibrous tissue, and neuroglia may be seen within the cyst wall. It may be that the recently described testicular "pilomatrixoma" is a variant of a dermoid cyst (260a). Metastasis from a pure dermoid cyst has not been reported. This situation contrasts with mature teratoma which has metastatic potential, and, for this reason, "mature teratoma" is an unacceptable substitute for "dermoid cyst." We have not identified IGCNU in the few cases of dermoid cyst we have seen, and the occurrence of IGCNU argues against a diagnosis of dermoid cyst.

Immature Teratoma. Immature teratomas contain elements that resemble normal embryonic tissues. Mildly immature tissues commonly include adipose tissue, often with a myxoid background and prominent vascular pattern (fig. 4-89); fetal-type intestinal glands; and a nonspecific, spindle cell stroma that encircles glands in an apparent recapitulation of developing gastrointestinal or respiratory tract (fig. 4-90). This stroma usually has a modestly cellular, low-grade character (fig. 4-91) but may also be more cellular, mitotically active, and unassociated with a glandular component. Fetal-type hepatic cords may sometimes be identified, often with erythroblasts. More immature elements commonly include neuroepithelium, resembling that of the developing neural tube and embryonic nervous system, and blastomatous tissue resembling the blastema and embryonic tubules of the developing kidney or lung. The neuroepithelium consists of small cells arranged in tubules and rosettes (fig. 4-92), with foci of more diffuse growth. Blastema consists of oval to spindle cells with scant cytoplasm in generally nodular arrays; such foci are often intermingled with primitive-appearing tubules consisting of cuboidal to columnar cells with high nuclear to cytoplasmic ratios and a scant amount of clear to lightly staining cytoplasm (fig. 4-93). Foci may resemble Wilms' tumor (fig 4-94). Sometimes primitive-appearing tubules occur in the absence of blastema (fig. 4-95). Embryonic rhabdomyoblastic tissue is sometimes identified (fig. 4-96), as well as more mature-appearing, fetal-type skeletal muscle. As expanded upon

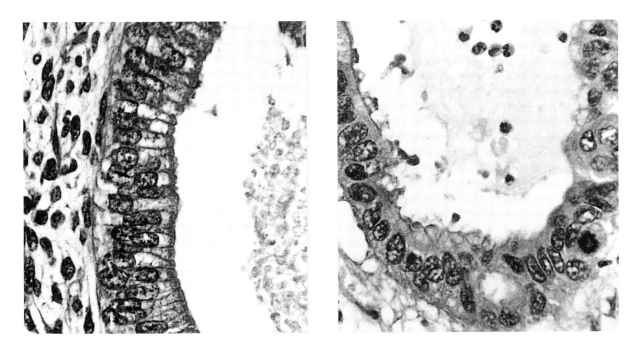

Figure 4-86
TERATOMA

Left: Portion of a teratomatous gland lined by mildly atypical columnar cells and surrounded by a modestly cellular, immature stroma.

Right: Portion of a teratomatous gland showing atypia of the lining epithelium with some loss of polarity, hyperchromasia, and mitotic activity.

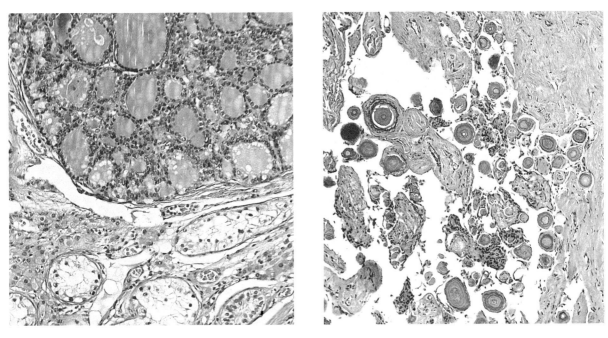

Figure 4-87
TERATOMA

Left: Thyroid tissue is present.
Right: Meningeal tissue with psammoma bodies.

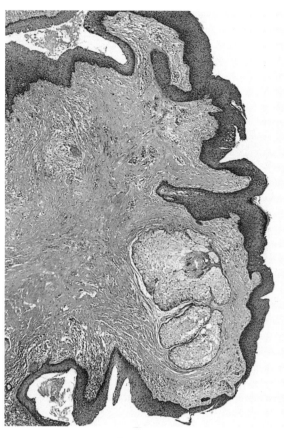

Figure 4-88
DERMOID CYST
The wall of a dermoid cyst consists of a squamous epithelial lining, sebaceous glands, and fibrous stroma.

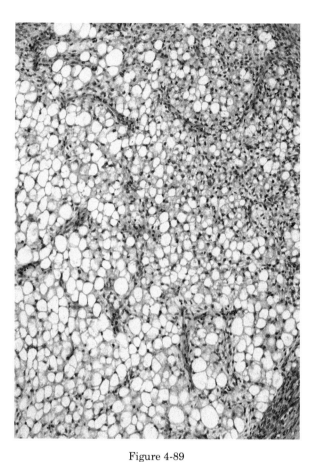

Figure 4-89
TERATOMA
Immature adipose tissue with lipoblastic cells and prominent vascularity.

Figure 4-90
TERATOMA
This immature teratoma has a cellular, spindle cell stroma encircling small, immature glands.

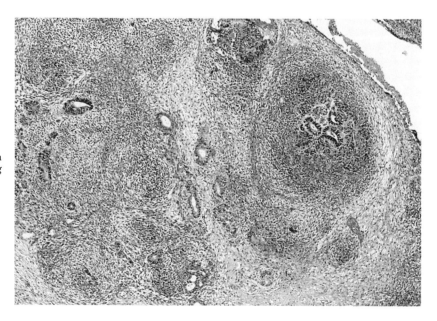

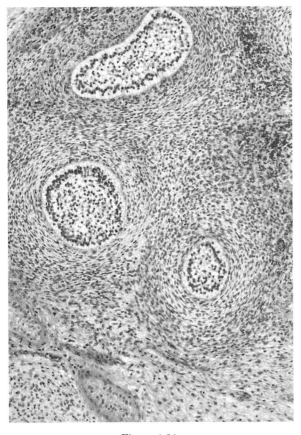

Figure 4-91
TERATOMA
This teratoma of low-grade immaturity has hypercellular, concentric arrays of spindle cells arranged around nests of epithelium.

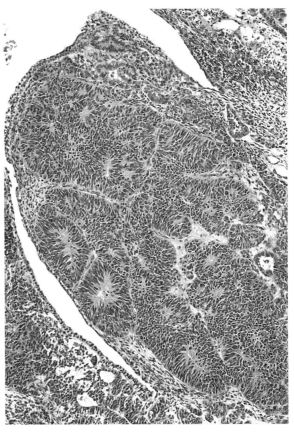

Figure 4-92
TERATOMA
Immature teratoma containing embryonic-appearing neuroepithelium consisting of hyperchromatic cells with lightly eosinophilic cytoplasm arranged in rosettes.

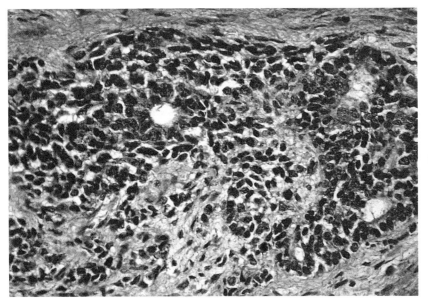

Figure 4-93
TERATOMA
Blastema with primitive-appearing tubules in an immature teratoma.

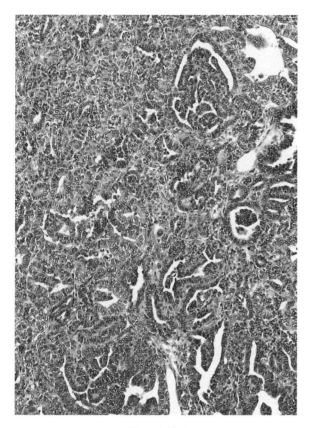

Figure 4-94
BLASTOMATOUS TUMOR IN TERATOMA

There is a large area of primitive, embryonal-type tubules, similar to a monomorphous, well-differentiated tubular pattern of Wilms' tumor.

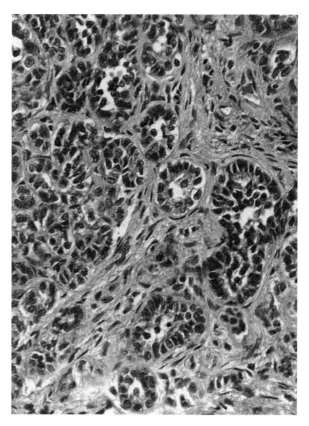

Figure 4-95
TERATOMA
Embryonal tubules in an immature teratoma.

later in this chapter, minor foci resembling primitive neuroectodermal tumor (PNET) (fig. 4-97) do not merit a separate diagnosis unless larger than most of a low-power (4X objective) microscopic field (259).

We grade the degree of immaturity as either high grade (when highly cellular and mitotically active immature elements are identified) or low grade (when less cellular and less mitotically active elements are identified). An estimate of their extent is also given: focal, multifocal, or diffuse. It is has not been shown, however, that this provides any clinically useful information.

Teratoma with a Secondary Malignant Component. This rare lesion is most commonly encountered in adult patients with immature teratomas who develop various tumors of nongerminal type. We prefer to avoid the term "teratoma with malignant transformation" because it implies that teratomas lacking this change are benign, which is

not the case. This phenomenon is much less common in the testis than the ovary where a sizable number of teratomas, particularly in postmenopausal patients, develop squamous cell carcinoma. In the testis, the very rare squamous cell carcinomas are usually of other origins (see chapter 7), although we have seen a case of sarcomatoid squamous cell carcinoma of apparent teratomatous origin. The most commonly identified type of secondary malignant neoplasm in the testis is rhabdomyosarcoma, which may have either an embryonal or alveolar appearance (fig. 4-98), with the usual features of those neoplasms (277b). (Although PNETs are somewhat more common, they are, by the convention established for ovarian tumors, considered a monodermal teratoma [see page 163]). Angiosarcoma is rare (243a). We diagnose such neoplasms when they form a pure nodule of "substantial size" (on the order of half to a whole field viewed with a 4X objective). As long as such elements are scattered

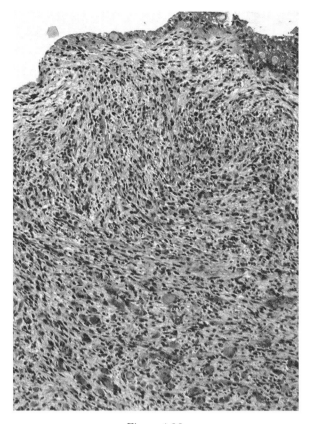

Figure 4-96
TERATOMA

Embryonic rhabdomyoblastic tissue is adjacent to glandular epithelium (top) in an immature teratoma. Distinction of such foci from embryonal rhabdomyosarcoma is made on the basis of their size (see text).

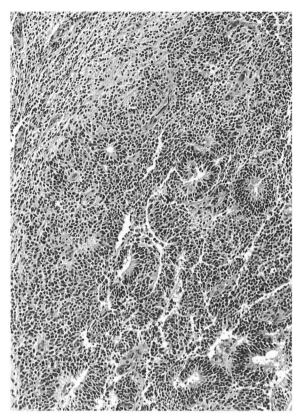

Figure 4-97
FOCUS OF PRIMITIVE NEUROECTODERMAL
TISSUE IN TERATOMA

There is a proliferation of primitive neuroepithelium in sheets, rosettes, and tubules.

among other teratomatous elements, we regard them as immature teratoma.

In rare instances, somatic-type carcinomas develop from the epithelium of mature teratomatous elements, such as adenocarcinomas derived from enteric-type glandular structures. Such carcinomas are recognizable by their pattern of stromal invasion. This occurs less commonly in testicular teratomas than it does in ovarian teratomas.

The significance of a secondary malignant component in a teratoma depends on its location. Ahmed et al. (220) identified five primary testicular tumors with "malignant transformation of teratomatous elements." All of these patients were disease-free following treatment on follow-up ranging from 22 to 120 months. This situation contrasts with 12 patients having "teratoma with malignant transformation" at metastatic sites following chemotherapy, 9 of whom had progres-

sive disease. Comiter et al. (229a) also reported an aggressive course in their study of 18 patients with testicular teratomas "with malignant transformation," but 17 presented with metastatic disease. Motzer and co-workers (263a) reported a poor outcome for patients with incomplete resections. The most common malignancies were sarcomas of various histologic types, although enteric adenocarcinoma and squamous carcinoma also occurred (220,229a). The i(12p) chromosomal anomaly occurs in many of these cases, despite the diverse histologies of the secondary malignant components (263a).

The importance of this lesion has become enhanced due to effective chemotherapy of the usual malignant germ cell elements. Ulbright et al. (282) reported a series of 11 male patients in whom "nongerm cell" malignancies occurred, usually at metastatic sites following chemotherapy directed

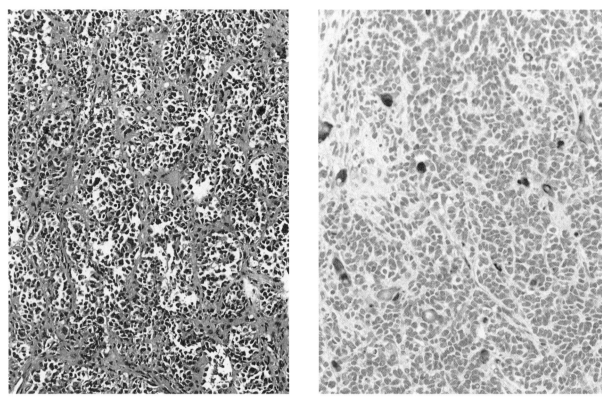

Figure 4-98
RHABDOMYOSARCOMA IN TERATOMA
Left: Rhabdomyoblasts with discohesion and scattered tumor giant cells with the overall features of alveolar rhabdomyosarcoma.
Right: A focus of embryonal rhabdomyosarcoma from a different case consists of small, hyperchromatic, primitive skeletal muscle cells arranged in cords and nests. Scattered cells are reactive for desmin (immunoperoxidase stain with anti-desmin).

against nonseminomatous germ cell tumors. It was felt that the most likely explanation for this phenomenon was selective overgrowth of chemoresistant clones of frankly malignant teratomatous elements following chemotherapy. A variety of malignant phenotypes occurred, although various sarcomas, especially rhabdomyosarcoma, were the most common (258a). More recently it has been suggested that some of these sarcomatous elements may derive from the stromal elements of yolk sac tumor (255,283). Mostofi (262) suggested that small foci of "malignant transformation" of teratomatous elements may be identified in the testicular primary of most, if not all, patients in whom such elements are identified within the metastases, supporting a chemoselection phenomenon. Comiter et al. (229a) found such foci in 52 percent of the primary tumors in their series. The prognosis for patients with metastases containing sarcomatous elements is generally poor (220,229a,255),

in contrast to that of patients having mature teratoma following chemotherapy.

Grading. The grading of immature testicular teratomas remains of unproven value, unlike the situation with immature teratomas of the ovary (265,278). This is because most pure teratomas of the testis occur in children and have a uniformly good prognosis regardless of the presence of immature elements. Additionally, most testicular teratomas in adults, although much more commonly having immature elements than childhood cases, are intermixed with other, aggressively acting germ cell tumor components. The grading of the teratomatous elements in such cases is therefore rendered meaningless. A large series of pure teratomas in adults is difficult to assemble, and the utility of grading in such a series is not ascertained. The prognostic impact of grading would furthermore be complicated by the possibility of discrepant histology in a metastatic lesion (see page 147 and Table 1-3).

Immunohistochemical Findings. The immunohistochemical findings in teratomas reflect those normally found in the components that it reproduces (260,280), and only those of differential diagnostic importance are mentioned here. AFP may be focally positive in the glandular structures of some teratomas; such AFP-positive glands may have either enteric- or respiratory-type epithelium (244). AFP may also be present in cells showing hepatic differentiation (263). Mostofi and Sesterhenn (263) reported AFP positivity in 19 percent of testicular teratomas; Jacobsen et al. (245) reported AFP positivity of teratomatous epithelium in 5 of 14 (36 percent) cases. Alpha-1-antitrypsin is also identified in teratomatous epithelium, with 8 of 14 (57 percent) cases of teratoma reported positive by Jacobsen. CEA and ferritin are positive in about half the cases (245). PLAP is described in the glandular component of teratomas by several authors, with a reported frequency of 4 to 27 percent (226,257,281). The cellular stroma that commonly surrounds glands reacts for vimentin and variably for muscle markers (actin and desmin). p53 and retinoblastoma gene expression may also be identified in teratomatous components (223,277).

Special Diagnostic Techniques. Mature testicular teratomas are frequently aneuploid, with DNA values often in the hypotriploid range (261,266). Also, residual mature teratomatous lesions following chemotherapy have an aneuploid DNA index (261,266,272), with some cases showing further evolution of clones of cells with different aneuploid peaks from the primary tumor (261, 266). The i(12p) marker chromosome has been identified in testicular teratomas, as well as in the residual metastatic mature teratomas resected after chemotherapy (230). The presence of fewer chromosomes in such mature teratomatous metastases compared to the primary tumors argues that chemotherapy selects for a component with a capacity for differentiation (229). These data further emphasize that mature teratomas of postpubertal patients are malignant, although differentiated, neoplasms. Transformation to higher grade malignancies may therefore be an inherent tendency and is an argument for their surgical excision in metastatic sites (266).

Differential Diagnosis. The most important lesions that can be confused or misclassified as mature teratoma are dermoid and epidermoid cysts. While it is almost certain that dermoid cysts are of teratomatous origin, they should be separately subcategorized because of their benign behavior. Their entirely cystic gross appearance contrasts with that of the usual solid and cystic teratoma. Dermoid cysts lack immature elements in contrast to most teratomas in postpubertal patients. In our experience, they are also not associated with IGCNU.

Epidermoid cysts lack any component, including skin adnexal structures, other than a cyst composed of keratinizing squamous epithelium (see page 323). Their pathogenesis is still debated. Unlike teratomas in postpubertal patients, they are not associated with IGCNU (258) and behave in a uniformly benign fashion (268,273).

Spread and Metastasis. Dixon and Moore (232) identified local spread beyond the testis in 6 percent of cases of "teratoma" and metastases at presentation in 24 percent, but some cases were associated with seminoma. In a referral series of 41 adult patients with pure teratoma, 37 percent presented with clinically evident metastases, a higher than expected figure which likely reflects referral selection bias (254). The pattern of metastasis is similar to that of other germ cell tumors, with initial involvement of retroperitoneal lymph nodes. In autopsy studies of patients with metastatic testicular teratoma, 100 percent had involvement of para-aortic and iliac lymph nodes; 83 percent, the liver; 72 percent, bilateral lung; 36 percent, bone; 35 percent, pleura; and 25 percent, intestine (231).

As mentioned earlier (Table 1-3), metastatic involvement with discrepant histologies may occur, with the testis showing a pure teratoma and the metastasis containing a nonteratomatous germ cell tumor or vice versa (231,269). The possible reasons for this have been previously discussed (page 147). Because there may be an aggressively behaving component in a metastatic site, continued close follow-up is indicated. It is furthermore common to identify pure teratomatous metastases following the chemotherapeutic treatment of nonseminomatous germ cell tumors (234,235). Oosterhuis and colleagues and others (237,246, 267,270,276) have documented that this situation is highly associated with the presence of teratomatous elements in the testis, with the implication that either: 1) such teratomatous elements metastasized and were selected for by chemotherapy or 2) a precursor element metastasized but differentiated, because of an inherent tendency as evidenced by the testicular lesion, to teratoma, which was again selected for by chemotherapy. Regardless of the pathogenesis, teratomatous metastases are associated with a good prognosis following surgical excision (234,235), except in those rare instances in which a secondary malignant component has occurred (220,255,282). Disease-free survival rates of 87 to 94 percent are reported for patients with completely resected, pure teratomatous metastases (236,255,288). Surgical excision of such lesions is indicated because, as mentioned previously, they have a malignant genotype (261,266,272) and are susceptible to develop more aggressively behaving clones ("malignant transformation") (266). In addition, such mature teratomatous lesions, even in the absence of overt malignant transformation, can progressively enlarge and ultimately cause lethal complications due to their local effects, the "growing teratoma syndrome" (256,279).

The presence of mature teratomatous elements in the testicular tumors of patients with clinical disease limited to the testis correlates with a decreased likelihood of occult metastases (239,240,264,286).

Treatment and Prognosis. Pure testicular teratomas in childhood are benign, even when histologically immature, and are managed by orchiectomy alone (252,269,277a). Pure testicular teratomas in adults are rare; Johnson et al. (247) treated 18 patients with teratomas (some of whom also had associated seminomas) by orchiectomy followed by retroperitoneal lymph node dissection and achieved a 5-year survival rate of 100 percent. Forty-one adult patients with pure teratoma were treated at Indiana University with retroperitoneal lymphadenectomy and, in some cases, chemotherapy; 6 patients developed recurrences, 3 of whom were successfully treated, whereas 1 patient died of progressive tumor, another from treatment-related angiosarcoma, and a third had persistent tumor at last follow-up (254). There are no available data on the management of clinical stage I pure testicular teratoma. Pugh and Cameron (269), reporting the experience of the British Testicular Tumour Panel, identified 2 deaths due to tumor in 12 adult patients with pure testicular teratomas. Both patients died

due to metastases of nonteratomatous type (embryonal carcinoma and choriocarcinoma). In Dixon and Moore's studies (231), testicular teratomas, with or without seminoma, were associated with a 30 percent 5-year mortality.

MONODERMAL AND HIGHLY SPECIALIZED TUMORS

Carcinoid

General and Clinical Features. Primary carcinoid tumors may occur either as a pure testicular neoplasm (about 75 percent of the cases) or in association with a testicular teratoma (about 25 percent of the cases) (290,302,304). These tumors are rare; Berdjis and Mostofi (290) identified 12 cases among the files of testicular tumors at the Armed Forces Institute of Pathology, yielding a frequency of 0.17 percent.

Carcinoid tumors tend to occur in older patients than most other types of testicular germ cell tumor, with a mean and median age of 46 years (290,304) and a range of 10 to 83 years (301, 302,304). One carcinoid occurred in a cryptorchid testis (292), but this may be a coincidence. Most patients present with testicular enlargement that may or may not be associated with pain. Often the clinical history of a mass is long, with a mean of 38 months (304). Hydroceles are described in about 10 percent of patients (304). Carcinoid syndrome is unusual, occurring in about 12 percent of cases, but serotonin or its metabolites may be abnormally high in a greater number of patients (304); on the other hand, serotonin metabolites may be negative, even when serotonin is subsequently identified in the tumor by immunohistochemistry (298). A metastatic primary testicular carcinoid was associated with very high levels of 5-hydroxyindole acetic acid in the urine (293), and the presence of the carcinoid syndrome correlates with malignant behavior. This suggests that many tumors synthesize serotonin but in insufficient quantities to produce a carcinoid syndrome unless disseminated.

Gross Findings. Pure carcinoid tumors are usually solid, well-circumscribed, generally pale yellow to brown neoplasms (fig. 4-99). The reported size range is 0.5 to 11 cm, with a mean of 3.5 cm (304). Pure carcinoids tend to be larger than those associated with a teratoma (304). They do not invade surrounding structures.

Microscopic Findings. An insular pattern is usual, with small nests and acini separated by a fibrous to hyalinized stroma (fig. 4-100A). The cells have abundant eosinophilic cytoplasm, often with distinct granularity, and have round nuclei with coarse chromatin ("salt and pepper" chromatin) granules (fig. 4-100B). Both argyrophil and argentaffin stains are positive (fig. 4-100C); faint mucin staining may occur in glandular lumens. There is one report of a primary testicular carcinoid with extensive cutaneous metastases that had the trabecular growth pattern often seen in foregut carcinoids (301). There are no reports on the presence or absence of IGCNU adjacent to primary testicular carcinoids, and we have not identified it in the few pure carcinoids we have seen, but the experience is quite limited.

Special Diagnostic Studies. Few immuno-histochemical studies have been performed on primary testicular carcinoids. Those reported have usually shown positivity for chromogranin, neuron-specific enolase (NSE), serotonin, and cytokeratin (297,304), with some cases also being positive for gastrin, neurofilament, substance P, and vasoactive intestinal polypeptide (298,304). On ultrastructural examination, the pleomorphic neurosecretory granules characteristic of midgut-type carcinoid tumors are usually seen (298,302,304), although some cases may have more regular, round to oval granules (304). Flow cytometric study of three cases demonstrated near-diploid, aneuploid peaks and low S-phase values (less than 5 percent), consistent with indolent malignant tumors (304).

Differential Diagnosis. The major differential is with metastatic carcinoid. The presence of associated teratomatous elements indicates a primary nature. In the absence of associated teratoma, bilaterality, multifocal involvement, and lymphatic/vascular invasion all favor metastasis. Clinical evidence of extratesticular involvement is also important in making this determination, as is the history of a known primary carcinoid tumor at another site. Confusion with a Sertoli cell tumor may also occur because of its nested and diffuse growth patterns, the abundant eosinophilic cytoplasm of some cases, and the usual bland cytologic features and low mitotic activity. The coarse chromatin and frequently prominent

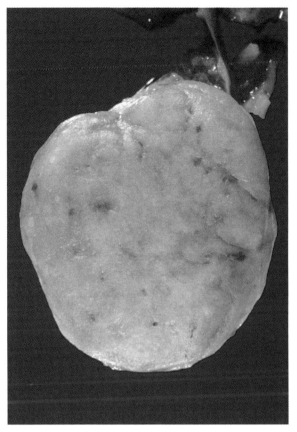

Figure 4-99
CARCINOID
The tumor has a solid, tan cut surface.

cytoplasmic granularity, however, are not features of Sertoli cell tumor. Also, the nests of carcinoid tumor appear different from the tubules of Sertoli cell tumors in most cases. Immunostains directed against inhibin A may be helpful since Sertoli cell tumors are frequently positive (293a,b), and we would anticipate that testicular carcinoids would prove negative, although we are aware of only one case that has been specifically studied (Kommoss F, unpublished observations, 1998). Since Sertoli cell tumors have been positive in one study for chromogranin and synaptophysin (293a), immunostains for these markers may be less useful in the differential with carcinoid tumor.

Treatment and Prognosis. Fatal metastatic disease developed in only 1 of the 12 patients in the series of Berdjis and Mostofi (290), while a second had a clinical diagnosis of metastatic involvement. Zavala-Pompa et al. (304), in a thorough review,

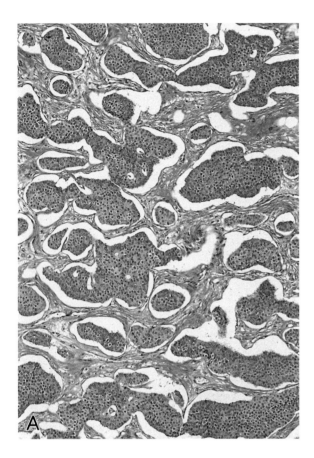
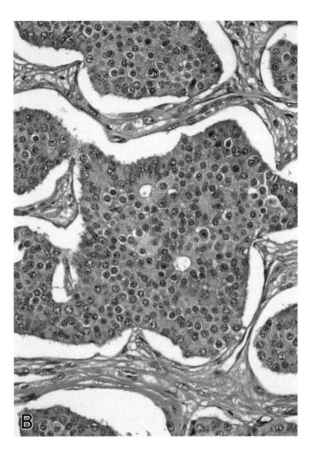
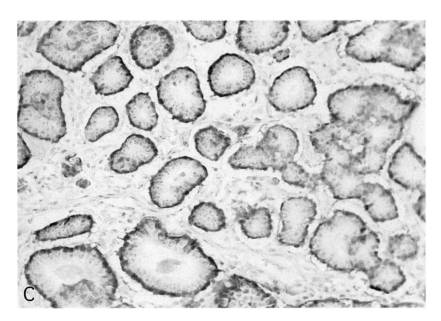

Figure 4-100
CARCINOID

A: Well-defined acini and solid islands of cells are separated by a fibrous stroma.
B: The cells have abundant eosinophilic cytoplasm and round nuclei with coarsely granular chromatin.
C: Positive Masson-Fontana reaction. (Fig. 3.45 from Young RH, Scully RE. Testicular tumors. Chicago: ASCP Press, 1990:70.)

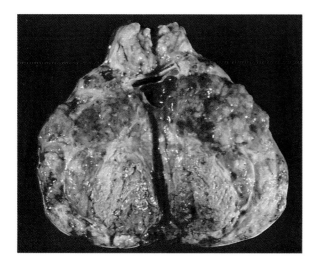

Figure 4-101
PRIMITIVE NEUROECTODERMAL TUMOR
The highly malignant nature of the tumor is suggested by the necrosis and hemorrhage within this large mass that replaced the testis. (Fig. 3.46 from Young RH, Scully RE. Testicular tumors. Chicago: ASCP Press, 1990.)

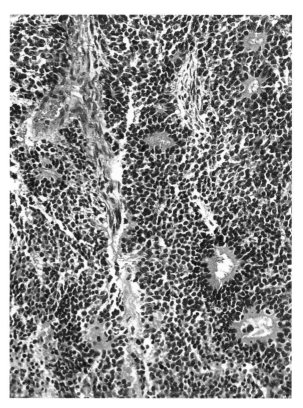

Figure 4-102
PRIMITIVE
NEUROECTODERMAL TUMOR
True rosettes in an otherwise solid area.

identified metastatic disease in 4 of 50 (8 percent) patients. One case of possible metastasis from a carcinoid tumor occurred after a 17-year interval. Features that correlate with malignant behavior include large tumor size (average, 7.3 cm) and the occurrence of the carcinoid syndrome; tumor necrosis, mitotic rate, and vascular invasion did not correlate with malignancy (304). Small tumor size (less than 4 cm) and an association with teratomatous elements generally indicate an indolent course (304). It is also likely that metastatic cases are disproportionately reported; most primary testicular carcinoids are cured by orchiectomy which, with clinical follow-up, is the usual form of therapy.

Primitive Neuroectodermal Tumor

There are isolated reports of primitive neuroectodermal tumor (PNET) of the testis, as well as a series of 35 PNETs, either in the testis or in metastatic sites (289,294–296,303). Some cases represent relatively pure PNET (figs. 4-101, 4-102) (289,295,296), whereas the majority of testicular PNETs are a small component of a mixed germ cell tumor (294,303). In the latter case, distinction from immature teratoma is based on the size of the primitive neural component (see page 156).

These tumors occur in young adult patients and are typically gray-white and partially necrotic (fig. 4-101) (289,295). Microscopically, there are areas of small, poorly differentiated malignant cells (289, 295), with most cases having foci of overt neural differentiation in the form of primitive neural-type tubules lined by stratified epithelium, ependymal-type rosettes, or neuroblastic cells in an eosinophilic, fibrillary neuropil (fig. 4-102) (289,294). A melanotic variant resembles the paratesticular retinal anlage tumor (see page 256) (289b). Ultrastructural examination of one case showed neurosecretory granules (295).

In the absence of light microscopic evidence of neural differentiation, confusion may occur with other small cell tumors of the testis such as lymphoma, embryonal rhabdomyosarcoma, or metastatic small cell carcinoma (295). This differential diagnosis is aided by using immunohistochemical markers directed against neural and neuroendocrine markers as well as lymphoid and muscle markers (299,300). Electron microscopy may be of additional help (300). Desmoplastic small round cell tumor may rarely demonstrate tubules and rosettes, but it is based in the paratestis and shows the characteristic poly-immunophenotype (291) (see chapter 7).

In the series of Michael et al. (294), no poor prognosis could be attributed to testicular PNET in the absence of known metastases, but these cases represented focal PNETs in germ cell tumors. However, there was a high mortality when PNETs occurred in metastatic sites, always in patients previously treated with chemotherapy.

Other Monodermal Teratomas

In theory, overgrowth of any teratomatous element may result in a monodermal teratoma. The distinction of a monodermal teratoma from a similar appearing tumor derived from nongerminal cells is important given the metastatic potential of teratomas. This differential may hinge upon the identification of associated IGCNU in the monodermal teratoma, as in a recently described pure cartilaginous teratoma (300a). In contrast to the ovary, overgrowth of thyroid tissue in the testis (struma testis) is very rare as noted earlier. One case of a papillary carcinoma (298a) and one of an atypical follicular adenoma (302b) have been described in "struma testis," but without immunohistochemical confirmation. Tumors resembling nephroblastoma are also rare but are seen with greater frequency in metastatic sites following chemotherapy (294a). As noted on page 147, epidermoid cysts are not considered in the category of teratoma and, unlike teratomas in adult patients, are not associated with IGCNU.

REFERENCES

Embryonal Carcinoma

1. Albers P, Miller GA, Orazi A, et al. Immunohistochemical assessment of tumor proliferation and volume of embryonal carcinoma identify patients with clinical stage A nonseminomatous testicular germ cell tumor at low risk for occult metastasis. Cancer 1995;75:844–50.

2. Albers P, Ulbright TM, Albers J, et al. Tumor proliferative activity is predictive of pathological stage in clinical stage A nonseminomatous testicular germ cell tumors. J Urol 1996;155:579–86.

3. Allhoff EP, Liedkes S, Wittekind C, et al. DNA content in NSGCT/CSI: a new prognosticator for biologic behaviour [Abstract]. J Cancer Res Clin Oncol 1990;1(Suppl):592.

4. Aronsohn RS, Nishiyama RH. Embryonal carcinoma. An unexpected cause of sudden death in a young adult. JAMA 1974;229:1093–4.

5. Balslev E, Francis D, Jacobsen GK. Testicular germ cell tumors. Classification based on fine needle aspiration biopsy. Acta Cytol 1990;34:690–4.

6. Bartkova J, Bartek J, Lukas J, et al. p53 protein alterations in human testicular cancer including preinvasive intratubular germ-cell neoplasia. Int J Cancer 1991;49:196–202.

7. Battifora H, Sheibani K, Tubbs RR, Kopinski MI, Sun TT. Antikeratin antibodies in tumor diagnosis. Distinction between seminoma and embryonal carcinoma. Cancer 1984;54:843–8.

8. Boseman FT, Giard RW, Kruseman AC, Knijenenburg G, Spaander PJ. Human chorionic gonadothropin and alpha-fetoprotein in testicular germ cell tumors: a retrospective immunohistochemical study. Histopathology 1980;4:673–84.

9. Bosl GJ, Lange PH, Nochomovitz LE, et al. Tumor markers in advanced non-seminomatous testicular cancer. Cancer 1981;47:572–6.

10. Burke AP, Mostofi FK. Placental alkaline phosphatase immunohistochemistry of intratubular malignant germ cells and associated testicular germ cell tumors. Hum Pathol 1988;19:663–70.

11. Castedo SM, de Jong B, Oosterhuis JW, et al. i(12p)-negative testicular germ cell tumors. A different group? Cancer Genet Cytogenet 1988;35:171–8.

12. Costello AJ, Mortensen PH, Stillwell RG. Prognostic indicators for failure of surveillance management of stage I non-seminomatous germ cell tumours. Aust NZ J Surg 1989;59:119–22.

13. Damjanov I, Andrews PW. Ultrastructural differentiation of a clonal human embryonal carcinoma cell line in vitro. Cancer Res 1983;43:2190–8.

14. Damjanov I, Clark RK, Andrews PW. Cytoskeleton of human embryonal carcinoma cells. Cell Differ 1984; 15:133–9.

15. Damjanov I, Fox N, Knowles BB, Solter D, Lange PH, Fraley EE. Immunohistochemical localization of stage-specific embryonic antigens in human testicular germ cell tumors. Am J Pathol 1982;108:225–30.

16. de Bruin MJ, Oosterhof GO, Debruyne FM. Nerve-sparing retroperitoneal lymphadenectomy for low stage testicular cancer. Br J Urol 1993;71:336–9.

17. de Graaff WE, Sleijfer DT, de Jong B, Dam A, Schraffordt Koops H, Oosterhuis JW. Significance of aneuploid stemlines in testicular nonseminomatous germ cell tumors. Cancer 1993;72:1300–4.

18. de Riese WT, Albers P, Walker EB, et al. Predictive parameters of biologic behavior of early stage nonseminomatous testicular germ cell tumors. Cancer 1994;74:1335–41.

19. De Riese WT, De Riese C, Ulbright TM, et al. Flow-cytometric and quantitative histologic parameters as prognostic indicators for occult retroperitoneal disease in clinical-stage-I non-seminomatous testicular germ-cell tumors. Int J Cancer 1994;57:628–33.

20. Delozier-Blanchet CD, Walt H, Engel E, Vuagnat P. Cytogenetic studies of human testicular germ cell tumours. Int J Androl 1987;10:69–77.

21. Dixon FJ, Moore RA. Tumors of the male sex organs. Atlas of Tumor Pathology, 1st Series, Fascicles 31b and 32. Washington, D.C.: Armed Forces Institute of Pathology, 1952.

22. Dunphy CH, Ayala AG, Swanson DA, Ro JY, Logothetis C. Clinical stage I nonseminomatous and mixed germ cell tumors of the testis. A clinicopathologic study of 93 patients on a surveillance protocol after orchiectomy alone. Cancer 1988;62:1202–6.

23. Einhorn LH. Cancer of the testis: a new paradigm. Hosp Pract 1986;15:165–78.

24. Einhorn LH. Chemotherapy of disseminated testicular cancer. In: Skinner DG, Lieskovsky G, eds. Diagnosis and management of genitourinary cancer. Philadelphia: WB Saunders, 1988:526–31.

25. Fernandez EB, Sesterhenn IA, McCarthy WF, Mostofi FK, Moul JW. Proliferating cell nuclear antigen expression to predict occult disease in clinical stage I nonseminomatous testicular germ cell tumors. J Urol 1994;152:1133–8.

26. Ferreiro JA. Ber-H2 expression in testicular germ cell tumors. Hum Pathol 1994;25:522–4.

27. Ferry JA, Ulbright TM, Young RH. Anaplastic large cell lymphoma presenting in the testis. J Urol Pathol 1997;5:139–47.

29. Fossä SD, Aass N, Kaalhus O. Testicular cancer in young Norwegians. J Surg Oncol 1988;39:43–63.

30. Fossä SD, Nesland JM, Waehre H, Amellem O, Pettersen EO. DNA ploidy in the primary tumor from patients with nonseminomatous testicular germ cell tumors clinical stage I. Cancer 1991;67:1874–7.

28. Fossä SD, Qvist H, Stenwig AE, Lien HH, Ous S, Giercksky KE. Is postchemotherapy retroperitoneal surgery necessary in patients with nonseminomatous testicular cancer and minimal residual tumor masses? J Clin Oncol 1992;10:569–73.

31. Freedman LS, Parkinson MC, Jones WG, et al. Histopathology in the prediction of relapse of patients with stage I testicular teratoma treated by orchidectomy alone. Lancet 1987;2:294–8.

32. Friedman NB, Moore RA. Tumors of the testis: a report on 922 cases. Milit Surgeon 1946;99:573–93.

33. Fukuda M, Ikuma S, Setoyama C, Shimada K. Decrease in the c-myb gene transcript during differentiation of mouse teratocarcinoma stem cells. Biochem Int 1987;15:73–9.

34. Fung CY, Kalish LA, Brodsky GL, Richie JP, Garnick MB. Stage I nonseminomatous germ cell testicular tumor: prediction of metastatic potential by primary histopathology. J Clin Oncol 1988;6:1467–73.

35. Geller NL, Bosl GJ, Chan EY. Prognostic factors for relapse after complete response in patients with metastatic germ cell tumors. Cancer 1989;63:440–5.

36. Gels ME, Hoekstra HJ, Sleijfer DT, et al. Detection of recurrence in patients with clinical stage I nonseminomatous testicular germ cell tumors and consequences for further follow-up: a single-center 10-year experience. J Clin Oncol 1995;13:1188–94.

37. Hawkins EP, Finegold MJ, Hawkins HK, Krischer JP, Starling KA, Weinberg A. Nongerminomatous malignant germ cell tumors in children: a review of 89 cases from the Pediatric Oncology Group, 1971–1984. Cancer 1986;58:2579–84.

38. Highman WJ, Oliver RT. Diagnosis of metastases from testicular germ cell tumours using fine needle aspiration cytology. J Clin Pathol 1987;40:1324–33.

39. Hittmair A, Rogatsch H, Hobisch A, Mikuz G, Feichtinger H. CD30 expression in seminoma. Hum Pathol 1996;27:1166–71.

40. Jacobsen GK. Histogenetic considerations concerning germ cell tumours. Morphological and immunohistochemical comparative investigation of the human embryo and testicular germ cell tumours. Virchows Arch [A] 1986;408:509–25.

41. Jacobsen GK, Barlebo H, Olsen JK, et al. Testicular germ cell tumours in Denmark 1976–1980: pathology of 1058 consecutive cases. Acta Radiol Oncol 1984;23:239–47.

42. Jacobsen GK, Jacobsen M, Clausen PP. Distribution of tumor-associated antigens in the various histologic components of germ cell tumors of the testis. Am J Surg Pathol 1981;5:257–66.

43. Jacobsen GK, Rorth M, Osterlind K, et al. Histopathological features in stage I non-seminomatous testicular germ cell tumours correlated to relapse. Danish Testicular Cancer Study Group. APMIS 1990;98:377–82.

44. Jacobsen GK, Talerman A. Atlas of germ cell tumours. Copenhagen: Munksgaard, 1989

45. Javadpour N. The role of biologic tumor markers in testicular cancer. Cancer 1980;45:1755–61.

46. Javadpour N, Canning DA, O'Connell KJ, Young JD. Predictors of recurrent clinical stage I nonseminomatous testicular cancer. A prospective clinicopathologic study. Urology 1986;27:508–11.

47. Koss LG, Zajicek J. Aspiration biopsy. In: Koss LG, ed. Diagnostic cytology and its histopathologic basis. 4th ed. Philadelphia: JB Lippincott, 1992:1234–402.

48. Kratzik C, Aiginger P, Kuzmits R, et al. HLA-antigen distribution in seminoma, HCG-positive seminoma and non-seminomatous tumours of the testis. Urol Res 1989;17:377–80.

49. Lifschitz-Mercer B, Fogel M, Moll R, et al. Intermediate filament protein profiles of human testicular non-seminomatous germ cell tumors: correlation of cytokeratin synthesis to cell differentiation. Differentiation 1991;48:191–8.

50. Manivel JC, Jessurun J, Wick MR, Dehner LP. Placental alkaline phosphatase immunoreactivity in testicular germ cell tumors. Am J Surg Pathol 1987;11:21–9.

51. Marrett LD, Weir HK, Clarke EA, Magee CJ. Rates of death from testicular cancer in Ontario from 1964-82: analysis by major histologic subgroups. Can Med Assoc J 1986;135:999–1002.

51a. McCluggage WG, Ashe P, McBride H, Maxwell P, Swan JM. Localization of the cellular expression of inhibin in trophoblastic tissue. Histopathology 1998;32:252–6.

52. Mead GM, Stenning SP, Parkinson MC, et al. The Second Medical Research Council study of prognostic factors in nonseminomatous germ cell tumors. Medical Research Council Testicular Tumour Working Party. J Clin Oncol 1992;10:85–94.

53. Misaki H, Shuin T, Yao M, Kubota Y, Hosaka M. Expression of myc family oncogenes in primary human testicular cancer. Nippon Hinyokika Gakkai Zasshi 1989;80:1509–13.

54. Moriyama N, Daly JJ, Keating MA, Lin CW, Prout GR Jr. Vascular invasion as a prognosticator of metastatic disease in nonseminomatous germ cell tumors of the testis. Importance in "surveillance only" protocols. Cancer 1985;56:2492–8.

55. Morse MJ, Whitmore WF. Neoplasms of the testis. In: Walsh PC, Gittes RF, Perlmutter AD, Stamey TA, eds. Campbell's urology. Philadelphia: WB Saunders, 1986:1535–82.

56. Mostofi FK. Pathology of germ cell tumors of testis: a progress report. Cancer 1980;45:1735–54.

57. Mostofi FK, Price EB Jr. Tumors of the male genital system. Atlas of Tumor Pathology, 2nd Series, Fascicle 8. Washington, D.C.: Armed Forces Institute of Pathology, 1973.

58. Mostofi FK, Sesterhenn IA, Davis CJ Jr. Immunopathology of germ cell tumors of the testis. Semin Diagn Pathol 1987;4:320–41.

59. Mostofi FK, Sesterhenn IA, Davis CJ Jr. Developments in histopathology of testicular germ cell tumors. Semin Urol 1988;6:171–88.

60. Mostofi FK, Sobin LH. Histological typing of testicular tumors (International histological classification of tumors, No. 16). Geneva: World Health Organization, 1977.

61. Motoyama T, Watanabe H, Yamamoto T, Sekiguchi M. Human testicular germ cell tumors in vitro and in athymic nude mice. Acta Pathol Jap 1987;37:431–48.

62. Motzer RJ, Rodriguez E, Reuter VE, et al. Genetic analysis as an aid in diagnosis for patients with midline carcinomas of uncertain histologies. JNCI 1991;83:341–6.

63. Moul JW, Foley JP, Hitchcock CL, et al. Flow cytometric and quantitative histological parameters to predict occult disease in clinical stage I nonseminomatous testicular germ cell tumors. J Urol 1993;150:879–83.

64. Moul JW, McCarthy WF, Fernandez EB, Sesterhenn IA. Percentage of embryonal carcinoma and of vascular invasion predicts pathological stage in clinical stage I nonseminomatous testicular cancer. Cancer Res 1994;54:362–4.

65. Moul JW, Theune SM, Chang EH. Detection of RAS mutations in archival testicular germ cell tumors by polymerase chain reaction and oligonucleotide hybridization. Genes Chrom Cancer 1992;5:109–18.

66. Murakami SS, Said JW. Immunohistochemical localization of lactate dehydrogenase isoenzyme 1 in germ cell tumors of the testis. Am J Clin Pathol 1984;81:293–6.

67. Nazeer T, Ro JY, Kee KH, Ayala AG. Spermatic cord contamination in testicular cancer. Mod Pathol 1996;9:762–6.

68. Nicolai N, Pizzocaro G. A surveillance study of clinical stage I nonseminomatous germ cell tumors of the testis: 10-year followup. J Urol 1995;154:1045–9.

69. Niehans GA, Manivel JC, Copland GT, Scheithauer BW, Wick MR. Immunohistochemistry of germ cell and trophoblastic neoplasms. Cancer 1988;62:1113–23.

70. Oosterhuis JW, Castedo SM, de Jong B, et al. Ploidy of primary germ cell tumors of the testis. Pathogenetic and clinical relevance. Lab Invest 1989;60:14–21.

71. Pallesen G, Hamilton-Dutoit SJ. Ki-1 (CD30) antigen is regularly expressed in tumor cells of embryonal carcinoma. Am J Pathol 1988;133:446–50.

72. Peckham M. Testicular cancer. Acta Oncol 1988;27:439–53.

73. Pera MF, Blasco Lafita MJ, Mills J. Cultured stem-cells from human testicular teratomas: the nature of human embryonal carcinoma, and its comparison with two types of yolk-sac carcinoma. Int J Cancer 1987;40:334–43.

74. Pera MF, Cooper S, Mills J, Parrington JM. Isolation and characterization of a multipotent clone of human embryonal carcinoma cells. Differentiation 1989;42:10–23.

75. Pizzocaro G, Zanoni F, Salvioni R, Milani A, Piva L, Pilotti S. Difficulties of a surveillance study omitting retroperitoneal lymphadenectomy in clinical stage I nonseminomatous germ cell tumors of the testis. J Urol 1987;138:1393–6.

76. Pugh RC. Testicular tumours–introduction. In: Pugh RC, ed. Pathology of the testis. Oxford: Blackwell Scientific, 1976:139–59.

77. Rabes HM. Proliferation of human testicular tumours. Int J Androl 1987;10:127–37.

78. Raghavan D, Vogelzang NJ, Bosl GJ, et al. Tumor classification and size in germ-cell testicular cancer: influence on the occurrence of metastases. Cancer 1982;50:1591–5.

79. Richie JP, Kantoff PW. Is adjuvant chemotherapy necessary for patients with stage B1 testicular cancer? J Clin Oncol 1991;9:1393–6.

80. Rodriguez PN, Hafez GR, Messing EM. Nonseminomatous germ cell tumor of the testicle: does extensive staging of the primary tumor predict the likelihood of metastatic disease? J Urol 1986;136:604–8.

80a. Roth LM, Gillespie JJ. Ultrastructure of testicular tumors. In: Talerman A, Roth LM, eds. Pathology of the testis and its adnexa. New York: Churchill-Livingstone, 1986:155–68.

81. Rowland RG, Donohue JP. Scrotum and testis. In: Gillenwater JY, Grayhack JT, Howards SS, Duckett JW, eds. Adult and pediatric urology. 2nd ed. St. Louis: Mosby-Year Book, 1991:1565–98.

82. Samaniego F, Rodriguez E, Houldsworth J, et al. Cytogenetic and molecular analysis of human male germ cell tumors: chromosome 12 abnormalities and gene amplification. Genes Chrom Cancer 1990;1:289–300.

83. Saukko P, Lignitz E. Sudden death caused by malignant testicular tumors. Zeit Rechtsmed 1990;103:529–36.

84. Shah VI, Amin MB, Linden MD, Zarbo RJ. Utility of a selective immunohistochemical (IHC) panel in the detection of components of mixed germ cell tumors (GCT) of testis [Abstract]. Mod Pathol 1998;11:95A.

85. Shah VI, Amin MB, Linden MD, Zarbo RJ. Immunohistologic profile of spindle cell elements in non-seminomatous germ cell tumors (NSGCT): histogenetic implications [Abstract]. Mod Pathol 1998;11:96A.

86. Shuin T, Misaki H, Kubota Y, Yao M, Hosaka M. Differential expression of protooncogenes in human germ cell tumors of the testis. Cancer 1994;73:1721–7.

87. Sledge GW Jr, Eble JN, Roth BJ, Wuhrman BP, Fineberg N, Einhorn LH. Relation of proliferative activity to survival in patients with advanced germ cell cancer. Cancer Res 1988;48:3864–8.

88. Sogani PC, Fair WR. Surveillance alone in the treatment of clinical stage I nonseminomatous germ cell tumor of the testis (NSGCT). Semin Urol 1988;6:53–6.

89. Srigley JR, Mackay B, Toth P, Ayala A. The ultrastructure and histogenesis of male germ neoplasia with emphasis on seminoma with early carcinomatous features. Ultrastruc Pathol 1988;12:67–86.

90. Stiller D, Bahn H, Pressler H. Immunohistochemical demonstration of alpha-fetoprotein in testicular germ cell tumors. Acta Histochem Suppl (Jena) 1986;33:225–31.

91. Stoter G, Sylvester R, Sleijfer DT, et al. Multivariate analysis of prognostic variables in patients with disseminated non-seminomatous testicular cancer: results from an EORTC multi-institutional phase III study. Int J Androl 1987;10:239–46.

92. Sturgeon JF, Jewett MA, Alison RE, et al. Surveillance after orchidectomy for patients with clinical stage I nonseminomatous testis tumors. J Clin Oncol 1992;10:564–8.

93. Tainsky MA, Cooper CS, Giovanella BC, Vande Woude GF. An activated rasN gene: detected in late but not early passage human PA1 teratocarcinoma cells. Science 1984;225:643–5.

94. Tesch H, Fürbass R, Casper J, et al. Cellular oncogenes in human teratocarcinoma cell lines. Int J Androl 1990;13:377–88.

95. Uchida T, Shimoda T, Miyata H, et al. Immunoperoxidase study of alkaline phosphatase in testicular tumor. Cancer 1981;48:1455–62.

96. Ulbright TM, Goheen MP, Roth LM, Gillespie JJ. The differentiation of carcinomas of teratomatous origin from embryonal carcinoma. A light and electron microscopic study. Cancer 1986;57:257–63.

97. Ulbright TM, Orazi A, de Riese W, et al. The correlation of P53 protein expression with proliferative activity and occult metastases in clinical stage I non-seminomatous germ cell tumors of the testis. Mod Pathol 1994;7:64–8.

98. Ulbright TM, Roth LM. A pathologic analysis of lesions following modern chemotherapy for metastatic germ cell tumors. Pathol Annu 1990;25(Pt 1):313–40.

99. Ulbright TM, Roth LM, Brodhecker CA. Yolk sac differentiation in germ cell tumors. A morphologic study of 50 cases with emphasis on hepatic, enteric and parietal yolk sac features. Am J Surg Pathol 1986;10:151–64.

100. Visfeldt J, Giwercman A, Skakkebaek NE. Monoclonal antibody 43-9F: an immunohistochemical marker of embryonal carcinoma of the testis. APMIS 1992;100:63–70.

101. Vogelzang NJ. Prognostic factors in metastatic testicular cancer. Int J Androl 1987;10:225–37.

102. Wick MR, Swanson PE, Manivel JC. Placental-like alkaline phosphatase reactivity in human tumors: an immunohistochemical study of 520 cases. Hum Pathol 1987;18:946–54.

103. Williams SD, Einhorn LH. Neoplasms of the testis. In: Calabresi P, Schein PS, Rosenberg SA, eds. Medical oncology: basic principles and clinical management of cancer. New York: Macmillan, 1985:1077–88.

104. Wishnow KI, Johnson DE, Swanson DA, et al. Identifying patients with low-risk clinical stage I nonseminomatous testicular tumors who should be treated by surveillance. Urology 1989;34:339–43.

105. Wittekind C, Wichmann T, Von Kleist S. Immunohistological localization of AFP and HCG in uniformly classified testis tumors. Anticancer Res 1983;3:327–30.

106. Yamazawa K, Sekiya S, Kimura H, Kawata M, Inaba N, Takamizawa H. Cell biological characteristics of a human embryonal carcinoma cell line. Nippon Sanka Fujinka Gakkai Zasshi 1990;42:53–9.

107. Young RH, Scully RE. Testicular tumors. Chicago: ASCP Press, 1990.

Yolk Sac Tumor

108. Akhtar M, Ali MA, Sackey K, Jackson D, Bakry M. Fine-needle aspiration biopsy diagnosis of endodermal sinus tumor: histologic and ultrastructural correlations. Diagn Cytopathol 1990;6:184–92.

109. Balslev E, Francis D, Jacobsen GK. Testicular germ cell tumors: classification based on fine needle aspiration biopsy. Acta Cytol 1990;34:690–4.

110. Bartkova J, Bartek J, Lukas J, et al. p53 protein alterations in human testicular cancer including preinvasive intratubular germ-cell neoplasia. Int J Cancer 1991;49:196–202.

111. Bradfield JS, Hagen RO, Ytredal DO. Carcinoma of the testis: an analysis of 104 patients with germinal tumors of the testis other than seminoma. Cancer 1973;31:633–40.

112. Brosman SA. Testicular tumors in prepubertal children. Urology 1979;13:581–8.

113. Brown LM, Pottern LM, Hoover RN, Devesa SS, Aselton P, Flannery JT. Testicular cancer in the United States: trends in incidence and mortality. Int J Epidemiol 1986;15:164–70.

114. Brown NJ. Yolk-sac tumour ("orchioblastoma") and other testicular tumours of childhood. In: Pugh RC, ed. Pathology of the testis. Oxford: Blackwell Scientific, 1976:356–70.

115. Burke AP, Mostofi FK. Placental alkaline phosphatase immunohistochemistry of intratubular malignant germ cells and associated testicular germ cell tumors. Hum Pathol 1988;19:663–70.

116. Carroll WL, Kempson RL, Govan DE, Freiha FS, Shochat SJ, Link MP. Conservative management of testicular endodermal sinus tumor in childhood. J Urol 1985;13:1011–4.

117. Chan JK, Chan VS, Mak KL. Congenital juvenile granulosa cell tumour of the testis: report of a case showing extensive degenerative changes. Histopathology 1990;17:75–80.

118. Clement PB, Young RH, Scully RE. Endometrioid-like variant of ovarian yolk sac tumor. A clinicopathological analysis of eight cases. Am J Surg Pathol 1987;11:767–78.

119. Cohen MB, Friend DS, Molnar JJ, Talerman A. Gonadal endodermal sinus (yolk sac) tumor with pure intestinal differentiation: a new histologic type. Pathol Res Pract 1987;182:609–16.

120. Czaja JT, Ulbright TM. Evidence for the transformation of seminoma to yolk sac tumor, with histogenetic considerations. Am J Clin Pathol 1992;97:468–77.

121. de Jong B, Oosterhuis JW, Castedo SM, Vos A, te Meerman GJ. Pathogenesis of adult testicular germ cell tumors. A cytogenetic model. Cancer Genet Cytogenet 1990;48:143–67.

122. de Peralta-Venturina MN, Ro JY, Ordonez NG, Ayala AG. Diffuse embryoma of the testis. An immunohistochemical study of two cases. Am J Clin Pathol 1994;102:402–5.

123. Dominguez-Franjo P, Vargas J, Rodriguez-Peralto JL, et al. Fine needle aspiration biopsy findings in endodermal sinus tumors. A report of four cases with cytologic, immunocytochemical and ultrastructural findings. Acta Cytol 1993;37:209–15.

124. Drago JR, Nelson RP, Palmer JM. Childhood embryonal carcinoma of testes. Urology 1978;12:499–504.

124a. Fernandes ET, Etcubanas E, Rao BN, Kumar AP, Thompson EI, Jenkins JJ. Two decades of experience with testicular tumors in children at St. Judes Children's Research Hospital. J Pediatr Surg 1989;24:677–82.

125. Ferreiro JA. Ber-H2 expression in testicular germ cell tumors. Hum Pathol 1994;25:522–4.

126. Freedman LS, Parkinson MC, Jones WG, et al. Histopathology in the prediction of relapse of patients with stage I testicular teratoma treated by orchidectomy alone. Lancet 1987;2:294–8.

127. Fujimoto J, Hata J, Ishii E, et al. Differentiation antigens defined by mouse monoclonal antibodies against human germ cell tumors. Lab Invest 1987;57:350–8.

128. Gonzalez-Crussi F, Roth LM. The human yolk sac and yolk sac carcinoma: an ultrastructural study. Hum Pathol 1976;7:675–91.

129. Grady RW, Ross JH, Kay R. Patterns of metastatic spread in prepubertal yolk sac tumor of the testis. J Urol 1995;153:1259–61.

130. Harms D, Janig U. Germ cell tumours of childhood: report of 170 cases including 59 pure and partial yolk-sac tumours. Virchows Arch [A] 1986;409:223–9.

131. Hawkins EP, Finegold MJ, Hawkins HK, Krischer JP, Starling KA, Weinberg A. Nongerminomatous malignant germ cell tumors in children: a review of 89 cases from the Pediatric Oncology Group, 1971-1984. Cancer 1986;58:2579–84.

132. Jacobsen GK. Alpha-fetoprotein (AFP) and human chorionic gonadotropin (HCG) in testicular germ cell tumours. A comparison of histologic and serologic occurrence of tumour markers. Acta Pathol Microbiol Immunol Scand [A] 1983;91:183–90.

133. Jacobsen GK. Histogenetic considerations concerning germ cell tumours. Morphological and immunohistochemical comparative investigation of the human embryo and testicular germ cell tumours. Virchows Arch [A] 1986;408:509–25.

134. Jacobsen GK, Jacobsen M. Alpha-fetoprotein (AFP) and human chorionic gonadotropin in testicular germ cell tumours: a prospective immunohistochemical study. Acta Pathol Microbiol Scand [A] 1983;91:165–76.

135. Jacobsen GK, Jacobsen M. Possible liver cell differentiation in testicular germ cell tumours. Histopathology 1983;7:537–48.

136. Jacobsen GK, Jacobsen M, Clausen PP. Distribution of tumor-associated antigens in the various histologic components of germ cell tumors of the testis. Am J Surg Pathol 1981;5:257–66.

137. Jacobsen GK, Talerman A. Atlas of germ cell tumours. Copenhagen: Munksgaard, 1989.

138. Jenderny J, Koster E, Meyer A, et al. Detection of chromosome aberrations in paraffin sections of seven gonadal yolk sac tumors of childhood. Hum Genet 1995;96:644–50.

139. Kaplan GW, Cromie WC, Kelalis PP, Silber I, Tank ES Jr. Prepubertal yolk sac testicular tumors–report of the testicular tumor registry. J Urol 1988;140:1109–12.

140. Kaplan WE, Firlit CF. Treatment of testicular yolk sac carcinoma in the young child. J Urol 1981;126:663–64.

140a. Kay R. Prepubertal Testicular Tumor Registry. J Urol 1993;150:671–4.

141. Koide O, Iwai S, Baba K, Iri H. Identification of testicular atypical germ cells by an immunohistochemical technique for placental alkaline phosphatase. Cancer 1987;60:1325–30.

142. Kramer SA. Pediatric urologic oncology. Urol Clin North Am 1985;12:31–42.

143. Kurman RJ, Norris HJ. Endodermal sinus tumor of the ovary: a clinical and pathologic analysis of 71 cases. Cancer 1976;38:2402–19.

144. Lawrence WD, Young RH, Scully RE. Juvenile granulosa cell tumor of the infantile testis. A report of 14 cases. Am J Surg Pathol 1985;9:87–94.

145. Loehrer PJ Sr, Williams SD, Einhorn LH. Testicular cancer: the quest continues. JNCI 1988;80:1373–82.

146. Logothetis CJ, Samuels ML, Trindade A, Grant C, Gomez L, Ayala A. The prognostic significance of endodermal sinus tumor histology among patients treated for stage III nonseminomatous germ cell tumors of the testes. Cancer 1984;53:122–8.

147. Manivel JC, Jessurun J, Wick MR, Dehner LP. Placental alkaline phosphatase immunoreactivity in testicular germ cell tumors. Am J Surg Pathol 1987;11:21–9.

148. Manivel JC, Reinberg Y, Niehans GA, Fraley EE. Intratubular germ cell neoplasia in testicular teratomas and epidermoid cysts. Correlation with prognosis and possible biologic significance. Cancer 1989;64:715–20.

149. Manivel JC, Simonton S, Wold SE, Dehner LP. Absence of intratubular germ cell neoplasia in testicular yolk sac tumors in children. Arch Pathol Lab Med 1988;112:641–5.

150. Marshall S, Lyon RP, Scott MP. A conservative approach to testicular tumors in children: 12 cases and their management. J Urol 1983;129:350–1.

151. Martinazzi M, Crivelli F, Zampatti C. Immunohistochemical study of hepatic and enteric structures in testicular endodermal sinus tumors. Bas Appl Histochem 1988;32:239–45.

152. Michael H, Ulbright TM, Brodhecker CA. The pluripotential nature of the mesenchyme-like component of yolk sac tumor. Arch Pathol Lab Med 1989;113:1115–9.

153. Miettinen M, Virtanen I, Talerman A. Intermediate filament proteins in human testis and testicular germ-cell tumors. Am J Pathol 1985;120:402–10.

154. Monaghan P, Raghavan D, Neville AM. Ultrastructure of xenografted human germ cell tumors. Cancer 1982;49:683–97.

155. Moran CA, Suster S. Yolk sac tumors of the mediastinum with prominent spindle cell features: a clinicopathologic study of three cases. Am J Surg Pathol 1997;21:1173–7.

156. Mostofi FK, Sesterhenn IA, Davis CJ Jr. Immunopathology of germ cell tumors of the testis. Semin Diagn Pathol 1987;4:320–41.

157. Mostofi FK, Sesterhenn IA, Davis CJ Jr. Developments in histopathology of testicular germ cell tumors. Semin Urol 1988;6:171–88.

158. Motoyama T, Watanabe H, Yamamoto T, Sekiguchi M. Human testicular germ cell tumors in vitro and in athymic nude mice. Acta Pathol Jap 1987;37:431–48.

159. Nakanishi I, Kawahara E, Kajikawa K, Miwa A, Terahata S. Hyaline globules in yolk sac tumor. Histochemical, immunohistochemical and electron microscopic studies. Acta Pathol Jap 1982;32:733–9.

160. Niehans GA, Manivel JC, Copland GT, Scheithauer BW, Wick MR. Immunohistochemistry of germ cell and trophoblastic neoplasms. Cancer 1988;62:1113–23.

161. Nogales-Fernandez F, Silverberg SG, Bloustein PA, Martinez-Hernandez A, Pierce GB. Yolk sac carcinoma (endodermal sinus tumor): ultrastructure and histogenesis of gonadal and extragonadal tumors in comparison with normal human yolk sac. Cancer 1977;39:1462–74.

162. Nseyo UO, Englander LS, Wajsman Z, Huben RP, Pontes JE. Histological patterns of treatment failures in testicular germ cell neoplasms. J Urol 1985;133:219–20.

163. Oosterhuis JW, Castedo SM, de Jong B, et al. Karyotyping and DNA flow cytometry of an orchidoblastoma. Cancer Genet Cytogenet 1988;36:7–11.

164. Pallesen G, Hamilton-Dutoit SJ. Ki-1 (CD30) antigen is regularly expressed in tumor cells of embryonal carcinoma. Am J Pathol 1988;133:446–50.

165. Perlman EJ, Cushing B, Hawkins E, Griffin CA. Cytogenetic analysis of childhood endodermal sinus tumors: a Pediatric Oncology Group study. Pediatr Pathol 1994;14:695–708.

166. Pierce GB, Bullock WK, Huntington RW. Yolk sac tumors of the testis. Cancer 1970;25:644–58.

167. Pow-Sang J, Sanchez J, Benavente V, Pow-Sang JM, Conroy L. Testicular yolk sac carcinoma in infants: natural history in 56 consecutive patients. Prog Clin Biol Res 1985;203:623–37.

168. Pugh RC, Parkinson C. The origin and classification of testicular germ cell tumours. Int J Androl 1981;4(Suppl):15–25.

169. Raghavan D, Heyderman E, Monaghan P, et al. Hypothesis: when is a seminoma not a seminoma? J Clin Pathol 1981;34:123–8.

170. Roth LM, Gillespie JJ. Pathology and ultrastructure of germinal neoplasia of the testis. In: Einhorn LH, ed. Testicular tumors: management and treatment. New York: Masson, 1980:1–28.

171. Sabio H, Burgert EO Jr, Farrow GM, Kelalis PP. Embryonal carcinoma of the testis in childhood. Cancer 1974;34:2118–21.

172. Shah VI, Amin MB, Linden MD, Zarbo RJ. Utility of a selective immunohistochemical (IHC) panel in the detection of components of mixed germ cell tumors (GCT) of testis [Abstract]. Mod Pathol 1998;11:95A.

173. Srigley JR, Mackay B, Toth P, Ayala A. The ultrastructure and histogenesis of male germ neoplasia with emphasis on seminoma with early carcinomatous features. Ultrastruc Pathol 1988;12:67–86.

174. Talerman A. Endodermal sinus (yolk sac) tumor elements in testicular germ-cell tumors in adults: comparison of prospective and retrospective studies. Cancer 1980;46:1213–7.

175. Talerman A. Germ cell tumors. In: Talerman A, Roth LM, eds. Pathology of the testis and its adnexa. New York: Churchill Livingstone, 1986:29–65.

176. Talerman A, Haije WG, Baggerman L. Serum alpha-fetoprotein (AFP) in patients with germ cell tumors of the gonads and extragonadal sites: correlation between endodermal sinus (yolk sac) tumor and raised serum AFP. Cancer 1980;46:380–5.

177. Teilum G. Gonocytoma: homologous ovarian and testicular tumors I: with discussion of "mesonephroma ovarii" (Schiller: Am J Cancer 1939). Acta Pathol Microbiol Scand 1946;23:242–51.

178. Teilum G. "Mesonephroma ovarii" (Schiller) - an extraembryonic mesoblastoma of germ cell origin in the ovary and the testis. Acta Pathol Microbiol Scand 1950;27:249–61.

179. Teilum G. Endodermal sinus tumors of the ovary and testis: comparative morphogenesis of the so-called mesonephroma ovarii (Schiller) and extraembryonic (yolk sac-allantoic) structures of the rat's placenta. Cancer 1959;12:1092–105.

180. Teilum G. Classification of endodermal sinus tumor (mesoblastoma vitellinum) and so-called "embryonal carcinoma" of the ovary. Acta Pathol Microbiol Scand 1965;64:407–29.

181. Teilum G. Special tumors of ovary and testis and related extragonadal lesions. Philadelphia: JB Lippincott, 1976.

182. Ulbright TM, Gersell DJ. Rete testis hyperplasia with hyaline globule formation. A lesion simulating yolk sac tumor. Am J Surg Pathol 1991;15:66–74.

183. Ulbright TM, Roth LM, Brodhecker CA. Yolk sac differentiation in germ cell tumors: a morphologic study of 50 cases with emphasis on hepatic, enteric and parietal yolk sac features. Am J Surg Pathol 1986;10:151–64.

184. Visfeldt J, Jørgensen N, Müller J, Møller H, Skakkebaek NE. Testicular germ cell tumours of childhood in Denmark, 1943–1989: incidence and evaluation of histology using immunohistochemical techniques. J Pathol 1994;174:39–47.

185. Vogelzang NJ, Bronson D, Savino D, Vessella RL, Fraley EF. A human embryonal-yolk sac carcinoma model system in athymic mice. Cancer 1985;55:2584–93.

186. Wu JT, Book L, Sudar K. Serum alpha fetoprotein (AFP) levels in normal infants. Pediatr Res 1981;15:50–2.

Choriocarcinoma and Other Trophoblastic Tumors

187. Barsky SH. Germ cell tumors of the testis. In: Javadpour N, Barsky SH, eds. Surgical pathology of urologic diseases. Baltimore: Williams & Wilkins, 1987:224–46.

188. Bartkova J, Bartek J, Lukas J, et al. p53 protein alterations in human testicular cancer including pre-invasive intratubular germ-cell neoplasia. Int J Cancer 1991;49:196–202.

189. Bosl GJ, Geller NL, Cirrincione C, et al. Multivariate analysis of prognostic variables in patients with metastatic testicular cancer. Cancer Res 1983;43:3403–7.

190. Bredael JJ, Vugrin D, Whitmore WF Jr. Autopsy findings in 154 patients with germ cell tumors of the testis. Cancer 1982;50:548–51.

191. Brigden ML, Sullivan LD, Comisarow RH. Stage C pure choriocarcinoma of the testis: a potentially curable lesion. CA Cancer J Clin 1982;32:82–4.

192. Chhieng DC, Jennings TA, Slominski A, Mihm MC Jr. Choriocarcinoma presenting as a cutaneous metastasis. J Cutan Pathol 1995;22:374–7.

193. Clark RK, Damjanov I. Intermediate filaments of human trophoblast and choriocarcinoma cell lines. Virchows Arch [A] 1985;407:203–8.

194. Damjanov I. Tumors of the testis and epididymis. In: Murphy WM, ed. Urological pathology. Philadelphia: W.B. Saunders, 1989:314–79.

195. Dixon FJ, Moore RA. Tumors of the male sex organs. Atlas of Tumor Pathology, 1st series, Fascicles 31b and 32. Washington, D.C.: Armed Forces Institute of Pathology, 1952.

196. Friedman NB, Moore RA. Tumors of the testis: a report on 922 cases. Milit Surgeon 1946;99:573–93.

197. Giralt SA, Dexeus F, Amato R, Sella A, Logothetis C. Hyperthyroidism in men with germ cell tumors and high levels of beta-human chorionic gonadotropin. Cancer 1992;69:1286–90.

198. Jacobsen GK, Barlebo H, Olsen J, et al. Testicular germ cell tumours in Denmark 1976–1980. Pathology of 1058 consecutive cases. Acta Radiol Oncol 1984;23:239–47.

199. Jacobsen GK, Jacobsen M. Alpha-fetoprotein (AFP) and human chorionic gonadotropin in testicular germ cell tumours: a prospective immunohistochemical study. Acta Pathol Microbiol Scand [A] 1983;91:165–76.

200. Jacobsen GK, Talerman A. Atlas of germ cell tumours. Copenhagen: Munksgaard, 1989.

201. Lind HM, Haghighi P. Carcinoembryonic antigen staining in choriocarcinoma. Am J Clin Pathol 1986;86:538–40.

202. Logothetis CJ, Samuels ML, Selig DE, et al. Cyclic chemotherapy with cyclophosphamide, doxorubicin, and cisplatin plus vinblastine and bleomycin in advanced germ cell tumors: results with 100 patients. Am J Med 1986;81:219–28.

203. Manivel JC, Niehans G, Wick MR, Dehner LP. Intermediate trophoblast in germ cell neoplasms. Am J Surg Pathol 1987;11:693–701.

204. Mazur MT, Lurain JR, Brewer JI. Fatal gestational choriocarcinoma. Clinicopathologic study of patients treated at a trophoblastic disease center. Cancer 1982;50:1833–46.

205. Mostofi FK, Price EB Jr. Tumors of the male genital system. Atlas of Tumor Pathology, 2nd Series, Fascicle 8. Washington, D.C.: Armed Forces Institute of Pathology, 1973.

206. Mostofi FK, Spaander P, Grigor K, Parkinson CM, Shakkebaek NE, Oliver RT. Consensus on pathological classifications of testicular tumours. Prog Clin Biol Res 1990;357:267–76.

207. Niehans GA, Manivel JC, Copland GT, Scheithauer BW, Wick MR. Immunohistochemistry of germ cell and trophoblastic neoplasms. Cancer 1988;62:1113–23.

208. Pierce GB Jr, Midgley AR Jr. The origin and function of human syncytiotrophoblastic giant cells. Am J Pathol 1963;43:153–73.

209. Pugh RC, Cameron KM. Teratoma. In: Pugh RC, ed. Pathology of the testis. Oxford: Blackwell Scientific, 1976:199–244.

210. Rabes HM. Proliferation of human testicular tumours. Int J Androl 1987;10:127–37.

211. Seguchi T, Iwasaki A, Sugao H, Nakano E, Matsuda M, Sonoda T. Clinical statistics of germinal testicular cancer. Nippon Hinyokika Gakkai Zasshi 1990;81:889–94.

212. Silva EG. Chorionic villous-like structures in metastatic testicular choriocarcinoma. Cancer 1987;60:207–10.

213. Srigley JR, Mackay B, Toth P, Ayala A. The ultrastructure and histogenesis of male germ neoplasia with emphasis on seminoma with early carcinomatous features. Ultrastruc Pathol 1988;12:67–86.

214. Stoter G, Sylvester R, Sleijfer DT, et al. A multivariate analysis of prognostic factors in disseminated non - seminomatous testicular cancer. Prog Clin Biol Res 1988;269:381–93.

215. Teilum G. Special tumors of ovary and testis and related extragonadal lesions. Philadelphia: JB Lippincott, 1976.

216. Ulbright TM, Loehrer PJ. Choriocarcinoma-like lesions in patients with testicular germ cell tumors. Two histologic variants. Am J Surg Pathol 1988;12:531–41.

217. Ulbright TM, Young RH, Scully RE. Trophoblastic tumors of the testis other than classic choriocarcinoma: "monophasic" choriocarcinoma and placental site trophoblastic tumor: a report of two cases. Am J Surg Pathol 1997;21:282–8.

218. Vaeth M, Schultz HP, von der Maase H, et al. Prognostic factors in testicular germ cell tumours: experiences with 1058 consecutive cases. Acta Radiol Oncol 1984;23:271–85.

219. Young RH, Kurman RJ, Scully RE. Proliferations and tumors of intermediate trophoblast of the placental site. Semin Diagn Pathol 1988;5:223–37.

Teratoma: Mature, Immature, and with a Secondary Malignant Component

220. Ahmed T, Bosl GJ, Hajdu SI. Teratoma with malignant transformation in germ cell tumors in men. Cancer 1985;56:860–3.

221. Assaf G, Mosbah A, Homsy Y, Michaud J. Dermoid cyst of testis in five-year-old child. Urology 1983;22:432–4.

222. Barsky SH. Germ cell tumors of the testis. In: Javadpour N, Barsky SH, eds. Surgical pathology of urologic diseases. Baltimore: Williams & Wilkins, 1987:224–46.

223. Bartkova J, Bartek J, Lukas J, et al. p53 protein alterations in human testicular cancer including pre-invasive intratubular germ-cell neoplasia. Int J Cancer 1991;49:196–202.

223a. Bell FG. Tumours of the testis: the teratoid group. Brit J Surg 1925;13:7–38.

224. Broggi G, Appetito C, di Leone L, et al. Dermoid cyst in undescended testis in a 9-year-old boy. Urol Int 1991;47:110–2.

225. Brosman SA. Testicular tumors in prepubertal children. Urology 1979;13:581–8.

226. Burke AP, Mostofi FK. Placental alkaline phosphatase immunohistochemistry of intratubular malignant germ cells and associated testicular germ cell tumors. Hum Pathol 1988;19:663–70.

227. Burt AD, Cooper G, MacKay C, Boyd JF. Dermoid cyst of the testis. Scot Med J 1987;32:146–8.

228. Cameron-Strange A, Horner J. Differentiated teratoma of testis metastasizing as differentiated teratoma in adult. Urology 1989;33:481–2.

229. Castedo SM, Oosterhuis JW, de Jong B, et al. A residual mature teratoma with a more balanced karyotype than the primary testicular nonseminoma? Cancer Genet Cytogenet 1988;32:51–7.

229a. Comiter CV, Kibel AS, Richie JP, Nucci MR, Renshaw AA. Prognostic features of teratomas with malignant transformation: a clinicopathologic study of 21 cases. J Urol 1998;159:359–63.

230. Delozier-Blanchet CD, Walt H, Engel E, Vuagnat P. Cytogenetic studies of human testicular germ cell tumours. Int J Androl 1987;10:69–77.

231. Dixon FJ, Moore RA. Tumors of the male sex organs. Atlas of Tumor Pathology, 1st Series, Fascicles 31b & 32. Washington, D.C.: Armed Forces Institute of Pathology, 1952.

232. Dixon FJ, Moore RA. Testicular tumors: a clinicopathologic study. Cancer 1953;6:427–54.

233. Dockerty MB, Priestly JT. Dermoid cysts of the testis. J Urol 1942;48:392–400.

234. Donohue JP, Roth LM, Zachary JM, Rowland RG, Einhorn LH, Williams SD. Cytoreductive surgery for metastatic testis cancer: tissue analysis of retroperitoneal masses after chemotherapy. J Urol 1982;127:1111–4.

235. Einhorn LH, Williams SD, Mandelbaum I, Donohue JP. Surgical resection in disseminated testicular cancer following chemotherapeutic cytoreduction. Cancer 1981;48:904–8.

236. Fossä SD, Aass N, Ous S, et al. Histology of tumor residuals following chemotherapy in patients with advanced nonseminomatous testicular cancer. J Urol 1989;142:1239–42.

237. Foster RS, Baniel J, Leibovitch I, et al. Teratoma in the orchiectomy specimen and volume of metastasis are predictors of retroperitoneal teratoma in low stage nonseminomatous testis cancer. J Urol 1996;155:1943–5.

238. Friedman NB, Moore RA. Tumors of the testis: a report on 922 cases. Milit Surgeon 1946;99:573–93.

239. Fung CY, Kalish LA, Brodsky GL, Richie JP, Garnick MB. Stage I nonseminomatous germ cell testicular tumor: prediction of metastatic potential by primary histopathology. J Clin Oncol 1988;6:1467–73.

240. Gels ME, Hoekstra HJ, Sleijfer DT, et al. Detection of recurrence in patients with clinical stage I nonseminomatous testicular germ cell tumors and consequences for further follow-up: a single-center 10-year experience. J Clin Oncol 1995;13:1188–94.

241. Gilman PA. The epidemiology of human teratomas. In: Damjanov I, Knowles BB, Solter D, eds. The human teratomas: experimental and clinical biology. Clinton, NJ: Humana Press, 1983:81–104.

241a. Grady RW, Ross JH, Kay R. Epidemiological features of testicular teratoma in a prepubertal population. J Urol 1997;158:1191–2.

242. Gupta AK, Gupta MK, Gupta K. Dermoid cyst of the testis (a case report). Indian J Cancer 1986;23:21–3.

243. Hawkins E, Heifetz SA, Giller R, Cushing B. The prepubertal testis (prenatal and postnatal): its relationship to intratubular germ cell neoplasia: a combined Pediatric Oncology Group and Children's Cancer Study Group. Hum Pathol 1997;28:404–10.

243a. Hughes DF, Alen DC, O'Neill JJ. Angiosarcoma arising in a testicular teratoma. Histopathology 1991;18:81–3.

244. Jacobsen GK, Jacobsen M. Alpha-fetoprotein (AFP) and human chorionic gonadotropin in testicular germ cell tumours: a prospective immunohistochemical study. Acta Pathol Microbiol Scand [A] 1983;91:165–76.

245. Jacobsen GK, Jacobsen M, Clausen PP. Distribution of tumor-associated antigens in the various histologic components of germ cell tumors of the testis. Am J Surg Pathol 1981;5:257–66.

246. Jaeger N, Weissbach L, Bussar-Maatz R. Size and status of metastases after inductive chemotherapy of germ-cell tumors. Indication for salvage operation. World J Urol 1994;12:196–9.

247. Johnson DE, Bracken RB, Blight EM. Prognosis for pathologic stage I non-seminomatous germ cell tumors of the testis managed by retroperitoneal lymphadenectomy. J Urol 1976;116:63–8.

248. Jorgensen N, Muller J, Giwercman A, Visfeldt J, Moller H, Skakkebaek NE. DNA content and expression of tumour markers in germ cells adjacent to germ cell tumours in childhood: probably a different origin for infantile and adolescent germ cell tumours. J Pathol 1995;176:269–78.

249. Kashiwagi A, Nagamori S, Toyota K, Maeno K, Koyanagi T. DNA ploidy of testicular germ cell tumors in childhood; difference from adult testicular tumors. Nippon Hinyokika Gakkai Zasshi 1993;84:1655–9.

250. Kay R. Prepubertal Testicular Tumor Registry. J Urol 1993;150:671–4.

251. Kedia K, Fraley EE. Adult teratoma of the testis metastasizing as adult teratoma: case report and review of literature. J Urol 1975;114:636–9.

252. Kooijman CD. Immature teratomas in children. Histopathology 1988;12:491–502.

253. Kusuda L, Leidich RB, Das S. Mature teratoma of the testis metastasizing as mature teratoma. J Urol 1986;135:1020–2.

254. Leibovitch I, Foster RS, Ulbright TM, Donohue JP. Adult primary pure teratoma of the testis. The Indiana experience. Cancer 1995;75:2244–50.

255. Loehrer PJ, Hui S, Clark S, et al. Teratoma following cisplatin-based combination chemotherapy for nonseminomatous germ cell tumors: a clinicopathological correlation. J Urol 1986;135:1183–9.

256. Logothetis CJ, Samuels ML, Trindade A. The growing teratoma syndrome. Cancer 1982;50:1629–35.

257. Manivel JC, Jessurun J, Wick MR, Dehner LP. Placental alkaline phosphatase immunoreactivity in testicular germ cell tumors. Am J Surg Pathol 1987;11:21–9.

258. Manivel JC, Reinberg Y, Niehans GA, Fraley EE. Intratubular germ cell neoplasia in testicular teratomas and epidermoid cysts. Correlation with prognosis and possible biologic significance. Cancer 1989;64:715–20.

258a. Michael H. Nongerm cell tumors arising in patients with testicular germ cell tumors. J Urol Pathol 1998;9:39–60.

259. Michael H, Hull MT, Ulbright TM, Foster RS, Miller KD. Primitive neuroectodermal tumors arising in testicular germ cell neoplasms. Am J Surg Pathol 1997;21:896–904.

260. Miettinen M, Virtanen I, Talerman A. Intermediate filament proteins in human testis and testicular germ-cell tumors. Am J Pathol 1985;120:402–10.

260a.Minkowitz G, Lee M, Minkowitz S. Pilomatricoma of the testicle. An ossifying testicular tumor with hair matrix differentiation. Arch Pathol Lab Med 1995;119:96–9.

261. Molenaar WM, Oosterhuis JW, Meiring A, Sleyfer DT, Koops HS, Cornelisse CJ. Histology and DNA contents of a secondary malignancy arising in a mature residual lesion six years after chemotherapy for a disseminanted non-seminomatous testicular tumor. Cancer 1986;58:264–8.

262. Mostofi FK. Histological change ostensibly induced by therapy in the metastasis of germ cell tumors of testis. Prog Clin Biol Res 1985;203:47–60.

263. Mostofi FK, Sesterhenn IA. Pathology of germ cell tumors of testes. Prog Clin Biol Res 1985;203:1–34.

263a.Motzer RJ, Amsterdam A, Prieto V, et al. Teratoma with malignant transformation: diverse malignant histologies arising in men with germ cell tumors. J Urol 1998;159:133–8.

264. Moul JW, McCarthy WF, Fernandez EB, Sesterhenn IA. Percentage of embryonal carcinoma and of vascular invasion predicts pathological stage in clinical stage I nonseminomatous testicular cancer. Cancer Res 1994;54:362–4.

265. Norris HJ, Zirkin HJ, Benson WL. Immature (malignant) teratoma of the ovary: a clinical and pathologic study of 58 cases. Cancer 1976;37:2359–72.

266. Oosterhuis JW, de Jong B, Cornelisse CJ, et al. Karyotyping and DNA flow cytometry of mature residual teratoma after intensive chemotherapy of disseminated non-seminomatous germ cell tumor of the testis: a report of two cases. Cancer Genet Cytogenet 1986;22:149–57.

267. Oosterhuis JW, Suurmeyer AJ, Sleyfer DT, Koops HS, Oldhoff J, Fleuren G. Effects of multiple-drug chemotherapy (cis-diammine-dichloroplatinum, bleomycin and vinblastine) on the maturation of retroperitoneal lymph node metastases of nonseminomatous germ cell tumors of the testis: no evidence for de novo induction of differentiation. Cancer 1983;51:408–16.

268. Price EB Jr. Epidermoid cysts of the testis: a clinical and pathologic analysis of 69 cases from the testicular tumor registry. J Urol 1969;102:708–13.

269. Pugh RC, Cameron KM. Teratoma. In: Pugh RC, ed. Pathology of the testis. Oxford: Blackwell Scientific, 1976:199–244.

270. Rabbani F, Gleave ME, Coppin CM, Murray N, Sullivan LD. Teratoma in primary testis tumor reduces complete response rates in the retroperitoneum after primary chemotherapy. The case for primary retroperitoneal lymph node dissection of stage IIb germ cell tumors with teratomatous elements. Cancer 1996;78:480–6.

271. Renedo DE, Trainer TD. Intratubular germ cell neoplasia (ITGCN) with p53 and PCNA expression and adjacent mature teratoma in an infant testis. An immunohistochemical and morphologic study with a review of the literature. Am J Surg Pathol 1994;18:947–52.

272. Ro J, Sella A, El-Naggar A, Ayala A. Mature growing teratoma: clinicopathologic and DNA flow cytometric analysis [Abstract]. Lab Invest 1990;62:83A.

273. Shah KH, Maxted WC, Chun B. Epidermoid cysts of the testis: a report of three cases and an analysis of 141 cases from the world literature. Cancer 1981;47:577–82.

274. Simmonds PD, Lee AH, Theaker JM, Tung K, Smart CJ, Mead GM. Primary pure teratoma of the testis. J Urol 1996;155:939–42.

275. Stevens MJ, Norman AR, Fisher C, Hendry WF, Dearnaley DP, Horwich A. Prognosis of testicular teratoma differentiated. Br J Urol 1994;73:701–6.

276. Steyerberg EW, Keizer HJ, Stoter G, Habbema JD. Predictors of residual mass histology following chemotherapy for metastatic non-seminomatous testicular cancer: a quantitative overview of 996 resections. Eur J Cancer 1994;30A:1231–9.

277. Strohmeyer T, Reissmann P, Cordon-Cardo C, Hartmann M, Ackermann R, Slamon D. Correlation between retinoblastoma gene expression and differentiation in human testicular tumors. Proc Nat Acad Sci USA 1991;88:6662–6.

277a.Tapper D, Lack EE. Teratomas in infancy and childhood. A 54-year experience at the Children's Hospital. Ann Surg 1983;198:398–410.

277b.Terrier-Lacombe MJ, Martinez-Madrigal F, Porta W, Rahal J, Droz JP. Embryonal rhabdomyosarcoma arising in a mature teratoma of the testis: a case report. J Urol 1990;143:1232–4.

278. Thurlbeck WM, Scully RE. Solid teratoma of the ovary. Cancer 1960;13:804–11.

279. Tongaonkar HB, Deshmane VH, Dalal AV, Kulkarni JN, Kamat MR. Growing teratoma syndrome. J Surg Oncol 1994;55:56–60.

280. Trojanowski JQ, Hickey WF. Human teratomas express differentiated neural antigens: an immunohistochemical study with anti-neurofilament, anti-glial filament, and anti-myelin basic protein monoclonal antibodies. Am J Pathol 1984;115:383–9.

281. Uchida T, Shimoda T, Miyata H, et al. Immunoperoxidase study of alkaline phosphatase in testicular tumor. Cancer 1981;48:1455–62.

282. Ulbright TM, Loehrer PJ, Roth LM, Einhorn LH, Williams SD, Clark SA. The development of non-germ cell malignancies within germ cell tumors. A clinicopathologic study of 11 cases. Cancer 1984;54:1824–33.

283. Ulbright TM, Michael H, Loehrer PJ, Donohue JP. Spindle cell tumors resected from male patients with germ cell tumors: a clinicopathologic study of 14 cases. Cancer 1990;65:148–56.

284. von Hochstetter AR, Hedinger CE. The differential diagnosis of testicular germ cell tumors in theory and practice: a critical analysis of two major systems of classification and review of 389 cases. Virchows Arch [A] 1982;396:247–77.

285. Wegner HE, Herbst H, Loy V, Dieckmann KP. Testicular dermoid cyst in a 10-year-old child: case report and discussion of etiopathogenesis, diagnosis, and treatment. Urol Int 1995;54:109–11.

286. Wishnow KI, Johnson DE, Swanson DA, et al. Identifying patients with low-risk clinical stage I non-seminomatous testicular tumors who should be treated by surveillance. Urology 1989;34:339–43.

287. Wogalter H, Scofield GF. Adult teratoma of the testicle metastasizing as adult teratoma. J Urol 1962;87:573–6.

288. Zuk RJ, Jenkins BJ, Martin JE, Oliver RT, Baithun SI. Findings in lymph nodes of patients with germ cell tumours after chemotherapy and their relation to prognosis. J Clin Pathol 1989;42:1049–54.

Monodermal Teratomas

289. Aguirre P, Scully RE. Primitive neuroectodermal tumor of the testis. Report of a case. Arch Pathol Lab Med 1983;107:643–5.

289a. Amin MB, Young RH, Scully RE. Immunohistochemical profile of Sertoli and Leydig cell tumors of the testis [Abstract]. Mod Pathol 1998;11:76A.

289b. Anagnostaki l, Jacobsen GK, Horn T, Sengeløv, Braændstrup O. Melanotic neuroectodermal tumour as a predominant component of an immature testicular teratoma. APMIS 1992;100:809–16.

290. Berdjis CC, Mostofi FK. Carcinoid tumors of the testis. J Urol 1977;118:777–82.

291. Cummings OW, Ulbright TM, Young RH, Dei Tos AP, Fletcher CD, Hull MT. Desmoplastic small round cell tumors of the para-testicular region: a report of six cases. Am J Surg Pathol 1997;21:219–25.

292. Finci R, Gunhan O, Celasun B, Gungor S. Carcinoid tumor of undescended testis. J Urol 1987;137:301–2.

293. Hosking DH, Bowman DM, McMorris SL, Ramsey EW. Primary carcinoid of the testis with metastases. J Urol 1981;125:255–6.

293a. Iczkowski KA, Bostwick DG, Cheville JC. Inhibin is a sensitive and specific marker for testicular sex cord–stromal tumors. Mod Pathol 1998;11:774–9.

293b. McCluggage WG, Shanks JH, Whiteside C, Maxwell P, Banerjee SS, Biggart JD. Immunohistochemical study of testicular sex cord–stromal tumors, including staining with anti-inhibin antibody. Am J Surg Pathol 1998;22:615–9.

294. Michael H, Hull MT, Ulbright TM, Foster RS, Miller KD. Primitive neuroectodermal tumors arising in testicular germ cell neoplasms. Am J Surg Pathol 1997;21:896–904.

294a. Michael H, Hull MT, Foster RS, Sweeny CJ, Ulbright TM. Nephroblastoma-like tumors in patients with testicular germ cell tumors. Am J Surg Pathol 1998;22:1107–14.

295. Nistal M, Paniagua R. Primary neuroectodermal tumour of the testis. Histopathology 1985;9:1351–9.

296. Nocks BN, Dann JA. Primitive neuroectodermal tumor (immature teratoma) of testis. Urology 1983;22:543–4.

297. Ogawa A, Sugihara S, Nakazawa Y, et al. A case of primary carcinoid tumor of the testis. Gan No Rinsho 1988;34:1629–34.

298. Ordonez NG, Ayala AG, Sneige N, Mackay B. Immunohistochemical demonstration of multiple neurohormonal polypeptides in a case of pure testicular carcinoid. Am J Clin Pathol 1982;78:860–4.

298a. Pal AK, Chopra SK, Kalra AS. Calcifying malignant struma of the testis: a case report. Ind J Cancer 1975; 12:210–3.

299. Parham DM, Webber B, Holt H, Williams WK, Maurer H. Immunohistochemical study of childhood rhabdomyosarcomas and related neoplasms. Results of an Intergroup Rhabdomyosarcoma Study Project. Cancer 1991;67:3072–80.

300. Schmidt D, Harms D, Pilon VA. Small-cell pediatric tumors: histology, immunohistochemistry, and electron microscopy. Clin Lab Med 1987;7:63–89.

300a. Singh N, Cumming J, Theaker JM. Pure cartilaginous teratoma differentiated of the testis. Histopathology 1997;20:373–4.

301. Sullivan JL, Packer JT, Bryant M. Primary malignant carcinoid of the testis. Arch Pathol Lab Med 1981;105:515–7.

302. Talerman A, Gratama S, Miranda S, Okagaki T. Primary carcinoid tumor of the testis: case report, ultrastructure and review of the literature. Cancer 1978;42:2696–706.

302a. Unger PD, Cohen EL, Talerman A. Mixed germ cell tumor of the testis: a unique combination of seminoma and teratoma composed predominantly of prostatic tissue. J Urol Pathol 1998;9:257–63.

302b. Waxman M, Vuletin JC, Pertschuk LP, Bellamy J, Enu K. Pleomorphic atypical thyroid adenoma arising in struma testis: light microscopic, ultrastructural and immunofluorescent studies. Mount Sinai J Med 1982;49:13–7.

303. Young RH, Scully RE. Testicular tumors. Chicago: ASCP Press, 1990.

304. Zavala-Pompa A, Ro JY, El-Naggar A, et al. Primary carcinoid tumor of testis. Immunohistochemical, ultrastructural, and DNA flow cytometric study of three cases with a review of the literature. Cancer 1993;72:1726–32.

❖❖❖

5

MIXED GERM CELL, REGRESSED GERM CELL, AND GERM CELL–SEX CORD–STROMAL TUMORS

MIXED GERM CELL TUMORS

Definition. These neoplasms contain more than one germ cell tumor component. Cases of seminoma with syncytiotrophoblast cells are, by convention, excluded from this category.

General Features. In a study of 1,053 cases, Jacobsen et al. (11) found that mixed germ cell tumors comprised 69 percent of all non-seminomatous germ cell tumors and 32 percent of testicular germ cell tumors. In another study of 513 testicular germ cell tumors, Barsky (1) reported an even higher percentage of mixed type (91 percent of nonseminomatous tumors and 60 percent of all testicular germ cell tumors), perhaps due to the referral nature of that material and the inclusion of cases of seminoma with syncytiotrophoblast giant cells. Most of the more common combinations of tumor types are shown in Table 5-1; a common pattern is embryonal carcinoma with one or more components of tera-toma, seminoma, and yolk sac tumor, but virtu-ally any combination can be seen.

For diagnosis, these tumors should be termed "mixed germ cell tumor, composed of . . ." fol-lowed by a tabulation of the components, with an estimate of their percentage; for example, "mixed germ cell tumor composed of embryonal carcinoma (60 percent), yolk sac tumor (25 per-cent), seminoma (15 percent), and rare syn-cytiotrophoblast cells."

Clinical Features. The clinical features of mixed germ cell tumors are similar to those of the nonseminomatous category as a whole, with the usual mode of presentation being testicular enlargement, sometimes associated with pain. The tumors occur at an average age of 30 years, with patients who have a predominance of em-bryonal carcinoma averaging 28 years and those with a predominance of seminoma 33 years (3). Prepubertal patients rarely have mixed germ cell tumors. Serum marker elevations are com-mon and reflect the components of the tumors. Alpha-fetoprotein (AFP) elevation occurs in about 60 percent and human chorionic gonado-tropin (hCG) in about 55 percent of patients with metastatic disease (20).

Gross Findings. The tumors are variegated (fig. 5-1): solid white to gray areas may reflect a seminomatous component (fig. 5-2) whereas non-seminomatous elements more frequently are asso-ciated with areas of necrosis, hemorrhage, and cystic degeneration (fig. 5-1A,B). Teratomatous ele-ments may be suspected when cysts that are non-degenerative in appearance are seen (fig. 5-1C).

Microscopic Findings. The individual com-ponents are identical to those seen in pure germ cell tumors. The combination of embryonal car-cinoma and teratoma (fig. 5-3) has been termed

Table 5-1

COMBINATIONS OF NEOPLASTIC GERM CELL TUMOR TYPES IN 352 MIXED GERM CELL TUMORS*

Tumor Types	Number	(%)
EC + T**	90	(26)
EC + S	55	(16)
EC + YST + T	39	(11)
EC + T + CC	26	(7)
EC + T + S	22	(6)
T + S	20	(6)
EC + YST	15	(4)
EC + YST + T + CC	15	(4)
EC + CC	13	(4)
EC + YST + T	12	(3)
EC + YST + S	9	(3)
Other combinations	36	(10)

*Adapted from Jacobsen GK, Barlebo H, Olsen J, et al. Testicular germ cell tumours in Denmark 1976-1980: pathology of 1058 consecutive cases. Acta Radiol Oncol 1984; 23:239-47.
**EC = embryonal carcinoma; CC = choriocarcinoma; S = seminoma; T= teratoma; YST = yolk sac tumor.

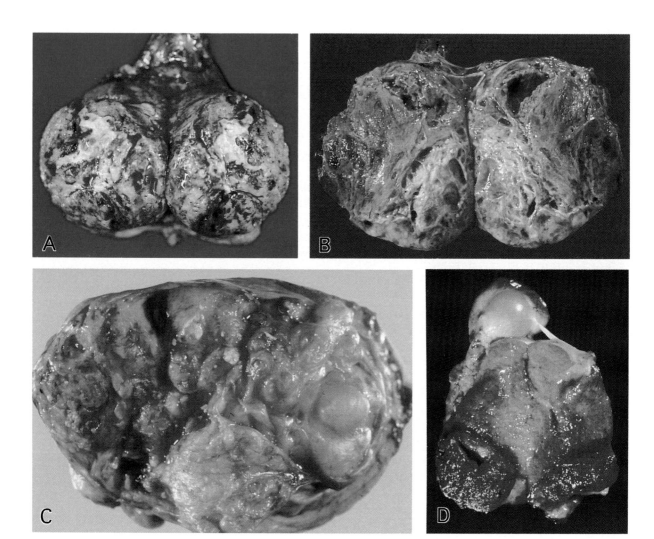

Figure 5-1
MIXED GERM CELL TUMORS

A: Typical variegated sectioned surface with areas of necrosis. This tumor had immature teratoma, yolk sac tumor, and embryonal carcinoma components. (Courtesy of Dr. P.R. Faught, Indianapolis, IN.)

B: Prominent cystic degeneration in a tumor composed of yolk sac tumor and embryonal carcinoma.

C: Cysts, representing a teratomatous component, are present in a neoplasm that also contained embryonal carcinoma.

D: Beefy red areas are conspicuous in this tumor that had a prominent choriocarcinoma component as well as embryonal carcinoma.

"teratocarcinoma," but it is preferable to list the components separately. Commonly overlooked is a focal reticular or myxomatous pattern of yolk sac tumor contiguous with embryonal carcinoma (fig. 5-4A,B) or small foci of yolk sac tumor arising from embryoid bodies (see below). The contrasting cytologic features of seminoma cells and those of embryonal carcinoma are such that they usually stand out in marked contrast to each other, but occasionally the two cell types appear to merge (fig. 5-4C). Liver-like cells may be seen in association with yolk sac tumor elements (fig. 5-4D). We have seen a single

case, courtesy of Dr. V. E. Reuter, where multiple small foci of squamous differentiation occurred in an otherwise typical seminoma. The tumor was interpreted as seminoma and teratoma.

Two patterns of mixed germ cell tumor are sufficiently distinctive that they are separately subcategorized: the polyembryoma and diffuse embryoma.

Polyembryoma. This mixed germ cell tumor is composed of embryonal carcinoma and yolk sac tumor, sometimes with teratomatous components that are arranged in a pattern resembling the

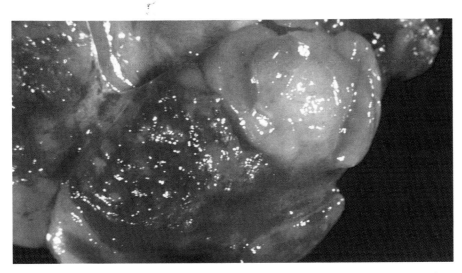

Figure 5-2
MIXED GERM CELL
TUMOR

Two distinct components, embryonal carcinoma (lower left) and seminoma (upper right) were present, as could be suspected on gross examination.

Figure 5-3
MIXED GERM CELL
TUMOR

An admixture of columnar embryonal carcinoma cells (right) and mature teratomatous cartilage.

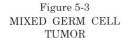

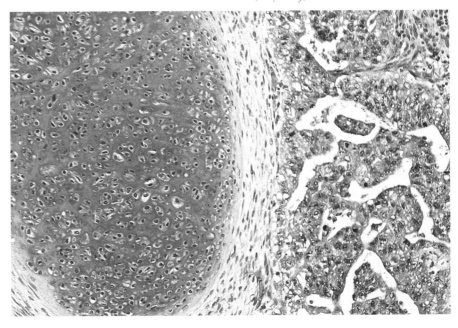

presomitic embryo prior to day 18 of development (6). Because of its highly organized nature, some authorities consider it a separate, unique form of nonseminomatous germ cell neoplasm and do not classify it as a "mixed" germ cell tumor. They argue that it lacks the random admixture that is usually seen in other mixed germ cell tumors and that it recapitulates a very early stage of embryonic development. According to this viewpoint, it therefore qualifies as an extremely immature form of immature teratoma. While there is merit to these views, in our opinion it is preferable to consider the polyembryoma as a unique and

highly organized form of mixed germ cell tumor, given that it behaves and is treated like other mixed germ cell tumors with similar components (16). Also, polyembryomatous foci always comprise a portion of a mixed germ cell tumor, and have not been reported in pure form in the testis to our knowledge. There is most often an associated component of teratoma. The patients' age range is that for nonseminomatous germ cell tumors (6,16). Substantial AFP elevations occur (16).

The tumors are solid and cystic (reflecting a frequent associated component of teratoma), with foci of hemorrhage and necrosis (16).

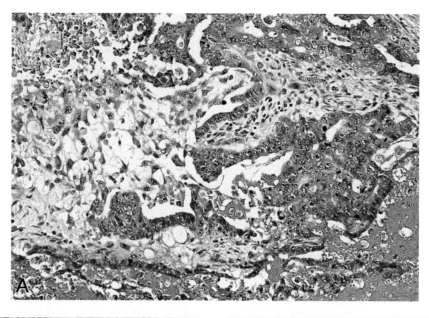

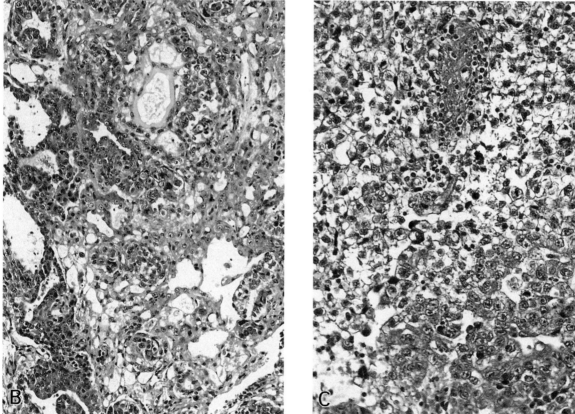

Figure 5-4
MIXED GERM CELL TUMORS

A: The loosely arranged, focally vacuolated cells in this field represent focal yolk sac tumor associated with an embryonal carcinoma component (the larger, more darkly staining foci with focal glandular differentiation [right]).

B: In this area the yolk sac tumor and embryonal carcinoma components do not contrast with each other to the degree seen in A, although they can still be distinguished in most areas.

C: Seminoma (top) merges with embryonal carcinoma (bottom right).

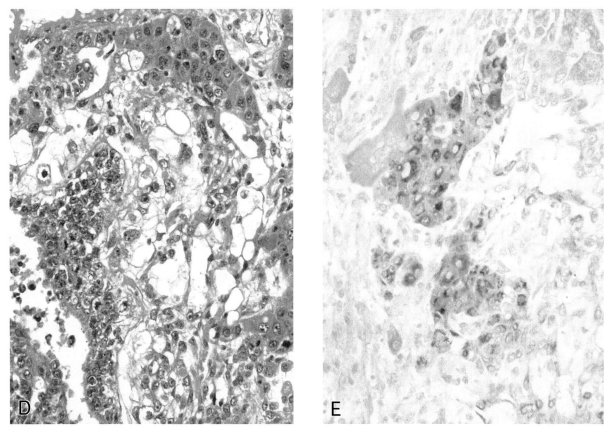

Figure 5-4 (Continued)
D: Liver-like cells (top) in a mixed germ cell tumor. Note embryonal carcinoma (lower left) and reticular yolk sac tumor (right).
E: Liver-like cells in a mixed germ cell tumor react for alpha-fetoprotein (anti-alpha-fetoprotein immunostain).

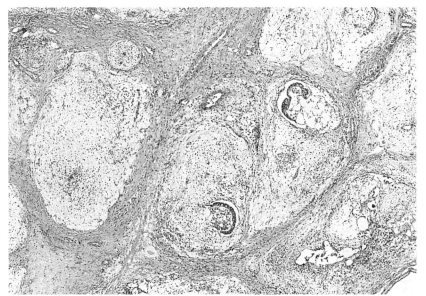

Figure 5-5
POLYEMBRYOMA
Embryoid bodies are scattered in a loose mesenchyme analogous to the extraembryonic mesenchyme.

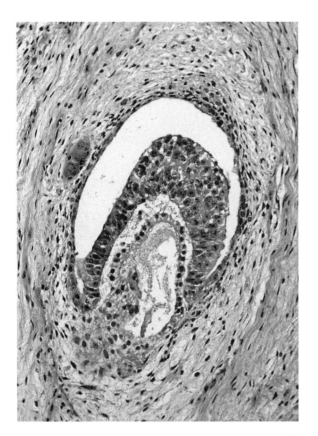 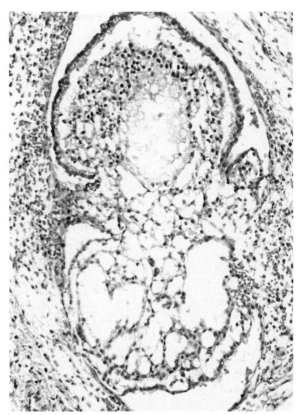

Figure 5-6
POLYEMBRYOMA

Left: A high magnification of an embryoid body shows a central core of embryonal carcinoma mimicking the embryonic plate, with a "dorsal" amnion-like cavity and a "ventral" yolk sac-like structure. A syncytiotrophoblastic cell is also apparent close to the "amnion."

Right: Two embryoid bodies are fused, and there is a central aggregate of yolk sac tumor epithelium. Invasion beyond the embryoid body has not occurred and this appearance does not merit the separate diagnosis of yolk sac tumor.

There are scattered embryo-like bodies ("embryoid bodies") (fig. 5-5) with a central plate of cuboidal to columnar embryonal carcinoma cells of one to four layers thickness, a "dorsal" amnion-like cavity typically lined by flattened epithelium, and a "ventral" yolk sac–like vesicle composed of reticular and myxomatous yolk sac tumor (fig. 5-6). These bodies are from 0.2 to 0.7 mm in greatest dimension and are surrounded by a myxoid, embryonic-type of mesenchyme, giving rise to a very distinctive low-power appearance (fig. 5-5).

The "amnion" is usually composed of flattened cells, but Nakashima et al. (16) have described both intestinal and squamous differentiation arising from the amniotic epithelium. Argyrophilic cells may be identified in the intestinal structures. Yolk sac structures appear to derive from proliferation of the cells of the embryonic disc, which migrate as stellate cells. Hepatic differentiation may then develop in this "embryonic yolk sac." Syncytiotrophoblastic giant cells may be identified in close proximity to the amnion and yolk sac (6). Immunohistochemically, the yolk sac–like areas stain for AFP (16). Sometimes the microscopic foci of yolk sac tumor elements that are seen in the embryoid bodies merge imperceptibly with larger foci to justify a separate diagnosis of yolk sac tumor. The latter diagnosis is recommended when the yolk sac foci exceed 3 mm (22). Not all embryoid bodies are perfectly organized as described above (fig. 5-7), and blastocyst-like structures may occur in embryonal carcinoma, probably representing an ontogenetically earlier form of similar differentiation (12,13). Polyembryomas behave like other nonseminomatous tumors and are treated similarly.

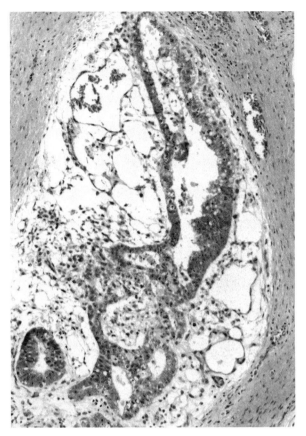

Figure 5-7
MIXED GERM CELL TUMOR
This mixed germ cell tumor has a poorly formed embryoid body with a central core of embryonal carcinoma around which is a haphazard arrangement of yolk sac tumor epithelium.

Diffuse Embryoma. This tumor is characterized by an intimate admixture of orderly arranged embryonal carcinoma and yolk sac tumor in roughly equal proportions (fig. 5-8) (4,5); minor trophoblastic or teratomatous elements are also occasionally present, and liver-like cells may occur. The yolk sac tumor elements may "garland" foci of embryonal carcinoma as a parallel layer of flattened epithelium, a pattern that has been described as ribbon- or necklace-like (fig. 5-8). This pattern is similar to that described as a "double-layered" pattern of embryonal carcinoma (10,17), said to be present in 7 percent of "embryonal carcinomas" (10), which we consider in the diffuse embryoma category and a form of mixed germ cell tumor. The flattened cell layer in such cases generally stains for AFP, supporting its yolk sac tumor nature (fig. 5-9).

Treatment and Prognosis. The treatment of mixed germ cell tumors is similar to that of nonseminomatous tumors in general. The presence of some elements appears to modify the behavior of other components. Brawn (2) has shown that the presence of a teratomatous component in conjunction with embryonal carcinoma significantly lowers the metastatic rate compared to a pure embryonal carcinoma; this was not attributable to the lower volume of embryonal carcinoma in the mixed germ cell tumor. The occurrence of different potentials for differentiation in human embryonal carcinoma cell lines (14,18,19), in conjunction with this information, implies that embryonal carcinomas associated with teratoma have a greater inherent ability to differentiate than pure embryonal carcinomas and are therefore intrinsically less aggressive, a concept supported by the lower rate of occult metastases in patients with mixed germ cell tumors with a teratomatous component (8,9,15,21). The presence of yolk sac tumor elements within a testicular primary has also been associated with a lesser tendency to metastasize and may also reflect a greater inherent tendency of the neoplasm to differentiate (7).

REGRESSION OF TESTICULAR GERM CELL TUMORS ("BURNT-OUT" GERM CELL TUMORS)

General Features. In some patients who present with extragonadal germ cell tumors, careful clinical evaluation fails to reveal evidence of a testicular primary neoplasm (24,28, 29,34). Some of these tumors may represent primary germ cell tumors of extragonadal origin, presumably developing from misplaced germ cells. There is convincing evidence, however, that a considerable proportion of such patients have primary testicular neoplasms that have partially or completely regressed and therefore are not detected by clinical examination. Indeed, some patients may only develop a clinically evident testicular tumor after metastatic disease is apparent (23). An occult testicular origin is most likely for apparent extragonadal tumors developing in the retroperitoneum (28,31). With isolated mediastinal involvement there is a much higher probability of a true extragonadal origin (31).

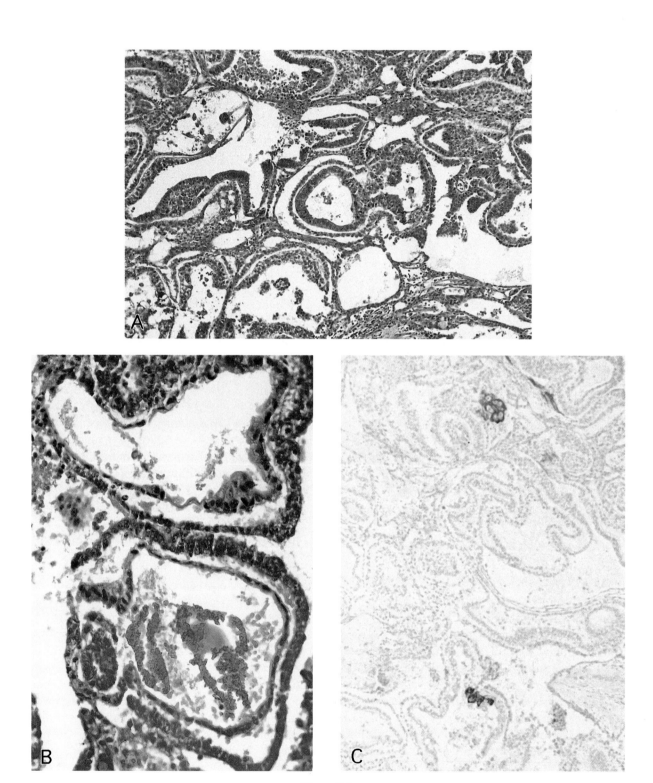

Figure 5-8
DIFFUSE EMBRYOMA

A: Embryonal carcinoma and yolk sac tumor show a diffuse, orderly admixture in ribbons and circular patterns.

B: Higher magnification showing an approximate equal proportion of embryonal carcinoma and yolk sac tumor arranged like a necklace.

C: Syncytiotrophoblast cells are highlighted by an immunostain for hCG. Note the still perceptible orderly arrangement. (Fig. 3.63 from Young RH, Scully RE. Testicular tumors. Chicago, ASCP Press, 1990:79.)

The concept of spontaneous regression in testicular germ cell tumors is based on studies of patients who died of metastatic germ cell tumor and were found to have testicular abnormalities only at autopsy (35). In their autopsy series of 61 cases, Bar and Hedinger (27) found "burnt-out" testicular primaries in 6 (10 percent) of their patients. Azzopardi and co-workers (26) documented 70 cases of complete or partial regression in patients with metastatic, nonseminomatous germ cell tumors. Patients with metastatic choriocarcinoma probably have the highest proportion of regressed primary neoplasms (33), but regression has also been identified in patients with metastatic embryonal carcinoma, mixed germ cell tumors, and, less commonly, seminoma (25,26,29). There appears, therefore, to be a general correlation between the tendency to regress and the tendency to spontaneously necrose. The common persistence of teratomatous elements is a likely consequence of their resistance to spontaneous (and, indeed, chemotherapy-induced) necrosis. Azzopardi and Hoffbrand (25) identified an early case of regression in a seminoma in which foci of coagulative necrosis with ghost-like remnants of tumor cells were surrounded by a fibrohistiocytic reaction. Because a testicular primary may regress at the same time metastases grow, huge metastatic deposits may occur with only microscopic testicular lesions (fig. 5-10).

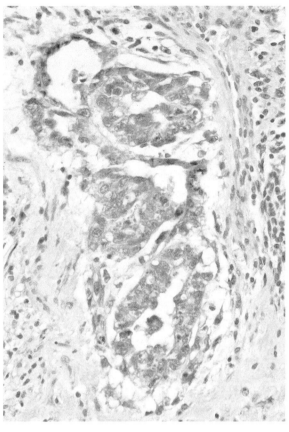

Figure 5-9
MIXED GERM CELL TUMOR
AFP is positive in the flattened cells representing a yolk sac tumor component intermingled with embryonal carcinoma cells which are negative.

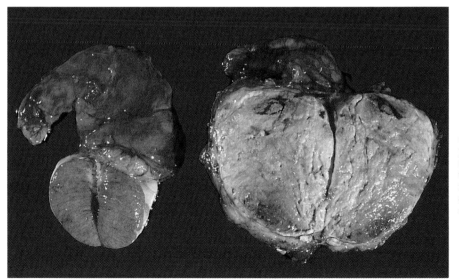

Figure 5-10
REGRESSED
("BURNT-OUT")
GERM CELL TUMOR
The patient presented with a large, mostly necrotic retroperitoneal tumor composed of seminoma and mature teratoma (right). The grossly normal testis (left) contained a microscopic area of scarring and mature teratoma.

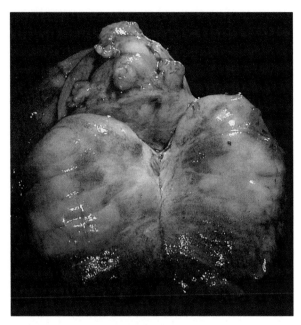

Figure 5-11
REGRESSED ("BURNT-OUT") GERM CELL TUMOR
An irregularly outlined, firm, white zone of scarring is seen in the testis of a patient with extensive retroperitoneal seminoma.

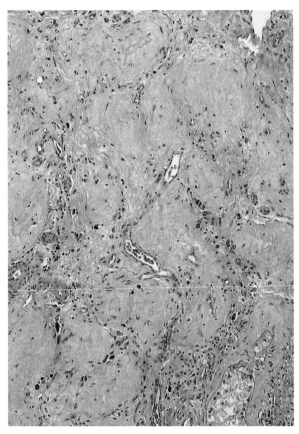

Figure 5-12
REGRESSED ("BURNT-OUT") GERM CELL TUMOR
Scarred area with numerous hemosiderin-laden macrophages.

Gross Findings. Gross examination of regressed germ cell tumors may reveal one or more poorly demarcated zones of firm, white scar tissue (fig. 5-11). Cysts reflecting teratomatous glands or small, hard islands of cartilage may also be identified.

Microscopic Findings. On microscopic examination the scarred zones consist of irregularly outlined, dense deposits of collagen that often contain hemosiderin-laden macrophages, scattered lymphocytes, and xanthoma cells (fig. 5-12). Round deposits of hematoxyphilic material in and around the scarred areas are common (fig. 5-13). Such "hematoxylin-staining" bodies contain both calcium and deoxyribonucleic acid (DNA) (26) and correspond to regressed, intratubular, necrotic tumor with dystrophic calcification. Hematoxylin-staining bodies do not commonly occur in patients with regressed seminoma since intratubular necrosis of seminoma is unusual (25,32). Intratubular germ cell neoplasia, unclassified (IGCNU) may be seen (31), as well as minute amounts of residual invasive tumor, teratomatous glands and cysts (fig. 5-14), and cartilage.

Histologic discrepancies between the metastatic tumor and the residual, partially regressed testicular neoplasm are common (27). For instance, patients may present with metastatic embryonal carcinoma and only have microscopic foci of seminoma and scarring in the testis (34). Such cases may well represent mixed germ cell tumors in which the disseminated element regressed in the testis while other testicular components persisted. Another explanation for discrepancy between the morphology of the testicular tumor and the metastasis is transformation of tumor types (30).

GERM CELL–SEX CORD–STROMAL TUMORS

These tumors consist of both neoplastic germ cell and sex cord–stromal elements. There are two types of germ cell-sex cord-stromal tumor: gonadoblastoma and unclassified type.

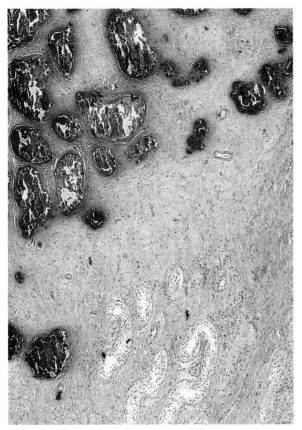

Figure 5-13
REGRESSED ("BURNT-OUT") GERM CELL TUMOR
A scarred zone contains numerous round foci of dystrophic calcification with central necrotic debris. Such foci have been described as "hematoxylin-staining bodies" and correspond to necrotic intratubular germ cell tumor.

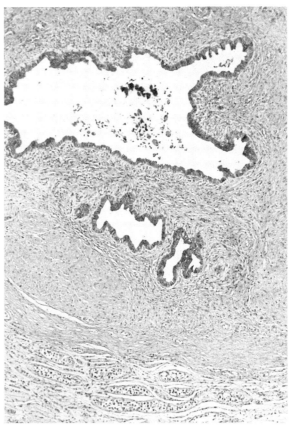

Figure 5-14
REGRESSED ("BURNT-OUT") GERM CELL TUMOR
Teratomatous glands and cysts are present within the scarred zones.

Gonadoblastoma

General Features. About 20 percent of gonadoblastomas occur in phenotypic males, usually under 20 years of age, who also often have cryptorchidism, hypospadias, and gynecomastia, which usually cause the clinical presentation (44). An initially reported association with the Beckwith-Wiedemann syndrome has been retracted (45). Surgical exploration of the cryptorchid gonads often reveals female internal genitalia (uterus and fallopian tubes) that result from failure of the mullerian duct to involute (42). The gonads usually have the features of mixed gonadal dysgenesis (unilateral streak gonad or streak testis and contralateral testis or bilateral streak testis) and karyotypic analysis almost always reveals the presence of a Y chromosome, usually as 45,X/46,XY mosaicism or 46,XY (42). One study, using fluorescence in situ hybridization in cases of gonadoblastoma in patients with 45,X/46,XY mosaicism, showed a higher proportion of tumor nuclei with a Y chromosome compared to non-neoplastic stromal nuclei, supporting a role for the Y chromosome in tumorigenesis (37b). Genetic marker studies have suggested a suspect gene close to the centromere (41a,47). In a series of 101 tumors, 18 occurred in a recognizable testis (44). Overall, about 40 percent of gonadoblastomas are bilateral, but the frequency of bilaterality in phenotypic males may be less (44).

Many consider gonadoblastoma a form of in situ germ cell tumor since, at the time of diagnosis, about half of the collective cases (including testicular, streak, and gonad of undetermined nature) have progressed to an invasive germinoma (seminoma or dysgerminoma) and 8 percent

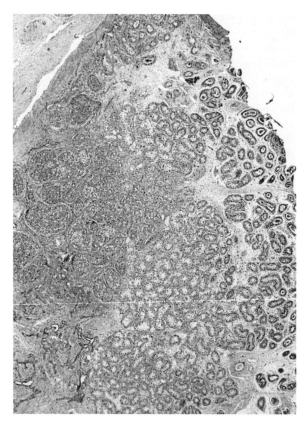

Figure 5-15
GONADOBLASTOMA
Nests of gonadoblastoma are present at left above the rete testis, with immature seminiferous tubules on the right.

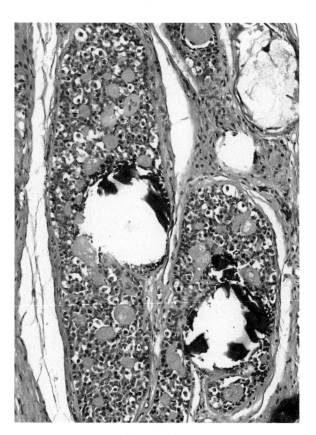

Figure 5-16
GONADOBLASTOMA
Discrete nests are composed of dark sex cord cells that surround germ cells with clear cytoplasm. Note round deposits of basement membrane material and calcifications. (Fig. 6.2 from Young RH, Scully RE. Testicular tumors. Chicago, ASCP Press, 1990:142.)

to another form of germ cell tumor such as embryonal carcinoma, yolk sac tumor, or teratoma (44). The exact number of invasive germ cell tumors that can be attributed as arising from gonadoblastoma is unknown because overgrowth often obliterates a preexisting gonadoblastoma; such cases, however, probably represent a very small minority of testicular germ cell tumors.

Gross Findings. About 25 percent of gonadoblastomas are microscopic; the remainder have measured up to 8 cm in diameter. They are brown to yellow to gray tumors, varying from soft and fleshy to firm and cartilage-like, often flecked with gritty calcifications and, less commonly, showing diffuse calcification (44). Large tumor size, fleshy areas, and hemorrhage or necrosis are suspicious for an invasive germ cell tumor that has arisen from the gonadoblastoma.

Microscopic Findings. The gonadoblastoma is composed of germ cells resembling seminoma cells, and immature Sertoli cells (figs. 5-15–5-18) that may contain Charcot-Böttcher filaments on ultrastructural examination (38,41). These two components are typically intermixed in rounded to irregular nests that often contain hyaline deposits of basement membrane surrounded by the sex cord cells (fig. 5-15). The sex cord cells may also have a peripheral arrangement around nests that largely consist of seminoma-like cells, or they may surround individual seminoma-like cells within the nests in a pattern similar to that of a primary ovarian follicle (44). Calcification occurs in 80 percent of the cases (fig. 5-16), starting in the basement membrane deposits; coalescence of calcifications may result in irregular, mulberry-shaped calcific islands devoid of tumor cells (44). Peripheral to the tumor nests, Leydig-like cells lacking Reinke crystals can be identified in two thirds of

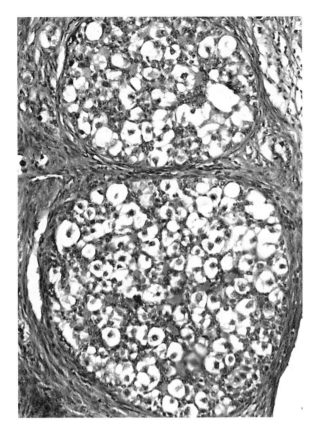

Figure 5-17
GONADOBLASTOMA

Neoplastic germ cells with clear cytoplasm, resembling seminoma cells, are surrounded by sex cord cells in two rounded nests. There are also interspersed deposits of eosinophilic basement membrane material. (Fig. 6.3 from Young RH, Scully RE. Testicular tumors. Chicago, ASCP Press, 1990:143.)

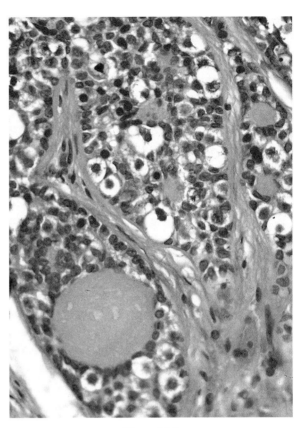

Figure 5-18
GONADOBLASTOMA

At higher magnification the seminoma-like features of the germ cells are apparent; the sex cord cells resemble immature Sertoli cells. Rounded deposits of basement membrane are apparent. A few Leydig-like cells are present in the stroma. (Fig. 6.4 from Young RH, Scully RE. Testicular tumors. Chicago, ASCP Press, 1990:143.)

cases but are more conspicuous in postpubertal patients (42,44). Invasive germ cell tumors developing from gonadoblastoma have typical features (see chapters 3 and 4). Coarse calcifications in an invasive germ cell tumor are suspicious for origin from a gonadoblastoma (44).

Immunohistochemical Findings. The seminoma-like cells stain for placental-like alkaline phosphatase (PLAP) as well as other markers of IGCNU (38b). The failure of some germ cells, however, to stain for these markers supports the presence of some intermixed, non-neoplastic germ cells and therefore a heterogeneous germ cell population (38b). Cytokeratins and vimentin are reactive in the Sertoli-like cells and laminin is positive in the basement membrane deposits (44). Inhibin marks the sex cord cells of some gonadoblastomas (37a,38c), and one study

showed positivity for the product of the Wilms' tumor gene (WT1) in the sex cord cells (37a).

Differential Diagnosis. Sertoli cell nodules, which commonly occur in cryptorchid testes (37,46), may be colonized by IGCNU and mimic gonadoblastoma (fig. 5-19). These lesions, however, occur in phenotypically normal males whose gonads lack dysgenetic features and who do not have internal mullerian genitalia, unlike many patients with gonadoblastoma. Their usual microscopic size and the frequently focal distribution of the malignant germ cells are distinct from gonadoblastoma. The distinction is important because the risk of bilaterality is considerably less, from 2 to 5 percent, than with gonadoblastoma.

Unlike gonadoblastoma, the unclassified form of mixed germ cell-sex cord-stromal tumor is not

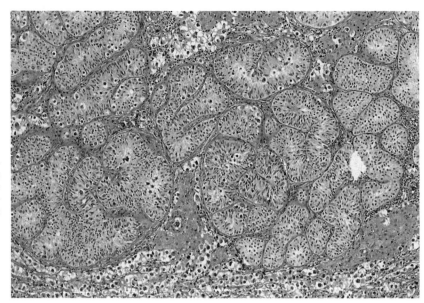

Figure 5-19
SERTOLI CELL NODULE
WITH IGCNU AND SEMINOMA
POTENTIALLY MIMICKING
GONADOBLASTOMA
IGCNU involves a Sertoli cell nodule. Note the focal distribution of the IGCNU cells in the Sertoli cell nodule in contrast to their diffuse distribution in gonadoblastoma. Seminoma is seen at the periphery.

characterized by the typical small nests with hyaline basement membrane deposits but forms larger, circumscribed to infiltrating nodules of sex cord tumor elements resembling any of the common types—Sertoli cell, granulosa cell, or unclassified sex cord-stromal elements—with admixed germ cells (see below).

Treatment and Prognosis. The usual treatment is bilateral gonadectomy because of the association with gonadal dysgenesis and the high frequency (at least 40 percent) of bilaterality. Such treatment is curative if prior to the development of an invasive germ cell tumor. If an invasive tumor is present, the treatment and prognosis are determined by its nature and stage.

Unclassified Germ Cell–Sex Cord–Stromal Tumors

These are rare tumors. The germ cells within these neoplasms have been considered neoplastic in the literature but most putative examples we have seen we have interpreted as sex cord-stromal tumors with entrapped, non-neoplastic germ cells (see below). The reported tumors have been in patients 30 to 69 years old who presented with a testicular mass, in the absence of hormonal symptoms or features of an intersex syndrome including gonadal dysgenesis (36,39,40). Usually, they are fleshy, solid, gray-white tumors that sometimes show cystic change. On microscopic examination, there is often a sheet-like pattern of sex cord cells with scant cytoplasm and usually angulated, sometimes grooved nuclei. Intertubular growth is often present at the periphery. Sertoli cell and granulosa cell differentiation may be apparent in the form of tubules, cords, or follicle-like structures, as seen in typical sex cord-stromal tumors (see chapter 6). Charcot-Böttcher filaments in one case confirmed Sertoli cell differentiation (36). The germ cell component most frequently occurs in distinct clusters (fig. 5-20), but rarely has a more diffuse arrangement. The germ cells are usually described as seminoma-like, with clear cytoplasm and round nuclei with prominent nucleoli (fig. 5-20) (38a), although glycogen was not identified in them in two cases (36,39), and one lacked reactivity for PLAP (39). In some of the reported cases, the germ cells have been described as appearing more mature than those of seminoma. Orchiectomy is standard therapy (39). No case is known to have metastasized, but the experience is limited because of their rarity.

A major lesion in the differential diagnosis is represented by cases noted above that we interpret as sex cord-stromal tumors with entrapped, non-neoplastic germ cells (48); in these the germ cells have round, uniform, euchromatic nuclei and are interspersed singly or in small nests, usually at the periphery of the tumor, but sometimes more centrally (fig. 5-21). They represent a small proportion of the tumor in most cases. The non-neoplastic nature of the germ cells in these cases is

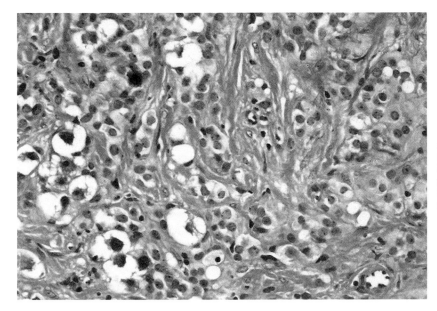

Figure 5-20
GERM CELL-SEX
CORD-STROMAL TUMOR,
UNCLASSIFIED VERSUS
"COLLISION TUMOR"
Neoplastic Sertoli cells admix with germ cells having the cytologic features of seminoma and IGCNU cells. Classification as a mixed germ cell–sex cord–stromal tumor or a collision tumor (Sertoli cell tumor and seminoma/IGCNU) may be problematic.

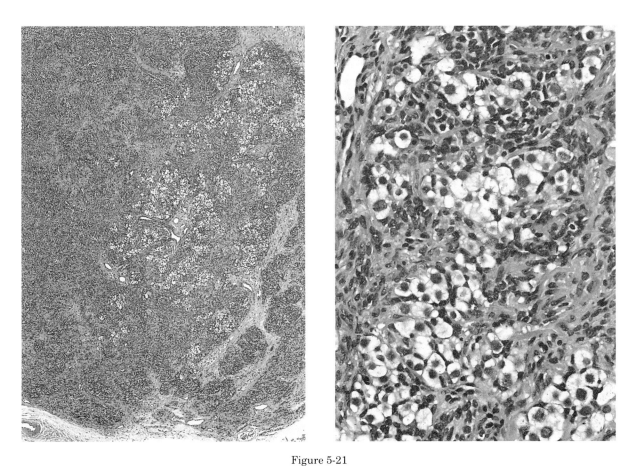

Figure 5-21
UNCLASSIFIED SEX CORD–STROMAL TUMOR WITH ENTRAPPED GERM CELLS
Left: A focus of light-staining germ cells is near the periphery of a tumor composed mainly of sex cord cells.
Right: High magnification shows the admixture of germ cells with sex cord cells. The germ cells have regular, round nuclei with a uniform, fine chromatin.

supported by their preferential peripheral location, bland nuclear features that are unlike those of the seminoma-like cells of gonadoblastoma, lack of PLAP and c-kit reactivity, and diploid DNA content on static cytophotometry (Ulbright TM, unpublished observations, 1998).

A "collision" tumor, with features of a sex cord-stromal tumor and a seminoma or IGCNU may rarely occur. Such a case should be regarded as two independent tumors, rather than a mixed germ cell-sex cord-stromal tumor, if pure populations of both types are evident. Sometimes this distinction, however, may be problematic (fig. 5-20).

The differential diagnosis with gonadoblastoma is discussed above. Prominent luteinized cells in a sex cord-stromal tumor may be misinterpreted as neoplastic germ cells, leading to misclassification as mixed germ cell-sex cord-stromal tumor. This differential is discussed on page 220.

REFERENCES

Mixed Germ Cell Tumors

1. Barsky SH. Germ cell tumors of the testis. In: Javadpour N, Barsky SH, eds. Surgical pathology of urologic diseases. Baltimore: Williams & Wilkins, 1987:224–46.
2. Brawn PN. The characteristics of embryonal carcinoma cells in teratocarcinomas. Cancer 1987;59:2042–6.
3. Brawn PN. The origin of germ cell tumors of the testis. Cancer 1983;51:1610–4.
4. Cardoso de Almeida PC, Scully RE. Diffuse embryoma of the testis. A distinctive form of mixed germ cell tumor. Am J Surg Pathol 1983;7:633–42.
5. de Peralta-Venturina MN, Ro JY, Ordonez NG, Ayala AG. Diffuse embryoma of the testis: an immunohistochemical study of two cases. Am J Clin Pathol 1994;101:402–5.
6. Evans RW. Developmental stages of embryo-like bodies in teratoma testis. J Clin Pathol 1957;10:31–9.
7. Freedman LS, Parkinson MC, Jones WG, et al. Histopathology in the prediction of relapse of patients with stage I testicular teratoma treated by orchidectomy alone. Lancet 1987;2:294–8.
8. Fung CY, Kalish LA, Brodsky GL, Richie JP, Garnick MB. Stage I nonseminomatous germ cell testicular tumor: prediction of metastatic potential by primary histopathology. J Clin Oncol 1988;6:1467–73.
9. Gels ME, Hoekstra HJ, Sleijfer DT, et al. Detection of recurrence in patients with clinical stage I nonseminomatous testicular germ cell tumors and consequences for further follow-up: a single-center 10-year experience. J Clin Oncol 1995;13:1188–94.
10. Jacobsen GK. Histogenetic considerations concerning germ cell tumours. Morphological and immunohistochemical comparative investigation of the human embryo and testicular germ cell tumours. Virchows Arch [A] 1986;408:509–25.
11. Jacobsen GK, Barlebo H, Olsen J, et al. Testicular germ cell tumours in Denmark 1976–1980: pathology of 1058 consecutive cases. Acta Radiol Oncol 1984;23:239–47.
12. Jacobsen GK, Talerman A. Atlas of germ cell tumours. Copenhagen: Munksgaard, 1989.
13. Melicow MM. Embryoma of testis: report of case and a classification of neoplasms of the testis. J Urol 1940;44:333–44.
14. Motoyama T, Watanabe H, Yamamoto T, Sekiguchi M. Human testicular germ cell tumors in vitro and in athymic nude mice. Acta Pathol Jap 1987;37:431–48.
15. Moul JW, McCarthy WF, Fernandez EB, Sesterhenn IA. Percentage of embryonal carcinoma and of vascular invasion predicts pathological stage in clinical stage I nonseminomatous testicular cancer. Cancer Res 1994;54:362–4.
16. Nakashima N, Murakami S, Fukatsu T, et al. Characteristics of "embryoid body" in human gonadal germ cell tumors. Hum Pathol 1988;19:1144–54.
17. Okamoto T. A human vitelline component in embryonal carcinoma of the testis. Acta Pathol Jap 1986;36:41–8.
18. Pera MF, Blasco Lafita MJ, Mills J. Cultured stem-cells from human testicular teratomas: the nature of human embryonal carcinoma, and its comparison with two types of yolk-sac carcinoma. Int J Cancer 1987;40:334–43.
19. Pera MF, Mills J, Parrington JM. Isolation and characterization of a multipotent clone of human embryonal carcinoma cells. Differentiation 1989;42:10–23.
20. Rustin GJ, Vogelzang NJ, Sleijfer DT, Nisselbaum JN. Consensus statement on circulating tumour markers and staging patients with germ cell tumours. Prog Clin Biol Res 1990;357:277–84.
21. Wishnow KI, Johnson DE, Swanson DA, et al. Identifying patients with low-risk clinical stage I nonseminomatous testicular tumors who should be treated by surveillance. Urology 1989;34:339–43.
22. Young RH, Scully RE. Testicular tumors. Chicago: ASCP Press, 1990.

Regression of Germ Cell Tumors

23. Abell MR, Fayos JV, Lampe I. Retroperitoneal germinomas (seminomas) without evidence of testicular involvement. Cancer 1965;18:273–90.

24. Asif S, Uehling DT. Microscopic tumor foci in testes. J Urol 1968;99:776–9.

25. Azzopardi JG, Hoffbrand AV. Retrogression in testicular seminoma with viable metastases. J Clin Pathol 1965;18:135–41.

26. Azzopardi JG, Mostofi FK, Theiss EA. Lesions of testes observed in certain patients with widespread choriocarcinoma and related tumors. Am J Pathol 1961;38:207–25.

27. Bär W, Hedinger C. Comparison of histologic types of primary testicular germ cell tumors with their metastases: consequences for the WHO and the British Nomenclatures? Virchows Arch [A] 1976;370:41–54.

28. Bohle A, Studer UE, Sonntag RW, Scheidegger JR. Primary or secondary extragonadal germ cell tumors. J Urol 1986;135:939–43.

29. Burt ME, Javadpour N. Germ-cell tumors in patients with apparently normal testes. Cancer 1981;47:1911–5.

30. Crook JC. Morphogenesis of testicular tumours. J Clin Pathol 1968;21:71–4.

31. Daugaard G, von der Maase H, Olsen J, Rorth M, Skakkebaek NE. Carcinoma-in-situ testis in patients with assumed extragonadal germ-cell tumours. Lancet 1987;2:528–30.

32. Holmes AS, Klimberg IW, Stonesifer KJ, Kramer BS, Wajsman Z. Spontaneous regression of testicular seminoma: case report. J Urol 1986;135:795–6.

33. Lopez JI, Angulo JC. Burned-out tumour of the testis presenting as retroperitoneal choriocarcinoma. Int Urol Nephrol 1994;26:549–53.

34. Meares EM Jr, Briggs EM. Occult seminoma of the testis masquerading as primary extragonadal germinal neoplasm. Cancer 1972;30:300–6.

35. Rottinto A, DeBellis H. Extragenital chorioma: its relation to teratoid vestiges in the testicles. Arch Pathol 1944;37:78–80.

Mixed Germ Cell-Sex Cord-Stromal Tumors

36. Bolen JW. Mixed germ cell-sex cord stromal tumor. A gonadal tumor distinct from gonadoblastoma. Am J Clin Pathol 1981;75:565–73.

37. Hedinger CE, Huber R, Weber E. Frequency of so-called hypoplastic or dysgenetic zones in scrotal and otherwise normal human testes. Virchows Arch Pathol Anat 1967;342:165–8.

37a. Hussong J, Crussi FG, Chou PM. Gonadoblastoma: immunohistochemical localization of müllerian-inhibiting substance, inhibin, WT-1, and p53. Mod Pathol 1997;10:1101–5.

37b. Iezzoni JC, von Kap-Herr C, Golden WL, Gaffey MJ. Gonadoblastomas in 45,X/46,XY mosaicism: analysis of Y-chromosome distribution by fluorescence in situ hybridization. Am J Clin Pathol 1997;108:197–201.

38. Ishida T, Tagatz GE, Okagaki T. Gonadoblastoma: ultrastructural evidence for testicular origin. Cancer 1976;37:1770–81.

38a. Jacobsen GK, Talerman A. Atlas of germ cell tumours. Copenhagen: Munksgaard, 1989.

38b. Jorgensen N, Muller J, Jaubert F, Clausen OP, Skakkebaek N. Heterogeneity of gonadoblastoma germ cells: similarities with immature germ cells, spermatogonia and testicular carcinoma in situ cells. Histopathology 1997;30:177–86.

38c. Kommoss F, Oliva E, Bhan A, Young RH, Scully RE. Inhibin expression in ovarian tumors and tumor-like lesions: an immunohistochemical study. Mod Pathol 1998;11:656–64.

39. Matoska J, Talerman A. Mixed germ cell-sex cord stromal tumor of the testis. A report with ultrastructural findings. Cancer 1989;64:2146–53.

40. Rames RA, Richardson M, Swiger F, Kaczmarek A. Mixed germ cell-sex cord stromal tumor of the testis: the incidental finding of a rare testicular neoplasm. J Urol 1995;154:1479.

41. Roth LM, Eglen DE. Gonadoblastoma. Immunohistochemical and ultrastructural observations. Int J Gynecol Pathol 1989;8:72–81.

42. Rutgers JL. Advances in the pathology of intersex syndromes. Hum Pathol 1991;22:884–91.

43. Salo P, Kääriäinen H, Petrovic V, Peltomäki P, Page DC, de la Chapelle A. Molecular mapping of the putative gonadoblastoma locus on the Y-chromosome. Genes Chrom Cancer 1995;14:210–4.

44. Scully RE. Gonadoblastoma. A review of 74 cases. Cancer 1970;25:1340–56.

45. Sotelo-Avila C, Gooch WM. Neoplasms associated with Beckwith-Wiedemann syndrome. Perspect Pediatr Pathol 1976;3:255–72.

46. Stalker AL, Hendry WT. Hyperplasia and neoplasia of the Sertoli cell. J Pathol Bacteriol 1952;64:161–8.

47. Tsuchiya K, Reijo R, Page DC, Disteche CM. Gonadoblastoma: molecular definition of the susceptibility region on the Y-chromosome. Am J Hum Genet 1995;57:1400–7.

48. Ulbright TM, Srigley JR, Reuter VE, Wojno K, Roth LM, Young RH. Sex cord-stromal tumors of the testis with entrapped germ cells: a mimic of mixed germ cell-sex cord-stromal tumor. Mod Pathol 1999;12:109A.

6

SEX CORD–STROMAL TUMORS

Sex cord–stromal tumors represent about 4 percent of all testicular neoplasms (3) but account for approximately 8 percent of those in prepubertal males (1). Their classification is presented in Table 6-1. The cells usually resemble, to varying degrees, the non-neoplastic Leydig cells (2), Sertoli cells, and nonspecific stromal cells of the testis in well-differentiated tumors. In more poorly differentiated tumors these similarities are generally less conspicuous, but the patterns of differentiation, such as tubular, that are usually focally present are diagnostic clues. Leydig cell tumor is the most common pure sex cord–stromal tumor, followed by Sertoli cell tumors, granulosa cell tumors, and pure stromal tumors. Rare tumors are morphologically reminiscent of the Sertoli–Leydig cell tumor of the ovary. The remaining neoplasms contain patterns of two or more of the above types or cannot be specifically placed into any clearly defined category. The former are categorized in the mixed group and the latter in the unclassified group, and, in combination, they account for a sizable number of all sex cord–stromal tumors.

Table 6-1

CLASSIFICATION OF SEX CORD–STROMAL TUMORS OF THE TESTIS

Sertoli–stromal cell tumors

   Sertoli cell tumor

      Variants: large cell calcifying

               sclerosing

   Sertoli-Leydig cell tumor

   Leydig cell tumor

Granulosa–stromal cell tumors

   Granulosa cell tumor

      Variants: adult

               juvenile

   Tumors in the fibroma-thecoma group

Mixed

Unclassified

SERTOLI–STROMAL CELL TUMORS

Sertoli Cell Tumors

General and Clinical Features. Sertoli cell tumors account for less than 1 percent of testicular neoplasms (9,15,17,25,32a). Although there are two pathologic subtypes, the large cell calcifying and sclerosing variants, only the former has sufficiently unique clinical features to merit separate coverage from the usual form, the Sertoli cell tumor, not otherwise specified (NOS). Although a "lipid-rich" variant of Sertoli cell tumor has been described in the literature, there are insufficient valid examples of pure, lipid-rich Sertoli cell tumors to consider them a separate subtype. Teilum's descriptions of this pattern appear to refer to foci within Sertoli–Leydig cell tumors (26-29).

Approximately 30 percent of reported "Sertoli cell tumors" have occurred in children, many under 1 year old (11). In our opinion, many of these cases have features of juvenile granulosa cell tumor, with the reports antedating the description of that entity. In support of this viewpoint, one recent pediatric series contained no Sertoli cell tumors, NOS, but there were four juvenile granulosa cell tumors (12). On the other hand, an element of subjectivity in the distinction of a juvenile granulosa cell tumor from a Sertoli cell tumor, particularly in the pediatric age group, is highlighted by another study that included 18 Sertoli cell tumors and 11 juvenile granulosa cell tumors (12a). The predominance of Sertoli cell tumors in that study, in contrast to our experience (32a) and that of Goswitz et al. (12), suggests that different criteria are being applied for the diagnosis of these tumors. In the largest series of Sertoli cell tumors, only 2 of 60 occurred in patients under 20 years of age (a 15-year-old and an 18-year-old), and the mean age was 46 years (32a). Only rarely, according to our criteria, do legitimate cases occur in children under 10 years of age (4,22,24).

Occasional tumors develop in patients with the androgen insensitivity syndrome (23). The large cell calcifying variant is associated with

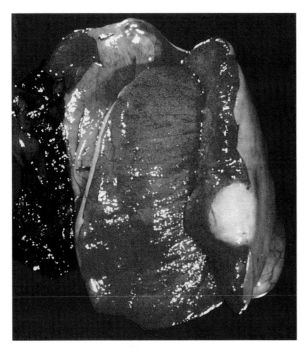

Figure 6-1
SERTOLI CELL TUMOR, SCLEROSING TYPE
The tumor is well circumscribed and white.

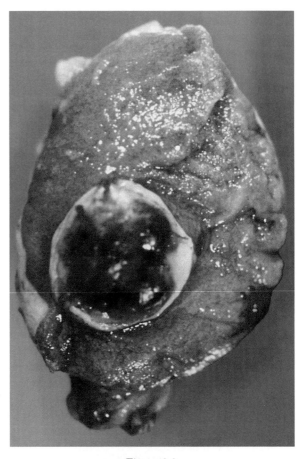

Figure 6-2
SERTOLI CELL TUMOR,
NOT OTHERWISE SPECIFIED
The tumor is well circumscribed and hemorrhagic.

Carney's syndrome (7), and its features (see page 202) may bring the patient to medical attention. Seven Sertoli cell tumors have occurred in boys from 1 1/2 to 8 years of age with the Peutz-Jeghers syndrome (5,6,8,10,32,34). All these boys had gynecomastia and elevated estradiol levels and many of their tumors had unusual microscopic features (see page 205). Despite these important associations, most patients with Sertoli cell tumors lack any known predisposing conditions and present with a testicular mass.

Based on a critical analysis of true Sertoli cell tumors in the literature, with the exclusion of Sertoli–Leydig cell tumors or unclassified sex cord–stromal tumors, only rare patients without the Peutz-Jeghers syndrome have endocrine manifestations such as gynecomastia. The latter is more common in patients with Leydig cell tumors, Sertoli–Leydig cell tumors, or tumors in the mixed and unclassified sex cord–stromal categories. Although the literature is difficult to evaluate, about 10 to 20 percent of all patients with sex cord–stromal tumors have gynecomastia. This manifestation is seen more often when the tumors are malignant.

Despite the association of some types of Sertoli cell tumor with endocrinologic abnormalities, studies of the hormonal production by these tumors are rare (10b). Gabrilove (11) reviewed 72 reported cases of Sertoli cell tumor and identified occasional patients with elevated serum testosterone, plasma estradiol, urinary estrogens, and urinary 17-ketosteroids. The exact nature, however, of many of these "Sertoli cell tumors" is not clear.

Gross Findings. Sertoli cell tumors are typically well-circumscribed, sometimes lobulated, yellow, tan, or white masses (figs. 6-1–6-3). Cysts are occasionally conspicuous (fig. 6-3). Sometimes foci of hemorrhage are present (fig. 6-2), but necrosis is rare. The mean diameter is approximately 3.5 cm, but the peculiar tumors in patients with the Peutz-Jeghers syndrome have typically been

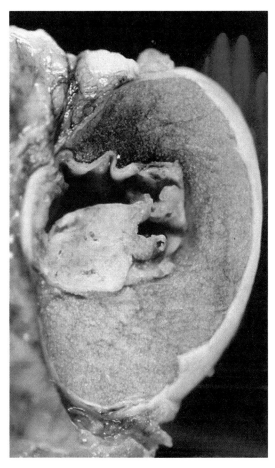

Figure 6-3
SERTOLI CELL TUMOR,
NOT OTHERWISE SPECIFIED
The sectioned surface shows conspicuous cysts.

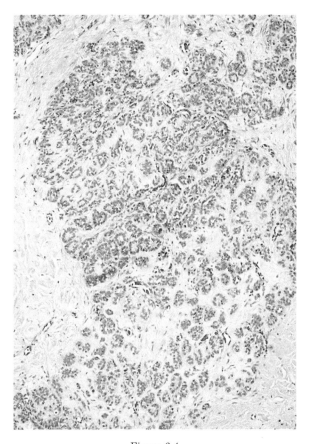

Figure 6-4
SERTOLI CELL TUMOR,
NOT OTHERWISE SPECIFIED
Nodular growth of small tubules separated by fibrous stroma.

smaller. With the exception of tumors in those patients or some of the large cell calcifying Sertoli cell tumors (see below), the neoplasms are almost invariably unilateral; there is only one apparently valid case of bilateral Sertoli cell tumor of otherwise conventional type (4). The vast majority are confined to the testis at presentation.

Microscopic Findings. These tumors may be of large cell calcifying (see below), sclerosing, or not otherwise specified (NOS) types (figs. 6-4–6-19). Reliable data on the frequency of the various subtypes are unavailable, since all the large series are based on consultation material. Our experience is that approximately 70 percent are in the NOS group, with most of the remainder evenly split between the large cell calcifying and sclerosing variants.

Microscopic examination usually shows enough tubular differentiation to permit categorization as Sertoli cell tumor, but the degree of tubular differentiation, and hence the overall low-power appearance of the tumor, is quite variable. Diffuse (fig. 6-7) and nodular (fig. 6-4) patterns often predominate on low power examination. Tubular differentiation in varying amounts is usually seen with ease in some areas of the tumor, and often is at least focally conspicuous. The tubules may be hollow and round or solid and elongated (figs. 6-8–6-11). Rarely they exhibit marked irregularity in size and shape (fig. 6-12) or have a retiform pattern (fig. 6-13). In some tumors, cords are prominent (fig. 6-18). Many Sertoli cell tumors have foci of solid growth (fig. 6-7), but tubular differentiation elsewhere facilitates the diagnosis. Rare neoplasms that have an entirely solid growth pattern can be diagnosed as Sertoli cell tumor when the

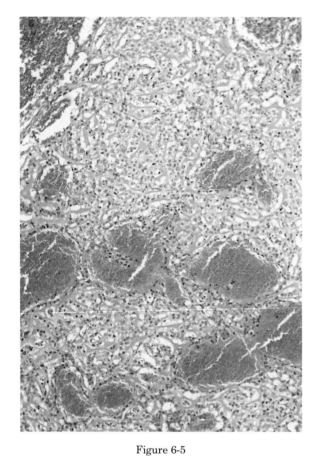

Figure 6-5
SERTOLI CELL TUMOR,
NOT OTHERWISE SPECIFIED
Engorged blood vessels are conspicuous. The tumor is forming small tubules and cords.

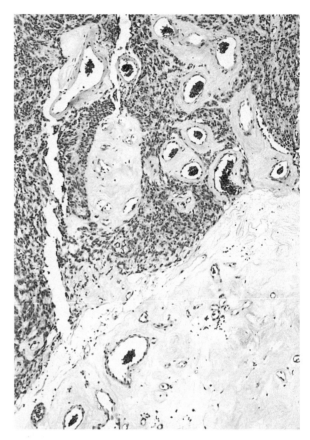

Figure 6-6
SERTOLI CELL TUMOR,
NOT OTHERWISE SPECIFIED
Prominent hyalinized stroma with many dilated blood vessels.

Figure 6-7
SERTOLI CELL TUMOR,
NOT OTHERWISE SPECIFIED
There is a diffuse growth of cells with appreciable eosinophilic cytoplasm resembling a Leydig cell tumor. Tubular differentiation was conspicuous in other areas.

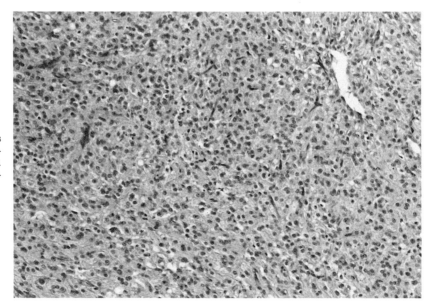

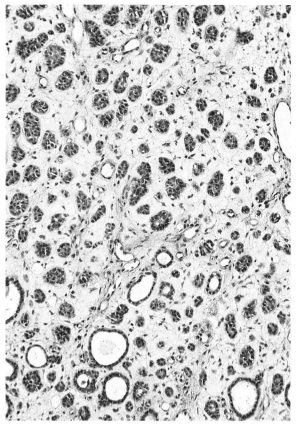

Figure 6-8
SERTOLI CELL TUMOR,
NOT OTHERWISE SPECIFIED
The solid and hollow tubules, some of which are dilated
and lined by a single layer of cells, are a common feature.

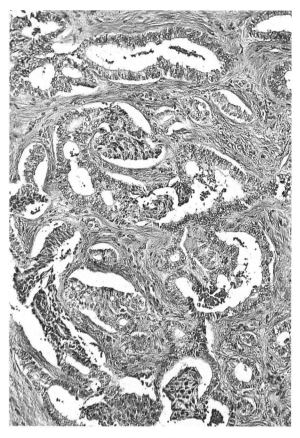

Figure 6-9
SERTOLI CELL TUMOR,
NOT OTHERWISE SPECIFIED
Hollow tubules lined by stratified cells resemble an en-
dometrioid neoplasm.

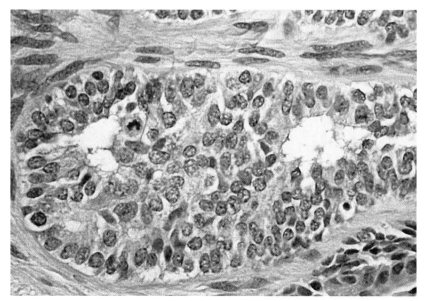

Figure 6-10
SERTOLI CELL TUMOR,
NOT OTHERWISE SPECIFIED
A tubule from the tumor in figure
6-9 is lined by stratified cells. Note the
mitotic figure.

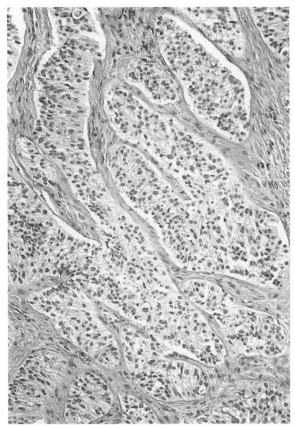

Figure 6-11
SERTOLI CELL TUMOR,
NOT OTHERWISE SPECIFIED
Solid tubular pattern.

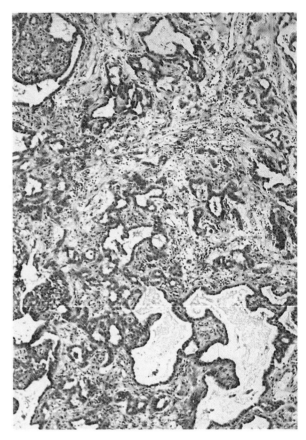

Figure 6-12
SERTOLI CELL TUMOR,
NOT OTHERWISE SPECIFIED
Many tubules are dilated and irregular in size and shape.

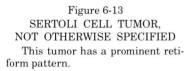

Figure 6-13
SERTOLI CELL TUMOR,
NOT OTHERWISE SPECIFIED
This tumor has a prominent reti-
form pattern.

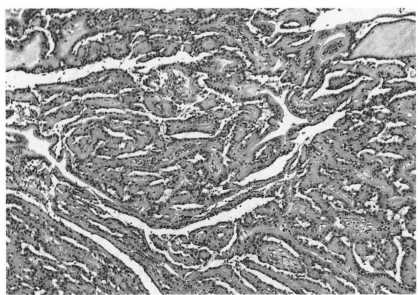

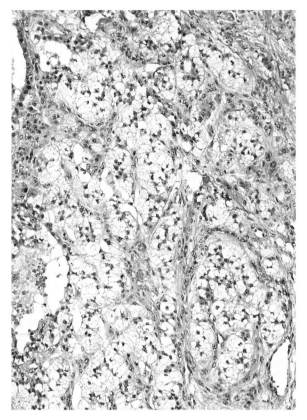

Figure 6-14
SERTOLI CELL TUMOR,
NOT OTHERWISE SPECIFIED
The tubules are composed of cells with abundant pale lipid-rich cytoplasm. This lipid-rich pattern of Sertoli cell neoplasia is almost always focal in our experience.

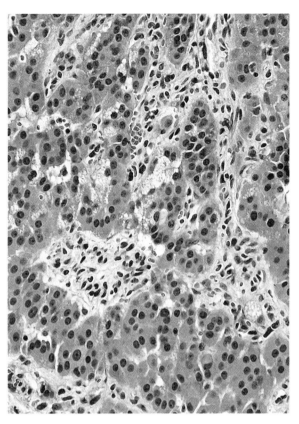

Figure 6-15
SERTOLI CELL TUMOR,
NOT OTHERWISE SPECIFIED
Tumor cells with abundant eosinophilic cytoplasm form solid tubules and cords.

appearance is inconsistent with any other plausible diagnosis and is buttressed by appropriate immunohistochemical findings.

The tumor cells usually have moderate to occasionally abundant, eosinophilic cytoplasm (fig. 6-15), but it may be pale due to lipid accumulation. This may take the form of fine droplets (fig. 6-16) or large vacuoles (fig. 6-17). The stroma may be scanty or composed of abundant, sometimes hyalinized fibrous tissue (fig. 6-6) which may contain prominent, occasionally dilated blood vessels (fig. 6-5). The majority of Sertoli cell tumors, NOS have bland cytologic features and little mitotic activity, but occasional tumors exhibit overt pleomorphism and conspicuous mitotic figures.

Some Sertoli cell tumors exhibit extensive sclerosis (fig. 6-20), placing the neoplasm in the descriptive category of a "sclerosing Sertoli cell tumor" (35). The tubules in these cases tend to

be small and solid, and the intensely sclerotic stroma is not as vascular as in many Sertoli cell tumors, NOS. With rare exceptions, these tumors have very bland cytologic features, and mitotic figures are typically infrequent. A common finding in the sclerosing variant is the presence of entrapped, non-neoplastic tubules that are reminiscent of the immature tubules seen in the Sertoli cell nodules often found in cryptorchid testes (see chapter 8). There is one case reported as a Sertoli cell tumor, supported by appropriate immunostains, which had a heterologous sarcomatous component (osteosarcoma) (11a) (see page 209).

Ultrastructural Findings. On ultrastructural examination, Sertoli cell tumors typically have a well-developed Golgi apparatus, variably prominent smooth endoplasmic reticulum, lipid droplets, lateral desmosomes, and a peripheral investment of basement membrane (fig. 6-21)

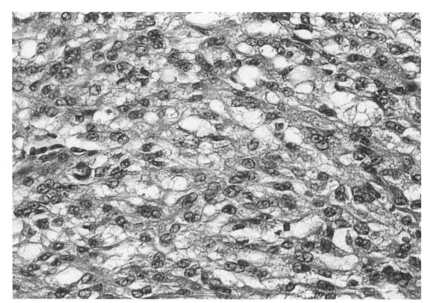

Figure 6-16
SERTOLI CELL TUMOR,
NOT OTHERWISE SPECIFIED
The tumor cells have finely vacuo-
lated cytoplasm.

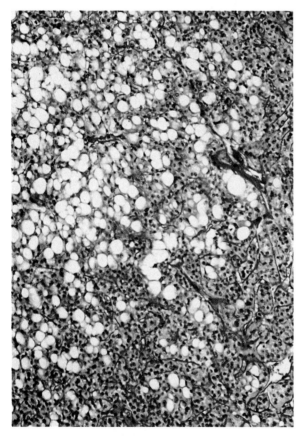

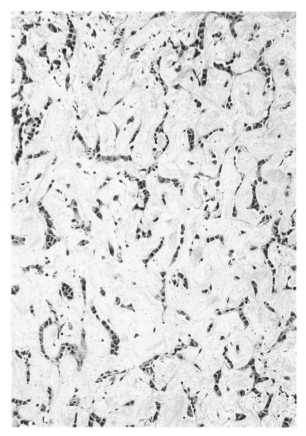

Figure 6-17
SERTOLI CELL TUMOR,
NOT OTHERWISE SPECIFIED
Many tumor cells have prominent lipid droplets.

Figure 6-18
SERTOLI CELL TUMOR,
NOT OTHERWISE SPECIFIED
Thin cords are separated by a prominent acellular stroma.

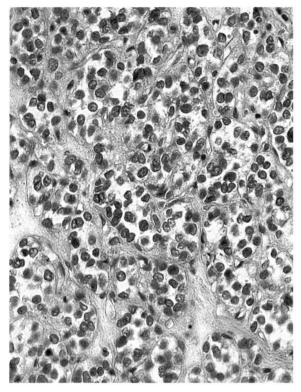

Figure 6-19
SERTOLI CELL TUMOR,
NOT OTHERWISE SPECIFIED

Tumor cells exhibit only mild atypicality. Note the tubular differentiation. This tumor was clinically malignant (see figure 6-22).

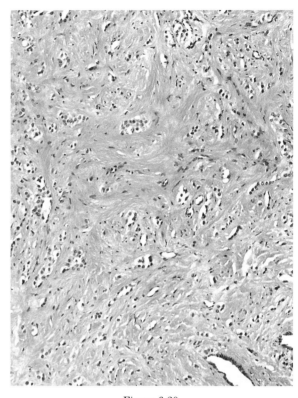

Figure 6-20
SERTOLI CELL TUMOR, SCLEROSING TYPE

Small tubules are separated by a conspicuous fibrous stroma.

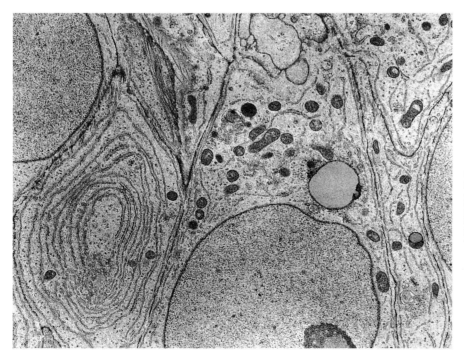

Figure 6-21
SERTOLI CELL TUMOR,
NOT OTHERWISE
SPECIFIED

A cluster of Sertoli cells shows tight junctions, prominent whorls of smooth and rough endoplasmic reticulum, lipid droplets, and interdigitating cell processes (top). (Courtesy of Dr. R. Erlandson, New York, NY.)

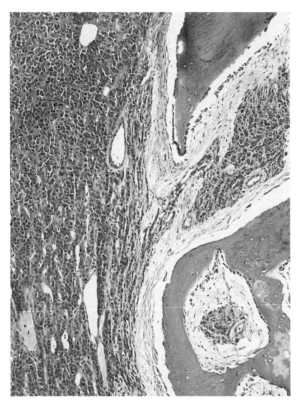

Figure 6-22
SERTOLI CELL TUMOR,
NOT OTHERWISE SPECIFIED
Bone metastasis (same case as figure 6-19).

inguinal lymph nodes, retroperitoneum, lung, bone, or liver. When the features of the malignant tumors were compared with those in patients with an uneventful follow-up of 5 or more years, the following pathologic features best correlated with a clinically malignant course: a tumor diameter of 5 cm or greater, necrosis, moderate to severe nuclear atypia, vascular invasion, and a mitotic rate over 5 mitotic figures per 10 high-power fields. Only 1 of 9 benign tumors with follow-up data of 5 years or longer had more than one of these features, whereas 5 of the 7 malignant tumors had at least three.

The initial treatment of a Sertoli cell tumor is radical orchiectomy. Retroperitoneal lymph node dissection is indicated if the patient has radiographically apparent retroperitoneal involvement. For cases judged to be likely malignant based on pathologic criteria alone, in the absence of known metastatic disease, it remains controversial if retroperitoneal lymph node dissection should be performed. At the minimum, close follow-up is indicated. Radiation and chemotherapy have not proved consistently effective, although there are sporadic cases that do respond to these modalities (16).

Large Cell Calcifying Sertoli Cell Tumor

Almost 50 large cell calcifying Sertoli cell tumors have been reported in patients from 2 to 51 years of age (average, 21 years) (13,16,18,19,21, 30,31). In approximately one third of the cases a variety of associated findings resulted in an interesting and unusual clinical situation; these included acromegaly, pituitary gigantism, hypercortisolemia, sexual precocity, sudden death, spotty mucocutaneous pigmentation, and the Peutz-Jeghers syndrome. (As noted below, many of the Sertoli cell tumors associated with the Peutz-Jeghers syndrome have unusual and distinctive "hybrid" microscopic features.) The correlating pathologic findings consisted of pituitary adenomas, bilateral primary adrenocortical hyperplasia, testicular Leydig cell tumors, cardiac myxomas, and lentigines (7).

Gross Findings. The tumors are usually 4 cm or less in diameter (mean, 2 cm) (fig. 6-23). They are often multifocal, and approximately 20 percent are bilateral. Multifocal and bilateral tumors are almost exclusively seen in patients with Carney's

(10a). Cisternae of rough endoplasmic reticulum may be prominent in some cases, but convincing Charcot-Böttcher filaments have not been identified in the relatively few cases in the NOS category that have been examined ultrastructurally, unlike the large cell calcifying variant (10a,30).

Prognosis and Treatment. No sclerosing Sertoli cell tumor or tumor in a patient with Peutz-Jeghers syndrome has proved clinically malignant to date. Large cell calcifying tumors are considered below.

In a recent study of 60 Sertoli cell tumors, NOS, 7 (12 percent) were clinically malignant (32a). Four patients had evidence of spread beyond the testis at the time of presentation; all 4 had lymph node involvement (1 inguinal, 1 retroperitoneal, 1 inguinal and retroperitoneal, 1 retroperitoneal and supraclavicular), and 1 patient also had lung and bone metastases (fig. 6-22). Three additional patients developed metastases 1.3, 4, and 12 years postoperatively, to

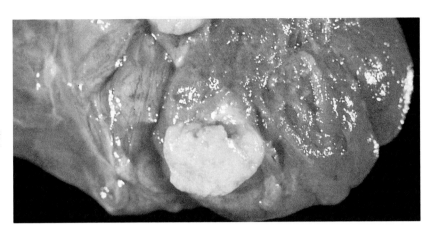

Figure 6-23
SERTOLI CELL TUMOR,
LARGE CELL CALCIFYING TYPE
A well-circumscribed tumor has a glistening, yellow-white sectioned surface.

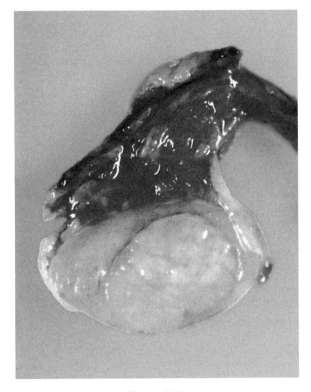

Figure 6-24
SERTOLI CELL TUMOR,
LARGE CELL CALCIFYING TYPE
A well-circumscribed, light tan tumor with a nodular cut surface. (Courtesy of Dr. J.Y. Ro, Houston, TX.)

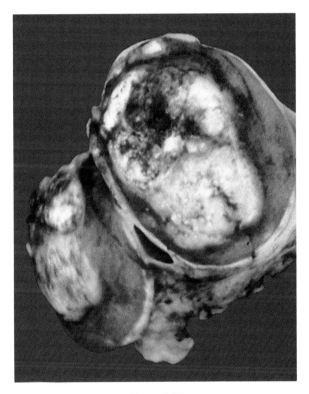

Figure 6-25
SERTOLI CELL TUMOR,
LARGE CELL CALCIFYING TYPE
This tumor is large and exhibits both hemorrhage and necrosis. It was clinically malignant.

syndrome. Sectioning reveals firm, yellow to tan to white tissue, often with granular, calcific foci. Most tumors are well circumscribed (fig. 6-24). Necrosis is occasionally seen (fig. 6-25).

Microscopic Findings. The tumor cells are arranged in sheets, nests, trabeculae, cords, small clusters, or solid tubules (figs. 6-26–6-29). Foci of intratubular tumor are found in approximately half of the cases, supporting their Sertoli cell origin (fig. 6-30). The stroma varies from loose and myxoid to densely collagenous. Some tumors exhibit a prominent neutrophilic infiltrate. The characteristic calcification is usually conspicuous (fig. 6-26) and sometimes massive, with

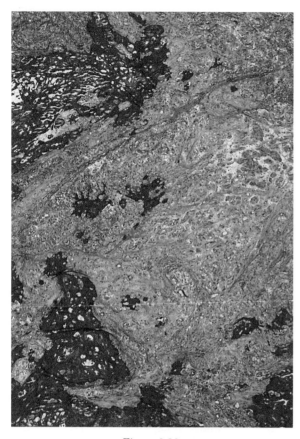

Figure 6-26
SERTOLI CELL TUMOR,
LARGE CELL CALCIFYING TYPE
Large, irregular, plaque-like foci of calcium are conspicuous on low-power examination.

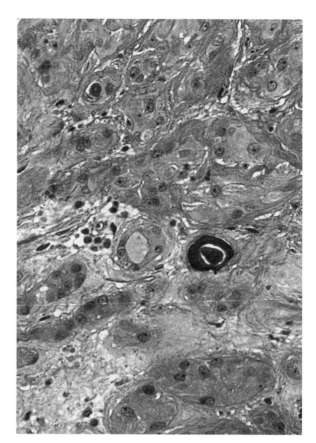

Figure 6-27
SERTOLI CELL TUMOR,
LARGE CELL CALCIFYING TYPE
Tumor cells have abundant eosinophilic cytoplasm.

Figure 6-28
SERTOLI CELL TUMOR, LARGE
CELL CALCIFYING TYPE
Tumor cells grow in cords and small clusters.

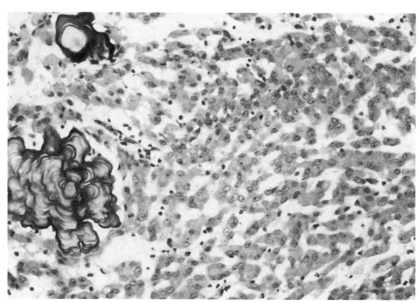

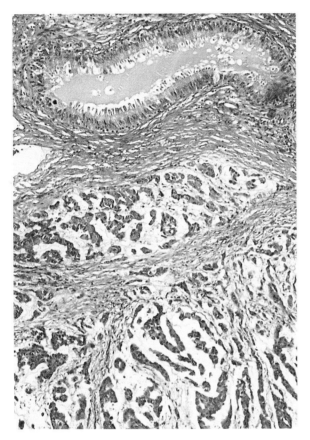

Figure 6-29
SERTOLI CELL TUMOR,
LARGE CELL CALCIFYING TYPE
Tumor has spread to involve the epididymis and was clinically malignant.

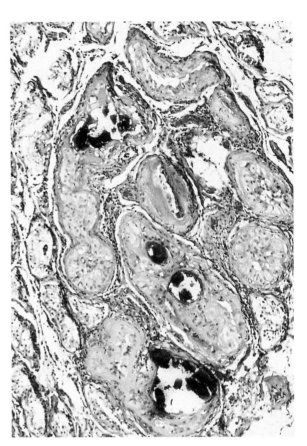

Figure 6-30
SERTOLI CELL TUMOR,
LARGE CELL CALCIFYING TYPE
Focus of intratubular growth.

large, wavy, laminated nodules. Small psammoma bodies occasionally are seen, as is ossification. The neoplastic cells are large and usually round, but are occasionally cuboidal or columnar, and rarely spindle shaped. In most cases the cytoplasm is abundant, eosinophilic, and finely granular (fig. 6-27), but occasionally it is amphophilic and slightly vacuolated. The nuclei are round or oval, with one or two small to moderate-sized nucleoli. Mitotic figures are generally rare. Ultrastructural studies support the Sertoli cell origin of the tumor, with the identification of Charcot-Böttcher filament bundles, the specific cytoplasmic inclusions of Sertoli cells, in occasional cases (fig. 6-31) (13,30,31).

The Sertoli cell tumors that occur in males with the Peutz-Jeghers syndrome often have some features of the large cell calcifying Sertoli cell tumor, but they frequently lack calcification

(figs. 6-32, 6-33) and, in some cases, resemble the sex cord tumor with annular tubules of the ovary (fig. 6-34) (33). Cysts may be present (fig. 6-33). Four of the reported tumors predominantly resembled the large cell calcifying Sertoli cell tumor, two the sex cord tumor with annular tubules, and one a Sertoli cell tumor, NOS (5,6,8, 10,32,34). The examples we have seen had appearances that can best be characterized as "hybrid" between the first two histologic types.

Differential Diagnosis. Sertoli cell tumors must be distinguished from the focal non-neoplastic clusters of tubules referred to as Sertoli cell nodules (see page 292). The latter are usually of microscopic size but are occasionally visible grossly as white nodules a few millimeters in diameter. On microscopic examination aggregates of closely clustered tubules with interspersed Leydig cells are seen; the tubules are lined by

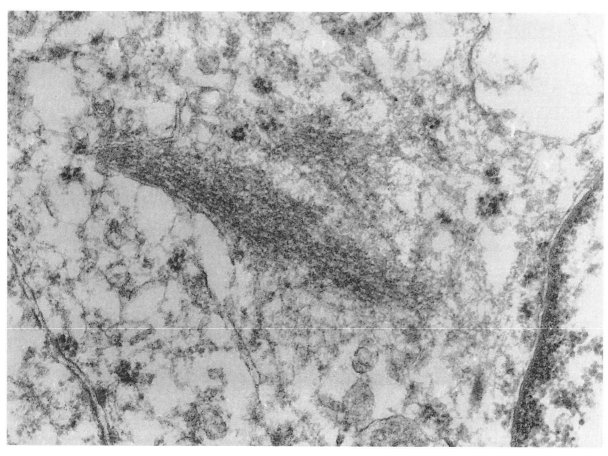

Figure 6-31
SERTOLI CELL TUMOR, LARGE CELL CALCIFYING TYPE
There is a perinuclear array of parallel cytoplasmic filaments (Charcot-Böttcher filaments), a feature of Sertoli cells. (Courtesy of Dr. B. Têtu, Québec, Canada.)

Figure 6-32
SERTOLI CELL TUMOR IN
PEUTZ-JEGHERS SYNDROME

Tumor cells grow in solid tubules and have abundant cytoplasm. The appearance is reminiscent of the large cell calcifying Sertoli cell tumor but calcification is lacking.

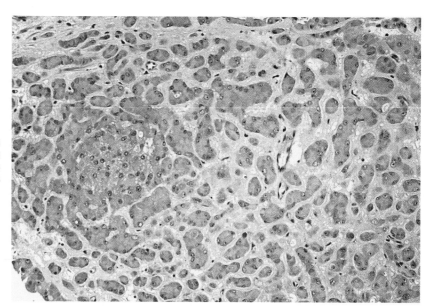

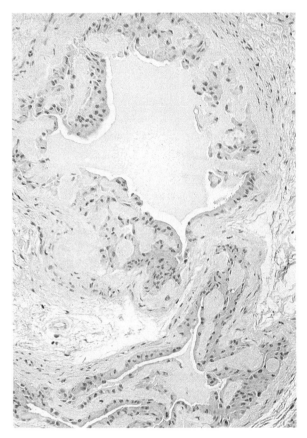

Figure 6-33
SERTOLI CELL TUMOR IN
PEUTZ-JEGHERS SYNDROME
Cysts are lined by Sertoli cells with abundant eosino-philic cytoplasm.

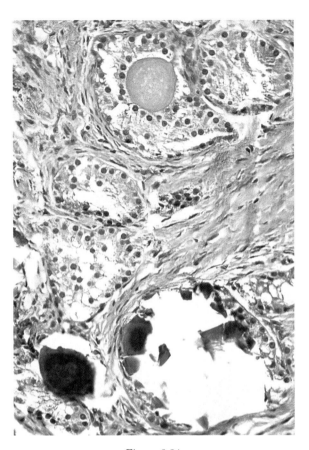

Figure 6-34
SERTOLI CELL TUMOR IN
PEUTZ-JEGHERS SYNDROME
An annular tubule at the top has the morphology of the sex cord tumor with annular tubules. Note the calcification at the bottom.

small, immature Sertoli cells and, in occasional cases, contain scattered spermatogonia as well. Some lesions have a radial arrangement of Sertoli cells around small hyaline bodies, resembling Call-Exner bodies; intratubular laminated calcified bodies may also be identified.

Pure Sertoli cell tumors are distinguished from mixed sex cord–stromal tumors on the basis of an often prominent, cellular stromal component in the latter (see page 210). This contrasts with the fibrotic to hyalinized, non-neoplastic appearance of the stroma in a pure Sertoli cell tumor.

Sertoli cell tumors lack the typical architectural features of the adult granulosa cell tumor, a much rarer neoplasm in the testis, and their cells generally have more conspicuous eosinophilic cytoplasm. Juvenile granulosa cell tumors, in contrast to the Sertoli cell tumor, NOS, exhibit prom-

inent follicle differentiation; the follicles are usually irregular in size and shape, in contrast to the tubular differentiation of the Sertoli cell tumors. Some juvenile granulosa cell tumors have little or no follicular differentiation, and, in such cases, intercellular basophilic fluid may impart a chondroid appearance suggestive of the diagnosis. The juvenile granulosa cell tumor typically has more immature-appearing nuclei with conspicuous mitotic activity than the majority of Sertoli cell tumors, NOS. Juvenile granulosa cell tumor typically occurs in the first few months of life; in contrast, in the largest series of Sertoli cell tumors, NOS, no patient was under 15 years of age (32a).

Areas in some Sertoli cell tumors, NOS, resemble Leydig cell tumors because of a diffuse growth of cells with appreciable eosinophilic cytoplasm. Despite this superficial similarity, many features help distinguish these tumors. Leydig cell tumors are more often yellow or brown on their sectioned surface. On microscopic examination the most helpful difference is the presence of tubular differentiation in most Sertoli cell tumors, a finding that excludes the diagnosis of Leydig cell tumor, although focal pseudotubules may be seen in rare Leydig cell tumors. Additionally, 30 to 40 percent of testicular Leydig cell tumors contain intracytoplasmic crystals of Reinke, which are absent in Sertoli cell tumors. Immunostaining for cytokeratin may assist, with typically stronger and more diffuse reactivity in Sertoli cell tumors and usually focal, weak, or absent reactivity in Leydig cell tumors; however, individual case variation limits the diagnostic utility of this stain. Inhibin immunoreactivity is typically much more intense and diffuse in Leydig cell tumors than in Sertoli cell tumors (4a,13a,16a).

Historically, the confusion between a Sertoli cell tumor in the large cell calcifying category and a Leydig cell tumor has been particularly problematic; before the former tumor was recognized it was often misdiagnosed as Leydig cell tumor. In addition to the features just reviewed that are helpful in the differential diagnosis, large cell calcifying Sertoli cell tumors often show intratubular growth and common bilaterality/ multifocality, in contrast to Leydig cell tumors. Although ossification has been rarely described in a Leydig cell tumor, the presence of calcification strongly favors a large cell calcifying Sertoli cell tumor.

Sertoli cell tumors may be potentially misdiagnosed as seminoma because of the common occurrence of seminoma and its frequently diffuse pattern. However, Sertoli cell tumors, although they may have a focal nonspecific chronic inflammatory cell infiltrate, generally lack a consistent sprinkling of lymphocytes in their stroma. We have seen, however, rare cases in which a diffuse and prominent lymphocytic infiltrate, in conjunction with cytoplasmic clarity, led to misinterpretation as seminoma. In such cases the lack of the following: granulomas, rounded nuclei with "flattened" edges, one to four prominent nucleoli, and glycogen-rich cytoplasm served in the distinction from seminoma. Rare seminomas (see chapter 3) have a well-developed, solid tubular pattern that on low-power examination suggests a Sertoli cell

tumor. This appears to have been the main confusing feature of five tumors whose distinction from Sertoli cell tumor was problematic, as mentioned by Collins and Symington over 30 years ago (9). However, tubular seminomas have the usual lymphocytes and cytologic features of seminoma, and typical seminoma is usually apparent in other areas. The presence of adjacent intratubular germ cell neoplasia provides additional evidence that a tubular tumor is a seminoma. Also, seminoma cells stain strongly for glycogen and placental-like alkaline phosphatase (in contrast to neoplastic Sertoli cells) and Sertoli cells stain for lipid, cytokeratins, and inhibin (in contrast to seminoma cells).

The rare endometrioid adenocarcinoma of the testis (see chapter 7) may enter into the differential diagnosis because the tubular glands of this tumor may simulate the hollow tubules seen in occasional Sertoli cell tumors. The patterns of the two neoplasms in other areas are so distinctive that this problem should be rare. Lack of staining of the Sertoli cell tubules for epithelial membrane antigen (4a,16a) may be helpful, as it has been in the distinction of "sertoliform" endometrioid carcinomas of the ovary from Sertoli cell tumors. Inhibin positivity in Sertoli cell tumors may also be helpful in this situation (4a,13a,16a,20).

The adenomatoid tumor may contain cells with conspicuous eosinophilic cytoplasm, like the Sertoli cell tumor, but the latter usually lacks the characteristic vacuolated cells typically seen in the adenomatoid tumor. Although adenomatoid tumors may involve the testis, they are primarily paratesticular, in contrast to the intratesticular Sertoli cell tumors. A rare neoplasm which could enter into the differential diagnosis on microscopic evaluation alone is the sertoliform rete cystadenoma (see page 239), but its usual confinement to the rete should make distinction easy in most instances. However, a rare tumor in this category of rete derivation that extensively involves the parenchyma may be impossible to distinguish from a Sertoli cell tumor of parenchymal origin. A metastatic adenocarcinoma with relatively regular tubular glands, such as one from the stomach, could mimic a Sertoli cell tumor, but such a neoplasm would tend to have a more variegated microscopic appearance than a Sertoli cell tumor, a prominent intertubular growth pattern, and

Table 6-2

COMPARISON BETWEEN THE REPORTED BENIGN AND MALIGNANT CASES OF LARGE CELL CALCIFYING SERTOLI CELL TUMOR

	Benign	Malignant
Number of reported cases	39	8
Mean age	17 years	39 years
Association with syndrome or congenital abnormality (see text)	36 %	12.5 %
Laterality/Focality	bilateral and/or multifocal (28%)	all unilateral and unifocal
Mean size	1.4 cm	5.4 cm
Histologic features	no extratesticular spread, size < 4 cm, mitoses rare, only mild nuclear atypia, no necrosis or lymphovascular invasion	contains 2 or more of the following: extratesticular spread size > 4 cm mitoses > 3/10 HPF significant nuclear atypia, necrosis, lymphovascular invasion

lymphatic involvement, and likely be associated with clinical evidence of tumor elsewhere. Epithelial membrane antigen positivity in most adenocarcinomas provides additional diagnostic aid in difficult cases, since this antigen is not expressed in Sertoli cell tumors (4a). Positivity for inhibin provides additional support for Sertoli cell tumor, since inhibin is negative in metastatic adenocarcinoma (20). The distinction of Sertoli cell tumor from carcinoid is discussed in chapter 4.

Prognosis and Treatment. Eight of the 47 reported cases of large cell calcifying Sertoli cell tumor have been clinically malignant (16). The mean age of patients with malignant tumors is 39 years, compared to 17 years for those with benign tumors. Only one patient with a malignant tumor had any of the unusual clinical findings of Carney's syndrome. In contrast to the benign tumors, a significant number of which are bilateral and multifocal, all the malignant tumors were unilateral and unifocal. Pathologic features which suggest a malignant course include large size and other features generally similar to those useful in determining prognosis in cases of Sertoli cell tumors, NOS. The features of the benign and malignant cases of large cell calcifying Sertoli cell tumor reported in the literature are contrasted in Table 6-2. The treatment is similar to that for other tumors in the NOS category; those

that are syndrome associated when bilateral or associated with multifocal disease may necessitate a more conservative approach.

Sertoli–Leydig Cell Tumor

Testicular tumors similar to the Sertoli–Leydig cell tumor of the ovary are rare. Six published cases had an unequivocal tubular component and/or patterns consistent with Sertoli–Leydig cell tumor of the ovary, with additionally a stromal component containing at least focal Leydig cells (36–41). One patient was 3.5 months of age; the others were 4, 53, 54, 63, and 66 years of age. Two patients had gynecomastia. One tumor with an unusual morphology (areas resembling osteosarcoma and malignant giant cell tumor) metastasized to the groin and lung 7 months after presentation (38). Another tumor with areas of osteosarcoma is perhaps best placed in the Sertoli-Leydig cell category because of the neoplastic stromal component although Leydig cells were not identified (37a) (see page 199).

Gross Findings. Testicular Sertoli–Leydig cell tumors have ranged from 1.8 to 12 cm in diameter. They are usually uniformly or dominantly solid, frequently yellow, and often have a lobulated sectioned surface. The single known malignant tumor had areas of hemorrhage and necrosis (38).

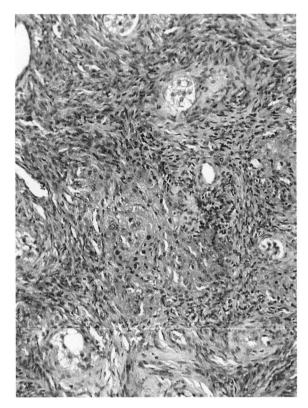

Figure 6-35
SERTOLI-LEYDIG CELL TUMOR
Sertoliform tubules are surrounded by a cellular neoplastic stroma that contains aggregates of Leydig cells.

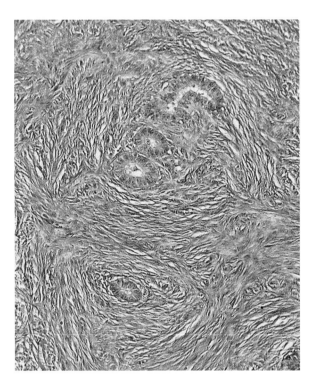

Figure 6-36
SERTOLI-LEYDIG CELL TUMOR
The stroma is cellular and neoplastic, a diagnostic feature of Sertoli-Leydig cell tumor, even in the absence of Leydig cells.

Microscopic Findings. Most of the tumors have tubules, cords, and trabeculae in haphazard arrangements in a background stroma that usually contains focal Leydig cells (fig. 6-35). However, we place a Sertoli–stromal cell tumor in the Sertoli-Leydig group, even if Leydig cells are absent, provided the stroma has a cellular, neoplastic appearance (fig. 6-36). The majority are of intermediate differentiation, according to the classification of ovarian cases, but some are poorly differentiated; there is only one report of a well-differentiated tumor (39). Retiform differentiation, with slit-like glands and cysts, is unusual (42). One tumor had areas of osteosarcoma and foci that resembled a malignant giant cell tumor (38). The metastases in that case were composed predominantly of osteosarcoma, but one lung lesion had the features of a malignant Leydig cell tumor with "unmistakable Reinke crystals." Typical heterologous elements, as seen in ovarian cases, have not been encountered to date.

Differential Diagnosis. The differential diagnosis for tumors with a prominent tubular pattern is similar to that of pure Sertoli cell tumors and is not repeated here. In general, the resemblance of these tumors to the rare, but well-known ovarian Sertoli–Leydig cell tumor should facilitate their recognition. The presence of a cellular, neoplastic stroma, sometimes with a Leydig cell component, separates the tumors from pure Sertoli cell tumors and, in contrast to unclassified tumors in the sex cord–stromal category, they have a less conspicuous fibrothecomatous stroma and lack areas of granulosa cell differentiation.

Leydig Cell Tumor

General and Clinical Features. Leydig cell tumors account for about 2 percent of testicular neoplasms (51a,56). Approximately 20 percent are detected in the first decade of life, 25 percent between 10 and 30 years, 30 percent between 30 and 50 years, and 25 percent beyond that age. Bilateral occurrence is rare.

Adults usually complain of testicular swelling, but gynecomastia causes the patient to seek medical attention in 15 percent of the cases (fig. 6-37) and is present in an additional 15 percent of patients on clinical evaluation (57). In several cases an impalpable tumor was detected by ultrasound examination of an adult with gynecomastia (55). A decrease in libido or potency may be an accompaniment in some cases. Children almost always present with isosexual pseudoprecocity, usually at 5 to 9 years of age (65), and more frequently have small tumors requiring special studies for detection. Approximately 10 percent of patients are asymptomatic and have tumors discovered on physical examination. The presence of an undescended testis or a history of it in 5 to 10 percent of the cases in one series (57) suggests that cryptorchidism may predispose to the development of Leydig cell tumors. Rare examples have occurred in patients with Klinefelter's syndrome but should be distinguished with particular care from the Leydig cell hyperplasia that is common in that disorder. One malignant "Leydig cell" tumor was associated with the adrenogenital syndrome (see page 293), but crystals of Reinke were absent in the tumor cells (50).

Testosterone is the major androgen produced by Leydig cell tumors, but secretion of androstenedione and dehydroepiandrosterone has also been reported (48,65). Urinary 17-ketosteroids may be normal or high. Elevated estrogen levels were recorded in patients with and without gynecomastia, and estradiol was present in high concentrations in spermatic vein blood in several cases (53). Testosterone levels and values for gonadotropins, particularly follicle-stimulating hormone (FSH), have been low in patients with gynecomastia and elevated estradiol levels (45,58); in a few other cases, plasma progesterone or urinary pregnanediol values were elevated (49,60). The abnormal hormonal levels may return to normal after removal of the tumor (44), but in some cases they persist.

Approximately 3 percent of Leydig cell tumors are bilateral, and the tumor has extended beyond the testis at the time of presentation in up to 15 percent of the cases (57).

Gross Findings. The tumors are typically sharply circumscribed, usually 3 to 5 cm in diameter, and sometimes lobulated by fibrous

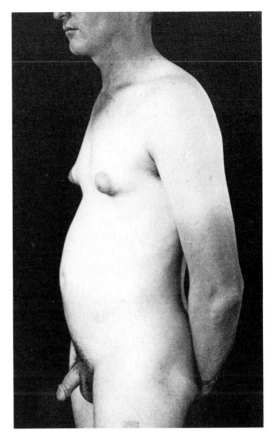

Figure 6-37
GYNECOMASTIA IN PATIENT WITH
LEYDIG CELL TUMOR
(Figure 76 from Fascicle 8, 2nd Series.)

septa (figs. 6-38, 6-39). They are usually uniformly solid and yellow (fig. 6-38) or yellow-tan, but occasionally are brown, green-brown (fig. 6-39), or gray-white. Foci of hemorrhage, necrosis, or both are present in approximately one quarter of the cases (fig. 6-40).

Microscopic Findings. The most common microscopic patterns are diffuse and nodular (figs. 6-41–6-51). In the former the stroma is typically inconspicuous and has a nondescript fibrous character. When the stroma is prominent, and in some cases extensively hyalinized, broad bands subdivide the tumor into isolated nodules. Occasionally the stroma is focally or conspicuously edematous or myxoid, and the tumor cells may be dispersed as relatively regular nests, irregular clusters (fig. 6-42), trabeculae, or cords. Rarely, a pseudotubular pattern is seen. In one

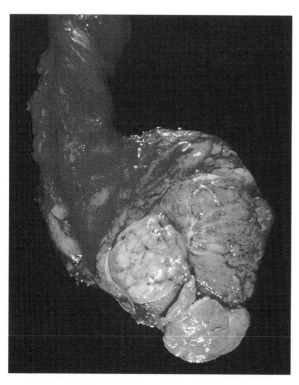

Figure 6-38
LEYDIG CELL TUMOR
The tumor is well demarcated and yellow. (Fig. 5.1 from Young RH, Scully RE. Testicular tumors. Chicago: ASCP Press, 1990:110.)

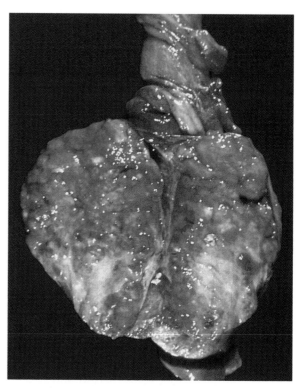

Figure 6-40
LEYDIG CELL TUMOR
The tumor is brown, nodular, and has a few small foci of yellow necrosis. Note the complete replacement of the testis by this tumor which was clinically malignant. (Fig. 5.3 from Young RH, Scully RE. Testicular tumors. Chicago: ASCP Press, 1990:112.)

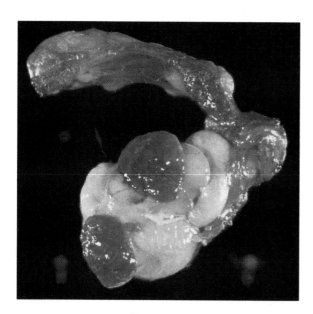

Figure 6-39
LEYDIG CELL TUMOR
This green-brown tumor from a prepubertal boy caused sexual precocity.

case, occasional psammoma bodies were scattered within the tumor (59), and in another there was ossification (43). One case in the literature (63) and three in our files showed adipose metaplasia (fig. 6-48).

The tumor cells are typically large and polygonal with abundant, slightly granular, eosinophilic cytoplasm (fig. 6-43). Occasionally, the cytoplasm is extensively vacuolated or spongy due to abundant lipid (fig. 6-44), and appears pale to clear. Focal, well-defined cytoplasmic vacuoles may impart a partial microcystic appearance in unusual cases (fig. 6-49). Rarely, the cells are small with scanty cytoplasm and have nuclei containing grooves, and exceptionally the tumor cells are spindle shaped (fig. 6-46) (62). These two cell types are usually associated with the characteristic polygonal cell type. Crystals of Reinke are identified in the cytoplasm in approximately one third of the cases (figs. 6-50, 6-51) (61), and lipochrome

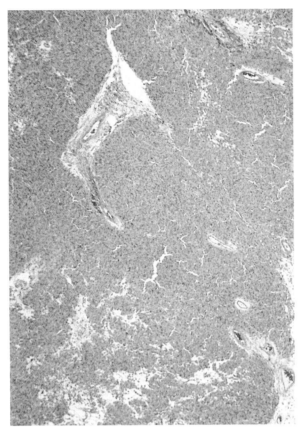

Figure 6-41
LEYDIG CELL TUMOR
Cells with abundant eosinophilic cytoplasm grow in lobular aggregates.

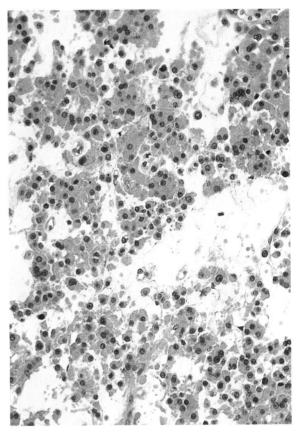

Figure 6-42
LEYDIG CELL TUMOR
Clusters of cells are separated by an edematous stroma.

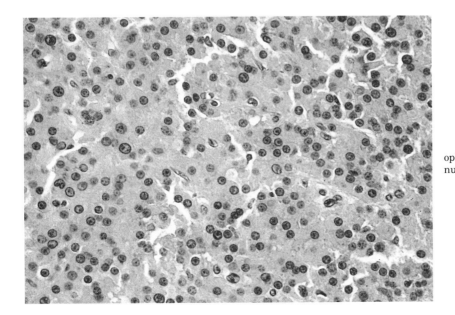

Figure 6-43
LEYDIG CELL TUMOR
Tumor cells have abundant eosinophilic cytoplasm and regular round nuclei, some with visible nucleoli.

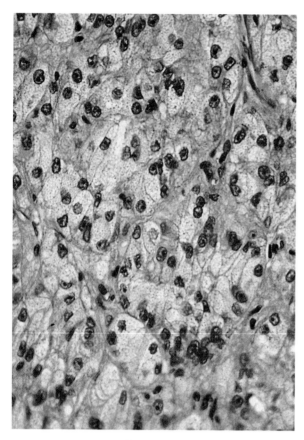

Figure 6-44
LEYDIG CELL TUMOR
Tumor cells have abundant pale cytoplasm due to lipid accumulation.

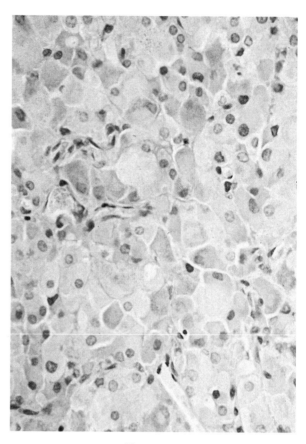

Figure 6-45
LEYDIG CELL TUMOR
Tumor cells contain abundant brown lipochrome pigment.

Figure 6-46
LEYDIG CELL TUMOR
Tumor cells are spindle shaped.

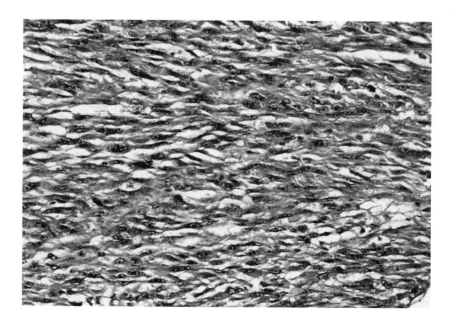

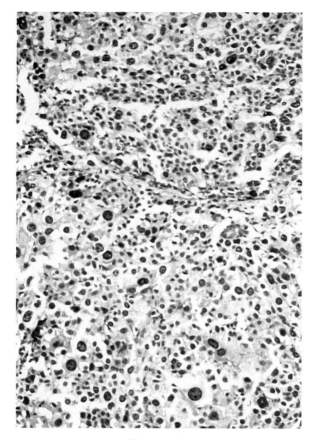

Figure 6-47
LEYDIG CELL TUMOR
Marked nuclear pleomorphism in a tumor which was clinically malignant.

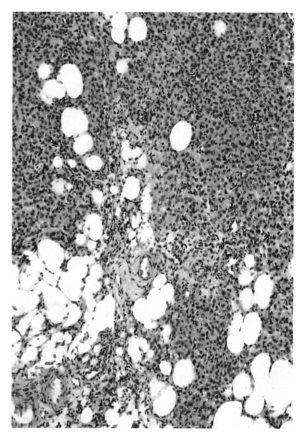

Figure 6-48
LEYDIG CELL TUMOR
Prominent fatty metaplasia, a rare feature.

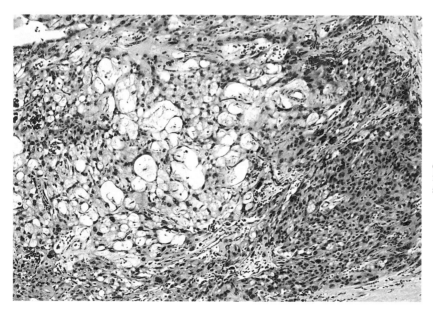

Figure 6-49
LEYDIG CELL TUMOR
Prominent cytoplasmic vacuoles create a microcystic pattern, mimicking yolk sac tumor. Tumor at right shows the usual appearance.

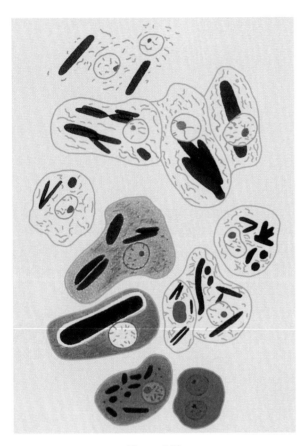

Figure 6-50
REINKE CRYSTALS
Reinke's drawing of the intracytoplasmic crystalloids in Leydig cells (1896) at high magnification. Absolute alcohol fixation and Weigert's fibrin stain were used. The crystalloids stain bright royal blue and the cytoplasm light claret lake. (Legend and photograph courtesy of the late Dr. W. Ober.)

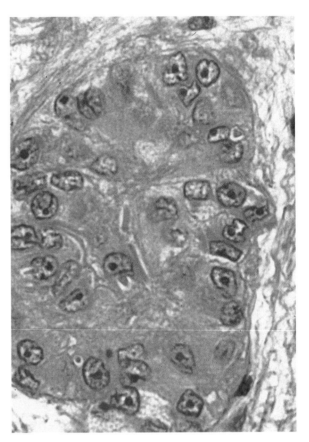

Figure 6-51
LEYDIG CELL TUMOR
Rod-shaped crystals of Reinke are seen in the middle of the illustration.

pigment in 10 to 15 percent (fig. 6-45). The nuclei are typically round and contain a single prominent nucleolus. Nuclear atypicality is usually absent or slight, but is marked in approximately 30 percent of the cases. The mitotic rate varies greatly: it is usually low, in accord with the bland cytology of most tumors, but is typically appreciable in cases with striking nuclear atypia.

Ultrastructural Findings. Ultrastructurally there are features of steroid-secreting cells, including prominent vesicles of smooth endoplasmic reticulum that are sometimes arranged in concentric whorls around lipid droplets (fig. 6-52) (51), mitochondria with either tubular or lamellar cristae, and lipid droplets (51b). In some cases, Reinke crystals, showing the distinctive periodicity, are identified (fig. 6-53).

Differential Diagnosis. A Leydig cell tumor may be confused with three non-neoplastic lesions. The first of these is Leydig cell hyperplasia, which may be florid, particularly in cryptorchid testes. However, the usual lack of a discrete mass on gross inspection and the presence of atrophic tubules in the midst of the Leydig cells should suggest the correct diagnosis. When grossly apparent, Leydig cell hyperplasia is usually multifocal, and the nodules are small. Malakoplakia is more likely to be a problem because it may result in the formation of a single, homogeneous, yellow or brown mass that may be grossly indistinguishable from a Leydig cell tumor, although in many cases the presence of an abscess is a major clue to the diagnosis of malakoplakia. On low-power microscopic examination the eosinophilic histiocytes (von Hansemann cells) of malakoplakia may be misconstrued as Leydig cells, but they

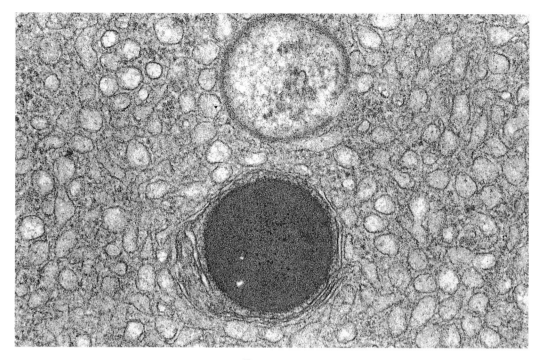

Figure 6-52
LEYDIG CELL TUMOR
There are numerous vesicles of smooth endoplasmic reticulum, occasionally surrounding lipid droplets. (Courtesy of Dr. R. Erlandson, New York, NY.)

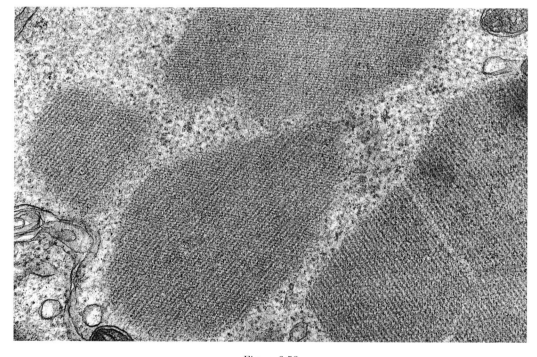

Figure 6-53
LEYDIG CELL TUMOR
Geometrically shaped Reinke crystals have a striking periodicity. (Courtesy of Dr. R. Erlandson, New York, NY.)

typically involve tubules as well as the interstitium and are admixed with other inflammatory cells. The presence of Michaelis-Gutmann bodies is diagnostic of malakoplakia.

The testicular "tumors" that may develop in patients with the adrenogenital syndrome closely resemble Leydig cell tumors but differ from them in their usual bilaterality, multifocality, and dark brown color, although occasional Leydig cell tumors, which are more often yellow or yellow-tan, may also be brown. More reliable than color is the fact that seminiferous tubules may be present within the non-neoplastic lesion (see page 295) but are found only rarely within a Leydig cell tumor. The cells of the "adrenogenital tumor" tend to be larger, with more abundant cytoplasm, than seen in Leydig cell tumors and contain lipochrome pigment (responsible for the dark color) more frequently and in greater amounts. Crystals of Reinke have not been identified within the cells of the "tumors" of the adrenogenital syndrome. Similar criteria are helpful for differentiating Leydig cell tumor from the hyperplastic nodules of steroid cells that may be seen in patients with Nelson's syndrome (see page 297).

Leydig cell tumors are generally relatively easily distinguished from Sertoli cell tumors and other tumors in the sex cord–stromal category because the resemblance of the neoplastic cells to Leydig cells is usually sufficiently striking to suggest the correct diagnosis. The specific differential diagnosis with Sertoli cell tumors, including the large cell calcifying subtype, is discussed on page 207. The rare Leydig cell tumor that contains cells with nuclear grooves and focally resembles a granulosa cell tumor has other areas characteristic of Leydig cell tumor that are easily found.

Leydig cell tumors may be confused with malignant lymphomas, particularly when their cells have scant cytoplasm and atypical nuclei. Lymphomas have a much higher frequency of bilaterality, common involvement of the epididymis and spermatic cord, characteristic intertubular infiltration of the tumor cells, invasion of the tubules in one third of the cases, and the distinctive cytologic features of the neoplastic cells. Appropriate immunostains can also resolve this differential, but they are rarely necessary. The differential diagnosis with plasmacytoma is considered on page 279.

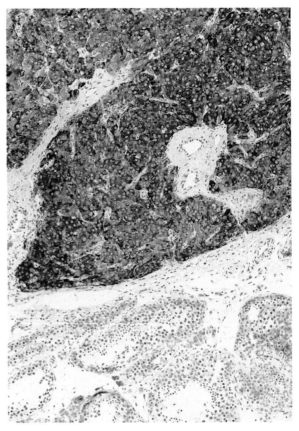

Figure 6-54
LEYDIG CELL TUMOR
Strong positivity for inhibin in a Leydig cell tumor. Non-neoplastic Sertoli cells and Leydig cells (bottom) also are reactive (anti-inhibin immunoperoxidase stain).

Occasional Leydig cell tumors have foci with small cytoplasmic vacuoles, and rare cases have prominent large vacuoles that may be confused with the microcystic pattern of yolk sac tumor (fig. 6-49) (46a). The presence of areas of typical Leydig cell tumor, the generally low mitotic rate, the occurrence of cells with foamy cytoplasm, and the absence of other patterns reminiscent of yolk sac tumor are helpful distinguishing features in these cases. Additional support can be obtained with immunostains: inhibin is positive in Leydig cell tumor (fig. 6-54), AFP is negative, and cytokeratins (AE1/AE3) are weak or negative (55a,57a); opposite patterns of reactivity are expected in yolk sac tumor.

The one Leydig cell tumor we have seen with a prominent spindle cell component and a single example of "sarcomatoid Leydig cell tumor" reported in the literature (62) each had conventional foci that were crucial in establishing their nature. If these are not present in initial sections, a mistaken diagnosis of sarcoma might result, with a more ominous prognosis. Such cases may also be misinterpreted as mixed sex cord–stromal tumors if the spindled cells are not recognized as Leydig cell variants, although this is not an important distinction from the clinical standpoint.

Metastatic carcinoma, particularly from the prostate, may be mistaken for a Leydig cell tumor when the former has a diffuse pattern and cells with appreciable eosinophilic cytoplasm. In such cases the clinical history is usually helpful, and, in the rare cases with an occult primary, other areas characteristic of prostatic adenocarcinoma are usually present. Immunostaining for prostate-specific acid phosphatase and prostate-specific antigen should be diagnostic. Inhibin positivity in Leydig cell tumor (42a,45a,55a,57b,57c) and its expected negativity in metastatic adenocarcinoma based on the experience in the ovary (62a) should clarify the diagnosis. The history, presence of melanin pigment, and immunostaining with HMB-45 aid in the rare differential with metastatic malignant melanoma. S-100 protein is sometimes demonstrated in Leydig cell tumors and therefore not helpful in this situation (55a,57a,61a).

Prognosis and Treatment. In the largest series of Leydig cell tumors, 5 of 30 patients with follow-up (17 percent) developed metastases (57). There is one report of bilateral malignant Leydig cell tumors (63a). A number of features viewed in aggregate are helpful in assessing the likelihood of a malignant course. The average age of patients with malignant tumors is 63 years, in contrast to 40 years for Leydig cell tumors in general (57). Only an occasional patient with a malignant tumor has presented with endocrine manifestations (43,64), despite frequently elevated levels of various hormones or their metabolites. A malignant course in a prepubertal patient with a Leydig cell tumor is exceptional (52). Tumors that metastasize are typically larger than those with a benign course. In one series, benign tumors had an average diameter of 2.7 cm, compared to 6.9 cm for malignant ones (57). The latter characteristically have infiltrative margins, invade lymphatics or blood vessels, and contain foci of necrosis. They also have a high mitotic rate (over 3 per 10 high-power fields) and significant nuclear

atypicality much more often than benign tumors. All 5 clinically malignant tumors in a series of 40 reported by Kim et al. (57) had four or more of the above features; 12 of the 14 tumors that were benign on the basis of follow-up of 2 or more years had none of them. Two additional studies confirmed the predictive value of these features for malignant behavior and found that an aneuploid DNA content and high proliferative fraction as assessed by the MIB-1 antibody also correlated with malignant behavior (48a,57a)

Malignant Leydig cell tumors spread most commonly to regional lymph nodes (72 percent), lung (43 percent), liver (38 percent), and bone (28 percent) (54). About 20 percent of the patients with clinically malignant tumors have metastases at the time of diagnosis (54). The treatment of a Leydig cell tumor is inguinal orchiectomy. If the gross or histologic features indicate a likelihood of malignancy, a retroperitoneal lymphadenectomy should be considered. The treatment of metastatic Leydig cell tumor has been generally unsatisfactory (46,47,54). Most patients with a clinically malignant Leydig cell tumor die within 5 years, but occasionally there is a prolonged course.

GRANULOSA–STROMAL CELL TUMORS

Granulosa cell tumors, like their ovarian counterparts, are now subdivided into two categories, adult and juvenile. It is impossible to make any conclusive statement concerning the relative frequency of the two because the juvenile type is only recently recognized, and criteria for distinguishing the adult type from unclassified sex cord–stromal tumors are subjective and therefore inconsistently applied. However, in our consultation material we have seen more cases of the juvenile type than the adult type; both are rare in the testis.

Adult-Type Granulosa Cell Tumor

Clinical Features. Less than two dozen adult granulosa cell tumors are well documented (68,69,72-74,78). The tumors typically occur in adults with an average age of 42 years. Twenty percent of the reported cases were associated with gynecomastia (fig. 6-55). Some patients have a history of testicular enlargement of several years' duration.

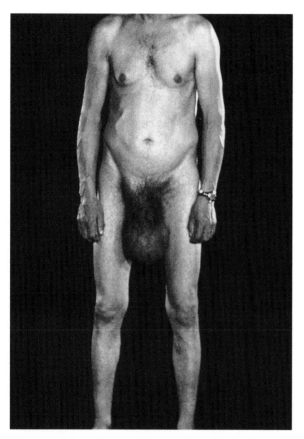

Figure 6-55
PROMINENT SCROTAL ENLARGEMENT AND
GYNECOMASTIA IN PATIENT WITH
GRANULOSA CELL TUMOR OF ADULT TYPE
ILLUSTRATED IN FIGURE 6-56

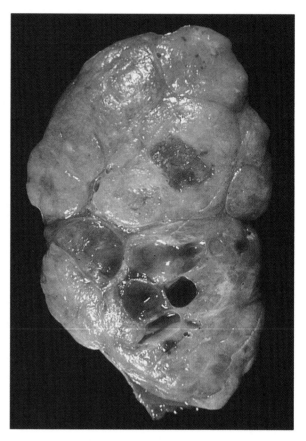

Figure 6-56
GRANULOSA CELL TUMOR, ADULT TYPE
The tumor is lobulated, brownish yellow, and mostly solid with focal hemorrhage. (Fig. 5.33 from Young RH, Scully RE. Testicular tumors. Chicago: ASCP Press, 1990:127.)

Gross Findings. The tumors measure up to 13 cm in diameter and typically are homogeneous, yellow to yellow-gray or white, firm, and lobulated (fig. 6-56). Cysts are sometimes present.

Microscopic Findings. The patterns are usually either microfollicular, with Call-Exner bodies (fig. 6-57), or diffuse (fig. 6-58), but other patterns, as seen in the ovary, may be observed. The cytoplasm is typically scanty, and the nuclei are pale with variably prominent grooves (fig. 6-59). If the architectural features are typical of adult granulosa cell tumor, a paucity of nuclear grooves is still consistent with the diagnosis. The mitotic rate is generally low, but a high rate has been seen in at least one tumor (69). These tumors may have the prominent fibrous to thecomatous stroma that characterizes the better known ovarian counterpart. In occasional cases the stromal cells have

abundant pale to eosinophilic cytoplasm (fig. 6-60). Immunohistochemistry has been performed in only occasional cases, with positivity for vimentin but not for cytokeratin (69).

Differential Diagnosis. Unclassified tumors in the sex cord–stromal category often have a focal appearance compatible with a granulosa cell tumor, but a specific diagnosis of granulosa cell tumor should only be made when all, or almost all, the neoplasm has granulosa cell features. As mentioned earlier, rare Leydig cell tumors also contain cells with nuclear grooves, but other features of Leydig cell tumor are present. Abundant pale cytoplasm in the cells of the stromal component of an adult granulosa cell tumor may simulate the germ cell component of the rare mixed germ cell-sex cord-stromal tumor. However, the nuclei in the sex cord–stromal tumors

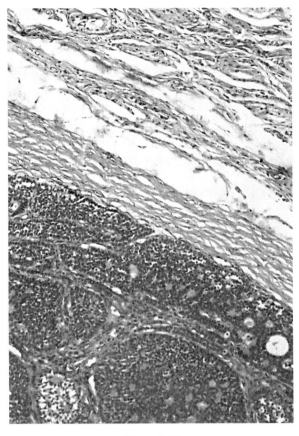

Figure 6-57
GRANULOSA CELL TUMOR, ADULT TYPE
The tumor is well circumscribed and contains numerous Call-Exner bodies. (Courtesy of Dr. A. Talerman, Philadelphia, PA.)

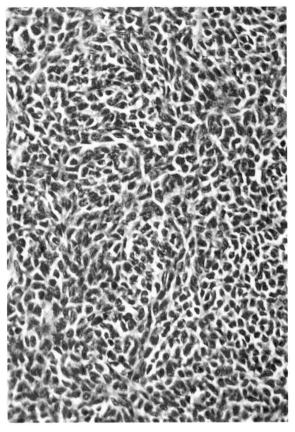

Figure 6-58
GRANULOSA CELL TUMOR, ADULT TYPE
The tumor has a diffuse pattern.

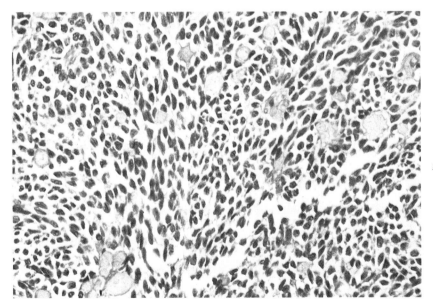

Figure 6-59
GRANULOSA CELL TUMOR, ADULT TYPE
Many of the nuclei have nuclear grooves. Note the Call-Exner bodies.

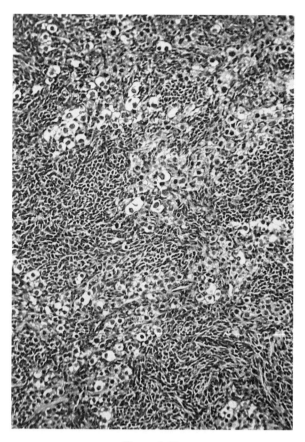

Figure 6-60
GRANULOSA CELL TUMOR, ADULT TYPE

Many tumor cells have abundant cytoplasm that ranges from eosinophilic to pale. The juxtaposition of these lutein-type cells with typical granulosa cells with scant cytoplasm may cause the erroneous diagnosis of a mixed germ cell-sex cord-stromal tumor to be made, with the lutein-type cells misinterpreted as germ cells because of their abundant pale cytoplasm.

are typically smaller and may be irregular, unlike the larger, round nuclei of germ cells. Since we have seen such cells lead to the erroneous diagnosis of a mixed germ cell-sex cord-stromal tumor, it is ideal that the putative neoplastic germ cell nature of such cells be confirmed by staining for periodic acid–Schiff (PAS) and appropriate immunoreactivity for placental-like alkaline phosphatase (PLAP). As detailed in chapter 5, we believe many other of these supposed "mixed" tumors actually represent a sex cord–stromal tumor with entrapped, non-neoplastic germ cells.

Prognosis and Treatment. Four patients with granulosa cell tumor had metastases. In

two, retroperitoneal lymph node spread was present at presentation (69,72). One patient was alive 14 months, and the other 14 years later. One received radiation therapy and the other chemotherapy. The other two patients with malignant tumors died of disease, at 5 months (73) and just over 11 years (69). A size greater than 7 cm, vascular or lymphatic invasion, and hemorrhage or necrosis are features of malignant tumors (69). Treatment is similar to that outlined for Sertoli cell tumors, NOS.

Juvenile-Type Granulosa Cell Tumor

General and Clinical Features. This is the most common neoplasm of the testis in the first 6 months of life (66,67,68a,70,75–77,79–81). The tumor is occasionally seen in older children but is rare in adults. Occasional juvenile granulosa cell tumors occur in undescended testes of infants with intersexual disorders (77,81), and one developed in a patient with the Drash syndrome (71). A testicular mass is the invariable presenting feature. All the reported cases had a benign outcome.

Gross Findings. The tumors measure up to 6 cm in diameter. They may be solid, cystic, or both (figs. 6-61, 6-62). The solid tissue may be nodular and yellow-orange (fig. 6-61) or tan-white (fig. 6-62). The cysts are usually thin-walled and contain viscid or gelatinous fluid, or clotted blood.

Microscopic Findings. Microscopic examination reveals variably prominent follicular and solid patterns (figs. 6-63–6-68). The follicles vary from large and round to oval, to small and irregular. They typically contain basophilic (fig. 6-64) or eosinophilic fluid that is stained by mucicarmine (fig. 6-65). In nonfollicular areas the cells grow in sheets, nodules (fig. 6-66), and irregular clusters (fig. 6-67). Hyalinization is sometimes extensive, and in some cases intercellular basophilic mucinous fluid is conspicuous and may result in a vaguely "chondroid" appearance (fig. 6-63). In some cases the tumor cells are dispersed loosely in the stroma, simulating, to a degree, the reticular pattern of yolk sac tumor. The tumor cells have moderate to large amounts of pale to occasionally eosinophilic cytoplasm and hyperchromatic, round to oval nuclei, some of which contain nucleoli (fig. 6-68). Mitotic activity is usually evident and often prominent (fig. 6-68).

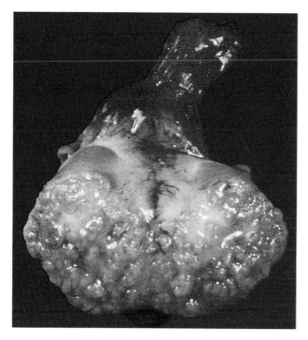

Figure 6-61
GRANULOSA CELL TUMOR, JUVENILE TYPE
The tumor is solid, lobulated, and orange-tan. (Courtesy of Dr. J. Henley, Indianapolis, IN.)

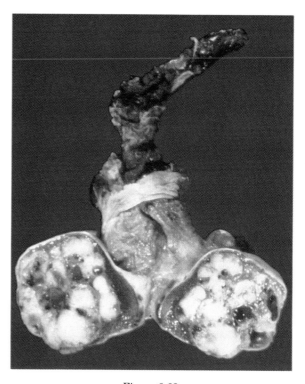

Figure 6-62
GRANULOSA CELL TUMOR, JUVENILE TYPE
The sectioned surface of the tumor is composed of multiple nodules of solid white tissue with several interspersed cysts. (Fig. 5.36 from Young RH, Scully RE. Testicular tumors. Chicago: ASCP Press, 1990:128.)

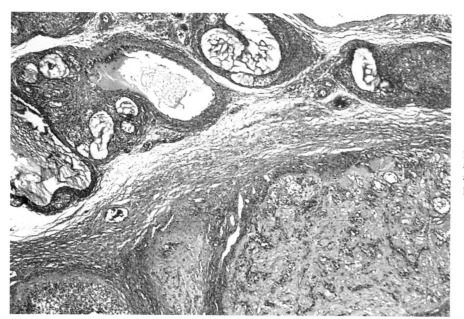

Figure 6-63
GRANULOSA CELL TUMOR, JUVENILE TYPE
Mixed follicular and solid patterns. A predominantly solid area (bottom right) is basophilic and has a vaguely chondroid appearance.

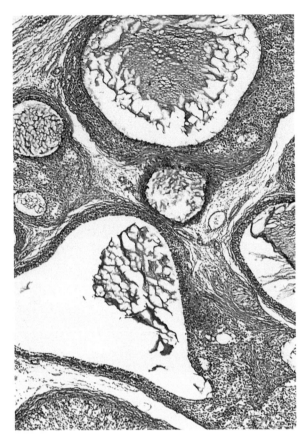

Figure 6-64
GRANULOSA CELL TUMOR, JUVENILE TYPE
Large follicles contain basophilic intraluminal material.

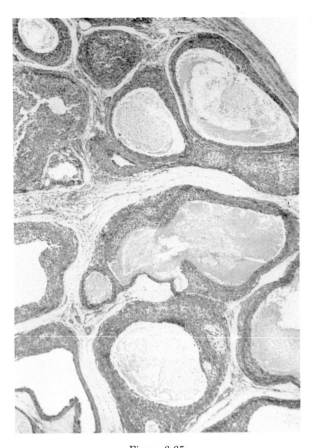

Figure 6-65
GRANULOSA CELL TUMOR, JUVENILE TYPE
Material within follicles of the type seen in the previous illustration is positive with the mucicarmine stain.

Figure 6-66
GRANULOSA CELL TUMOR,
JUVENILE TYPE
Tumor cells grow in large nodular aggregates.

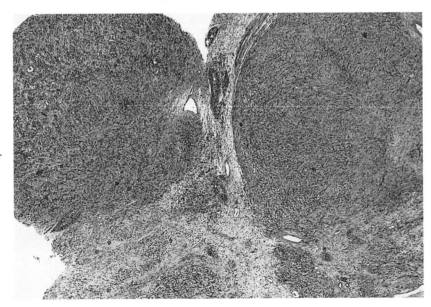

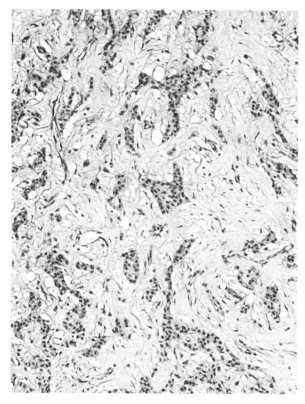

Figure 6-67
GRANULOSA CELL TUMOR, JUVENILE TYPE
Small clusters of tumor cells and single cells are irregularly distributed in a stroma that varied from hyaline to slightly basophilic.

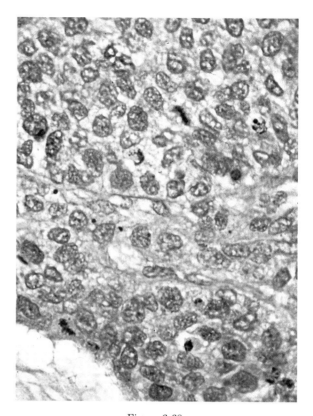

Figure 6-68
GRANULOSA CELL TUMOR, JUVENILE TYPE
Nuclei are immature and exhibit brisk mitotic activity.

Differential Diagnosis. The juvenile granulosa cell tumor may be misinterpreted as a yolk sac tumor, one of the other relatively frequent tumors of infants, particularly when it exhibits a "reticular" pattern and brisk mitotic activity. The presence of follicles in most juvenile granulosa cell tumors, the absence of the various characteristic patterns of yolk sac tumor, the lack of strong and diffuse immunohistochemical staining for cytokeratin, and the absence of reactivity for alphafetoprotein should help avoid this mistake. Yolk sac tumors are usually seen beyond 6 months of age.

Juvenile granulosa cell tumors are distinguished from the adult form by the greater degree of irregularity in size and shape of the follicles, which usually show intraluminal basophilic fluid that is typically absent in the adult tumors. Also the juvenile cases have more abundant cytoplasm, a more immature nuclear appearance, and a greater degree of mitotic activity. The age of the patient is again helpful

because of the great tendency for the juvenile variant to be found in the first year of life.

The differential with Sertoli cell tumors has been discussed in that section, and, as noted, there are a number of "Sertoli cell" tumors in the literature that probably represent juvenile granulosa cell tumors according to our criteria.

The primitive nuclei, mitotic activity, and eosinophilic cytoplasm of the juvenile granulosa cell tumor may raise a concern for embryonal rhabdomyosarcoma with scattered rhabdomyoblastic cells. Embryonal rhabdomyosarcoma, however, is almost always a paratesticular tumor and usually found in older children (mean age, 7 years). Rare testicular cases do occur, probably representing sarcomatous overgrowth in teratomas, but have not, to our knowledge, been reported in infants. Although cystic degeneration may occur, the characteristic fluid-filled follicles of juvenile granulosa cell tumor are not a feature. Immunostains for markers of skeletal muscle could resolve this differential.

TUMORS IN THE
FIBROMA-THECOMA GROUP

Tumors in this category are uncommon, and, in most cases, resemble either the typical ovarian fibroma or the cellular variant (88). We have not personally seen a convincing example of testicular thecoma, and the one tumor reported in the literature as "thecoma" (89) is best placed in the fibroma category according to our criteria. Collins and Symington (83), who reported four tumors of the testicular parenchyma in this group and noted a resemblance to ovarian fibroma, commented, however, that "the analogy not be too far pressed." It is certainly possible that some cases are not of gonadal stromal origin but arise from nonspecific soft tissue fibroblasts (see page 259), but it is convenient to consider them all together here.

Clinical Findings. The 14 patients whose tumors appear to definitely or probably fit in this category ranged from 5 to 52 (mean, 30) years of age. They typically presented with a testicular mass (82–87,89,90). Although follow-up is limited, it has been unremarkable.

Gross Findings. The tumors range from 0.5 to 7.0 (mean, 3.0) cm in maximum dimension and are typically well circumscribed and firm, and tan-white to, more commonly, yellow. Hemorrhage and necrosis are absent.

Microscopic Findings. These tumors are by definition indistinguishable from a typical or cellular fibroma of the ovary. They are characterized by spindle-shaped fibroblasts associated with variable amounts of collagen that often grow in a storiform pattern, sometimes associated with mild degrees of edema and modest vascularity (fig. 6-69). The cellular tumors are often strikingly so, and occasional cellular tumors have up to 2 mitotic figures per 10 high-power fields. Ultrastructural studies show fibroblastic or myofibroblastic differentiation, with the tumor cells containing filaments, subplasmalemmal electron-dense bodies, pinocytotic vesicles, discontinuous basal lamina, and intercellular desmosomes. Immunohistochemical studies yield variable results. The most consistently positive immunostains include vimentin and actin, however, focal desmin, keratin, and S-100 reactivity is reported. Although ultrastructural and immunohistochemical studies are of academic interest, in our opinion they are not indicated for routine evaluation.

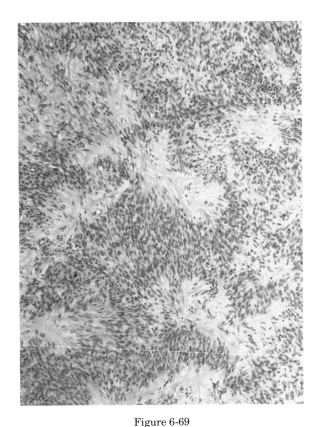

Figure 6-69
CELLULAR FIBROMA
Note the identity with the ovarian tumor of the same name.

Differential Diagnosis. Noncellular fibromas are similar to fibromatous tumors of the testicular tunics and are distinguished from them on the basis of gross characteristics (see chapter 7, Table 7-1). Cellular fibromas may bring into the differential diagnosis the exceptionally rare fibrosarcoma of the testis (see chapter 7). There are no established criteria for the distinction of these two tumors in the testis, but it appears reasonable to apply similar criteria to those used in the ovary (88). The tumors are distinguished from leiomyomas of both typical and cellular type (each exceptionally rare in the testis) using criteria applicable in the ovary and soft tissues. We have not found actin staining reliable in this differential. Unclassified sex cord–stromal tumors may have prominent fibromatous areas but, by definition, have at least some focal epithelial differentiation that permits distinction from pure fibromas. This distinction is important because of the benign course of all reported fibromas, whereas occasional tumors in the sex cord–stromal, unclassified category are malignant. Although experience is limited, unclassified sex cord–stromal tumors with a predominance of spindle cells are frequently positive for both S-100 protein and smooth muscle actin, whereas fibromas are smooth muscle actin positive but negative for S-100 protein (88a).

SEX CORD–STROMAL TUMORS, MIXED AND UNCLASSIFIED

General and Clinical Features. Some testicular sex cord–stromal tumors have patterns of two or more of the above discussed specific subtypes, but distinguishing them in the literature from cases in the unclassified category is often impossible. It is therefore unrealistic to cover separately the mixed and unclassified tumors on the basis of the available information. All patterns in a mixed tumor should be recorded, and the behavior of the tumor is most likely to be that of the predominant pattern or that which is most histologically atypical. Tumors in the unclassified category frequently lack specific differentiation or contain patterns and cells resembling to varying degrees both testicular and ovarian elements (91,93). Unclassified sex cord–stromal tumors occur at all ages. In a registry of tumors in children, 62 percent of sex cord tumors were considered unclassified (92). From another viewpoint, approximately one third of the reported tumors have been from children. The most common clinical symptom is painless testicular enlargement, but gynecomastia is present in about 10 percent of patients.

Gross Findings. The tumors vary greatly in size, with many replacing most or all of the testis. They are usually well circumscribed (fig. 6-70) and composed of white to yellow, often lobulated tissue, sometimes traversed by gray-white fibrous septa. Cysts are occasionally present; hemorrhage and necrosis are uncommon.

Microscopic Findings. The appearance of the individual patterns in mixed tumors is similar to that observed when such patterns are seen in pure form, as discussed above.

A spectrum of patterns is seen in the unclassified tumors, ranging from predominantly epithelial to predominantly stromal (figs. 6-71–6-73). The better differentiated tumors typically contain solid to hollow tubules or cords composed of, or lined by,

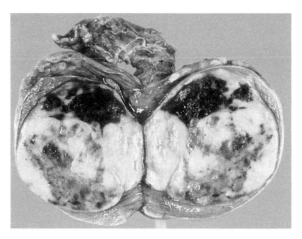

Figure 6-70
SEX CORD–STROMAL TUMOR, UNCLASSIFIED
The well-circumscribed tumor is white with focal hemorrhage.

cells resembling Sertoli cells. Islands and masses of cells resembling granulosa cells (fig. 6-71) and containing Call-Exner–like bodies may also be present, but usually the nuclei lack grooves and, although often suggestive of granulosa cell tumor, the overall architectural and cytologic features are usually not typical of that tumor. The cytoplasm of cells lining sertoliform tubules varies from scanty to abundant, and may be eosinophilic, amphophilic, or vacuolated and lipid-laden; the nuclei are round to oval and often vesicular, and sometimes contain single small nucleoli; mitotic figures are variably prominent. The stromal component may be densely cellular or fibromatous (fig. 6-72). Leydig cells may be seen. Some stromal cells may have abundant vacuolated or eosinophilic cytoplasm. The less differentiated tumors exhibit varying degrees of nuclear pleomorphism and mitotic activity. Diffuse and sarcomatoid patterns are frequent, and in some areas it may be difficult or impossible to distinguish the epithelial and stromal components on routine staining. Reticulum stains may help delineate the two components (93a). Spindle cell–predominant cases are often reactive for S-100 protein and smooth muscle actin, similar to granulosa cell tumors (93a).

Differential Diagnosis. It should be readily evident in most cases that these tumors are in the sex cord–stromal category as opposed to, for example, any other more common form of testicular neoplasm in the germ cell tumor group. The

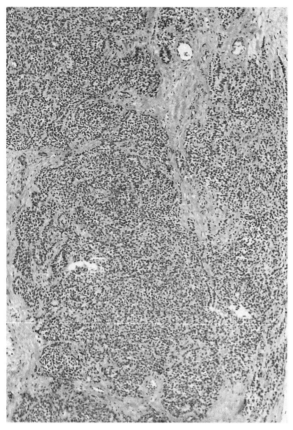

Figure 6-71
SEX CORD–STROMAL TUMOR, UNCLASSIFIED
Epithelial pattern in a tumor which in other areas had a predominant stromal pattern (see figure 6-72).

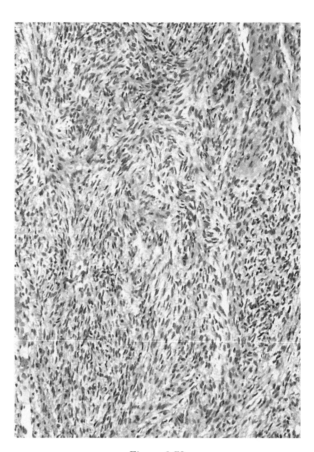

Figure 6-72
SEX CORD–STROMAL TUMOR, UNCLASSIFIED
Prominent cellular mesenchymal growth in other areas of tumor seen in figure 6-71.

Figure 6-73
SEX CORD–STROMAL
TUMOR, UNCLASSIFIED
The epithelial component of this tumor exhibited a prominent microcystic pattern.

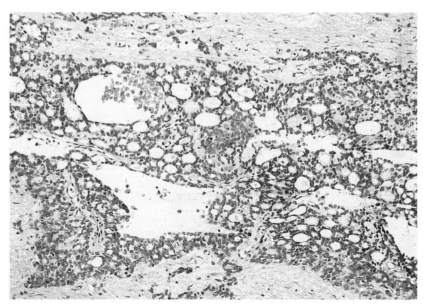

greatest problem is the distinction of tumors in the unclassified and mixed category from pure tumors of the various subtypes discussed earlier. However, strict adherence to the morphologic features and criteria discussed in those sections should, in the majority of cases, enable the pure tumors to be separated from those in the mixed and unclassified categories. Of particular note is the prominent cellular stromal component of many unclassified tumors and the typical presence of both granulosa-like and Sertoli-like areas. When the epithelial component is small, areas of the tumor may resemble one or other form of pure sarcoma of the testis, and such a diagnosis should only be made after thorough sampling, supplemented by reticulum stains, has ruled out epithelial elements that are consistent with a sex cord nature.

Prognosis. An important aspect of these tumors is the rarity of malignant behavior in children compared to an approximately 25 percent frequency of malignancy in adults. Features that generally correlate with aggressive behavior are similar to those that suggest malignant behavior in pure sex cord–stromal tumors, namely, large size, extratesticular spread, necrosis, vascular invasion, marked nuclear pleomorphism, and brisk mitotic activity. The patterns of spread are predominantly to inguinal and retroperitoneal lymph nodes, but visceral metastases are not rare. In cases with overt malignant features on microscopic examination, a staging lymph node dissection is indicated.

IMMUNOHISTOCHEMISTRY OF SEX CORD–STROMAL TUMORS

Certain specific situations in which immunohistochemistry may be helpful in the differential diagnosis of sex cord–stromal tumors of the testis have been mentioned in the previous sections, but we have included here a brief summary of the growing information on this topic (94–104). Important findings that may aid in diagnosing Leydig cell tumors include their positivity for inhibin, negativity for epithelial membrane antigen and HMB-45, and usually negative or weak and focal staining for cytokeratin. The tumors are vimentin positive which, in conjunction with inhibin positivity, negative staining for epithelial membrane antigen, and variable cytokeratin im-

munoreactivity, is helpful in the differential diagnosis with metastatic carcinoma. Some Leydig cell tumors are S-100 protein positive, so this stain has limited value when considering melanoma (95,97,98,100), although a negative result favors Leydig cell tumor. An antibody to melan-A has stained a small number of Leydig cell tumors and has proved to be a diagnostic aid (94a).

Sertoli cell tumors, NOS, are usually positive for cytokeratin and vimentin, and negative for epithelial membrane antigen (94,95,98). Inhibin is usually positive, although often focal, and such positivity favors Sertoli cell tumor over germ cell tumor or metastatic carcinoma. It may also help to identify the Sertoli nature of peculiar biphasic neoplasms in which the nature of the epithelial component is uncertain (94b). A recent study has shown that the large cell calcifying variant of Sertoli cell tumor often stains for S-100 protein (96), as do some Sertoli cell tumors, NOS (94,95,98).

Within the granulosa cell group, staining for cytokeratin is usually either absent or only focally positive, and vimentin is usually strongly positive. S-100 protein and smooth muscle actin may be demonstrated in both the juvenile and adult types (100,101), and desmin has also been demonstrated in the juvenile variant (100). Based on the experience with ovarian cases, we would expect both the adult and juvenile forms of granulosa cell tumor to stain for inhibin (102). While this has been demonstrated for the juvenile granulosa cell tumor of the testis (Kommoss F, unpublished observations, 1998), we are not aware of inhibin studies on the pure adult form of testicular tumor. The spindle cell areas of granulosa cell tumors may stain for desmin, while these areas in unclassified tumors may be S-100 protein and smooth muscle actin immunoreactive, and focally positive for cytokeratin, in keeping with the myoepithelial or myofibroblastic differentiation of some of the cells.

Immunohistochemical staining of fibromatous tumors is rarely indicated, but a potential finding of note is usual negativity for desmin, which provides evidence against a smooth muscle tumor. Weak desmin staining and actin staining has to be interpreted in light of the overall microscopic findings. As noted earlier, we have not found actin staining reliable in the distinction of fibromatous from myogenic tumors.

REFERENCES

General References

1. Kaplan GW, Cromie WJ, Kelalis PP, Silber I, Tank ES. Gonadal stromal tumors: a report of the prepubertal testicular tumor registry. J Urol 1986;136:300–2.
2. Ober WB, Sciagura C. Leydig, Sertoli, and Reinke: three anatomists who were on the ball. Pathol Annu 1981;16(Pt. 1):1–13.

3. Scully RE. Testicular tumors with endocrine manifestiatons. In: De Groot LJ, ed. Endocrinology, 3rd ed. Philadelphia: WB Saunders Co., 1995:2442–8.

Sertoli Cell Tumors

4. Adlington SR, Salm R. A case of bilateral tubular adenoma of the testis. Brit J Surg 1960;48:152–5.
4a. Amin MB, Young RH, Scully RE. Immunohistochemical profile of Sertoli and Leydig cell tumors of the testis [Abstract]. Mod Pathol 1998;11:76A.
5. Caccamea A, Cozzi F, Farragiana T, Boscherini B, Pierro A. Feminizing Sertoli cell tumor associated with Peutz-Jeghers syndrome. Tumori 1985;71:379–85.
6. Cantu JM, Rivera H, Ocampo-Campos R, et al. Peutz-Jeghers syndrome with feminizing Sertoli cell tumor, NOS. Cancer 1980;46:223–8.
7. Carney JA, Gordon H, Carpenter PC, Shenoy BV, Go VL. The complex of myxomas, spotty pigmentation, and endocrine overactivity. Medicine 1985;64:270–83.
8. Coen P, Kulin H, Ballantine T, et al. An aromatase-producing sex-cord tumor resulting in prepubertal gynecomastia. N Engl J Med 1991;324:317–22.
9. Collins DH, Symington T. Sertoli-cell tumor. Brit J Urol 1964;36:52–61.
10. Dubois RS, Hoffman WH, Krishnan TH, et al. Feminizing sex cord tumor with annular tubules in a boy with Peutz-Jeghers syndrome. J Pediatr 1982;101:568–71.
10a. Erlandson RA. Diagnostic transmission electron microscopy of tumors with clinicopathological, immunohistochemical, and cytogenetic correlations. New York: Raven Press, 1994.
10b. Freeman DA. Steroid hormone-producing tumors in man. Endocr Rev 1986;7:204–20.
11. Gabrilove JL, Freiberg EK, Leiter E, Nicolis GL. Feminizing and non-feminizing Sertoli cell tumors. J Urol 1980;124:757–67.
11a. Gilcrease MZ, Delgado R, Albores-Saavedra J. Testicular Sertoli cell tumor with a heterologous sarcomatous component: immunohistochemical assessment of Sertoli cell differentiation. Arch Pathol Lab Med 1998;122:907–11.
12. Goswitz JJ, Pettinato G, Manivel JC. Testicular sex cord–stromal tumors in children: clinicopathologic study of sixteen children with review of literature. Pediatr Pathol Lab Med 1996;16:451–70.
12a. Harms D, Kock LR. Testicular juvenile granulosa cell and Sertoli cell tumours: a clinicopathologic study of 29 cases from the Kiel Paediatric Tumor Registry. Virchows Arch 1997;430:301–9.
13. Horn T, Jao W, Keh PC. Large-cell calcifying Sertoli cell tumor of the testis: a case report with ultrastructural study. Ultrastruct Pathol 1983;4:359–64.
13a. Iczkowski KA, Bostwick DG, Cheville JC. Inhibin is a sensitive and specific marker for testicular sex cord-stromal tumors. Mod Pathol 1998;11:774–9.
14. Jacobsen GK. Malignant Sertoli cell tumors of the testis. J Urol Pathol 1993;1:233–55.
15. Kaplan GW, Cromie WJ, Kelalis PP, Silber I, Tank ES. Gonadal stromal tumors: a report of the Prepubertal Testicular Tumor Registry. J Urol 1986;136:300–2.
16. Kratzer SS, Ulbright TM, Talerman A, et al. Large cell calcifying Sertoli cell tumor of the testis: contrasting features of six malignant and six benign tumors and a review of the literature. Am J Surg Pathol 1997;21:1271–80.
16a. McCluggage WG, Shanks JH, Whiteside C, Maxwell P, Banerjee SS, Biggart JD. Immunohistochemical study of testicular sex cord-stromal tumors, including staining with anti-inhibin antibody. Am J Surg Pathol 1998;22:615–9.
17. Mostofi FK, Theiss EA, Ashley DJ. Tumors of specialized gonadal stroma in human male subjects. Cancer 1959;12:944–57.
18. Plata C, Algaba F, Anjudar M. Large cell calcifying Sertoli cell tumour of the testis. Histopathology 1995;26:255–9.
19. Proppe KH, Scully RE. Large-cell calcifying Sertoli cell tumor of the testis. Am J Clin Pathol 1980;74:607–19.
20. Rishi M, Howard LN, Bratthauer GL, Tavassoli FA. Use of monoclonal antibody against human inhibin as a marker of sex cord-stromal tumors of the ovary. Am J Surg Pathol 1997;21:583–9.
21. Rosenzweig JL, Lawrence DA, Vogel DL, et al. Adrenocorticotropin-independent hypercortisolemia and testicular tumors in a patient with a pituitary tumor and gigantism. J Clin Endocrinol Metab 1982;55:421–7.
22. Rosvoll RV, Woodard JR. Malignant Sertoli cell tumor of the testis. Cancer 1968;22:8–13.
23. Rutgers JL, Scully RE. The androgen insensitivity syndrome (testicular feminization): a clinicopathologic study of 43 cases. Int J Gynecol Pathol 1991;10:126–44.
24. Sharma S, Seam RK, Kapoor HL. Malignant Sertoli cell tumour of the testis in a child. J Surg Oncol 1990;44:129–31.
25. Talerman A. Malignant Sertoli cell tumor of the testis. Cancer 1971;28:446–55.
26. Teilum G. Arrhenoblastoma—androblastoma. Homologous ovarian and testicular tumors. II. Including the so-called luteomas and adrenal tumors of the ovary and the interstitial cell tumors of the testis. Acta Pathol Microbiol Scand 1943;23:252–64.
27. Teilum G. Classification of testicular and ovarian androblastoma and Sertoli cell tumors. A survey of comparative studies with consideration of histogenesis, endocrinology, and embryological theories. Cancer 1958;11:769–82.
28. Teilum G. Estrogen producing Sertoli-cell tumors (androblastoma tubulare lipoides of the human testis and ovary). Homologous ovarian and testicular tumors, III. J Clin Endocrinol 1949;9:301–18.

29. Teilum G. Homologous tumors in the ovary and testis. Contributions to classification of the gonadial tumors. Acta Obstet Gynecol 1944;24:480–503.

30. Têtu B, Ro JY, Ayala AG. Large cell calcifying Sertoli cell tumor of the testis. A clinicopathologic, immunohistochemical and ultrastructural study of two cases. Am J Clin Pathol 1991;96:717–22.

31. Waxman M, Damjanov I, Khapra A, Landal SJ. Large cell calcifying Sertoli tumor of testis. Light microscopic and ultrastructural study. Cancer 1984;54:1574–81.

32. Wilson DM, Pitts WC, Hintz RL, Rosenfeld RG. Testicular tumors with Peutz-Jeghers syndrome. Cancer 1986;57:2238–40.

32a. Young RH, Koelliker DD, Scully RE. Sertoli cell tumors of the testis, not otherwise specified. A clinicopathologic analysis of 60 cases. Am J Surg Pathol 1998;22:709–21.

33. Young RH, Welch WR, Dickersin GR, Scully RE. Ovarian sex cord tumor with annular tubules: review of 74 cases including 27 with Peutz-Jeghers syndrome and four with adenoma malignum of the cervix. Cancer 1982;50:1384–402.

34. Young S, Gooneratne S, Straus FH, Zeller WP, Bulun SE, Rosenthal IM. Feminizing Sertoli cell tumors in boys with Peutz-Jeghers syndrome. Am J Surg Pathol 1995;19:50–8.

35. Zukerberg LR, Young RH, Scully RE. Sclerosing Sertoli cell tumor of the testis: a report of 10 cases. Am J Surg Pathol 1991;15:829-34.

Sertoli-Leydig Cell Tumors

36. Fam A, Ishak KG. Androblastoma of the testicle: report of a case in an infant 3 1/2 months old. J Urol 1958;79:859–62.

37. Fuglsang F, Ohlse NS. Androblastoma predominantly feminizing. With report of a case. Acta Chir Scand 1957;112:405–10.

37a. Gilcrease MZ, Delgado R, Albores-Saavedra J. Testicular Sertoli cell tumor with a heterologous sarcomatous component. Immunohistochemical assessment of Sertoli cell differentiation. Arch Pathol Lab Med 1996;122:907–11.

38. Oosterhuis JW, Castedo SM, de Jong B, et al. A malignant mixed gonadal stromal tumor of the testis with heterologous components and i(12p) in one of its metastases. Cancer Genet Cytogenet 1989;41:105–14.

39. Perito PE, Ciancio G, Civantos F, Politano VA. Sertoli-Leydig cell testicular tumor: case report and review of sex cord/gonadal stromal tumor histogenesis. J Urol 1992;148:883–5.

40. Teilum G. Arrhenoblastoma-androblastoma. Homologous ovarian and testicular tumors. II. Including the so-called luteomas and adrenal tumors of the ovary and the interstitial cell tumors of the testis. Acta Pathol Microbiol Scand 1943;23:252–64.

41. Teilum G. Homologous tumors in the ovary and testis. Contributions to classification of the gonadial tumors. Acta Obstet Gynecol 1944;24:480–503.

42. Young RH, Scully RE. Ovarian Sertoli-Leydig cell tumors with a retiform pattern: a problem in histopathologic diagnosis. A report of 25 cases. Am J Surg Pathol 1983;7:775–1.

Leydig Cell Tumors

42a. Amin MB, Young RH, Scully RE. Immunohistochemical profile of Sertoli and Leydig cell tumors of the testis [Abstract]. Mod Pathol 1998;11:76A.

43. Balsitis M, Sokol M. Ossifying malignant Leydig (interstitial) cell tumour of the testis. Histopathology 1990;16:597–601.

44. Bercovici P, Nahoul K, Ducasse M, et al. Leydig cell tumor with gynecomastia: further studies–the recovery after unilateral orchidectomy. J Clin Endocrinol Metab 1985;61:957–62.

45. Bercovici P, Nahoul K, Tater D, et al. Hormonal profile of Leydig cell tumors with gynecomastia. J Clin Endocrinol Metab 1984;59:625–30.

45a. Bergh A, Cajander S. Immunohistochemical localization of inhibin-alpha in the testes of normal men and in men with testicular disorders. Int J Androl 1990;13:463–9.

46. Bertrem KA, Bratloff B, Hodges GF, Davidson H. Treatment of malignant Leydig cell tumor. Cancer 1991;68:2324–9.

46a. Billings SD, Roth LM, Ulbright TM. Microcystic Leydig cell tumors mimicking yolk sac tumor: a report of four cases. Am J Surg Pathol 1999;23:546–51.

47. Bokemeyer C, Harstrick A, Gonnermann O, et al. Metastatic Leydig cell tumours of the testis: report of four cases and review of the literature. Int J Oncol 1993;2:241–4.

48. Boulanger P, Somma M, Chevalier S, Bleau G, Roberts KD, Chapdelaine A. Elevated secretion of androstenedione in a patient with a Leydig cell tumour. Acta Endocrinol 1984;107:104–9.

48a. Cheville JC, Sebo TJ, Lager DJ, Bostwick DG, Farrow GM. Leydig cell tumor of the testis: a clinicopathologic, DNA content and MIB-1 comparison of non-metastasizing and metastasizing tumors. Am J Surg Pathol 1998;22:1361–7.

49. Czernobilsky H, Czernobilsky B, Schneider HG, et al. Characterization of a feminizing testicular Leydig cell tumor by hormone profile, immunocytochemistry, and tissue culture. Cancer 1985;56:1667–76.

50. Davis JM, Woodroff J, Sadasivan R, Stephens R. Case report: congenital adrenal hyperplasia and malignant Leydig cell tumor. Am J Med Sci 1995;309:63–5.

51. Dickersin GR. Diagnostic electron microscopy: a text/atlas. New York: Igaku-Shoin, 1988.

51a. Dilworth JP, Farrow GM, Oesterling JE. Non-germ cell tumors of testis. Urology 1991;37:399–417.

51b. Erlandson RA. Diagnostic transmission electron microscopy of tumors with clinicopathological, immunohistochemical, and cytogenetic correlations. New York: Raven Press, 1994.

52. Freeman DA. Steroid hormone-producing tumors in man. Endocrine Reviews 1986;7:204–20.

53. Gabrilove JL, Nicolis GL, Mitty HA, Sohval AR. Feminizing interstitial cell tumor of the testis. Personal observations and review of the literature. Cancer 1975;35:1184–202.

54. Grem JL, Robins I, Wilson KS, Gilchrist K, Trump DK. Metastatic Leydig cell tumor of the testis. Report of three cases and review of the literature. Cancer 1986;58:2116–9.

55. Haas GP, Pittabiga S, Gomella L, et al. Clinically occult Leydig cell tumor presenting with gynecomastia. J Urol 1989;142:1325–7.

55a. Iczkowski KA, Bostwick DG, Cheville JC. Inhibin is a sensitive and specific marker for testicular sex cord-stromal tumors. Mod Pathol 1998;11:774–9.

56. Kay R. Prepubertal Testicular Tumor Registry. J Urol 1993;150:671–4.

57. Kim I, Young RH, Scully RE. Leydig cell tumors of the testis. A clinicopathological analysis of 40 cases and review of the literature. Am J Surg Pathol 1985;9:177–92.

57a. McCluggage WG, Shanks JH, Arthur K, Banerjee SS. Cellular proliferation and nuclear ploidy assessments augment prognostic factors in predicting malignancy in testicular Leydig cell tumours. Histopathology 1998;33:361–8.

57b. McCluggage WG, Shanks JH, Whiteside C, Maxwell P, Banerjee SS, Biggart JD. Immunohistochemical study of testicular sex cord-stromal tumors, including staining with anti-inhibin antibody. Am J Surg Pathol 1998;22:615–9.

57c. Mehta MK, Garde SV, Sheth AR. Occurrence of FSH, inhibin and other hypothalamic-pituitary-intestinal hormones in normal fertility, subfertility, and tumors of human testes. Int J Fertil Menopausal Stud 1995;40:39–46.

58. Mineur P, DeCooman S, Hustin J, Verhoeven G, Der Hertogh R. Feminizing testicular Leydig cell tumor: hormonal profile before and after unilateral orchidectomy. J Clin Endocrinol Metab 1987;64:686–91.

59. Minokowitz S, Soloway H, Soscia J. Ossifying interstitial cell tumor of the testis. J Urol 1965;94:592–5.

60. Perez C, Novoa J, Alcaniz J, Salto L, Barcelo B. Leydig cell tumour of the testis with gynaecomastia and elevated oestrogen, progesterone and prolactin levels: case report. Clin Endocrinol 1980;13:409–12.

61. Reinke F. Beiträge zur Histologie des Menschen. Arch Mikr Anat 1896;47:34–44.

61a. Renshaw AA, Gordon M, Corless CL. Immunohistochemistry of unclassified sex cord-stromal tumors of the testis with a predominance of spindle cells. Mod Pathol 1997;10:693–700.

62. Richmond I, Banerjee SS, Eyden BP, Sissons MC. Sarcomatoid Leydig cell tumor of testis. Histopathology 1995;27:578–80.

62a. Rishi M, Howard LN, Bratthauer GL, Tavassoli FA. Use of monoclonal antibody against human inhibin as a marker of sex cord-stromal tumors of the ovary. Am J Surg Pathol 1997;21:583–9.

63. Santonja C, Varona C, Burgos FJ, Nistal M. Leydig cell tumor of testis with adipose metaplasia. Appl Pathol 1989;7:201–4.

63a. Sugimura J, Suzuki Y, Tamura G, Funaki H, Fujioka T, Satodate R. Metachronous development of malignant Leydig cell tumor. Hum Pathol 1997;28:1318–20.

64. Shapiro CM, Sankovitch A, Yoon WJ. Malignant feminizing Leydig cell tumor. J Surg Oncol 1984;27:73–5.

65. Wilson BE, Netzloff ML. Primary testicular abnormalities causing precocious puberty. Leydig cell tumor, Leydig cell hyperplasia and adrenal rest tumor. Ann Clin Lab Sci 1983;13:315–20.

Granulosa Cell Tumors

66. Chan JK, Chan VS, Mak KL. Congenital juvenile granulosa cell tumour of the testis: report of a case showing extensive degenerative changes. Histopathology 1990;17:75–80.

67. Crump WD. Juvenile granulosa cell (sex cord-stromal) tumor of fetal testis. Urology 1983;129:1057–8.

68. Gaylis FD, August C, Yeldandi A, Nemcek A, Garnett J. Granulosa cell tumor of the adult testis: ultrastructural and ultrasonographic characteristics. J Urol 1989;141:126–7.

68a. Harms D, Kock LR. Testicular juvenile granulosa cell and Sertoli cell tumours: a clinicopathologic study of 29 cases from the Kiel Paediatric Tumor Registry. Virchows Arch 1997;430:301–9.

69. Jimenez-Quintero LP, Ro JY, Zavala-Pompa A, et al. Granulosa cell tumor of the adult testis: a clinicopathologic study of seven cases and a review of the literature. Hum Pathol 1993;24:1120–5.

70. Lawrence WD, Young RH, Scully RE. Juvenile granulosa cell tumor of the infantile testis. A report of 14 cases. Am J Surg Pathol 1985;9:87–94.

71. Manivel JC, Sibley RK, Dehner LP. Complete and incomplete Drash syndrome: a clinicopathologic study of five cases of a dysontogenetic neoplastic complex. Hum Pathol 1987;18:80–9.

72. Matoska J, Ondrus D, Talerman A. Malignant granulosa cell tumor of the testis associated with gynecomastia and long survival. Cancer 1992;69:1769–72.

73. Mostofi FK, Theiss EA, Ashley DJ. Tumors of specialized gonadal stroma in human male subjects. Cancer 1959;12:944–57.

74. Nistal M, Lázaro R, García J, Paniagua R. Testicular granulosa cell tumor of the adult type. Arch Pathol Lab Med 1992;116:284–7.

75. Nistal M, Redondo E, Paniagua R. Juvenile granulosa cell tumor of the testis. Arch Pathol Lab Med 1988; 112:1129–32.

76. Pinto MM. Juvenile granulosa cell tumor of the infant testis: case report with ultrastructural observations. Pediatr Pathol 1985;4:277–89.

77. Raju U, Fine G, Warrier R, Kini R, Weiss L. Congenital testicular juvenile granulosa cell tumor in a neonate with X/XY mosaicism. Am J Surg Pathol 1986;10:577–83.

78. Talerman A. Pure granulosa cell tumor of the testis. Report of a case and review of the literature. Appl Pathol 1985;3:117–22.

79. Uehling DT, Smith JE, Logan R, Hafez GR. Newborn granulosa cell tumor of the testis. J Urol 1987;138:385–6.

80. White JM, McCarthy MP. Testicular gonadal stromal tumors in newborns. Urology 1982;20:121–4.

81. Young RH, Lawrence WD, Scully RE. Juvenile granulosa cell tumor—another neoplasm associated with abnormal chromosomes and ambiguous genitalia. A report of three cases. Am J Surg Pathol 1985;9:737–43.

Tumors in the Fibroma-Thecoma Group

82. Allen PR, King AR, Sage MD, Sorrel VF. A benign gonadal stromal tumor of the testis of spindle fibroblastic type. Pathology 1990;22:227–9.

83. Collins DH, Symington T. Sertoli-cell tumor. Br J Urol 1964;36:52–61.

84. Greco MA, Feiner HD, Theil KS, Muffarrij AA. Testicular stromal tumor with myofilaments: ultrastructural comparison with normal gonadal stroma. Hum Pathol 1984;15:228–43.

85. Jones MA, Young RH, Scully RE. Benign fibromatous tumors of the testis and paratesticular region: a report of 9 cases with a proposed classification of fibromatous tumors and tumor-like lesions. Am J Surg Pathol 1997;7:47–53.

86. Miettinen M, Salo J, Virtanen I. Testicular stromal tumor: ultrastructural, immunohistochemical, and gel electrophoretic evidence of epithelial differentiation. Ultrastruct Pathol 1986;10:515–28.

87. Nistal M, Puras A, Perna C, Guarch R, Paniagua R. Fusocellular gonadal stromal tumour of the testis with epithelial and myoid differentiation. Histopathology 1996;29:259–64.

88. Prat J, Scully RE. Cellular fibromas and fibrosarcomas of the ovary: a comparative clinicopathological analysis of seventeen cases. Cancer 1981;47:2663–70.

88a. Renshaw AA, Gordon M, Corless CL. Immunohistochemistry of unclassified sex cord-stromal tumors of the testis with a predominance of spindle cells. Mod Pathol 1997;10:693–700.

89. Schenkman NS, Moul JW, Nicely ER, Maggio MI, Ho CK. Synchronous bilateral testis tumor: mixed germ cell and theca cell tumors. Urology 1993;42:593–5.

90. Weidner N. Myoid gonadal stromal tumor with epithelial differentiation (? testicular myoepithelioma). Ultrastruct Pathol 1991;15:409–16.

Sex Cord-Stromal Tumors, Unclassified

91. Eble JN, Hull MT, Warfel KA, Donohue JP. Malignant sex cord-stromal tumor of testis. J Urol 1984;131:546–50.

92. Kay R. Prepubertal Testicular Tumor Registry. J Urol 1993;150:671–4.

93. Mostofi FK, Theiss EA, Ashley DJ. Tumors of specialized gonadal stroma in human male patients. Cancer 1959;12:944–57.

93a. Renshaw AA, Gordon M, Corless CL. Immunohistochemistry of unclassified sex cord-stromal tumors of the testis with a predominance of spindle cells. Mod Pathol 1997;10:693–700.

Immunohistochemistry

94. Amin MB, Young RH, Scully RE. Immunohistochemical profile of Sertoli and Leydig cell tumors of the testis [Abstract]. Mod Pathol 1998;11:76A.

94a. Busam KJ, Iversen K, Coplan KA, et al. Immunoreactivity for A103, an antibody to Melan-A (Mart-1), in adrenocortical and other steroid tumors. Am J Surg Pathol 1998;22:57–61.

94b. Gilcrease MZ, Delgado R, Albores-Saavedra J. Testicular Sertoli cell tumor with a heterologous sarcomatous component. Immunohistochemical assessment of Sertoli cell differentiation. Arch Pathol Lab Med 1996;122:907–11.

95. Iczkowski KA, Bostwick DG, Cheville JC. Inhibin is a sensitive and specific marker for testicular sex cord-stromal tumors. Mod Pathol 1998;11:774–9.

96. Kratzer SS, Ulbright TM, Talerman A, et al. Large cell calcifying Sertoli cell tumor of the testis: contrasting features of six malignant and six benign tumors and a review of the literature. Am J Surg Pathol 1997;21:1271–80.

97. McClaren K, Thomson D. Localization of S-100 protein in a Leydig and Sertoli cell tumour of testis. Histopathology 1989;15:649–52.

98. McCluggage WG, Shanks JH, Whiteside C, Maxwell P, Banerjee SS, Biggart JD. Immunohistochemical study of testicular sex cord-stromal tumors, including staining with anti-inhibin antibody. Am J Surg Pathol 1998;22:615–9.

99. Nielsen K, Jacobsen GK. Malignant Sertoli cell tumor of the testis. An immunohistochemical study and a review of the literature. APMIS 1988;96:755–60.

100. Perez-Atayde AR, Joste N, Mulhern H. Juvenile granulosa cell tumor of the infantile testis: evidence of a dual epithelial-smooth muscle differentiation. Am J Surg Pathol 1996;20:72–9.

101. Renshaw AA, Gordon M, Corless CL. Immunohistochemistry of unclassified sex cord-stromal tumors of the testis with a predominance of spindle cells. Mod Pathol 1997;10:693–700.

102. Rishi M, Howard LN, Bratthauer GL, Tavassoli FA. Use of monoclonal antibody against human inhibin as a marker of sex cord-stromal tumors of the ovary. Am J Surg Pathol 1997;21:583–9.

103. Sasano H, Nakashima N, Matsuzaki O, et al. Testicular sex cord-stromal lesions: immunohistochemical analysis of cytokeratin, vimentin and steroidogenic enzymes. Virchows Arch [A] 1992;421:163–9.

104. Ventura T, Discepoli S, Coletti G, et al. Light microscopic, immunohistochemical and ultrastructural study of a case of Sertoli cell tumor of the testis. Tumori 1987;73:649–53.

7

MISCELLANEOUS PRIMARY TUMORS OF THE TESTIS, ADNEXA, AND SPERMATIC CORD
HEMATOPOIETIC TUMORS
SECONDARY TUMORS

MISCELLANEOUS PRIMARY TUMORS OF THE TESTIS, ADNEXA, AND SPERMATIC CORD

Ovarian-Type Epithelial Tumors

General and Clinical Features. Most ovarian-type epithelial tumors that occur in and around the testis resemble serous tumors of borderline malignancy (figs. 7-1, 7-2) (3,8,11,15,16), with fewer serous carcinomas (figs. 7-3, 7-4) (6), and rare cases of other types, including endometrioid adenocarcinoma (figs. 7-5, 7-6) (16), mucinous cystadenoma (7), mucinous cystic tumor of borderline malignancy (personal observations), mucinous cystadenocarcinoma (figs. 7-7, 7-8) (4,9), clear cell adenocarcinoma (16), and Brenner tumor (figs. 7-9, 7-10) (1,2,5,10,13). The number of reported tumors does not exceed 10 in any category other than serous. It is possible that the serous tumors may be more common than the literature suggests, as a critical review of the reported cases of "carcinoma of the rete testis" by Nochomovitz and Orenstein (9a) uncovered nine cystic tumors that closely resembled ovarian serous borderline tumors on both gross and microscopic examination.

Most ovarian-type epithelial tumors occur in adults, who are typically relatively young; the average age in one series of six patients with serous carcinoma was 31 years (6). The symptoms are the usual ones of a testicular mass; there may be an associated hydrocele. One serous carcinoma was associated with elevation of the serum CA-125 level (6). One tumor, which we reviewed and felt represented an endometrioid carcinoma (figs. 7-5, 7-6), arose at the site of the appendix testis in a man treated for many years with estrogen, suggesting its possible role in the genesis of the tumor (8). The mucinous tumors may be associated with prominent gelatinous deposits that distend the tunica vaginalis (fig.

7-8). In one case of mucinous cystadenocarcinoma of the testis a similar tumor involved the contralateral epididymis (9).

Some of these tumors appear to arise by mullerian metaplasia of the peritoneal lining of the tunica vaginalis, and others probably originate from the appendix testis (8) or mullerian remnants in the connective tissue between the testis

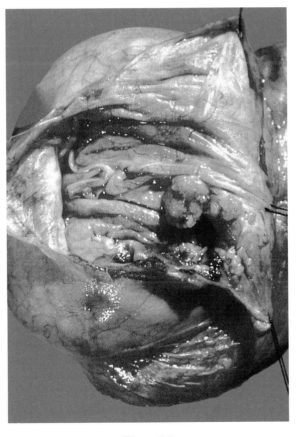

Figure 7-1
SEROUS PAPILLARY CYSTIC TUMOR
OF BORDERLINE MALIGNANCY
Overlying a smooth tunica vaginalis is a unilocular cyst with several small foci of velvety nodular tumor tissue arising from the cyst lining.

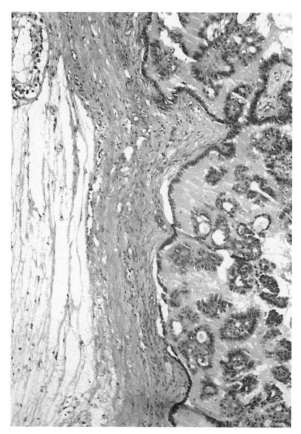

Figure 7-2
SEROUS PAPILLARY CYSTIC TUMOR
OF BORDERLINE MALIGNANCY
An intratesticular cyst is lined by tubal-type epithelium from which arise many papillae that exhibit the characteristic pattern of this tumor.

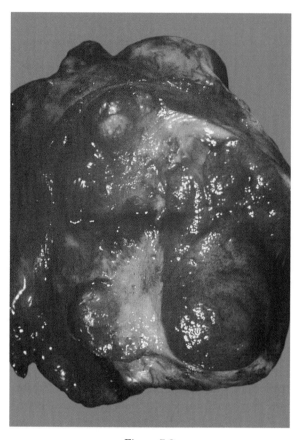

Figure 7-3
SEROUS CARCINOMA OF
PARATESTICULAR REGION
Yellow-white sclerotic tumor tissue lies between the testis and epididymis in the testiculoepididymal groove.

and epididymis or in the spermatic cord (14). An origin from the appendix testis is supported by a recent study of six serous carcinomas (6) which included four tumors centered on the epididymotesticular groove, the location of the appendix testis in the majority of the cases (12). Still others, particularly intratesticular mucinous types, may represent monodermal teratomas, analogous to the presumed germ cell origin of a subset of mucinous cystic tumors of the ovaries. At least some Brenner tumors probably arise from the common Walthard nests of the tunica vaginalis (12). A final possible origin is the ovarian component of an ovotestis or the ovarian streak component of a dysgenetic gonad. This was considered the possible explanation of one tumor, a mucinous cystadenoma, that was associated with adjacent tubal tissue (7). In accord with their vari-

able histogenesis, some of these tumors may be entirely intratesticular, whereas others may be confined to the tunica vaginalis or beyond.

Gross Findings. The gross features of these tumors are variable. The serous tumors of borderline malignancy are typically cystic, with fleshy papillae lining their inner aspects (fig. 7-1). The serous carcinomas are usually firm, gritty masses with indistinct margins (fig. 7-3). The mucinous tumors are prominently cystic; the rare clear cell and endometrioid tumors have no specific features; and the one Brenner tumor we have seen had a solid and cystic sectioned surface (fig. 7-9).

Microscopic Findings. The features of these neoplasms, by definition, are identical to those of their well-known ovarian counterparts and will not be reiterated in detail here (figs. 7-2, 7-4–7-8, 7-10)

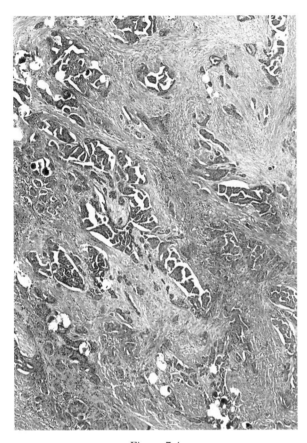

Figure 7-4
SEROUS CARCINOMA OF TESTIS
Small clusters of neoplastic serous cells infiltrate irregularly in a desmoplastic stroma. Note the psammomatous calcification.

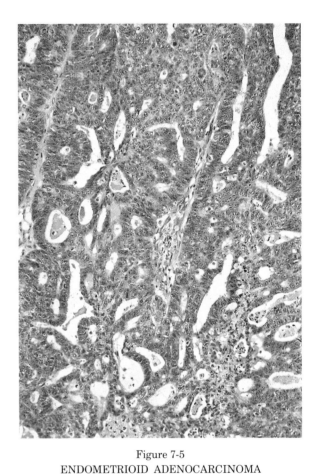

Figure 7-5
ENDOMETRIOID ADENOCARCINOMA
OF PARATESTICULAR REGION
Note the typical glandular pattern of this neoplasm. (Courtesy of Dr. N.M. Kernohan, Aberdeen, UK.) (Same tumor as figure 7-6.)

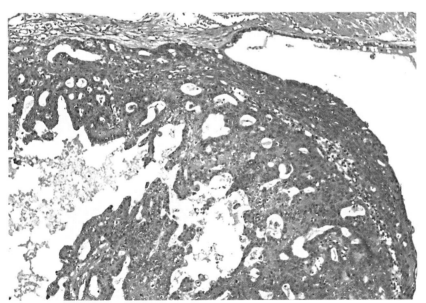

Figure 7-6
ENDOMETRIOID
ADENOCARCINOMA
OF PARATESTICULAR REGION
This tumor projected into a cyst, the lining of which is seen at the top right. The tumor in this region is composed of cells with appreciable eosinophilic cytoplasm, and some of the tumor cells were spindle shaped. (Courtesy of Dr. N.M. Kernohan, Aberdeen, UK.)

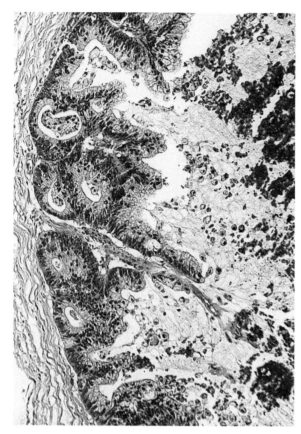

Figure 7-7
MUCINOUS CYSTADENOCARCINOMA
OF TESTIS, LOW GRADE

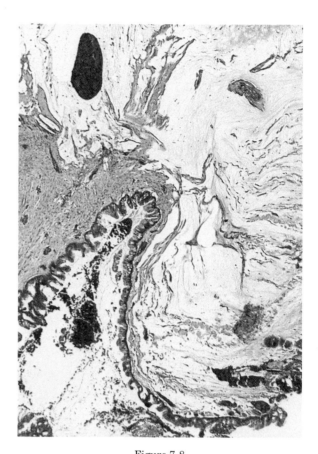

Figure 7-8
MUCINOUS CYSTADENOCARCINOMA OF TESTIS
There is prominent extravasated mucin, and abundant mucoid tissue filled the scrotal sac.

(11a). Occasional serous tumors are predominantly borderline with only small foci of invasion (6,11). One endometrioid carcinoma which we examined had typical areas as well as other foci with spindle cells felt to represent abortive squamous differentiation (fig. 7-6)(8). Potentially, the sex cord–like foci so common in endometrioid carcinoma of the ovary might be encountered in a tumor of the testis or paratestis. One Brenner tumor was associated with an adenomatoid tumor (10), and another had areas of malignant degeneration (squamous cell and transitional cell carcinoma) and paraaortic lymph node metastases (2).

Differential Diagnosis. As the literature review cited above (9a) indicates, serous tumors are particularly apt to be confused with carcinomas of the rete testis, and they may also be misinterpreted as mesotheliomas. The typical location of carcinomas of the rete testis in the hilus and the presence on microscopic examination of tumor nests in the rete are helpful in the differential diagnosis, as is the characteristic papillary budding of serous borderline tumors, which are composed of cells that are less atypical than those of carcinoma of the rete. Although serous borderline tumors of the tunica vaginalis may be grossly indistinguishable from mesotheliomas, the papillae in well-differentiated mesotheliomas are not as broad as those of serous borderline tumors, do not exhibit the same degree of cellular budding and cellular stratification, and are lined by more uniform cuboidal cells containing eosinophilic cytoplasm; psammoma bodies are typically rare, and cilia are absent. Similar general features distinguish mesothelioma from a serous carcinoma. Immunohistochemistry may be helpful in this differential as the serous papillary tumors are frequently positive for Leu M1, TAG 72 (B72.3), and carcinoembryonic antigen (CEA) whereas mesotheliomas

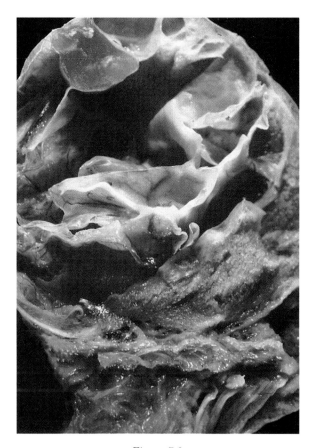

Figure 7-9
BRENNER TUMOR OF TESTIS
Sectioned surface of multiloculated cystic neoplasm that replaced the testis. (Courtesy of Dr. J.R. Srigley, Toronto, Canada.)

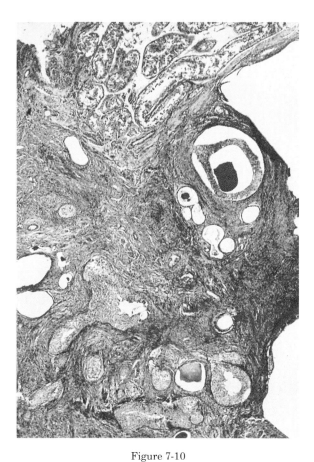

Figure 7-10
BRENNER TUMOR OF TESTIS
Nests of transitional cell epithelium, some with central lumen formation, lie in a fibrous stroma. Note the unremarkable seminiferous tubules at the top.

are negative. Mucinous and endometrioid carcinomas must be distinguished on the basis of both clinical and pathologic findings from metastatic adenocarcinomas. Clear cell carcinoma should be differentiated from the rare clear cell adenocarcinoma of the epididymis (see page 255); the distinction depends on careful gross evaluation and is not always resolvable with certainty.

Prognosis and Treatment. There is not enough information to make any firm conclusions concerning prognosis and therapy other than to note the good prognosis of typical serous borderline tumors and, as expected, the Brenner tumors without atypical features. One serous borderline tumor with focal invasion was associated with abdominal metastases after 7 years (6), indicating that even minimal invasion may be clinically consequential.

Benign Tumors of the Rete Testis

Six benign tumors of the rete testis, designated adenoma, cystadenoma, and adenofibroma, have been reported in patients from 12 to 51 years old who presented with palpable masses (17,21,22). The tumors were solid, cystic (fig. 7-11, left), or both on gross examination. Microscopic examination showed continuity with the rete testis and cystic and papillary patterns, with the cysts and papillae lined by benign-appearing epithelium (fig. 7-11, right). Two tumors were noteworthy because of a prominent component of sertoliform tubules (fig. 7-12) (21). The gross features of these lesions distinguish them from real or apparent hyperplasia of the rete (18,23) (see page 322) and also help distinguish those with Sertoli-like tubules from Sertoli cell tumors, which are centered in the testis proper and not the rete (although they may extend to it).

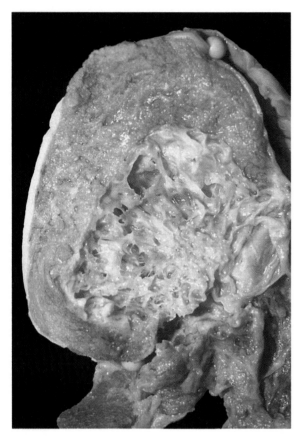
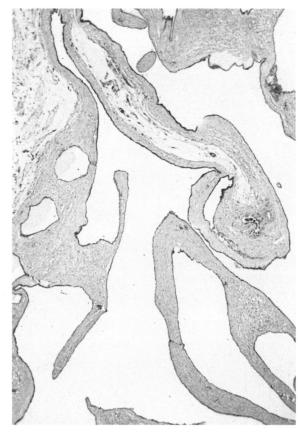

Figure 7-11
CYSTADENOMA OF RETE TESTIS
Left: A multilocular cystic mass involves the rete.
Right: The locules are lined by a single layer of epithelial cells.

Carcinoma of the Rete Testis

General and Clinical Features. Rete carcinomas typically occur in men over 30 years of age who present with scrotal pain and swelling (20, 24,25); approximately half the tumors are associated with a hydrocele, and the occurrence of tumor nodules on the scrotal skin is relatively common. The symptoms are occasionally of long duration. One tumor occurred 10 years after excision of a hydrocele that contained foci of adenomatous hyperplasia of the rete (20a).

As summarized by Nochomovitz and Orenstein (25), five criteria should ideally be met before a tumor is placed in the category of a rete testis carcinoma: 1) absence of histologically similar extratesticular tumor; 2) tumor centered in testicular hilus; 3) morphology incompatible with any other type of testicular or paratesticu-

lar tumor; 4) demonstration of a transition between the unaffected rete testis and the tumor; and 5) a predominantly solid gross appearance. Those authors added the last criterion because most of the cystic "carcinomas of the rete" are more compatible with a serous tumor. However, this criterion should not be applied too rigorously as not all valid rete carcinomas are predominantly solid (fig. 7-13). We believe that criterion 4 can also be ignored, if all other features fit; large tumors might well obliterate preexistent benign structures. Also, a transition was demonstrated in only two thirds of the cases that Nochomovitz and Orenstein accepted. Carcinomas of the rete initially spread locally and then via lymphatics to para-aortic and iliac lymph nodes. Hematogenous spread to many sites, particularly the lungs, may be seen. The tumor has a poor prognosis, with an approximate 40 percent disease-free survival rate (25a).

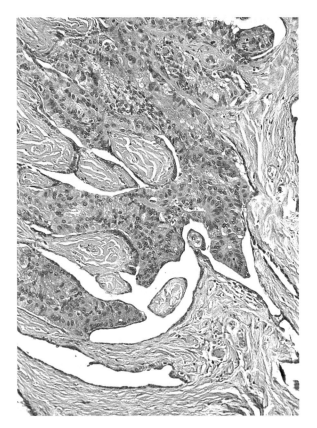 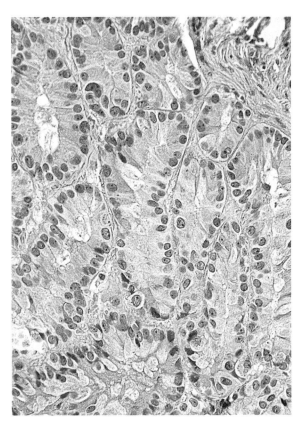

Figure 7-12
SERTOLIFORM CYSTADENOMA OF RETE TESTIS
Left: An epithelial proliferation exhibiting tubular differentiation protrudes into dilated rete channels.
Right: High-power view demonstrates the resemblance of the tubules to those of a Sertoli cell tumor.

Gross Findings. The tumors range from 1 to 10 cm and are typically solid, firm, and rubbery but may have a minor cystic component and, rarely, are predominantly cystic (fig. 7-13). The tumor tissue is usually white. In addition to the dominant mass, smaller tumor nodules may be present on the tunica albuginea, and, in 30 percent of the cases, there is gross involvement of the spermatic cord.

Microscopic Findings. Microscopic examination reveals tubular, papillary, and solid patterns. Low-power magnification often shows large, cellular nodules and smaller, irregular clumps. The tubules are typically elongated, compressed, and slit-like (fig. 7-14). The papillae, which are present in three quarters of the cases, may project into cysts, and may be small or large with fibrous or hyalinized cores (fig. 7-15). In some cases they resemble the chordae retis of the non-neoplastic rete testis (fig. 7-15). Varying

amounts of necrosis may be present. The residual rete may be cystically dilated and contain intraluminal nests of tumor. There may be solid areas with a nonspecific appearance and focal tubular differentiation. Infrequently, a sertoliform appearance may occur (26a). Occasional tumors have a cellular spindle cell component that results in a biphasic pattern (19,26). The stroma is often prominent and may be extensively hyalinized. The neoplastic cells are typically small and cuboidal with scanty cytoplasm; nuclear stratification and at least moderate nuclear pleomorphism and mitotic activity are usually present. Spread into the parenchyma may be conspicuous (25b).

Differential Diagnosis. Metastatic adenocarcinomas from various sites may simulate adenocarcinoma of the rete and, as noted under the diagnostic criteria, an extratesticular primary must be excluded before the latter is diagnosed.

241

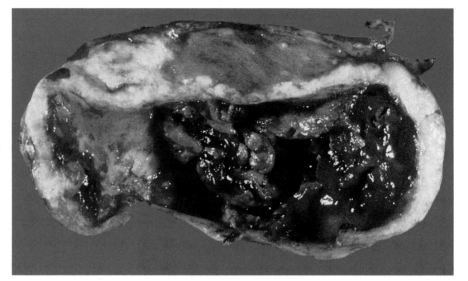

Figure 7-13
CARCINOMA
OF RETE TESTIS
Abundant hemorrhagic tumor fills most of this cystic neoplasm. (Courtesy of J.Y. Ro, Houston, TX.)

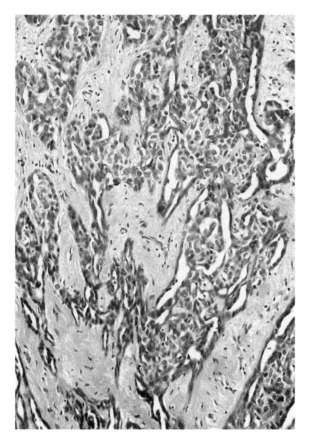

Figure 7-14
ADENOCARCINOMA OF RETE TESTIS
Note the typical slit-like glandular pattern.

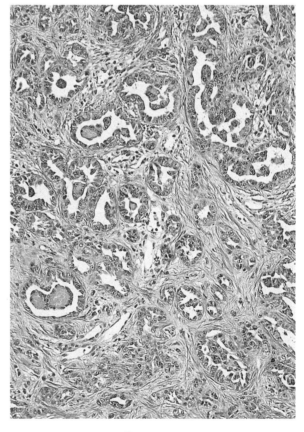

Figure 7-15
ADENOCARCINOMA OF RETE TESTIS
This metastatic focus of tumor shows distinctive papillae with hyalinized cores.

Carcinoma of the lung and prostate are the two that may be most problematic; immunostains for prostate specific antigen and prostatic acid phosphatase are helpful with regard to the second consideration. Rete adenocarcinomas must be distinguished from serous tumors of the testis (see page 235). Mesotheliomas may also simulate rete carcinomas because, like the latter, they may have elongated, slit-like tubules. The distribution of mesothelioma and the presence of other distinctive patterns, however, should help in the differential diagnosis. Histochemical and immunostains assist with this differential diagnosis, since mesotheliomas are almost always negative for neutral mucins, CEA, Leu-M1, and TAG 72 (B72.3), and some rete adenocarcinomas stain for one or more of these (25,25a). A new, relatively specific mesothelioma marker, calretinin, may also prove helpful, but we are not aware that it has been studied in rete carcinoma (19a). The presence of long microvilli on ultrastructural examination is considered diagnostic of mesothelioma in this context (25,25a). In some atrophic testes a relatively prominent and seemingly hyperplastic rete may result in an erroneous suspicion of adenoma or carcinoma. Rarely, true hyperplasia of the rete testis occurs, but this is usually a consequence of invasion of the rete by some other tumor and cytologic features of malignancy are lacking in the rete epithelium in such cases (see page 322).

Adenomatoid Tumor

General and Clinical Features. This tumor is of mesothelial origin and represents the most common benign neoplasm of the testicular adnexa, accounting for about 60 percent of the cases. It may occur at essentially any age but is rare in children (28). Although it usually is located in the epididymis, often at the lower pole, it may also arise in or beneath the tunica albuginea and extend into the testicular parenchyma (35,38), or rarely, arise in the spermatic cord (33). Despite the infiltrative borders of some tumors, the clinical course is invariably benign (27–41).

Gross Findings. The adenomatoid tumor is almost always unilateral and solitary, and rarely exceeds 5 cm in diameter (figs. 7-16, 7-17). Although typically round or oval and well demarcated (fig. 7-16), it may be plaque-like (fig. 7-17) and have ill-defined margins. It is composed of

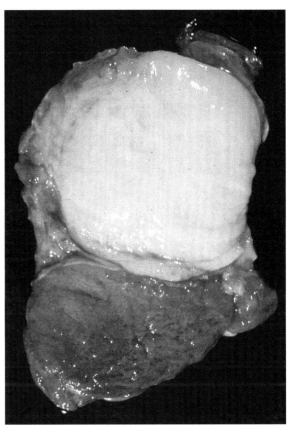

Figure 7-16
ADENOMATOID TUMOR
The epididymis is replaced by a large, cream colored, bulging mass. (Fig. 8.1 from Young RH, Scully RE. Testicular tumors. Chicago: ASCP Press, 1990:169.)

solid, white, tan to gray-white, glistening tissue (figs. 7-16, 7-17); when it involves the testis prominently, it may resemble a seminoma.

Microscopic Findings. The cardinal features are small to cystic, round, oval, or slit-like tubules; small cords and clusters of cells; and individual cells, often containing large intracytoplasmic vacuoles (figs. 7-18, 7-19). The neoplastic cells lining the tubules vary from flat to columnar and contain moderate to large amounts of dense eosinophilic or vacuolated cytoplasm. When arranged as cords or nests, the cytoplasm is typically abundant and eosinophilic and the characteristic vacuoles may be inconspicuous, thereby imparting a more cellular appearance to the tumor (fig. 7-20). The stroma, which is often prominent (figs. 7-21, 7-22), is usually fibrous and sometimes hyalinized (fig. 7-21); it may contain smooth muscle (fig. 7-22),

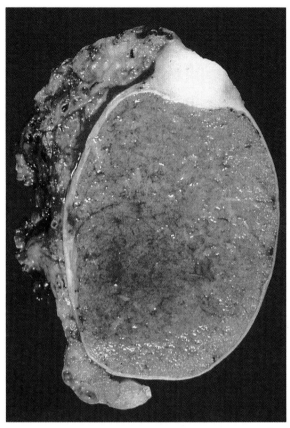

Figure 7-17
ADENOMATOID TUMOR
A cap-like grayish white tumor involves and expands the tunica albuginea. (Courtesy of Dr. F.B. Askin, Baltimore, MD.)

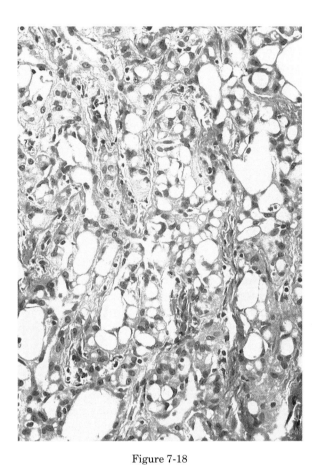

Figure 7-18
ADENOMATOID TUMOR
The neoplasm is made up of gland-like structures, tubules, and vacuoles in a fibrous stroma.

Figure 7-19
ADENOMATOID TUMOR
The tubules in this neoplasm are focally cystic.

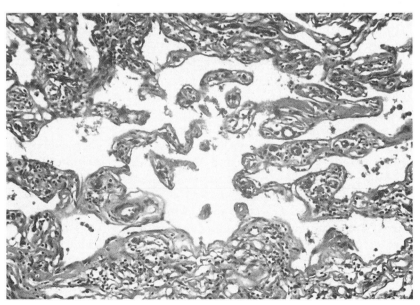

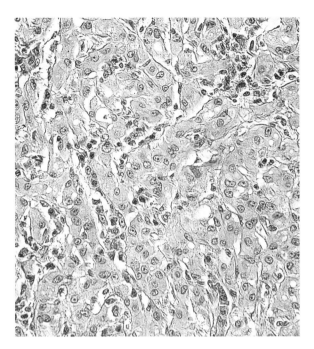

Figure 7-20
ADENOMATOID TUMOR
There is a solid proliferation of cells with appreciable eosinophilic cytoplasm and lack of the characteristic conspicuous vacuoles.

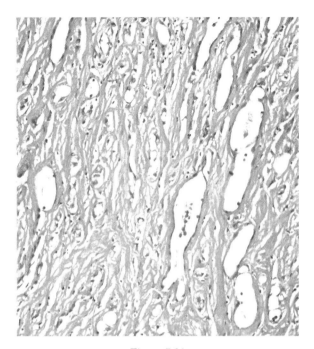

Figure 7-21
ADENOMATOID TUMOR
There is prominent stromal hyalinization.

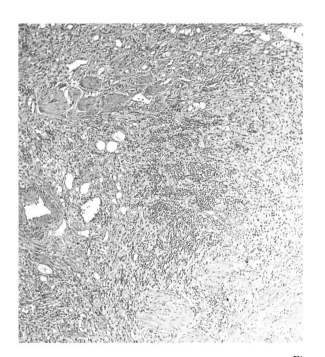

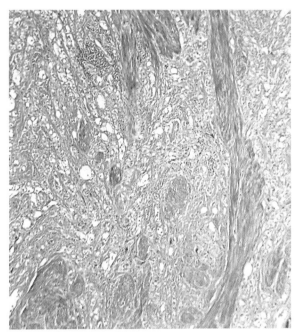

Figure 7-22
ADENOMATOID TUMOR
Left: This low-power illustration shows a focally prominent lymphoid infiltrate and scattered bundles of smooth muscle.
Right: A Masson trichrome stain shows the stroma to contain both smooth muscle and collagen.

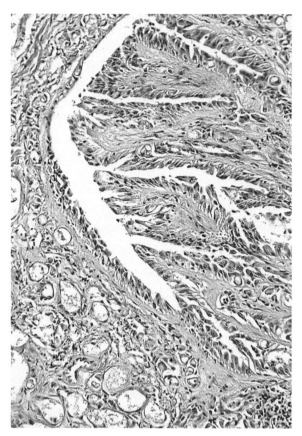

Figure 7-23
ADENOMATOID TUMOR
This unusual example has focal papillae, with areas of typical appearance (bottom) elsewhere.

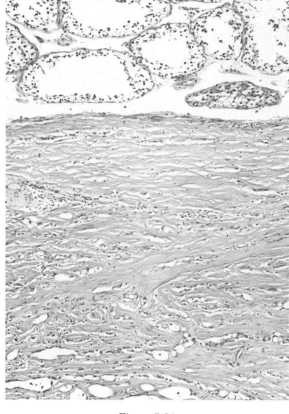

Figure 7-24
ADENOMATOID TUMOR
There is a sharp interface with the adjacent seminiferous tubules.

which rarely predominates, and lymphoid aggregates may be prominent (fig. 7-22). Focal papillae are rare (fig. 7-23). One unusual tumor had a cellular mesenchymal component with atypical cytologic features (28). The interface with adjacent testicular tissue may be sharp (fig. 7-24) or irregular (fig. 7-25).

Differential Diagnosis. The plethora of histologic patterns of adenomatoid tumors may raise diverse considerations in differential diagnosis, ranging from sex cord tumors (see chapter 6), to vascular tumors, to signet-ring cell tumors, to benign mesenchymal neoplasms (for stroma-predominant cases), to malignant mesothelioma, and even other very rare considerations. Entirely removed adenomatoid tumors are only occasionally the source of diagnostic problems because of their typically innocuous gross appearance and awareness of their common occurrence in this

region. If an adenomatoid tumor is only biopsied, usually in the frozen section setting, initial confusion with malignant mesothelioma may occur and the gross features of the tumor should be ascertained. It is helpful that malignant mesotheliomas are often large and typically diffuse in contrast to adenomatoid tumors. The biphasic pattern of some mesotheliomas is incompatible with an adenomatoid tumor, and the atypia and diffuse papillae of many mesotheliomas exceeds that of an adenomatoid tumor. The vacuolated cells and gland-like differentiation of the adenomatoid tumor may raise the question of a yolk sac tumor, but the cells do not have the primitive nuclear features or other patterns of the latter; in rare cases where doubt persists immunohistochemical positivity of the yolk sac tumor for alpha-fetoprotein is helpful. Also, yolk sac tumor is rarely primary in the paratestis, although we

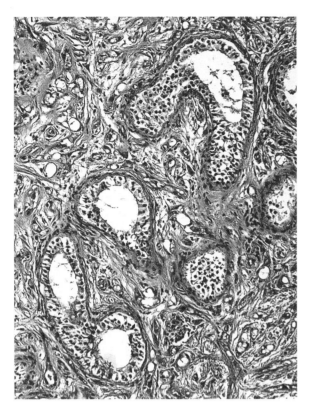

Figure 7-25
ADENOMATOID TUMOR
This tumor infiltrated irregularly between the seminiferous tubules.

have seen one such case. The vacuoles and gland-like differentiation may also simulate a metastatic adenocarcinoma, particularly signet-ring cell adenocarcinoma. Appreciation of the overall pattern of the tumor is almost invariably helpful in this regard, and the quiescent appearance of the stroma in an adenomatoid tumor contrasts with the desmoplasia often seen in the stroma of a metastatic signet-ring cell carcinoma. Also adenomatoid tumors are only weakly reactive in luminal spaces for neutral mucins and in only a minority of cases (40), whereas signet-ring carcinomas are frequently strongly positive for them.

The adenomatoid tumor should be distinguished from the rare examples of histiocytoid (epithelioid) hemangioma that involve the testis (see page 260). It is probable that some of the reported cases of "adenomatoid tumor" that exhibited immunohistochemical staining for vascular markers are examples of this neoplasm. Distinction between the two may be difficult on routine

microscopic examination, but the cells lining the spaces in a histiocytoid hemangioma typically are plumper than in adenomatoid tumor, and their nuclei frequently have a very irregular, cleaved contour. Some histiocytoid hemangiomas are associated with a prominent infiltrate of eosinophils. Finally, in some of the vascular tumors, one can appreciate that the lesional spaces are clearly vessel lumens filled with blood, unlike spaces in the adenomatoid tumor. In a problematic case immunohistochemical staining for vascular markers resolves the dilemma.

Appreciation of the primarily paratesticular location of the adenomatoid tumor is particularly important in cases that simulate primary tumors of the testicular parenchyma because of their prominently solid, cellular growth with inconspicuous vacuoles. If such a tumor is thought "testicular" rather than paratesticular, problems may ensue. Furthermore, some adenomatoid tumors can involve the testicular parenchyma to an appreciable degree and it may not be obvious whether the tumor actually arose in the testis or paratestis. The two primary testicular tumors that are occasionally simulated because of a diffuse growth of cells with eosinophilic cytoplasm are the Leydig cell tumor and Sertoli cell tumor (see chapter 6). Careful scrutiny of well-sampled adenomatoid tumors always shows at least a few typical vacuoles. Prominent lipofuscin favors Leydig cell tumor over adenomatoid tumor, as does foamy cytoplasm; Reinke crystals are pathognomonic. Focal sertoliform tubules and, rarely, intratubular growth favor Sertoli cell tumor. The strong and diffuse cytokeratin reactivity in adenomatoid tumors contrasts with its usual absence in Leydig cell tumors. We expect that inhibin would prove useful in this differential diagnosis since it is positive in most Leydig cell tumors and also is frequently positive in Sertoli cell tumors; we are not aware, however, that it has been studied in adenomatoid tumors.

Malignant Mesothelioma

General and Clinical Features. Although typically tumors of middle-aged to elderly men (mean age, 53.5 years), 20 percent of the approximately 66 reported cases occurred in patients in the first three decades, with at least two patients in the first decade (42,43,46–51).

247

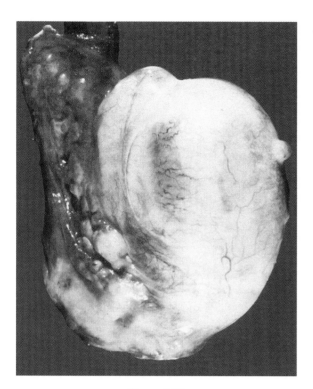

Figure 7-26
MALIGNANT MESOTHELIOMA

The tunica vaginalis is diffusely thickened by white tumor tissue which extends irregularly into the adjacent epididymis and surrounding soft tissue. (Fig. 14-18 from Ro JY, Grignon DJ, Amin MB, Ayala A. Atlas of surgical pathology of the male reproductive tract. Philadelphia: W.B. Saunders, 1997:177.)

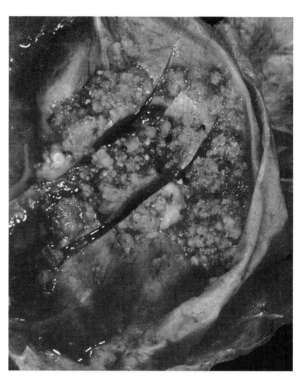

Figure 7-27
MALIGNANT MESOTHELIOMA

The tunica vaginalis is studded by focally confluent papillary tumor tissue. (Fig. 8.7 from Young RH, Scully RE. Testicular tumors. Chicago: ASCP Press, 1990:172.)

Malignant mesotheliomas of the tunica vaginalis are often associated with a hydrocele, which may recur repeatedly after tapping; in several patients with recurrent hydrocele, the mesothelioma had been overlooked for months, or rarely, even years (46,48). The tumor occasionally presents as an incidental finding in a hernia sac. A mass or ill-defined firmness may be palpated, but the diagnosis of a neoplasm is often not apparent until the time of exploration. A history of asbestos exposure is present in 40 percent of the patients in whom information on exposure, or lack thereof, is available (47).

Gross Findings. Gross examination typically reveals tumor coating the tunica vaginalis (fig. 7-26) or multiple nodules studding it (fig. 7-27), but an associated hydrocele and reactive changes may result in gross features that are inconclusive for a neoplasm. Tumor may infiltrate into the adjacent soft tissues of the spermatic cord, epididymis, or testis (fig. 7-26).

Microscopic Findings. Microscopic examination reveals patterns similar to those encountered in malignant mesotheliomas of the pleura and peritoneal cavity (figs. 7-28–7-37). Approximately 75 percent of the tumors are epithelial and 25 percent biphasic (fig. 7-32) (47). The epithelial tumors are typically papillary (figs. 7-28, 7-29) or tubulopapillary (fig. 7-30). Occasionally they resemble so-called well-differentiated papillary mesothelioma of the female peritoneum (44,45). Although often predominantly exophytic and noninvasive, at least focal infiltration of the wall of a hydrocele sac or the tunica occurs in most cases. The papillae often have thick fibrovascular cores which are occasionally hyalinized. The infiltrating tubules vary from large and oval to small and round or slit-like (fig. 7-31). Rare tumors contain occasional psammoma bodies. When the tumor involves the testis proper, it usually effaces tubules but may infiltrate between them (fig. 7-35) and, rarely, exhibits a striking intratubular pattern of growth (fig. 7-36).

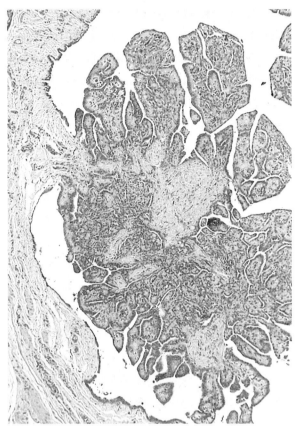

Figure 7-28
MALIGNANT MESOTHELIOMA
A papillary neoplasm arises from the tunica vaginalis.

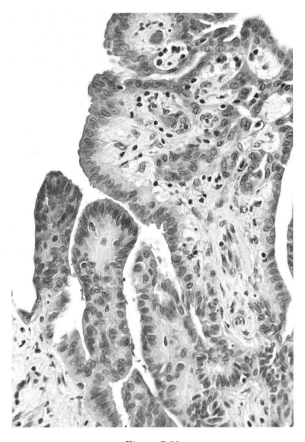

Figure 7-29
MALIGNANT MESOTHELIOMA
Papillae are lined by a single layer of cells with relatively
bland cytologic features.

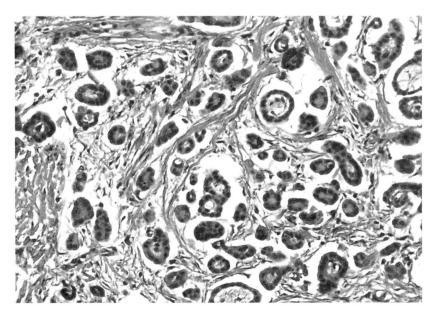

Figure 7-30
MALIGNANT MESOTHELIOMA
Tubulopapillary pattern.

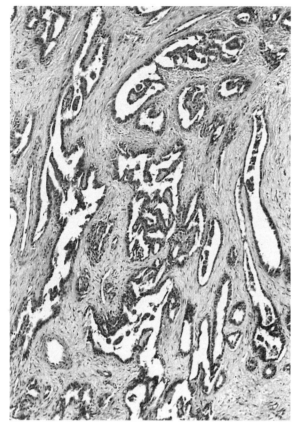

Figure 7-31
MALIGNANT MESOTHELIOMA
This slit-like pattern of glands is reminiscent of a carcinoma of the rete.

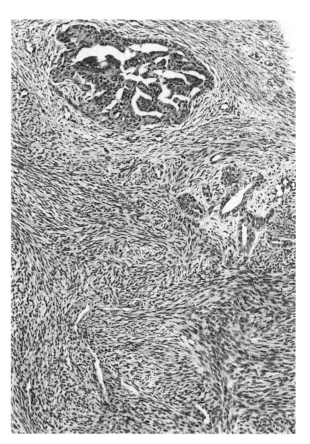

Figure 7-32
MALIGNANT MESOTHELIOMA
Biphasic pattern.

Figure 7-33
MALIGNANT MESOTHELIOMA
Sheet-like growth of cells with abundant eosinophilic cytoplasm.

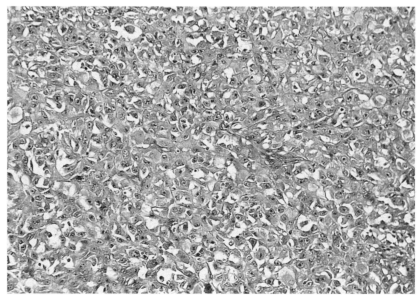

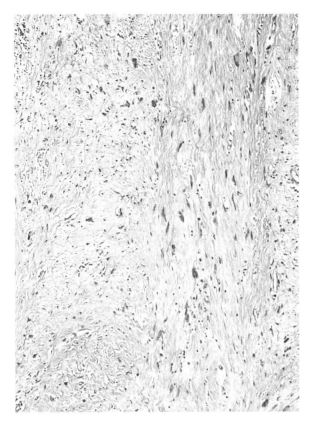

Figure 7-34
MALIGNANT MESOTHELIOMA
Sarcomatoid pattern. Note the cytologic atypia.

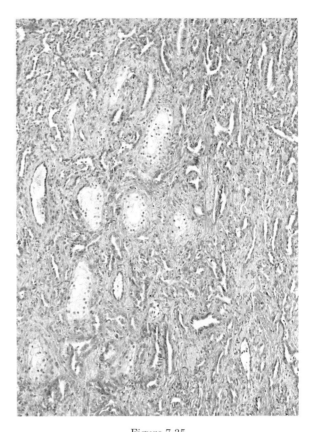

Figure 7-35
MALIGNANT MESOTHELIOMA
Tubular pattern with prominent infiltration into testicular parenchyma.

Involvement of the skin of the scrotum, penis, or suprapubic area may occur, and pagetoid involvement of the skin has been described.

The neoplastic cells are typically cuboidal and relatively uniform (fig. 7-28) with scant to moderate amounts of eosinophilic cytoplasm in well-differentiated tumors, but are highly malignant-appearing in other cases; they lack cilia. Occasionally the cytoplasm is abundant (fig. 7-33). Ultrastructural examination shows long, branching microvilli, cytoplasmic microfilaments, and desmosomes (50). Immunohistochemical staining in one series showed that all eight tumors were strongly positive for cytokeratin (AE1/AE3) in their epithelial component and in the spindle cells of the three biphasic tumors (47). Four of five tumors were at least focally positive for epithelial membrane antigen (EMA), and a similar number were positive for vimentin in both epithelial and spindle cell areas. Seven tumors were negative for CEA, and five of five were negative for TAG 72

(B72.3), Leu M1, and Ber-Ep4 (47). Calretinin is positive in malignant mesothelioma, including those of the tunica vaginalis, and is negative in most adenocarcinomas (45a).

Differential Diagnosis. Malignant mesothelioma must be distinguished from florid mesothelial hyperplasia (52) and from other neoplasms that it may resemble. The clinical presentation is helpful in the distinction from hyperplasia, which is more common in hernia sacs than hydrocele sacs. The presence of a mass with the typical studding of a hydrocele sac is incompatible with the diagnosis of mesothelial hyperplasia which is almost invariably a microscopic finding only. Nonetheless, as noted above, some mesotheliomas may have their gross features masked by inflammatory changes, and in such cases, microscopic findings are discriminatory (see also chapter 8, page 319). On microscopic examination mesothelial hyperplasia does not exhibit the

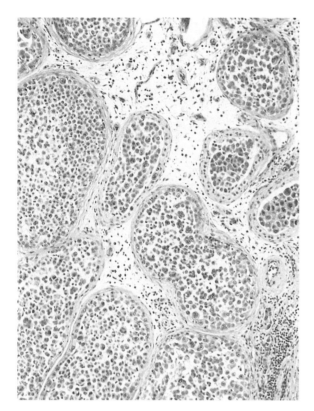

Figure 7-36
MALIGNANT MESOTHELIOMA
Prominent growth within seminiferous tubules.

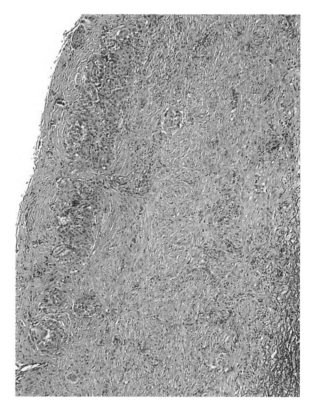

Figure 7-37
MALIGNANT MESOTHELIOMA
This illustration of a tumor within a hydrocele sac specimen shows, at the left, a prominent, almost confluent band-like proliferation of atypical mesothelial cells which focally infiltrate into the subjacent wall. On the basis of this field alone, establishing the diagnosis would be difficult.

complex, arborizing, papillary, fibrous stalks of papillary mesotheliomas. In mesothelial hyperplasia dominated by a tubular pattern, there is usually an intensely inflammatory background, an organized "layered" arrangement of the tubules, and lack of the overt invasion almost always appreciable in mesothelioma. The differential diagnosis with serous tumors is considered on page 238.

The clinical profile of carcinoma of the rete testis overlaps with that of mesothelioma, and, in addition, both tumors may have papillary and tubular patterns. Mesothelioma may also rarely have slit-like tubules (47) similar to those of carcinomas of the rete. Helpful features that distinguish rete carcinoma are a predominant or exclusive location within the rete testis and microscopic evidence of continuity with rete testis epithelium. Special stains may be useful ancillary diagnostic tools. Mesotheliomas produce hyaluronic acid (alcian blue positive, sensitive to hyaluronidase) and are negative for several im-

munohistochemical markers which are typically positive in adenocarcinoma, such as CEA, Leu M1, and TAG 72 (B72.3). Ultrastructural examination may also be helpful as the length/width ratio of microvilli in rete testis tumors is much lower than in mesothelioma (25). Additionally, there is a paucity of perinuclear tonofilaments in rete carcinomas. The grossly infiltrative growth of malignant mesothelioma helps distinguish it from the typically circumscribed adenomatoid tumor (see page 243). Also, the round, oval, or slit-like tubules and characteristic intracytoplasmic vacuoles of adenomatoid tumor are rarely prominent features of malignant mesothelioma.

Pleomorphic sarcomas with abundant eosinophilic cytoplasm, including pleomorphic rhabdomyosarcoma and malignant fibrous histiocytoma, may mimic mesothelioma, but appropriate immunostains can resolve this differential.

Prognosis and Treatment. Of patients with follow-up of over 2 years, 45 percent are dead of disease, 17 percent alive with disease, and 38 percent alive and apparently free of disease (47). Recurrence may occur over 6 years postoperatively. Even well-differentiated papillary tumors may be clinically malignant (47). The extent of disease at presentation has important prognostic implications. Six of 13 (46 percent) patients reported in the literature who had tumor confined to a hydrocele sac and who had at least a 2-year follow-up were disease free (47). In contrast, only 1 of 19 (5 percent) patients with either local invasion of the spermatic cord, skin, or testis or distant metastasis at the time of diagnosis was without disease. Aggressive therapy is required; radical orchiectomy is recommended. In about 15 percent of the cases, involvement of the scrotal skin at presentation has necessitated hemiscrotectomy. Various chemotherapeutic regimens are used to treat metastatic disease, but their efficacy has not been proven to date.

Desmoplastic Small Round Cell Tumor

Clinical Features. Eight examples of this distinctive neoplasm (54) have been described in the paratesticular region (53,55,56). They usually present as scrotal masses in patients of the typical young age (17 to 37 years) of this malignant neoplasm. Follow-up information is limited, but the tumor appears to have the same aggressive behavior it does in the peritoneum.

Gross Findings. The tumors usually range from 2.5 to 5.5 cm. They are typically bosselated or nodular, white to tan, firm masses that usually lack significant necrosis (fig. 7-38). In three of the eight cases, tumor studded the tunics away from the dominant mass, and in four there was extensive involvement of the epididymis.

Microscopic Findings. On microscopic examination the tumors are composed of multiple nodules, each made up of nests and islands of uniform-appearing, small cells that usually grow diffusely within the nests (fig. 7-39). Occasionally, short cords or small tubules are evident. The intervening stroma has a typical desmoplastic appearance, as denoted by the name of this tumor. The tumor cells typically have scant cytoplasm, with round to oval nuclei having finely stippled chromatin and indistinct nucleoli. Some

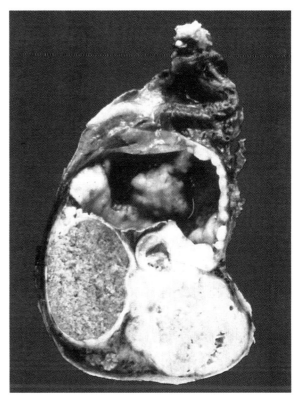

Figure 7-38
DESMOPLASTIC SMALL ROUND CELL TUMOR
The tunica vaginalis is distended and studded by a grayish white mass. (Courtesy of Dr. J. Prat, Barcelona, Spain.)

cells may have appreciable eosinophilic cytoplasm. Mitotic figures are frequent. One reported tumor contained scattered psammoma bodies, and another had focal pseudorosettes. Immunostains show the typical immunophenotype of this neoplasm: keratin, desmin, EMA, vimentin, and neuron-specific enolase (NSE) positivity. HBA-71, the antibody directed against the Ewing's sarcoma and primitive neuroectodermal tumor marker, is negative (53).

Differential Diagnosis. The desmoplastic small round cell tumor must be distinguished mainly from three other "small blue cell" tumors that may be primary, or at least present, in the paratesticular area: embryonal rhabdomyosarcoma, malignant lymphoma, and the retinal anlage tumor. Embryonal rhabdomyosarcoma occurs with rare exceptions at a much younger age (mean age, 6.6 years [see page 265]), and frequently has a myxoid to cellular stroma, unlike the uniformly desmoplastic stroma of this tumor. Occasional

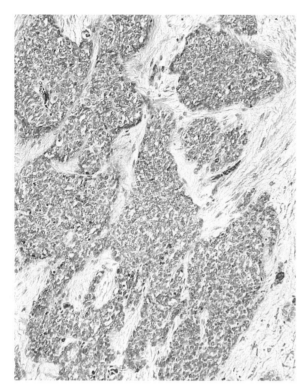

Figure 7-39
DESMOPLASTIC SMALL ROUND CELL TUMOR
Nests of cells with scant cytoplasm lie in a desmoplastic stroma.

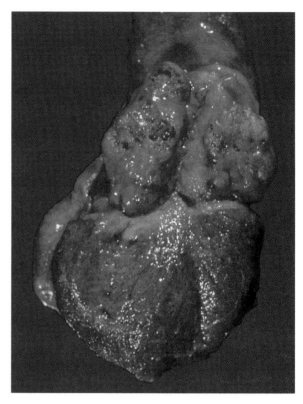

Figure 7-40
PAPILLARY CYSTADENOMA OF EPIDIDYMIS
The tumor is well circumscribed and yellow.

cells with striking eosinophilic cytoplasm or spindled cells point to rhabdomyoblastic differentiation. In conjunction with other features, their presence is helpful in establishing a diagnosis of rhabdomyosarcoma, and the demonstration of cytoplasmic cross striations is pathognomonic. Although cells with eosinophilic cytoplasm may be seen in the desmoplastic tumor, they lack the densely eosinophilic quality of rhabdomyoblasts. Malignant lymphomas may superficially appear similar but lack the characteristic nested pattern and desmoplastic stroma. In problematic cases an appropriate panel of immunohistochemical stains (leukocyte common antigen, cytokeratin, desmin, and NSE) is helpful, especially in limited samples of small round cell tumors of this region. As the morphologic spectrum of the desmoplastic small round cell tumor has expanded since its initial description, it should be borne in mind that it may have "variant" features, such as tubules and rosettes, that may cause initial confusion. The differential with retinal anlage tumor is discussed on page 257.

Papillary Cystadenoma of the Epididymis

Approximately 17 percent of patients with von Hippel-Lindau disease have epididymal papillary cystadenomas, which may be the initial manifestation of the disease (60). These lesions occur over a wide age range and are bilateral in about one third of the cases (61). Sporadic tumors, which are usually unilateral, occur in patients without this syndrome. A recent study demonstrated a somatic mutation in the von Hippel-Lindau gene of a sporadically occurring papillary cystadenoma of the epididymis (57). Rarely cystadenomas of this type are unassociated with the epididymis, and may occur high in the cord (56a).

The tumors vary in diameter up to 5 cm; they may be cystic, solid, or cystic and solid; some are bright yellow (fig. 7-40). Microscopic examination discloses tubules and cysts that often contain an eosinophilic colloid-like secretion; variably prominent papillae lined by cytologically benign

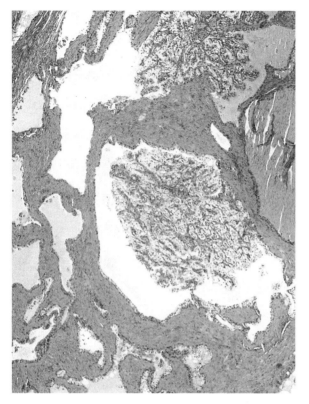

Figure 7-41
PAPILLARY CYSTADENOMA OF EPIDIDYMIS
Papillae project into several cysts.

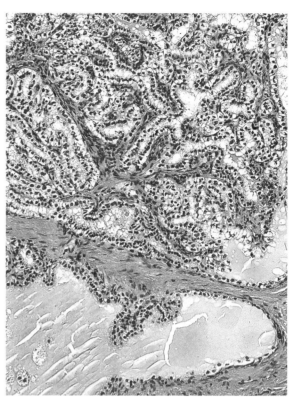

Figure 7-42
PAPILLARY CYSTADENOMA OF EPIDIDYMIS
The clear cytoplasm and bland cytologic features are evident.

columnar cells with clear, glycogen-rich cytoplasm (fig. 7-41) project into the cysts (fig. 7-42).

The features of epididymal papillary cystadenoma are unlike those of any other entity at this site, and, accordingly, there are few realistic considerations in the differential diagnosis. Spermatocele with proliferative epithelium ("mural papilloma") is distinguished from epididymal papillary cystadenoma based on its more focal nature, its more cuboidal or even flattened epithelium, and the association with degenerating spermatozoa (60a). Metastatic renal cell carcinoma generally exhibits a more heterogeneous microscopic appearance, greater cytologic atypia, or a striking sinusoidal vascular pattern.

Carcinoma of the Epididymis

General, Clinical, and Gross Features. Only eight epididymal adenocarcinomas hold up to close scrutiny (58,62). The tumors occurred in adults who had no distinctive clinical features.

Specifically, there was no evidence of von Hippel-Lindau disease in any patient. The gross characteristics were similarly nondiagnostic.

Microscopic Findings. These tumors are usually characterized by tubular (fig. 7-43) or tubulopapillary structures lined by clear cells that at least focally contain glycogen. Rarely, the tumor has the features of a squamous cell carcinoma (61a). The rare epididymal squamous metaplasia (see page 309) may provide the basis for squamous cell carcinoma at this site.

Differential Diagnosis. Adenocarcinoma of the epididymis may be confused primarily with clear cell papillary cystadenoma or metastatic adenocarcinoma. Although there are some shared architectural and cytologic features with the cystadenoma, specifically the tubulocystic aspect and focal clear cells, the obviously invasive glandular pattern, focal necrosis, and cytologic features of adenocarcinoma are differentiating features. As with any adenocarcinoma of the testicular and paratesticular regions, a metastasis should always

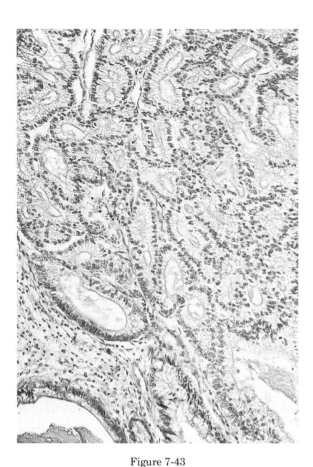

Figure 7-43
ADENOCARCINOMA OF EPIDIDYMIS
There is a confluent growth of glands lined by columnar cells with abundant pale cytoplasm.

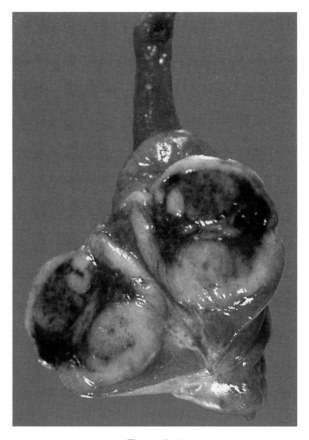

Figure 7-44
RETINAL ANLAGE TUMOR
There is prominent pigmentation of the neoplasm.

be carefully excluded by appropriate microscopic analysis and clinical investigation (see page 285). A similar comment pertains to squamous tumors. Finally, it should be remembered that the epithelium of the normal epididymis often shows a cribriform pattern and occasionally contains atypical cells similar to those seen more commonly in the seminal vesicle (59).

Retinal Anlage Tumor

Clinical Features. This rare tumor, also called *melanotic neuroectodermal tumor, melanotic hamartoma,* and *melanotic progonoma,* may occur in the epididymis (63–67), usually in children 10 months of age or less. Only one tumor of this type proved clinically malignant. It exhibited lymphatic invasion and microscopic foci of tumor were found in inguinal and retroperitoneal lymph nodes at the time of exploration (64).

Gross Findings. Most of the tumors are well circumscribed and round to oval. They are usually 4 cm or less in diameter. The sectioned surface is typically brown or black, at least focally (fig. 7-44), but may be predominantly or even exclusively cream colored (63) or gray (fig. 7-45).

Microscopic Findings. Microscopic examination reveals sheets, nests (figs. 7-46–7-48), cords, and spaces (fig. 7-49) composed of or lined by cells of two types: large columnar to cuboidal cells with vesicular nuclei and prominent nucleoli, often containing melanin pigment in their cytoplasm (fig. 7-47), and a predominant population of smaller cells with round to oval, hyperchromatic nuclei and scanty cytoplasm (fig. 7-48). The latter cells may exhibit considerable mitotic activity, and, when prominent, individual fields may resemble neuroblastoma, but Homer Wright rosettes are absent. The tumor cells, which may

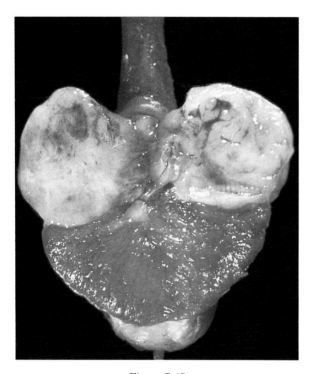

Figure 7-45
RETINAL ANLAGE TUMOR
Much of the sectioned surface of this neoplasm is white with only focal pigmentation.

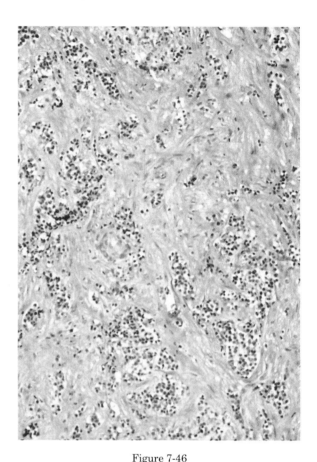

Figure 7-46
RETINAL ANLAGE TUMOR
Nests of cells lie in a fibrous stroma. At this magnification melanin pigmentation is inconspicuous.

infiltrate between the epididymal tubules (fig. 7-50), usually lie in a fibrous, rarely desmoplastic stroma (fig. 7-46). Performance of Masson-Fontana stains may aid in the identification of the melanin pigment which establishes the diagnosis. Both the large and small cells are positive immunohistochemically for NSE, synaptophysin, and HMB-45 (65a,66); S-100 protein may be identified in the large cells (66). There is less frequent, more variable reactivity for glial fibrillary acidic protein, desmin, EMA, and Leu 7. Occasional small cells are cytokeratin and vimentin positive (65a).

Differential Diagnosis. Because of its cellularity, mitotic activity, and small cells, the appearance of retinal anlage tumor may resemble other small cell malignant tumors that occur in this location in children, particularly embryonal rhabdomyosarcoma or undifferentiated sarcoma (63); desmoplastic small round cell tumor may also be a consideration when the two cell types and melanin pigment are inconspicuous. How-

ever, by definition, they must be present to establish the diagnosis of retinal anlage tumor and should be assiduously sought before making a more ominous, and erroneous, diagnosis (63). Differentiation from desmoplastic small round cell tumor may be particularly problematic in the rare case in which the retinal anlage tumor has a desmoplastic stroma. Appropriate immunostains, as discussed above and on page 253, may help in this circumstance. Malignant lymphoma may potentially enter the differential diagnosis but is unlikely to be a problem except perhaps in a biopsy specimen. The paratesticular location of the retinal anlage tumor and the absence of associated teratomatous elements distinguish it from the exceedingly rare melanotic neuroectodermal tumor of the testis (see chapter 4).

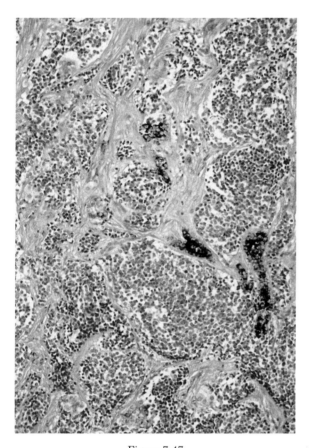

Figure 7-47
RETINAL ANLAGE TUMOR
Nests of nonpigmented cells are separated by stroma in which lie other cells that are overtly pigmented.

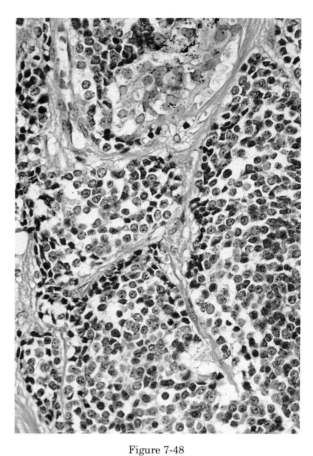

Figure 7-48
RETINAL ANLAGE TUMOR
Most of the cells in the nests are small with scant cytoplasm and resemble the cells of neuroblastoma, but occasional larger cells at the top have scant melanin pigment in their cytoplasm.

Figure 7-49
RETINAL ANLAGE TUMOR
Tubules and cysts are lined by cells with prominent melanin pigmentation.

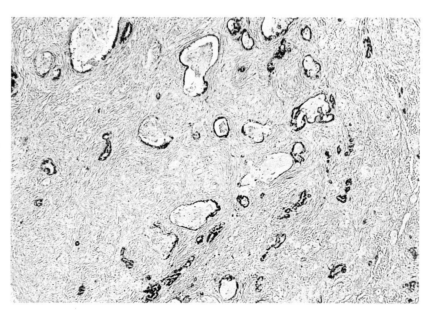

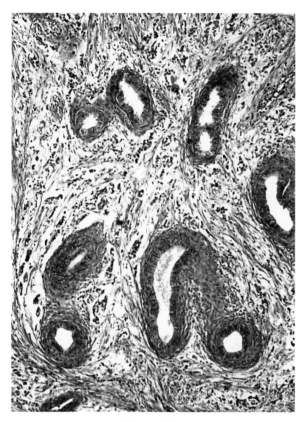

Figure 7-50
RETINAL ANLAGE TUMOR
The tumor infiltrates irregularly between epididymal tubules.

SOFT TISSUE TUMORS

Benign or Locally Aggressive Tumors

Benign soft tissue tumors are very rare in the testis but more common in the spermatic cord and epididymis. Leiomyoma and lipomas are the most common benign tumors in this region (96d), but essentially any soft tissue tumor may be seen in the paratesticular soft tissue or spermatic cord, and rarely in the testis itself (86a,97). In one general hospital series lipomas outnumbered leiomyomas about 4 to 1 (86a). Nonencapsulated accumulations of mature adipose tissue, scrotal lipomatosis, may mimic a lipoma and have been recorded to cause massive enlargement of the scrotum (85a). Occasionally, leiomyomas may have an epithelioid ("leiomyoblastoma") (97b) or plexiform appearance (70a). It remains controversial whether or not most of the lipomas are true neoplasms or examples of lipomatous hy-

Table 7-1

CLASSIFICATION OF BENIGN FIBROMATOUS TUMORS AND TUMOR-LIKE LESIONS OF TESTIS, ADNEXA, AND CORD

Tumors
    Parenchymal fibromas of gonadal stromal origin
    Fibromas of tunica albuginea*
    Paratesticular fibromas of soft tissue type*
    Angiomyofibroblastoma

Tumor-like Lesions
    Fibrous pseudotumor
    Inflammatory pseudotumor**

  *Some cases meet the criteria for "solitary fibrous tumor."
** Includes "proliferative funiculitis."

perplasia, and it may be difficult to distinguish those that develop from the cord from those that originate in the preperitoneal fat and invade the cord secondarily (71a). Rhabdomyomas are distinctly rare (97,97a), as are lipoblastomas in infants (98a). The features of the various soft tissue tumors are as seen elsewhere. Only lesions of particular interest, that cause significant diagnostic difficulty, or are recently described, are reviewed here.

Fibromatous Tumors. Fibromas of the testicular parenchyma are very rare if those of sex cord–stromal type (see chapter 6) are excluded (83,92). A classification of these lesions is presented in Table 7-1. One example we saw replaced almost the whole testis (fig. 7-51) and was extensively hyalinized (83). Another example in the literature simulated a seminoma grossly (70). More common, although still rare, are fibromas of the testicular tunics (fig. 7-52). Six examples are described in men from 22 to 74 years of age (83). Four were circumscribed, whorled, white masses, with variable areas of myxoid change, that arose from the tunica albuginea (fig. 7-52). One of these four was pedunculated (fig. 7-52), and the other three focally extended into the testis. The other two fibromas of the tunics in that series were unattached to the tunica albuginea and were circumscribed, white-tan, paratesticular masses partially covered by the tunica vaginalis. One probable and one possible fibroma of the tunics in the older literature

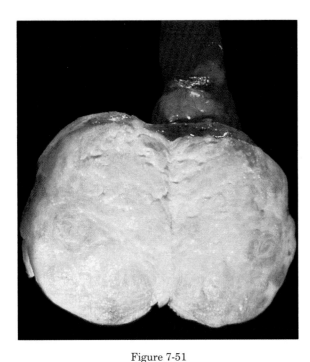

Figure 7-51
FIBROMA OF TESTIS
The testicular parenchyma is replaced by a large white mass that was firm.

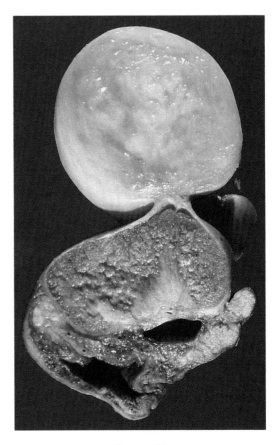

Figure 7-52
FIBROMA OF TUNICA ALBUGINEA
The pedunculated tumor is tethered to the tunica by a small stalk. The underlying testis is uninvolved. (Fig. 8.32 from Young RH, Scully RE. Testicular tumors. Chicago: ASCP Press, 1990:184.)

attained massive size (74) precluding determination of the origin of one (73).

On microscopic examination these neoplasms are typically mildly to moderately cellular, with bland, oval (fig. 7-53), spindle, or stellate cells lying in a myxoid or collagenous matrix (fig. 7-54) that is typically prominently vascular (fig. 7-55). Two of the six tumors were strongly immunoreactive for CD34, similar to the so-called solitary fibrous tumor that has been described at a variety of sites (83).

True fibromas of the paratesticular region may be confused with the reactive fibrous proliferations referred to by a variety of terms such as fibrous pseudotumor (see page 317). However, fibromas lack the association with a hydrocele, trauma, or inflammation that is often present in non-neoplastic proliferations; the latter are usually multinodular or diffuse hypocellular fibroblastic proliferations with abundant, often hyalinized collagen that is frequently calcified and may exhibit prominent inflammation. Fibromas lack the granulation tissue-like pseudosarcomatous cellularity and infiltration of so-called proliferative funiculitis (see page 313).

Vascular Tumors. Most subtypes of benign vascular tumor have been reported in the testis (figs. 7-56–7-61). In their report of histiocytoid hemangioma, Banks and Mills (68) reviewed the literature and found six additional cases that they interpreted as histiocytoid hemangioma, seven examples of cavernous hemangioma, and two of capillary hemangioma. Occasional hemangiomas of the testis are cellular (fig. 7-57) (79) and have an intertubular pattern of growth (fig. 7-57), sometimes causing diagnostic confusion until the vascular nature of the channels is appreciated. They may also be mitotically active (fig. 7-58). One rare case had a multifocal growth pattern (80a). The distinction of histiocytoid hemangioma (figs. 7-59–7-61) from adenomatoid tumor is discussed on page 247 (fig. 7-60). Since some histiocytoid hemangiomas stain for

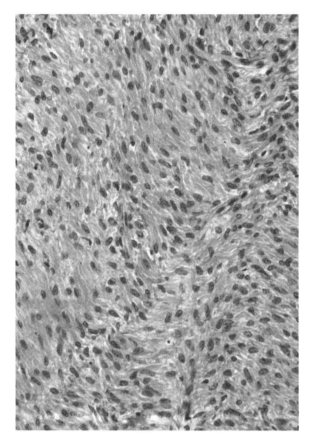

Figure 7-53
FIBROMA OF TUNICA ALBUGINEA
The tumor cells are regular without atypical cytologic features.

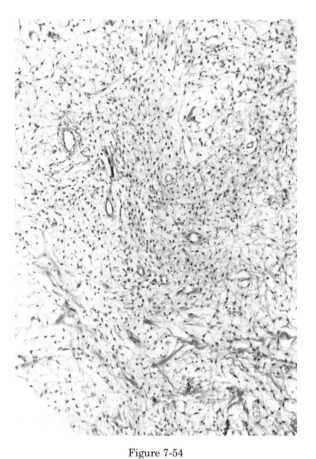

Figure 7-54
FIBROMA OF TUNICA ALBUGINEA
Round to stellate spindle cells lie within an edematous background.

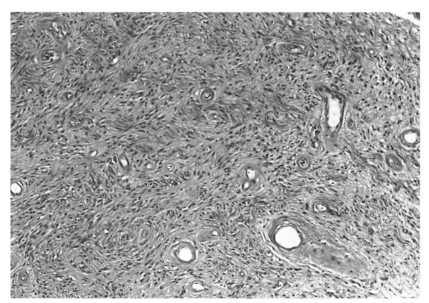

Figure 7-55
FIBROMA OF
TUNICA ALBUGINEA
This tumor is vascular and has features resembling those of the so-called solitary fibrous tumor.

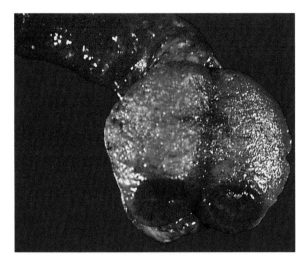

Figure 7-56
HEMANGIOMA OF TESTIS
The lesion is well circumscribed and red.

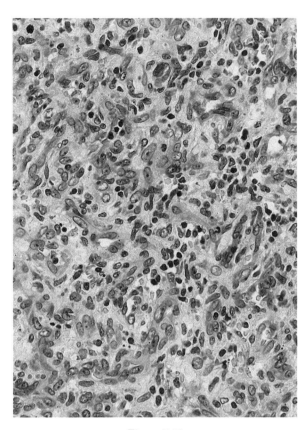

Figure 7-58
HEMANGIOMA OF TESTIS
High-power view of tumor in figure 7-57 showing a cellular neoplasm. A mitotic figure is present in the top left corner.

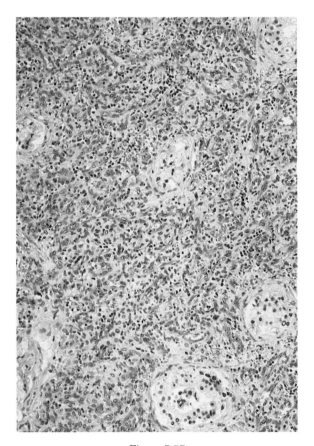

Figure 7-57
HEMANGIOMA OF TESTIS
The lesion infiltrates between the seminiferous tubules.

cytokeratin, such positivity should not be taken as evidence against a vascular tumor, although the intense and diffuse staining in adenomatoid tumors contrasts with the usually more focal reactivity in histiocytoid hemangiomas.

Aggressive Angiomyxoma, Angiomyofibroblastoma, and Calcifying Fibrous Pseudotumor. Examples of each of these three recently described soft tissue lesions have been described in the soft tissues of the scrotal sac and, rarely, within the scrotum proper; only a small number of each entity has been described to date. Aggressive angiomyxomas, like their vulvar counterparts, are characterized grossly by a nonencapsulated myxoid mass that often is large (fig. 7-62) (72,81,98). Microscopic examination shows spindled to stellate cells loosely dispersed in a myxoid stroma (fig. 7-63). The lesional cells have bland cytologic features, and mitotic activity is inconspicuous

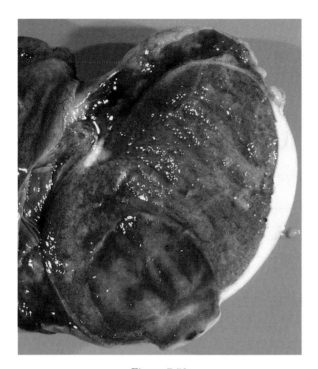

Figure 7-59
HISTIOCYTOID HEMANGIOMA OF TESTIS

Although the tumor is focally hemorrhagic, much of the sectioned surface has a fleshy-tan appearance. (Courtesy of Dr. R. Archibald, San Jose, CA.)

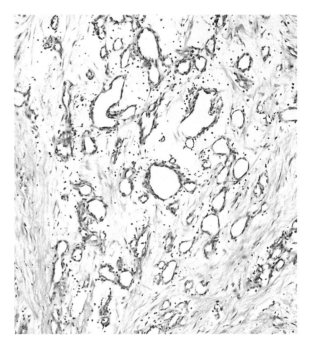

Figure 7-60
HISTIOCYTOID HEMANGIOMA OF TESTIS
Note the resemblance to an adenomatoid tumor.

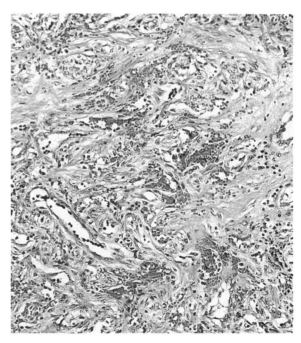

Figure 7-61
HISTIOCYTOID HEMANGIOMA OF TESTIS

Another area from the tumor in figure 7-60 showing abundant red blood cells within many of the lumens, which in this illustration are more characteristic of vascular channels than in the prior figure.

(fig. 7-63). A characteristic feature is the distinct vascular component of the tumor comprising randomly distributed, thin- to thick-walled vessels. Some of the vessel walls may be prominently hyalinized. Estrogen, progesterone, and androgen receptors have been demonstrated in the tumor cells, especially in the stellate cells of the more myxoid areas (96b). These tumors should be distinguished from benign myxoid soft tissue tumors because the aggressive angiomyxoma is infiltrative and has the potential for local recurrence.

Angiomyofibroblastoma occurs most commonly in middle-aged to older men (median age, 57 years) as a scrotal or inguinal mass that clinically is usually felt to represent a hernia (85c). The approximate mean diameter is 7 cm, and the cut surface is typically soft to rubbery and gray-white to yellow-brown (85c). In contrast to aggressive angiomyxoma, it is well circumscribed (fig. 7-64) and may have alternating hypercellular and hypocellular areas in which capillary-sized blood vessels are randomly distributed (fig. 7-65) (91). In some cases, but less commonly in

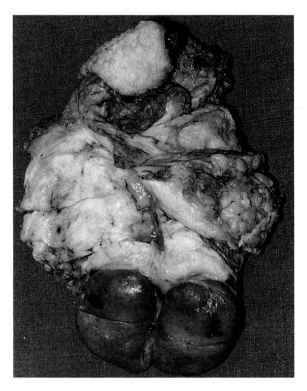

Figure 7-62
AGGRESSIVE ANGIOMYXOMA
An ill-defined mass of myxoid tissue fills the paratesticular region and extends to the scrotal skin (top). Note testis at bottom. (Courtesy of Dr. J.C. Iezzoni, Charlottesville, VA.)

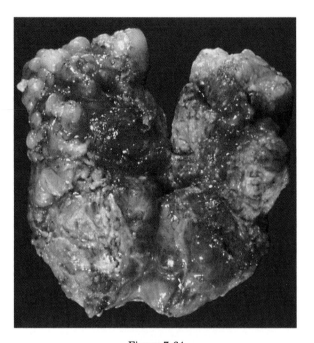

Figure 7-64
ANGIOMYOFIBROBLASTOMA
A lobulated, well-circumscribed, reddish tan mass. (Courtesy of Dr. W. Laskin, Chicago, IL.)

men than in women with vulvar involvement, the stromal cells aggregate around the blood vessels; in contrast to the tumors in women, those in men do not usually form nests or trabecular aggregates. The stroma varies from collagenous to myxoid, and there may be entrapped fat cells (85c). The tumor cells may have a plasmacytoid or epithelioid appearance and some of them may be binucleate or multinucleate. There is minimal nuclear atypia and scant mitotic activity. Immunohistochemical studies are positive for vimentin and may be positive for progesterone and estrogen receptors, CD34, actin, and desmin, but not S-100 protein (85c). These tumors have been invariably benign in the reported cases.

The calcifying fibrous pseudotumor occurs in children in contrast to aggressive angiomyxoma and angiomyofibroblastoma. The two "scrotal" examples measured 2.5 and 3.4 cm (77). Microscopic examination shows hyalinized fibrosclerotic tissue with a variable inflammatory component of lymphocytes and plasma cells and, with very rare exceptions, calcification of either psammomatous or dystrophic type.

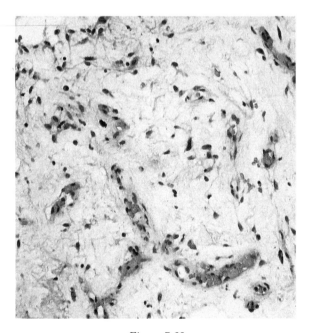

Figure 7-63
AGGRESSIVE ANGIOMYXOMA
Note the delicate blood vessels and myxoid background.

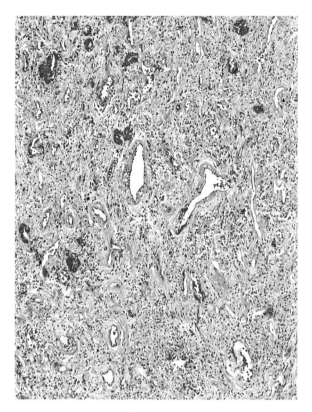

Figure 7-65
ANGIOMYOFIBROBLASTOMA
Note the prominent vascularity and cellular intervening stroma. (Courtesy of Dr. J. Fetsch, Washington, DC.)

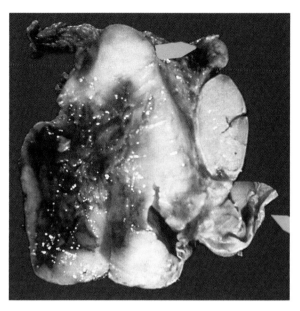

Figure 7-66
PARATESTICULAR EMBRYONAL
RHABDOMYOSARCOMA
Note the extensive hemorrhage and unremarkable testis (right).

Sarcomas

In a review of paratesticular tumors, the 34 sarcomas comprised 14 rhabdomyosarcomas, 9 liposarcomas, 7 leiomyosarcomas, and 4 malignant fibrous histiocytomas (97). The most common sarcoma in adults is liposarcoma (69,82,95) and in children is rhabdomyosarcoma (71,80,86, 87). Rarely rhabdomyosarcomas, or even more exceptionally other sarcomas, may originate in the testis of adults (88,93,94,99,100). Any malignant soft tissue tumor can be seen in the paratesticular tissues, as exemplified by reports of rhabdoid tumor of the spermatic cord (84), but most are rare and the features are as seen elsewhere (89,99,100). Fibromatosis of the cord has also been described (88).

Rhabdomyosarcoma. In a large study of paratesticular rhabdomyosarcomas from the Intergroup Rhabdomyosarcoma Study Group, the mean age of the patients was 6.6 years (86). The tumors ranged from 1 to 18 cm in maximum dimension,

with the majority from 4 to 6 cm. Most are of the embryonal subtype (figs. 7-66–7-71), including a recently described spindle cell variant with a more favorable prognosis (figs. 7-67, 7-69) (86). In the Intergroup study, almost 70 percent of the embryonal rhabdomyosarcomas were "conventional," approximately 27 percent were of the spindle cell subtype, and the small remainder were mixed spindle and non-spindle type (86).

Conventional embryonal rhabdomyosarcomas are typically lobulated, glistening, soft tumors that often show focal hemorrhage and necrosis (fig. 7-66). Spindle cell variants are firm, well demarcated, nonencapsulated, and may have a whorled "leiomyomatous" appearance (fig. 7-67). Typical embryonal rhabdomyosarcomas resemble their soft tissue and head and neck counterparts, and are characterized by primitive oval to elongate cells with uniform, hyperchromatic nuclei, often with myxoid areas (fig. 7-68). The spindle cell type (86) is characterized by elongated fusiform cells sometimes arranged in fascicles (fig. 7-69) with a variably prominent stroma that may be markedly collagenized. Some have a prominent storiform pattern. The cytoplasm in these cases is fibrillar, in contrast

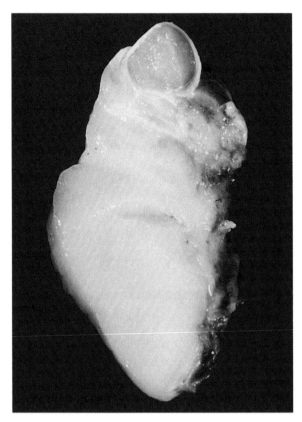

Figure 7-67
PARATESTICULAR EMBRYONAL
RHABDOMYOSARCOMA, SPINDLE CELL TYPE
This tumor, which was relatively firm, focally has a whorled appearance in contrast to the tumor in figure 7-66.

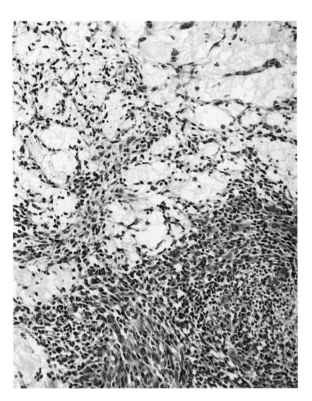

Figure 7-68
PARATESTICULAR EMBRYONAL
RHABDOMYOSARCOMA
Note the variable cellularity of the tumor and, in the cellular areas, the small hyperchromatic cells with scant cytoplasm and larger spindle-shaped cells with appreciable cytoplasm.

to the more dense eosinophilic cytoplasm of typical embryonal rhabdomyosarcoma. Classic areas of typical embryonal neoplasia are almost always found, albeit focally in some cases, at the periphery. Necrosis is infrequent in the spindle cell subtype.

About 6 percent of paratesticular rhabdomyosarcomas of childhood are of the alveolar subtype (86). This tumor has interlacing strands of fibrovascular stroma that create a honeycomb pattern of spaces containing solid or loose clusters of undifferentiated or slightly differentiated tumor cells with eosinophilic cytoplasm. Occasional giant tumor cells are present in some cases, as in other sites. Rarely, pleomorphic rhabdomyosarcomas occur in the paratesticular soft tissues, usually in the elderly (85b).

Although the diagnosis of rhabdomyosarcoma in the paratesticular region can usually be made on the basis of routinely stained sections, immu-

nohistochemical and ultrastructural studies may help in the distinction from other round cell and spindle cell tumors of this region. The neoplastic cells are positive for desmin, myoglobin (fig. 7-70), muscle-specific actin, vimentin, and, in the spindle cell variant, titin. The latter is a large molecular weight skeletal muscle protein that appears at a late stage of myogenesis, particularly in the postmitotic myoblasts and myotubules, and staining for it is consistent with the differentiated nature of the spindle cell subtype. The stellate and round cells of embryonal rhabdomyosarcoma are negative for titin. Antibodies directed against two myogenic regulatory proteins, myogenin and MyoD1, may provide an even more sensitive and specific means of identifying rhabdomyosarcoma (98c). Ultrastructural examination shows thick and thin filaments in the cytoplasm of most tumor cells, mainly as haphazard tangles or filaments but occasionally organized in the form of Z-bands (fig. 7-71).

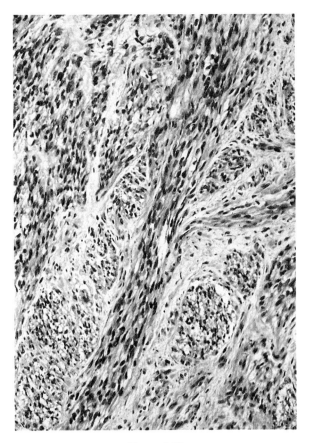

Figure 7-69
PARATESTICULAR EMBRYONAL
RHABDOMYOSARCOMA, SPINDLE CELL TYPE
There is a resemblance to leiomyosarcoma. (Courtesy of Dr.
J.Y. Ro, Houston, TX.)

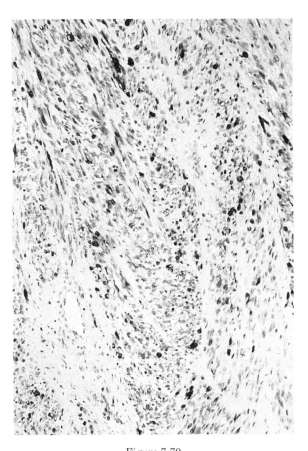

Figure 7-70
PARATESTICULAR EMBRYONAL
RHABDOMYOSARCOMA, SPINDLE CELL TYPE
An immunohistochemical stain for myoglobin is strongly
positive.

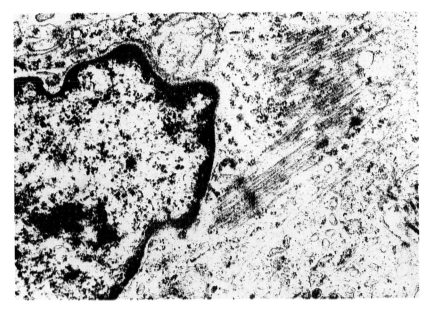

Figure 7-71
PARATESTICULAR EMBRYONAL
RHABDOMYOSARCOMA,
SPINDLE CELL TYPE:
ULTRASTRUCTURAL FEATURES
The cytoplasm contains thick and
thin filaments which occasionally are
oriented and inserted into perpendic-
ular densities (z-bands). (Courtesy of
Dr. J.Y. Ro, Houston, TX.)

The differential diagnosis of embryonal rhabdomyosarcoma of the conventional type includes malignant lymphoma, desmoplastic small round cell tumor (see page 253), and retinal anlage tumor (see page 256). Both malignant lymphoma and embryonal rhabdomyosarcoma have a fairly diffuse growth pattern, however, the presence of occasional cells with intensely eosinophilic cytoplasm is a helpful feature, as are their differing nuclear features and appropriate immunostains, if necessary. The differential diagnosis of the spindle cell variant of embryonal rhabdomyosarcoma includes leiomyosarcoma and fibrosarcoma; a review of paratesticular sarcomas that had been included in the original study of the British Testicular Tumour Panel verified that several cases of spindle cell rhabdomyosarcoma had been classified as either leiomyosarcoma or fibrosarcoma (96c). If pleomorphism is prominent, malignant fibrous histiocytoma is also a consideration. Although most errors regarding subclassification of spindle cell sarcomas, including malignant fibrous histiocytoma, leiomyosarcoma, or fibrosarcoma, are not therapeutically critical, this is not true for rhabdomyosarcoma which has specific treatment. The three former tumors occur in a much older age group than the younger patients with spindle cell embryonal rhabdomyosarcoma.

Leiomyosarcomas generally have a more consistent fascicular arrangement and are positive for smooth muscle actin, in addition to muscle-specific actin and desmin which also stain rhabdomyosarcomas. Spindle cell rhabdomyosarcomas, by definition, have a predominant spindle cell morphology, but there are often foci of conventional embryonal rhabdomyosarcoma. Markers specific for early skeletal muscle differentiation (myogenin, MyoD1) may also assist in the diagnosis.

Meconium periorchitis (see page 319) may surround atrophic skeletal muscle fibers, especially at the periphery, and may be misinterpreted as rhabdomyosarcoma. Unlike rhabdomyosarcoma, meconium periorchitis presents in neonates or infants, lacks cytologic features of malignancy, and has a more variegated appearance, with myxoid zones, lymphocytes, pigmented macrophages, foreign body giant cells, extracellular bile pigment, desquamated keratinocytes, and calcifications (75).

Patients with conventional embryonal rhabdomyosarcoma or the spindle cell subtype are treated with a multimodal regimen including chemotherapy, surgery, and/or radiation. The frequency of nodal metastases is generally higher than with other sarcomas; they occurred in 31 percent of the cases in the Intergroup Study, although in fewer patients with the spindle cell variant (16 percent) (86). The prognosis is relatively favorable, with a 5-year survival rate of approximately 80 percent for patients with conventional embryonal rhabdomyosarcoma and over 95 percent for patients with the spindle cell variant (86). One institution reported a worse outcome in postpubertal patients that was attributable to their presentation with more advanced stage disease (76a).

Liposarcoma. Approximately 65 cases of paratesticular liposarcoma, occurring in a wide age group from 16 to 90 years (mean, 56 years), have been reported (69,82,95,97). Grossly, the tumors are usually lobulated, relatively bulky, yellow masses often resembling a lipoma (fig. 7-72); pleomorphic liposarcomas are grey and white, fleshy and firm (fig. 7-73). Invasion of the testicular parenchyma may rarely occur. Histologically, liposarcomas of the paratesticular region display the spectrum observed elsewhere. The most common subtype is well differentiated, which may be lipoma-like with scattered lipoblasts or of the sclerosing type with prominent bands of fibrous tissue containing atypical cells (fig. 7-74). Myxoid liposarcomas, with their characteristic prominent plexiform vascular network, are the next most common; round cell, inflammatory, pleomorphic, and dedifferentiated liposarcomas may be seen less often.

The differential diagnosis of well-differentiated liposarcoma includes sclerosing lipogranuloma and large lipomas. Both of these lack atypical lipoblasts, and the former may be distinguished because of its association with a histiocytic, including giant cell, or granulomatous reaction to exogenous lipid. Other myxoid lesions of the paratesticular region may mimic a myxoid liposarcoma, including myxoid malignant fibrous histiocytoma, embryonal rhabdomyosarcoma, and aggressive angiomyxoma. Myxoid malignant fibrous histiocytoma lacks lipoblasts or the typical vascular pattern of liposarcoma; embryonal rhabdomyosarcoma has a more variable cellularity comprised of undifferentiated small cells with occasional forms suggesting rhabdomyoblastic

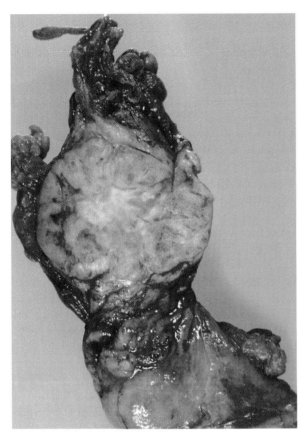

Figure 7-72
LIPOSARCOMA OF SPERMATIC CORD

A large yellow tumor that had the features of a pleomorphic liposarcoma on microscopic examination expands the cord. (Courtesy of Dr. J. Watts, Royal Oak, MI.)

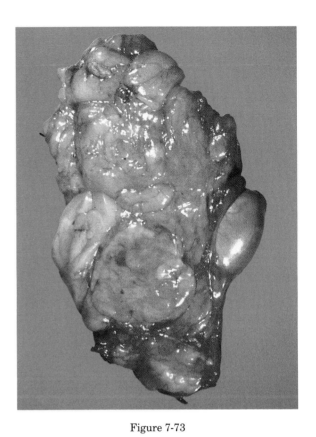

Figure 7-73
WELL-DIFFERENTIATED LIPOSARCOMA
OF SPERMATIC CORD

A well-circumscribed, large, golden yellow mass with a lobulated appearance is grossly suggestive of a fatty tumor. (Fig. 14-36 from Ro JY, Grignon DJ, Amin MB, Ayala A. Atlas of surgical pathology of the male reproductive tract. Philadelphia: W.B. Saunders, 1997:185.)

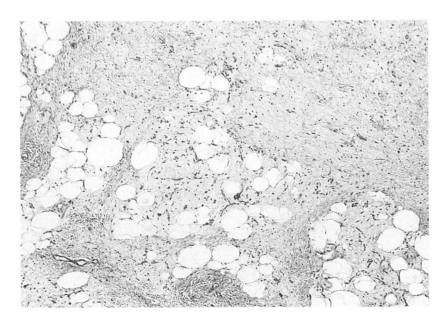

Figure 7-74
SCLEROSING LIPOSARCOMA
OF SPERMATIC CORD
Atypical lipoblasts are visible.

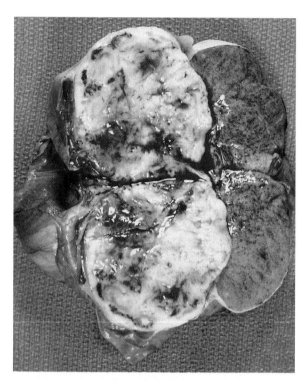

Figure 7-75
PARATESTICULAR LEIOMYOSARCOMA
Note the foci of hemorrhage and necrosis.

differentiation; and aggressive angiomyxoma lacks lipoblasts and, while having a prominent vascular component, lacks the plexiform vascular pattern of myxoid liposarcoma. The differential of inflammatory liposarcoma and inflammatory pseudotumor is discussed on page 316. Sometimes a retroperitoneal or abdominal liposarcoma may grow through the inguinal ring and present as a paratesticular lesion. The distinction of such cases from primary paratesticular liposarcoma depends on clinical and radiographic information concerning the extent of the tumor.

If the lesion is completely excised, with negative surgical margins, liposarcoma of the paratesticular lesion has a relatively favorable prognosis. Local recurrence is seen in less than one fourth of patients and about 10 percent, usually those with high-grade tumors, develop metastases.

Leiomyosarcoma. Leiomyosarcoma in the paratesticular region arises most often from the soft tissues of the spermatic cord, but may also arise from the epididymis (76a). The relative frequency of spermatic cord versus epididymal origin is approximately 5 to 1. Leiomyosarcomas occur in a wide age range, but more than 80 percent are in men over 40 years of age (78,97, 98). One was associated with paraneoplastic hCG production (96a).

Grossly, the tumors are solid, grayish white and may be whorled or, if high grade, hemorrhagic and necrotic (fig. 7-75). Microscopically, the diagnosis is usually relatively straightforward, with fascicles of spindled-shaped cells possessing cigar-shaped nuclei. Nuclear pleomorphism and anaplasia vary in individual cases, and tumors covering the entire spectrum of differentiation from low to high grade may be seen. The tumors immunohistochemically and ultrastructurally show evidence of smooth muscle differentiation.

The chief differential diagnostic consideration is separation of low-grade leiomyosarcoma from leiomyoma. The criteria for malignancy have not been standardized because of the relatively few cases reported, mostly as single case reports. We suggest that in addition to mitotic activity, cellularity, pleomorphism, and necrosis be taken into account and that the threshold for "leiomyosarcoma" be relatively low at this site. In the approximately 100 cases reported in the literature, approximately one third of the patients died of metastatic sarcoma, with or without local recurrence. The differential diagnosis also includes the spindle cell variant of embryonal rhabdomyosarcoma (see page 265).

Other Sarcomas. Approximately 20 cases of malignant fibrous histiocytoma of the spermatic cord have been described since 1972 (76,96,97). The mean age of these patients is 64 years (range, 15 to 81 years). Grossly, the neoplasms have a variegated gray-white appearance with necrosis, hemorrhage, and variable cystic change. The most frequent subtype is pleomorphic malignant fibrous histiocytoma, although tumors with inflammatory and myxoid features also occur. The follow-up information is somewhat sketchy, but approximately one third of patients have adverse outcomes in the form of local recurrence or distant metastasis. Fibrosarcomas of this region are rare. One malignant example of solitary fibrous tumor occurring at this site and with retroperitoneal metastases after 16 months has been documented (98b). The primary tumor in that case had a low mitotic rate and limited atypia but did exhibit necrosis. At least one case of Kaposi's sarcoma of the testis has been reported (85), and we have seen another unpublished example (fig. 7-76). Angiosarcomas of the testis or its adnexa are equally rare (88a).

Differential Diagnosis of Testicular Sarcomas. The diagnosis of a pure sarcoma of any type in the testis should only be made after thorough sampling to exclude an underlying tumor from which the sarcoma may have arisen, such as a teratoma or spermatocytic seminoma. Careful gross examination is required to exclude growth of sarcoma from the paratestis into the testis. Unclassified sex cord–stromal tumors may have a prominent and atypical spindle cell component that may mimic a sarcoma unless thorough sampling permits identification of its more distinctive epithelial features. Reticulum stains may prove useful in the distinction of some sex cord–stromal tumors from sarcomas, since the former may show reticulum fibers surrounding nests of sex cord elements that are not apparent in routinely stained sections.

OTHER RARE PRIMARY TUMORS

Wilms' Tumor. There are a few examples of extrarenal Wilms' tumor in the testicular adnexa or the testicular component of an ovotestis. Two cases occurred in children who were 6 months and 3.5 years of age, and the third in a 21-year-old (103, 105,107). The lesion in the latter patient, a true hermaphrodite, was an incidental microscopic finding on examination of a right-sided ovotestis. Although of microscopic size, it was highly mitotic, and the microscopic features were consistent with Wilms' tumor. The lesion from the 3.5-year-old boy was a 5-cm supratesticular mass that was histologically a characteristic Wilms' tumor. This patient developed a lung metastasis after 1 year but was well 18 months later, having received radiation therapy and chemotherapy. The lesion from the 6-month-old was a 3-cm tumor of the left spermatic cord. This patient was disease-free after 1 year. Despite its rarity, the diagnosis of extrarenal Wilms' tumor should be made with relative ease because of its distinctive features which are different from those of any other tumor in the testis or adnexa. It should also be distinguished from the equally rare examples of apparently benign metanephric hamartoma (see page 336). Occasional cases of Wilms' tumor-like foci in immature teratomas of the testis are distinguished from extrare-

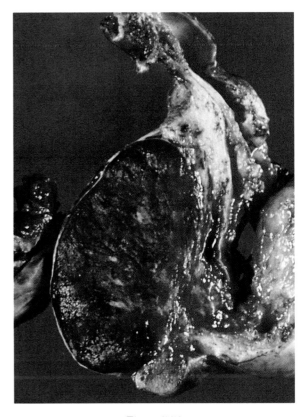

Figure 7-76
KAPOSI'S SARCOMA OF TESTIS
The testis is replaced by a hemorrhagic mass. (Courtesy of Dr. J. Henley, Indianapolis, IN.)

nal Wilms' tumor based on their association with other teratomatous components (see page 152).

Squamous Cell Carcinoma. One primary squamous cell carcinoma of the testis, thought to originate from an epidermoid cyst, was reported in a 64-year-old man (106). Such a lesion should, of course, be distinguished from a metastatic squamous cell carcinoma by appropriate clinical studies, although in this case the origin from the epidermoid cyst was convincing. One paratesticular squamous cell carcinoma arose in a hydrocele sac in an 85-year-old man (101); there was continuity between the invasive carcinoma and highly dysplastic squamous epithelium lining the hydrocele sac. A primary epididymal squamous cell carcinoma has been noted earlier (see page 255).

Paraganglioma. Approximately six paragangliomas of the spermatic cord have been described (102,104). None was associated with convincing evidence of function. They measured up to 10 cm and had the typical pathologic features.

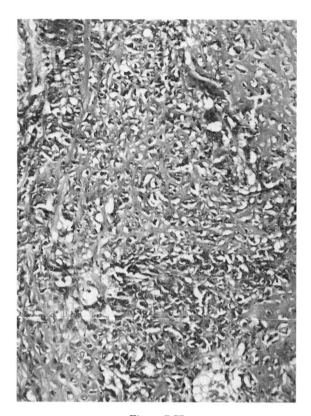

Figure 7-77
CARCINOSARCOMA OF TESTIS
Note the dark blue areas of carcinoma and prominent inter-
vening foci of osteosarcoma with conspicuous osteoid.

Carcinosarcoma. We have seen one unpublished example of carcinosarcoma of the testis in
an 84-year-old man. In this case, islands of poorly
differentiated carcinoma were admixed with areas
of osteosarcoma (fig. 7-77). This tumor did not have
epithelium that was recognizably of mullerian
type, in which instance the tumor would be classified as a mullerian carcinosarcoma, a convincing example of which has not been documented.
It also did not have features diagnostic of a
Sertoli nature although that was not investi-
gated by inhibin staining (see page 229).

**Testicular Tumor of Uncertain Cell Type
Associated with Cushing's Syndrome.** In one
remarkable case, a 3-year-old boy with signs and
symptoms of Cushing's syndrome had a massive
left testicular neoplasm that was considered responsible for the syndrome. The tumor, which
was malignant and caused the death of the patient, could not be classified with certainty but
had features suggestive of adrenal cortical type,

consistent with the clinical findings (102a). Potentially, the tumor may have arisen from adrenal cortical rests.

HEMATOPOIETIC TUMORS

Malignant Lymphoma

General and Clinical Features. Malignant
lymphomas account for about 5 percent of all
testicular neoplasms (108–110,112,114,116,118,
119,121,122,124,126–128,130,131,133,135–138)
and for about 50 percent of those in men over 60
years of age (108–118). Lymphomas are one of a
triad of tumors, along with spermatocytic seminoma and metastatic tumors, that pathologists
should particularly consider, assuming reason-
ably appropriate morphology, in older patients.

The mean age in the largest reported series of
testicular and paratesticular lymphomas was 56
years (114), with only rare cases in children
(130). Lymphoma is the most common bilateral
testicular tumor (fig. 7-78): bilaterality has occurred in up to 38 percent of the cases, although
the overall frequency is 12 to 18 percent. The
bilateral involvement is usually metachronous.
Approximately two thirds of patients have localized disease (Ann Arbor stage I or II), and the
remainder have involvement of lymph nodes or
extranodal sites, most commonly Waldeyer's
ring, the central nervous system, bones, or skin.
The latter are also common sites of relapse. Rare
intrascrotal lymphomas are apparently primary
in the epididymis or cord, or at least present at
those sites (114,127).

Gross Findings. Gross examination discloses
partial or complete replacement of the testis by a
fleshy to firm, often lobulated, cream-colored, tan,
pale yellow, or slightly pink homogeneous mass
(fig. 7-79). The median diameter is approximately 6 cm. There may be focal areas of necrosis. Epididymal involvement by lymphoma is
present on gross inspection in half of the cases
(fig. 7-79). The appearance closely resembles
that of a seminoma, but seminoma involves the
epididymis or spermatic cord much less often.

Microscopic Findings. In some cases low-
power microscopic examination shows predominant intertubular infiltration of tumor cells (fig.
7-80), but in others effacement of the tubules occurs, with the neoplastic cells invading and filling

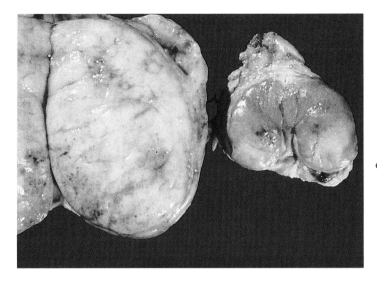

Figure 7-78
MALIGNANT LYMPHOMA
OF TESTIS
Both testes are involved by tumor with
one being much larger than the other.

Figure 7-79
MALIGNANT LYMPHOMA
OF TESTIS
The testis is effaced by creamy white
tissue that extensively involves the epi-
didymis. (Fig. 7.1 from Young RH, Scully
RE. Testicular tumors. Chicago: ASCP
Press, 1990:155.)

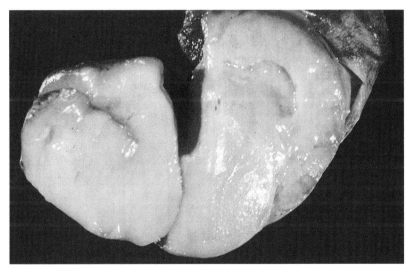

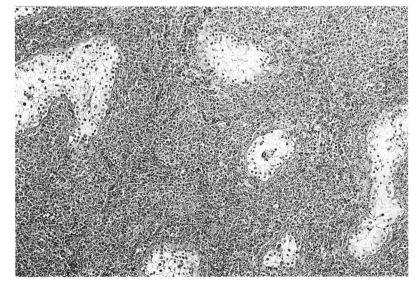

Figure 7-80
MALIGNANT LYMPHOMA
OF TESTIS
There is striking intertubular growth
on low-power examination.

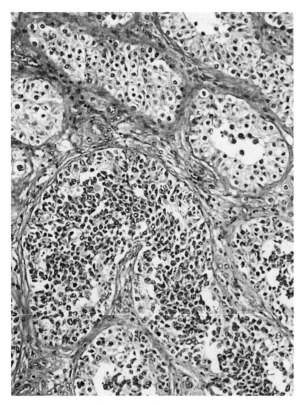

Figure 7-81
MALIGNANT LYMPHOMA
Several seminiferous tubules are filled by lymphoma cells with scant involvement of the intertubular tissue in this area.

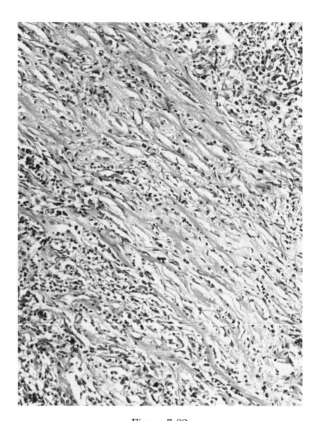

Figure 7-82
MALIGNANT LYMPHOMA
There is extensive sclerosis.

tubules within the tumor in as much as 80 percent of the cases (fig. 7-81). Staining for reticulum fibrils reveals separation of the fibrils in the walls of the tubules that have been invaded by lymphoma cells, in contrast to condensation of the fibrils in the walls of tubules invaded by seminoma cells. In 30 percent of the cases there is sclerosis that may be extensive (fig. 7-82). Testicular lymphoma involves the epididymis in 60 percent of the cases and the spermatic cord in 40 percent (114). Vascular invasion is seen in approximately 60 percent of the cases.

In one large study (114) the most common types of lymphoma were diffuse large cell (79 percent: 43 percent large noncleaved cell, 10 percent large cleaved cell, 3 percent multilobated, 9 percent not otherwise specified, 14 percent immunoblastic) and small noncleaved cell (9 percent) using the Working Formulation classification, and centroblastic (62 percent), immunoblastic (14 percent), and Burkitt's lymphoma (9 percent) using

the Kiel classification. Two cases of anaplastic (Ki-1) lymphoma involving the testis are reported (figs. 7-83–7-86) (109,116), one of them of the neutrophil-rich variant. One unusual type of lymphoma that rarely presents with testicular involvement is the lymphoma of T/natural killer (NK) cell origin that is most common in the midline facial region (nasal type T/NK cell lymphoma). This type of lymphoma, which is more common in Oriental populations, may be composed of small, medium-sized, or large cells and frequently shows angiocentric, angiodestructive growth (110). The nasal type T/NK cell lymphomas express a limited number of T-cell associated antigens as well as the NK cell-associated antigen CD56; nearly all contain Epstein Barr virus genetic material. Hodgkin's disease of the testis is extremely rare.

Nearly all lymphomas that present in the testis are B-cell lymphomas although there are exceptions (109,116,122). In one study, 33 tumors immunophenotyped were of B-cell lineage and 1 was

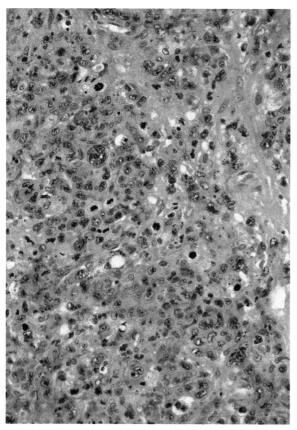

Figure 7-83
ANAPLASTIC LARGE CELL LYMPHOMA
Note the resemblance to a poorly differentiated carcinoma.

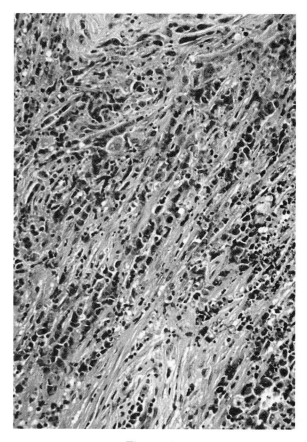

Figure 7-84
ANAPLASTIC LARGE CELL LYMPHOMA
The prominent growth in cords simulates an epithelial neoplasm.

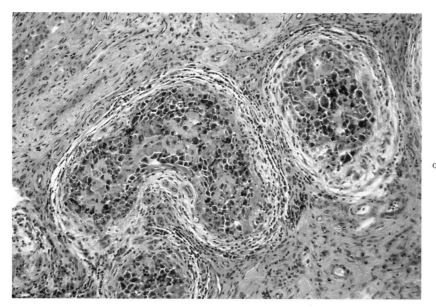

Figure 7-85
ANAPLASTIC LARGE
CELL LYMPHOMA,
INTRATUBULAR GROWTH
The pattern is reminiscent of that of intratubular embryonal carcinoma.

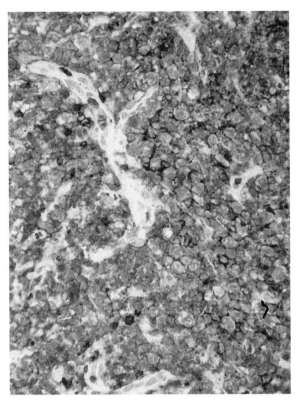

Figure 7-86
ANAPLASTIC LARGE CELL LYMPHOMA
The tumor cells are immunoreactive for CD43.

of T-cell lineage; the T-cell lymphoma was primary in the skin and involved the testis at relapse (114). In another study, however, 3 of 27 lymphomas (11 percent) were of T-cell type (131). The patient population and the lymphomas in this series differed from those of most other series. Children and adolescents were included and a relatively high proportion of the cases were of lymphoblastic type; two of the T-cell lymphomas were lymphoblastic lymphomas (131). A rare, low-grade peripheral T-cell lymphoma of testicular origin has also been reported (117a).

Differential Diagnosis. Testicular lymphomas are often confused with seminoma of the classic or spermatocytic type (128a). In general, lymphomas occur in an older age group than do typical seminomas. The characteristic intertubular pattern of growth of lymphoma is initially suggestive of the diagnosis in many cases but is not specific, and the diagnosis must be further supported by appreciation of the characteristic cyto-

morphologic features of lymphoma. Seminoma cells, unlike most lymphoma cells, have distinct cell membranes, abundant glycogen-rich cytoplasm, and rounded but focally flattened, central nuclei with one or a few prominent nucleoli. Some seminomas show, at their periphery, the prominent intertubular growth that is so typical of lymphoma, and this may, rarely, be a predominant pattern in seminoma. The cells of spermatocytic seminomas are glycogen free, polymorphous, and of three distinct types (see chapter 3). Immunohistochemical staining of lymphomas for leukocyte common antigen and B- and T-cell–associated antigens will help in problem cases.

Viral and granulomatous orchitis may be confused with lymphoma, but the heterogeneous and benign-appearing inflammatory cellular infiltrates of these lesions contrast with the more homogeneous and malignant-appearing infiltrate of lymphoma. Viral orchitis, additionally, has a patchy rather than diffuse distribution.

Distinction of lymphoma from embryonal carcinoma is rarely a problem except in the exceptional case of involvement of the testis by an anaplastic large cell lymphoma. In one case this differential diagnosis was difficult because of a striking presence in the lymphoma of epithelial-like formations which mimicked embryonal carcinoma (116). Further confusion was caused by the prominent intratubular growth of the tumor cells with necrosis, a picture similar to that of intratubular embryonal carcinoma. Absence of epithelial differentiation and intratubular germ cell neoplasia, unclassified, and the presence of markedly irregular, twisted nuclei suggested lymphoma and prompted appropriate immunohistochemical confirmation (positive for CD45, T-cell markers [CD3, CD45RO, CD43], and CD30, and negative for B-cell markers, placental alkaline phosphatase, and cytokeratin).

Prognosis. In a recent large series the actuarial 5-year disease-free survival rate for patients with malignant lymphoma of the testis was 35 percent, with a median of 13 months (114). Three favorable prognostic features were stage I disease, unilateral tumors, and sclerosis. The 5-year survival rate for stage I patients was 60 percent, compared to 17 percent for other stages combined; that for patients with unilateral disease was 40 percent compared to 0 percent for those with bilateral disease. Patients with tumors with sclerosis had a 5-year disease-free survival rate of 72 percent compared to 16 percent for patients whose tumors lacked sclerosis. Surprisingly, patients with right-sided tumors in that series had a better prognosis than those with left-sided tumors (55 versus 26 percent 5-year disease-free survival). In that study there was a better disease-free survival rate for patients with follicular mixed, diffuse mixed, and diffuse large cleaved cell lymphomas (compared to other categories in the Working Formulation) and for centroblastic-centrocytic lymphomas (compared to other categories in the Kiel classification), but the differences did not reach statistical significance.

Multiple Myeloma and Plasmacytoma

Clinical Features. Two percent of patients with multiple myeloma have testicular involvement but usually it is not detected until autopsy. Rarely, the involvement is clinically evident, and in a few cases testicular enlargement preceded recognition of the existence of the disease. Approximately 44 cases of testicular or epididymal plasmacytoma have now been reported in the English language literature (111,117,120,123,125,129, 137a). The patients ranged from 26 to 89 years of age (mean, 55 years). Almost half had a prior history of some form of plasma cell neoplasia. Of these, approximately 50 percent had multiple myeloma, while roughly equal numbers of the remainder had single osseous or extramedullary plasmacytomas, or both. Most have lesions at other sites when a testicular tumor is discovered, and the majority have progressive disease and die of myeloma. Rarely patients may have apparently isolated testicular plasmacytoma, but the follow-up has been short in some of these cases. In others, long-term follow-up has subsequently documented multiple myeloma. In one case, a patient with an epididymal plasmacytoma treated only by orchiectomy was alive at 5 years (118). In one remarkable case, a patient had multiple extramedullary plasmacytomas, including a testicular tumor on one side, followed 8 years later by an epididymal plasmacytoma on the opposite side. At the time of last follow-up, 26 years after initial presentation, he was well and had been disease free for 9 years (117).

Gross Findings. Testicular plasmacytomas are usually firm to soft, tan, golden tan, to gray-

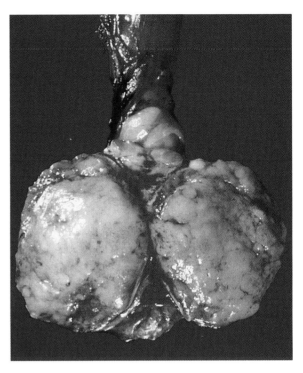

Figure 7-87
PLASMACYTOMA OF TESTIS
The testis is replaced by a creamy white mass.

white neoplasms (fig. 7-87) that measure up to 8 cm in greatest dimension and often replace most of the testicular parenchyma (117). They rarely have the characteristic fleshy white appearance and extratesticular involvement of lymphoma presenting in the testis. They may be extensively hemorrhagic (fig. 7-88).

Microscopic Findings. There is typically a central area of effacement of the underlying testicular tubules and a peripheral zone with intertubular growth of the neoplastic cells (fig. 7-89). Although in most cases a substantial component of the tumor cells consists of plasma cells (fig. 7-90), it is not rare for many of the tumor cells to have features which are deceptive with respect to their plasma cell nature. For example, they often do not have the characteristic cartwheel chromatin of the mature plasma cell but rather have vesicular nuclei with small or large central nucleoli and less chromatin along the nuclear membrane than normal plasma cells. Binucleate and multinucleate cells are often scattered among mononuclear tumor cells. Scattered anaplastic or bizarre cells may be present.

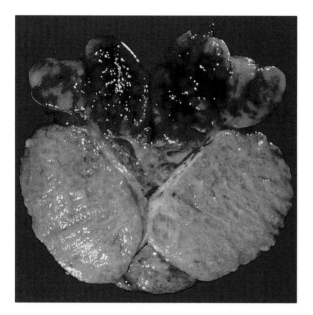

Figure 7-88
PLASMACYTOMA OF EPIDIDYMIS
The tumor is extensively hemorrhagic.

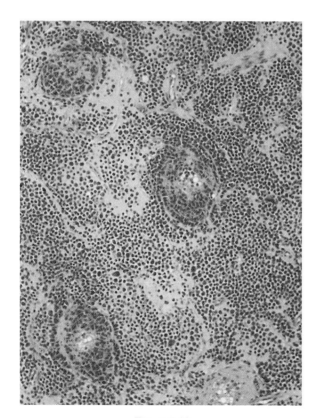

Figure 7-89
PLASMACYTOMA OF TESTIS
There is prominent intertubular growth but in addition
several tubules are invaded by the neoplastic plasma cells.

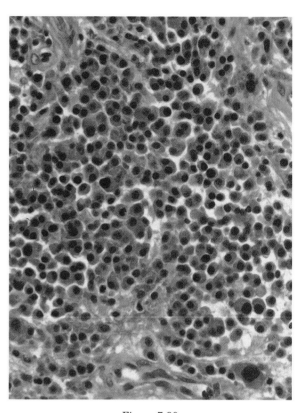

Figure 7-90
PLASMACYTOMA OF TESTIS
The plasmacytoid nature of the tumor cells is evident.

Differential Diagnosis. The most realistic considerations in the differential diagnosis are non-Hodgkin's lymphoma and seminoma of both typical and spermatocytic types. In a recent report of seven testicular plasmacytomas, three of the cases were submitted with these provisional diagnoses (117). The tumor cells in lymphoma typically have less abundant cytoplasm than plasma cells and lack a paranuclear hof. In addition, sclerosis is common in testicular lymphoma but rarely, if ever, seen in plasmacytoma. Clinical and gross features can provide some clues to the diagnosis. Most testicular lymphomas present with disease confined to the testis and paratestis whereas most testicular plasmacytomas are associated with widespread disease at diagnosis, although, as noted above, there are striking exceptions to this. Simultaneous involvement of both testes by a mass is much more common in cases of lymphoma than in cases of plasmacytoma. In problematic cases immunohistochemical staining can be helpful by demonstrating that plasmacytomas express cytoplasmic immunoglobulin of IgG or IgA type in contrast to surface immunoglobulin that is most often of IgM type in lymphoma. Plasmacytomas usually lack B-cell antigens and may lack leukocyte common antigen (CD45) but may stain for EMA, unlike most testicular lymphomas with the exception of the anaplastic large cell (Ki-1) variants. Distinction from seminoma should be straightforward on routine light microscopic examination because of the marked difference in the cytologic features of these two tumors; in a rare problematic case staining of seminoma for glycogen and differences in immunohistochemical staining of these tumors are diagnostic.

A more realistic problem may be the differential diagnosis with spermatocytic seminoma because of the various cell types of that neoplasm which are mimicked to some extent by the variations in cell size and shape seen in some cases of plasmacytoma. For example, the granular chromatin of some cells in plasmacytomas may suggest the "spireme" type chromatin seen in some cells of spermatocytic seminomas. However, careful high-power scrutiny in such cases should show many cells with the characteristic features of immature plasma cells: eccentric nuclei and amphophilic cytoplasm with a paranuclear hof.

Leydig cell tumor may enter the differential diagnosis because, like plasmacytoma, it has cells with appreciable eosinophilic cytoplasm. However, Leydig cell tumors are usually well-circumscribed, dark brown to tan tumors in which the neoplastic cells have more granular cytoplasm, lack a paranuclear hof, and have different nuclear characteristics.

Leukemia, Including Granulocytic Sarcoma

General and Clinical Features. The testis is involved on microscopic examination at autopsy in 64 percent of patients with acute leukemia, and 22 percent of those with chronic leukemia (117b). The testis is enlarged in 5 to 10 percent of the cases. Testicular swelling is evident during life in only 5 percent of patients with leukemia, and testicular enlargement as the presenting manifestation of the disease is exceptionally rare. Testicular leukemic involvement is now seen most commonly in biopsy specimens obtained to detect relapse after treatment of acute lymphoblastic leukemia. On microscopic examination the pattern of leukemic infiltration is similar to that of lymphoma, predominantly intertubular, with tubular invasion and effacement of the tubules in some cases. Growth in cords may be conspicuous and confusing.

Eight examples of granulocytic sarcoma (tumors composed of immature myeloid cells) of the testis have been reported in detail (113,115,120, 132,134). Two of the eight patients had a history of acute myeloid leukemia prior to developing the testicular disease, but two presented with testicular disease and subsequently developed the leukemia. Another patient presented with granulocytic sarcoma at another site and later had acute myeloid leukemia simultaneously with granulocytic sarcoma of the testis. In two additional patients the clinical background was that of a myelodysplastic syndrome. In one final unusual case the testicular disease was apparently localized and successfully treated by chemotherapy. This patient, who had worked at an atomic bomb test site, died of unrelated causes 12 years after development of the testicular granulocytic sarcoma without evidence of disease elsewhere (115). We have recently seen an example of epididymal granulocytic sarcoma.

Gross and Microscopic Findings and Differential Diagnosis. Granulocytic sarcomas are essentially indistinguishable from malignant lymphoma on gross examination, although, potentially, a green color may be suggestive of granulocytic sarcoma based on the experience with extratesticular cases; we are unaware, however, that this has been documented in a testicular example. The testicular granulocytic sarcomas we have seen were associated with particularly prominent extratesticular extension (fig. 7-91).

Microscopic evaluation of these tumors (fig. 7-92) may cause major diagnostic problems, as illustrated by the fact that four of the eight testicular tumors were misinterpreted as malignant lymphoma (three cases) (fig. 7-93) or plasmacytoma (one case) (fig. 7-94). Features favoring the diagnosis of granulocytic sarcoma rather than lymphoma include a slightly smaller cell size, more evenly dispersed chromatin, and less prominent nucleoli than found in immunoblasts or centroblasts. The nuclei of granulocytic sarcoma cells may be round or indented but usually lack the sharp angulation of cleaved lymphoid

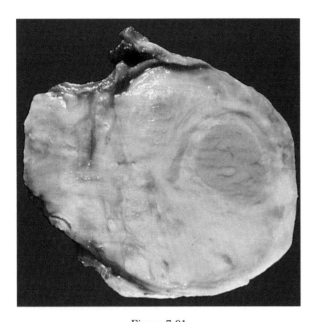

Figure 7-91
GRANULOCYTIC SARCOMA OF TESTIS
The compressed testis (yellow-orange tissue) is surrounded by a creamy tumor that extensively obliterates the paratesticular soft tissues.

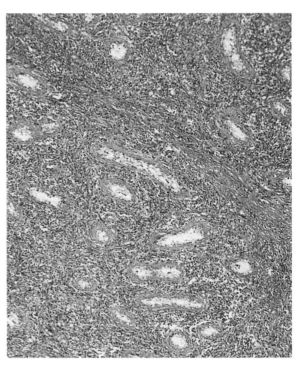

Figure 7-92
GRANULOCYTIC SARCOMA OF TESTIS
There is prominent intertubular growth of the tumor cells.

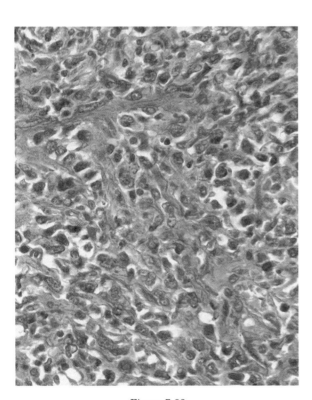

Figure 7-93
GRANULOCYTIC SARCOMA OF TESTIS
The tumor cells have prominently cleaved nuclei. Note the resemblance to a large cell lymphoma.

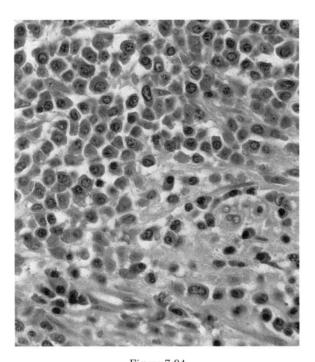

Figure 7-94
GRANULOCYTIC SARCOMA OF TESTIS
Most of the tumor cells have eccentric nuclei and abundant eosinophilic cytoplasm and simulate plasma cells.

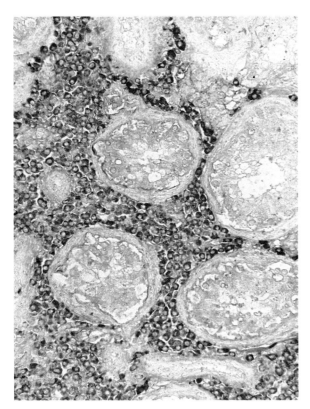

Figure 7-95
GRANULOCYTIC SARCOMA OF TESTIS
The tumor cells are positive when stained for chloroacetate esterase.

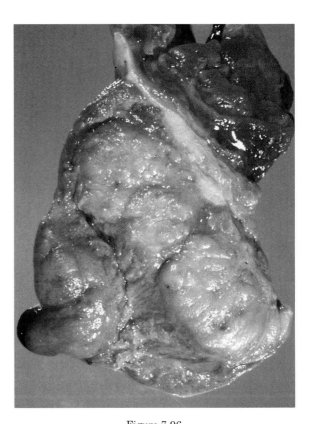

Figure 7-96
METASTATIC ADENOCARCINOMA
OF PROSTATE TO TESTIS
Much of the testis is replaced by a lobulated yellow-brown tumor.

cells. If immature cells with recognizable myeloid differentiation, such as eosinophilic myelocytes, are found, granulocytic sarcoma is strongly suggested. Enzyme histochemical stains for chloroacetate esterase (Leder's stain) (fig. 7-95) or immunohistochemical stains for lysozyme and myeloperoxidase should facilitate the diagnosis.

Plasmacytoma may be suggested because of large numbers of myelocytes with eccentric nuclei and moderate amounts of pink cytoplasm (fig. 7-94). An associated chronic inflammatory cell infiltrate, with small lymphocytes and mature plasma cells, may further complicate the interpretation. However, the predominant population in the tumor lacks the coarsely clumped chromatin, paranuclear hof, and more abundant nongranular cytoplasm characteristic of plasma cells. In addition, testicular granulocytic sarcomas often exhibit prominent intrascrotal, extratesticular spread, whereas testicular plasmacytomas are almost always confined to the testis.

SECONDARY TUMORS

General and Clinical Features. Although there were no nonhematopoietic metastases in over 600 autopsies of males dying of cancer at one center (161), metastases accounted for 3.6 percent of testicular tumors at another institution (154). The tumors are found most often in men over 50 years of age, but approximately one third of patients are under 40 years (146,156). They usually occur in patients with a known primary elsewhere, but the testicular mass is the presenting manifestation in 6 percent of cases (154). Carcinomas of the prostate (figs. 7-96–7-99) and lung most commonly metastasize to the testis, with the former accounting for one third and the latter for one fifth of the cases in the literature. Metastatic prostate cancer has been found in 6 percent of therapeutic orchidectomy specimens (148). The next most frequent sources of testicular

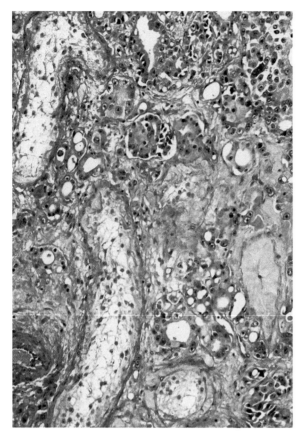

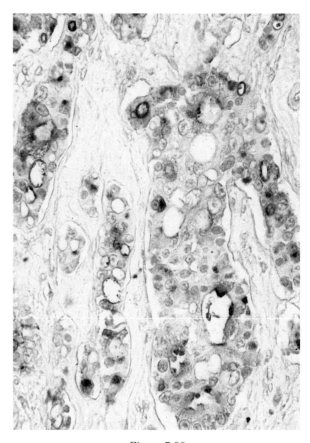

Figure 7-97
METASTATIC ADENOCARCINOMA
OF PROSTATE TO TESTIS
Clusters of tumor cells and a few neoplastic glands are present in the intertubular region.

Figure 7-98
METASTATIC ADENOCARCINOMA
OF PROSTATE TO TESTIS
The tumor in figure 7-97 exhibits a strong immunohistochemical reaction for prostate-specific antigen.

Figure 7-99
METASTATIC ADENOCARCINOMA
OF PROSTATE TO TESTIS

The appearance in this case caused confusion initially with a Leydig cell tumor.

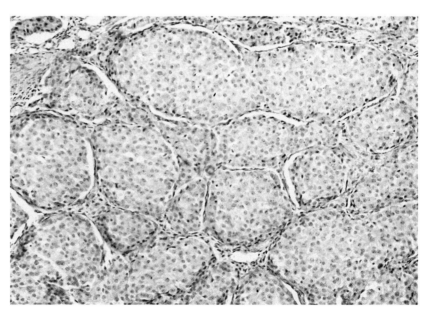

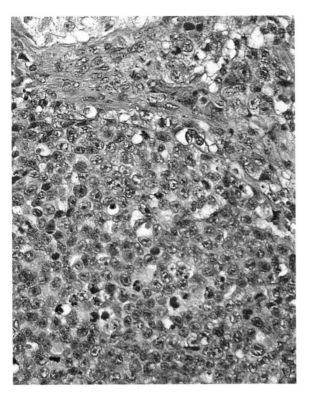

Figure 7-100
METASTATIC MALIGNANT MELANOMA TO TESTIS
The tumor cells are highly malignant, with prominent mitotic activity. Note a portion of a seminiferous tubule at the top.

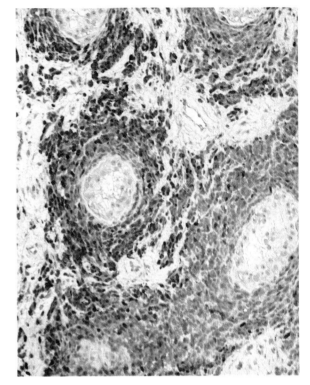

Figure 7-101
METASTATIC MALIGNANT MELANOMA TO TESTIS
The prominent intertubular growth in this case is highlighted by this immunohistochemical stain for S-100 protein.

metastases are malignant melanoma of the skin (8 percent of the cases) (figs. 7-100, 7-101) and carcinomas of the intestine, appendix and rectum (8 percent), kidney (6 percent), stomach, and pancreas (147,153,156, 157,162). Melanospermia may be present in cases of melanoma (144,152, 158). Occasional carcinoid tumors have metastasized to the testis (139). In one case (142), pressure on a probable testicular metastasis produced clinical manifestations of the carcinoid syndrome. Almost 4 percent of males with neuroblastoma had testicular metastases in one report (151). Testicular spread of many other tumors, including carcinomas of the bile duct, liver, thyroid, bladder, ureter, and penis; retinoblastoma; pleural mesothelioma; adenoid cystic carcinoma; Wilms' tumor; Merkel cell tumor (fig. 7-102); and occasional sarcomas (fig. 7-103) have been reported (140,141,143,145,149,155,159,160,164). Routes of spread include the vas deferens for prostatic carcinoma, spermatic veins for renal cell carcinoma, lymphatics for intestinal carci-

noma, and blood vessels for lung carcinoma. Testicular metastases are bilateral in approximately 20 percent of the cases.

Gross Findings. Sectioning usually reveals single or multiple nodules that may be confluent (fig. 7-96), but diffuse involvement is also seen. The presence of multiple nodules should raise the possibility of metastasis, particularly in a patient over 50 years of age.

Microscopic Findings. On microscopic examination the tumor is usually predominantly in the interstitium (fig. 7-97), but the neoplastic cells may also invade the tubules. There may be prominent involvement of blood vessels in the testis, epididymis, and cord which should suggest the diagnosis, assuming the morphology is inconsistent with a primary testicular neoplasm. The microscopic features of most metastatic tumors are incompatible with a primary testicular tumor, but nonetheless, occasionally significant errors in interpretation occur, as in one case of metastatic melanoma misdiagnosed as seminoma

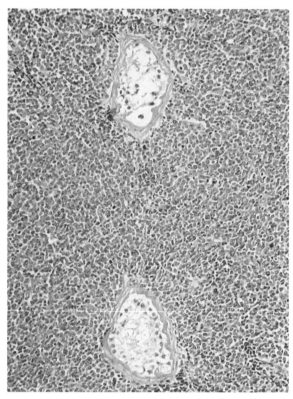

Figure 7-102
METASTATIC MERKEL CELL TUMOR TO TESTIS

There is a prominent intertubular pattern of growth and at this magnification the picture is indistinguishable from that of malignant lymphoma or certain other metastatic tumors such as melanoma.

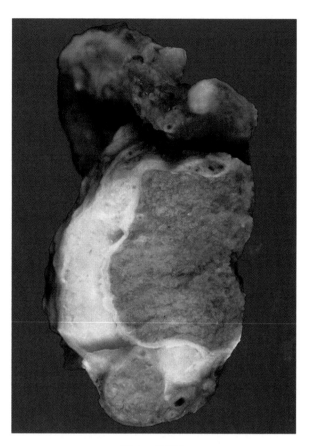

Figure 7-104
METASTATIC ADENOCARCINOMA FROM PANCREAS ENCASING EPIDIDYMIS
(Courtesy of Dr. J. Eble, Indianapolis, IN.)

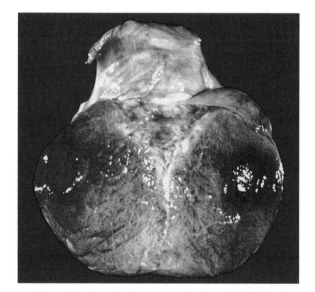

Figure 7-103
METASTATIC ANGIOSARCOMA TO TESTIS

(158). We have also seen metastatic renal cell carcinoma of the clear cell type misinterpreted as Sertoli cell tumor and seminoma. In occasional difficult cases, special stains, particularly for mucin, argyrophil granules, and melanin, and immunoperoxidase studies, particularly for prostatic carcinoma (fig. 7-98) and malignant melanoma (fig. 7-101), may help in the diagnosis. Markers to exclude germ cell or sex cord–stromal tumors may also be indicated if these are serious considerations based on the routine histology.

Metastases to the epididymis (fig. 7-104) (150) and cord (151a) may occasionally be challenging, both clinically and pathologically, when the tumor presents at these metastatic sites. Twenty-three metastatic tumors have presented as epididymal masses, with primary sites in the colon (7 cases), stomach (5 cases), pancreas (3 cases), prostate and kidney (2 cases each), ileum

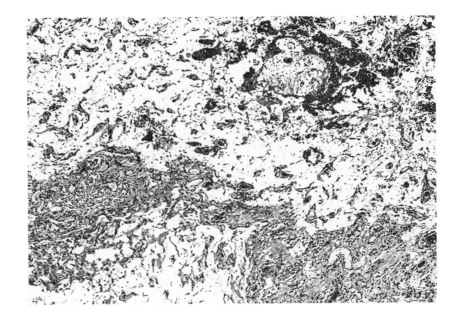

Figure 7-105
SECONDARY LOW-GRADE
MUCINOUS TUMOR OF
APPENDIX IN HERNIA SAC
Note the acellular mucin.

(carcinoid) (3 cases), and liver (150,151a). The morphologic differences from any primary tumor of the epididymis should suggest the possibility of a metastasis in most cases. Prominent vascular space invasion may also be helpful. In a series of malignant paratesticular and spermatic cord tumors from a general hospital, 10 tumors were primary and 9 metastatic (151a). Six of the metastases involved the spermatic cord, and four of these presented prior to the identification of the primary tumor. Rarely, appendiceal low-grade mucinous cystic neoplasms may present in a hernia sac prior to the discovery of the appendiceal lesion (fig. 7-105) (140a,163).

REFERENCES

Tumors of Ovarian Epithelial Type

1. Brennan MK, Srigley JR. Brenner tumor of the testis: case report and review of other intrascrotal examples. J Urol Pathol (in press).
2. Caccamo D, Socias M, Truchet C. Malignant Brenner tumor of the testis and epididymis. Arch Pathol Lab Med 1991;115:524–7.
3. DeNictolis M, Tommasoni S, Fabris G, Prat J. Intratesticular serous cystadenoma of borderline malignancy. A pathological, histochemical and DNA content study of a case with long-term follow-up. Virchows Arch [A] 1993;423:221–5.
4. Elbadawi A, Batchvarov MM, Linke CA. Intratesticular papillary mucinous cystadenocarcinoma. Urology 1979;14:280–4.
5. Goldman RL. A Brenner tumor of the testis. Cancer 1970;26:853–65.
6. Jones M, Young RH, Srigley JR, Scully RE. Paratesticular serous papillary carcinoma. A report of six cases. Am J Surg Pathol 1995;19:1359–66.
7. Kellert E. An ovarian type pseudomucinous cystadenoma in the scrotum. Cancer 1959;12:187–90.

8. Kernohan NM, Coutts AG, Best PV. Cystadenocarcinoma of the appendix testis. Histopathology 1990;17:147–54.
9. Nistal M, Revestido R, Paniagua R. Bilateral mucinous cystadenocarcinoma of the testis and epididymis. Arch Pathol Lab Med 1992;116:1360–3.
9a. Nochomovitz LE, Orenstein JM. Adenocarcinoma of the rete testis. Review and regrouping of reported cases and a consideration of miscellaneous entities. J Urogenit Pathol 1991;1:11–40.
10. Nogales FF Jr, Matilla A, Ortega I, Alvarez T. Mixed Brenner and adenomatoid tumor of the testis: an ultrastructural study and histogenetic considerations. Cancer 1979;43:539–43.
11. Remmele W, Kaiserling E, Zerban U, et al. Serous papillary cystic tumor of borderline malignancy with focal carcinoma arising in testis: case report with immunohistochemical and ultrastructural observations. Hum Pathol 1992;23:75–9.
11a. Scully RE, Young RH, Clement PB. Tumors of the ovary, maldeveloped gonads, fallopian tube, and broad ligament. Atlas of Tumor Pathology, 3rd Series, Fascicle 23. Washington D.C.: Armed Forces Institute of Pathology, 1998.

12. Sundarasivarao D. The mullerian vestiges and benign epithelial tumors of the epididymis. J Pathol Bacteriol 1953;66:417–31.

13. Uzoaru I, Ray VH, Nadimpalli V. Brenner tumor of the testis. Immunohistochemical comparison with its ovarian counterparts. J Urol Pathol 1995;3:249–53.

14. Walker AN, Mills SE, Glandular inclusions in inguinal hernia sacs and spermatic cords: müllerian-like remnants confused with functional reproductive structures. Am J Clin Pathol 1984;82:85–9.

15. Walker AN, Mills SE. Jones PF, Stanley CM III. Borderline serous cystadenoma of the tunica vaginalis testis. Surg Pathol 1988;1:431–6.

16. Young RH, Scully RE. Testicular and paratesticular tumors and tumor-like lesions of ovarian common epithelial and mullerian types. A report of four cases and review of the literature. Am J Clin Pathol 1986;86:146–52.

Tumors of the Rete

17. Altaffer LF, Dufour DR, Castleberry GM, Steele, SM. Coexisting rete testis adenoma and gonadoblastoma. J Urol 1982;127:332–5.

18. Channer JL, MacIver AG. Glandular changes in the rete testis: metastatic tumor or adenomatoid hyperplasia? [Letter] J Pathol 1989;157:81–3.

19. Crisp-Lindgren N, Travers H, Wells MM, Cawley LP. Papillary adenocarcinoma of rete testis. Autopsy findings, histochemistry, immunohistochemistry, ultrastructure, and clinical correlation. Am J Surg Pathol 1988;12:492–501.

19a. Doglioni C, Dei Tos AP, Laurino L, et al. Calretinin: a novel immunocytochemical marker for mesothelioma. Am J Surg Pathol 1996;20:1037–46.

20. Gisser SD, Nayak S, Kaneko M, Tchertkoff V. Adenocarcinoma of the rete testis: a review of the literature and report of a case with associated asbestosis. Hum Pathol 1977;8:219–24.

20a. Gruber H, Ratschek M, Pummer K, Breinl E, Spuller E, Hubmer G. Adenocarcinoma of the rete testis: report of a case with surgical history of adenomatous hyperplasia of the rete testis. J Urol 1997;158:1525–6.

21. Jones MA, Young RH. Sertoliform rete cystadenoma: a report of two cases. J Urol Pathol 1997;7:47–53.

22. Murad T, Tanahashi T. Adenofibroma of the rete testis. A case report with electron microscopy findings. Acta Pathol Jpn 1988;38:105–12.

23. Nistal M, Paniagua R. Adenomatous hyperplasia of the rete testis. J Path 1988;154:343–6.

24. Nochomovitz LE, Orenstein JM. Adenocarcinoma of the rete testis. Case report, ultrastructural observations, and clinicopathologic correlates. Am J Surg Pathol 1984;8:625–34.

25. Nochomovitz LE, Orenstein JM. Adenocarcinoma of the rete testis. Review and regrouping of reported cases and a consideration of miscellaneous entities. J Urogenit Pathol 1991;1:11–40.

25a. Nochomovitz LE, Orenstein JM. Adenocarcinoma of the rete testis: consolidation and analysis of 31 reported cases with a review of the literature. J Urol Pathol 1994;2:1–37.

25b. Samaratunga H, Kanowski P, Gloughlin B, Walker N, Searle J. Adenocarcinoma of the rete testis with intratubular invasion of the testis. J Urol Pathol 1994;2:291–300.

26. Visscher DW, Talerman A, Rivera LR, Mazur MT. Adenocarcinoma of the rete testis with a spindle cell component. A possible metaplastic carcinoma. Cancer 1989;64:770–5.

26a. Watson PH, Jacob VC. Adenocarcinoma of the rete testis with sertoliform differentiation. Arch Pathol Lab Med 1989;113:1169–71.

Adenomatoid Tumor

27. Barwick KW, Madri JA. An immunohistochemical study of adenomatoid tumors utilizing keratin and factor VIII antibodies. Evidence for a mesothelial origin. Lab Invest 1982;47:276–80.

28. Black WC, Benitez RE, Buesing OR, Hojnoski WS. Bizarre adenomatoid tumor of testicular tunics. Cancer 1964;17:1472–6.

29. Broth G, Bullock WK, Morrow J. Epididymal tumors: 1. Report of 15 new cases including review of literature. 2. Histochemical study of the so-called adenomatoid tumor. J Urol 1968;100:530–6.

30. Davy CL, Tang CK. Are all adenomatoid tumors adenomatoid mesotheliomas? Hum Pathol 1981;12:360–9.

31. De Klerk DP, Nime F. Adenomatoid tumors (mesothelioma) of testicular and paratesticular tissue. Urology 1975;6:635–41.

32. Glantz GM. Adenomatoid tumors of the epididymis: a review of 5 new cases, including a case report associated with hydrocele. J Urol 1966;95:227–33.

33. Golden A, Ash JE. Adenomatoid tumors of the genital tract. Am J Pathol 1945;21:63–79.

34. Jackson JR. The histogenesis of the "adenomatoid" tumor of the genital tract. Cancer 1958;11:337–50.

35. Kiely EA, Flanagan A, Williams G. Intrascrotal adenomatoid tumors. Br J Urol 1987;60:255–7.

36. Longo VJ, McDonald JR, Thompson GJ. Primary neoplasms of the epididymis. Special reference to adenomatoid tumors. JAMA 1951;147:937–41.

37. Mackay B, Bennington JL, Skoglund RW. The adenomatoid tumor: fine structural evidence for a mesothelial origin. Cancer 1971;27:109–15.

38. Miller F, Lieberman MK. Local invasion in adenomatoid tumors. Cancer 1968;21:933–9.

39. Stavrides A, Hutcheson JB. Benign mesotheliomas of testicular appendages: a morphologic and histochemical study of seven cases and review of theories of histogenesis. J Urol 1960;83:448–53.

40. Taxy JB, Battifora H, Oyasu R. Adenomatoid tumors: a light microscopic, histochemical, and ultrastructural study. Cancer 1974;34:306–16.

41. Yasuma T, Saito S. Adenomatoid tumor of the male genital tract. A pathological study of eight cases and review of the literature. Acta Pathol Jpn 1980;30:883–906.

Malignant Mesothelioma

42. Antman K, Cohen S, Dimitrov NV, Green M, Muggia F. Malignant mesothelioma of the tunica vaginalis testis. J Clin Oncol 1984;2:447–51.
43. Chen KT, Arhelger RB, Flam MS, Hanson JH. Malignant mesothelioma of the tunica vaginalis testis. Urology 1982;20:316–9.
44. Chetty R. Well differentiated (benign) papillary mesothelioma of the tunica vaginalis. J Clin Pathol 1992;45:1029-30.
45. Daya D, McCaughey WT. Well-differentiated papillary mesothelioma of the peritoneum. A clinicopathologic study of 22 cases. Cancer 1990;65:292–6.
45a. Doglioni C, Dei Tos AP, Laurino L, et al. Calretinin: a novel immunocytochemical marker for mesothelioma. Am J Surg Pathol 1996;20:1037–46.
46. Grove A, Jensen ML, Donna A. Mesotheliomas of the tunica vaginalis testis and hernia sacs. Virchows Arch [A] 1989;415:283–92.
47. Jones MA, Young RH, Scully RE. Malignant mesothelioma of the tunica vaginalis: A clinicopatho-

logic analysis of 11 cases with review of the literature. Am J Surg Pathol 1995;19:815–25.
48. Kasdon EJ. Malignant mesothelioma of the tunica vaginalis propria testis. Report of two cases. Cancer 1969;23:1144–50.
48a. Khan MA, Puri P, Devaney D. Mesothelioma of tunica vaginalis testis in a child. J Urol 1997;158:198–9.
49. Kuwabara H, Uda H, Sakamoto H, Sato A. Malignant mesothelioma of the tunica vaginalis testis. Report of a case and review of the literature. Acta Pathol Jpn 1991;41:857–63.
50. Mikuz G, Hopfel-Kreiner I. Papillary mesothelioma of the tunica vaginalis propria testis. A case report and ultrastructural study. Virchows Arch [A] 1982; 396:231–8.
51. Pizzolato P, Lamberty J. Mesothelioma of spermatic cord. Electron microscopic and histochemical characteristics of its mucopolysaccharides. Urology 1976;8:403–8.
52. Rosai J, Dehner LP. Nodular mesothelial hyperplasia in hernia sacs: a benign reactive condition simulating a neoplastic process. Cancer 1975;35:165–75.

Desmoplastic Small Round Cell Tumor

53. Cummings OW, Ulbright TM, Young RH, Dei Tos AP, Fletcher CD, Hull MT. Desmoplastic small round cell tumors of the para-testicular region: a report of six cases. Am J Surg Pathol 1997;21:219–25.
54. Gerald WL, Miller HK, Battifora H, Miettinen M, Silva EG, Rosai J. Intra-abdominal desmoplastic small round-cell tumor. Report of 19 cases of a distinctive type of high-grade polyphenotypic malignancy affecting young individuals. Am J Surg Pathol 1991;15:499–513.

55. Ordonez NG, el-Naggar AK, Ro JY, Silva EG, Mackay B. Intra-abdominal desmoplastic small cell tumor: a light microscopic, immunocytochemical, ultrastructural, and flow cytometric study. Hum Pathol 1993;24:850–65.
56. Prat J, Matias-Guiu X, Algaba F. Desmoplastic small round-cell tumor [Letter]. Am J Surg Pathol 1992;16:306–7.

Tumors of the Epididymis

56a. Ben-Izhak O. Solitary papillary cystadenoma of the spermatic cord presenting as an inguinal mass. J Urol Pathol 1997;7:55–61.
57. Gilcrease MZ, Schmidt L, Zbar B, Truong L, Rutledge M, Wheeler TM. Somatic von Hippel-Lindau mutation in clear cell papillary cystadenoma of the epididymis. Hum Pathol 1995;26:1341–6.
58. Jones MA, Young RH, Scully RE. Adenocarcinoma of the epididymis. A report of four cases and review of the literature. Am J Surg Pathol 1997;21:1474–80.
59. Kuo TT, Gomez LG. Monstrous epithelial cells in human epididymis and seminal vesicles. A pseudomalignant change. Am J Surg Pathol 1981;5:483–90.

60. Lamiell JM, Salazar FG, Hsia YE. von Hippel-Lindau disease affecting 43 members of a single kindred. Medicine 1989;68:1–29.
60a. Manivel JC. Pseudoneoplastic lesions of the male genitals. In: Wick MR, Humphrey PA, Ritter JH, eds. Pathology of pseudoneoplastic lesions. New York: Lippincott-Raven Press, 1997:247–63.
61. Price EB. Papillary cystadenoma of the epididymis. A clinicopathologic analysis of 20 cases. Arch Pathol 1971;91:456–70.
61a. Rowlands RD, Nicholson GW. A case of primary squamous-celled epithelioma of the epididymis. Lancet 1929;1:304–6.
62. Salm R. Papillary carcinoma of the epididymis. J Pathol 1969;97:253–9.

Retinal Anlage Tumor

63. Diamond D A, Breitfeld PP, Bur M, Gang D. Melanotic neuroectodermal tumor of infancy: an important mimicker of paratesticular rhabdomyosarcoma. J Urol 1992;147:673–5.
64. Johnson RE, Scheithauer BW, Dahlin DC. Melanotic neuroectodermal tumor of infancy. A review of seven cases. Cancer 1983;52:661–6.
65. Murayama T, Fujita K, Ohashi T, Matsushita T. Melanotic neuroectodermal tumor of the epididymis in infancy: A case report. J Urol 1989;141:105–6.
65a. Pettinato G, Manivel JC, d'Amore ES, Jasczc W, Gorlin RJ. Melanotic neuroectodermal tumor of infancy: a

reexamination of a histogenetic problem based on immunohistochemical, ultrastructural, and flow cytometric study of 10 cases. Am J Surg Pathol 1991;15:233–45.
66. Raju U, Zarbo RJ, Regezi JA, Krutchkoff DJ, Perrin EV. Melanotic neuroectodermal tumors of infancy: intermediate filament-, neuroendocrine-, and melanoma-associated antigen profiles. Appl Immunohistochem 1993;1:69–76.
67. Ricketts RR, Majmudarr B. Epididymal melanotic neuroectodermal tumor of infancy. Hum Pathol 1985;16:416–20.

Soft Tissue Tumors

68. Banks ER, Mills SE. Histiocytoid (epithelioid) hemangioma of the testis. The so-called vascular variant of "adenomatoid tumor." Am J Surg Pathol 1990;14:584–9.

69. Bellinger MF, Gibbons MD, Koontz WW Jr, Graff M. Paratesticular liposarcoma. Urology 1978;11:285–8.

70. Belville WD, Insalaco SJ, Dresner ML, Buck AS. Benign testis tumors. J Urol 1982;128:1198–200.

70a. Busmanis I. Paratesticular plexiform tumour of myofibroblastic origin. Histopathology 1991;18:178–80.

71. Cecchetto G, Grotto P, De Bernardi B, Indolfi P, Perilongo G, Carli M. Paratesticular rhabdomyosarcoma in childhood: experience of the Italian Cooperative Study. Tumori 1988;74:645–7.

71a. Cecil AB. Intrascrotal lipomata. J Urol 1927;17:557–66.

72. Clatch RJ, Drake WK, Gonzalez JG. Aggressive angiomyxoma in men. A report of two cases associated with inguinal hernias. Arch Pathol Lab Med 1993;117:911–3.

73. Collins DH, Symington T. Sertoli-cell tumour. Br J Urol 1964;36:52–61.

74. Dandia SD, Ojha DG. Giant fibroma of the epididymis: a case report. J Urol 1966;96:941–3.

75. Dehner LP, Scott D, Stocker JT. Meconium periorchitis: a clinicopathologic study of four cases with a review of the literature. Hum Pathol 1986;17:807–12.

76. Eltorky MA, O'Brien TF, Walzer Y. Primary paratesticular malignant fibrous histiocytoma. Case report and review of the literature. J Urol Pathol 1994;1:425–9.

76a. Farrell MA, Donnelly BJ. Malignant smooth muscle tumors of the epididymis. J Urol 1980;124:151–3.

76b. Ferrari A, Casanova M, Massimino M, Luksch R, Piva L, Fossati-Bellani F. The management of paratesticular rhabdomyosarcoma: a single institutional experience with 44 consecutive children. J Urol 1998;159:1031–4.

77. Fetsch JF, Montgomery EA, Meis JM. Calcifying fibrous pseudotumor. Am J Surg Pathol 1993;17:502–8.

78. Grey LF, Sorial RF, Shaw WH. Spermatic cord sarcoma. Leiomyosarcoma and retroperitoneal lymph node dissection. Urology 1986;27:28–31.

79. Hargreaves HK, Scully RE, Richie JP. Benign hemangioendothelioma of the testis: case report with electron microscopic documentation and review of the literature. Am J Clin Pathol 1982;77:637–42.

80. Horn RC, Enterline HT. Rhabdomyosarcoma: a clinicopathologic study and classification of 39 cases. Cancer 1958;11:181–99.

80a. Iczkowski KA, Kiviat J, Cheville JC, Bostwick DG. Multifocal capillary microangioma of the testis. J Urol Pathol 1997;7:113–9.

81. Iezzoni JC, Fechner RE, Wong LS, Rosai J. Aggressive angiomyxoma in males. A report of four cases. Am J Clin Pathol 1995;104:391–6.

82. Johnson DE, Harris JD, Ayala AG. Liposarcoma of the spermatic cord. Urology 1978;11:190–2.

83. Jones MA, Young RH, Scully RE. Benign fibromatous tumors of the testis and paratesticular region: a report of 9 cases with a proposed classification of fibromatous tumors and tumor-like lesions. Am J Surg Pathol 1997;21:296–305.

84. Kawanishi Y, Tamura M, Akiyama K, et al. Rhabdoid tumours of the spermatic cord. Br J Urol 1989;63:439–40.

85. Kneale BJ, Bishop NL, Britton JP. Kaposi's sarcoma of the testis. Brit J Urol 1993;72:116–7.

85a. Lander EB, Lee I. Giant scrotal lipomatosis. J Urol 1996;156:1773.

85b. Lanzafame S, Fragetta F, Emmanuele C, et al. Paratesticular pleomorphic rhabdomyosarcoma in the elderly. Int J Surg Pathol 1999;7:27–32.

85c. Laskin WB, Fetsch JF, Mostofi FK. Angiomyofibroblastoma-like tumor of the male genital tract: analysis of 11 cases with comparison to female angiomyofibroblastoma and spindle cell lipoma. Am J Surg Pathol 1998;22:6–16.

86. Leuschner I, Newton WA Jr, Schmidt D, et al. Spindle cell variants of embryonal rhabdomyosarcoma in the paratesticular region. A report of the Intergroup Rhabdomyosarcoma Study. Am J Surg Pathol 1993;17:221–30.

86a. Lioe TF, Biggart JD. Tumours of the spermatic cord and paratesticular tissue. A clinicopathological study. Br J Urol 1993;71:600–6.

87. Loughlin KR, Retik AB, Weinstein HJ, et al. Genitourinary rhabdomyosarcoma in children. Cancer 1989;63:1600–6.

88. Mac-Moune Lai F, Allen PW, Chan LW, Chan PS, Cooper JE, MacKenzie TM. Aggressive fibromatosis of the spermatic cord. A typical lesion in a "new" location. Am J Clin Pathol 1995;104:403–7.

88a. Mašera A, Ovcak Z, Mikuz G. Angiosarcoma of the testis. Virchows Arch 1999;434:351–3.

89. Matthew T. Osteosarcoma of the testis. Arch Pathol Lab Med 1981;105:38–9.

90. Mazzella FM, Sieber SC, Lopez V. Histiocytoid hemangioma of the testis: a case report. J Urol 1995;153:743–4.

91. Ockner DM, Sayadi H, Swanson PE, Ritter JH, Wick MR. Genital angiomyofibroblastoma. Comparision with aggressive angiomyxoma and other myxoid neoplasms of skin and soft tissue. Am J Clin Pathol 1997;107:36–44.

92. Parveen T, Fleischmann J, Petrelli M. Benign fibrous tumor of the tunica vaginalis testis. Report of a case with light, electron microscopic, and immunocytochemical study, and review of the literature. Arch Pathol Lab Med 1992;116:277–80.

93. Prince CL. Rhabdomyosarcoma of the testicle. J Urol 1942;48:187–95.

94. Ravich L, Lerman PH, Drabkin JW, Foltin E. Pure testicular rhabdomyosarcoma. J Urol 1965;94:596–9.

95. Schwartz SL, Swierzewski SJ III, Sondak VK, Grossman HB. Liposarcoma of the spermatic cord: report of 6 cases and review of the literature. J Urol 1995;153:154–7.

96. Sclama AO, Berger BW, Cherry JM, Young JD Jr. Malignant fibrous histiocytoma of the spermatic cord: the role of retroperitoneal lymphadenectomy in management. J Urol 1983;130:577–9.

96a. Seidl C, Lippert C, Grouls V, Jellinghaus W. Leiomyosarcoma des samenstranges mit paraneoplastischer b-hCG produktion. Pathologe 1998;19:146–50.

96b. Shah VI, Ro JY, Lee MW, et al. Angiomyxoid lesions of the spermatic cord including aggressive angiomyxoma (AAM): a morphologically heterogeneous group of tumorous lesions [Abstract]. Mod Pathol 1998;11:96A.

96c. Soosay GN, Parkinson MC, Paradinas J, Fisher C. Paratesticular sarcomas revisited: a review of cases in the British Testicular Tumour Registry. Br J Urol 1996;77:143–6.

96d. Spark RP. Leiomyoma of epididymis. Arch Pathol 1972;93:18–21.

97. Srigley JR, Hartwick RW. Tumors and cysts of the paratesticular region. Pathol Annu 1990;25(pt. 2):51–108.

97a. Tanda F, Cossu Rocca P, Bosincu L, Massarelli G, Cossu A, Manca A. Rhabdomyoma of the tunica vaginalis of the testis: a histologic, immunohistochemical, and ultrastructural study. J Urol Pathol 1997;10:608–11.

97b. Tokunaka S, Taniguchi N, Hashimoto H, Yachiku S, Fujita M. Leiomyoblastoma of the epididymis in a child. J Urol 1990;143:991–3.

98. Tsang WY, Chan JK, Lee KC, Fisher C, Fletcher CD. Aggressive angiomyxoma. A report of four cases occurring in men. Am J Surg Pathol 1992;16:1059–65.

98a. Turner DT, Shah SM, Jones R. Intrascrotal lipoblastoma. Br J Urol 1998;81:166–7.

98b. Vallat-Decouvelaere AV, Dry SM, Fletcher CD. Atypical and malignant solitary fibrous tumors in extrathoracic locations. Am J Surg Pathol 1998;22:1501–11.

98c. Wang NP, Marx J, McNutt MA, Rutledge JC, Gown AM. Expression of myogenic regulatory proteins (myogenin and MyoD1) in small blue round cell tumors of childhood. Am J Pathol 1995;147:1799–810.

99. Yachia D, Auslaender L. Primary leiomyosarcoma of the testis. J Urol 1989;141:955–6.

100. Zukerberg LR, Young RH. Primary testicular sarcoma: a report of two cases. Hum Pathol 1990;21:932–5.

Miscellaneous Rare Primary Tumors

101. Bryan RL, Liu S, Newman J, O'Brien JM, Considine J. Squamous cell carcinoma arising in a chronic hydrocoele. Histopathology 1990;17:178–80.

102. Dharkar D, Kraft JR. Paraganglioma of the spermatic cord. An incidental finding. J Urol Pathol 1994;2:89–93.

102a. Engel F, McPherson HT, Fetter BF, et al. Clinical, morphological, and biochemical studies on a malignant testicular tumor. J Clin Endocrinol Metab 1964;24:528–42.

103. Heyns CF, Van Niekerk JT, Rossouw DJ, Burger EC, De Klerk DP. Nephroblastoma in an ovotestis of a true hermaphrodite: a case report. J Urol 1987;137:1003–5.

104. Mashat F, Meccawi A, Garg S, Christian E. Paraganglioma of the spermatic cord [Letter]. Ann Saudi Med 1993;13:208–10.

105. Orlowski JP, Levin HS, Dyment PG. Intrascrotal Wilms' tumor developing in a heterotopic renal anlage of probable mesonephric origin. J Pediatr Surg 1980;15:679–82.

106. Shih DF, Wang JS, Tseng HH. Primary squamous cell carcinoma of the testis. J Urol 1996;156:1772.

107. Taylor WF, Myers M, Taylor WR. Extrarenal Wilms' tumour in an infant exposed to intrauterine phenytoin [Letter]. Lancet 1980;2:481–2.

Hematopoietic Diseases

108. Abell MR, Holtz F. Testicular and paratesticular neoplasms in patients 60 years of age and older. Cancer 1968;21:852–70.

109. Akhtar M, Al-Dayel F, Siegrist K, Ezzat A. Neutrophil-rich Ki-1-positive anaplastic large cell lymphoma presenting as a testicular mass. Mod Pathol 1996;9:812–5.

110. Chan JK, Tsang WY, Lau WH, et al. Aggressive T/natural killer cell lymphoma presenting as testicular tumor. Cancer 1996;77:1198–205.

111. Dolin S, Dewar JP. Extramedullary plasmacytoma. Am J Pathol 1956;32:83–103.

112. Doll DC, Weiss RB. Malignant lymphoma of the testis. Am J Med 1986;81:515–24.

113. Economopoulos T, Alexopoulos C, Anagnostou D, Stathakis N, Constantinidou M, Papageorgious E. Primary granulocytic sarcoma of the testis. Leukemia 1994;8:199–200.

114. Ferry JA, Harris NL, Young RH, Coen J, Zietman A, Scully RE. Malignant lymphoma of the testis, epididymis, and spermatic cord: a clinicopathological study of 69 cases with immunophenotypic analysis. Am J Surg Pathol 1994;18:376–90.

115. Ferry JA, Srigley JR, Young RH. Granulocytic sarcoma of the testis. A report of two cases of a neoplasm prone to misinterpretation. Mod Pathol 1997;10:320–5.

116. Ferry JA, Ulbright TM, Young RH. Anaplastic large cell lymphoma of the testis: a lesion that may be confused with embryonal carcinoma. J Urol Pathol 1996;5:139–47.

117. Ferry JA, Young RH, Scully RE. Testicular and epididymal plasmacytoma: a report of 7 cases, including three that were the initial manifestation of plasma cell myeloma. Am J Surg Pathol 1997;21:590–8.

117a. Froberg MK, Hamati H, Kant JA, Addya K, Salhany KE. Primary low-grade T-helper cell testicular lymphoma. Arch Pathol Lab Med 1997;121:1096–9.

117b. Givler RL. Testicular involvement in leukemia and lymphoma. Cancer 1969;23:1290–5.

118. Gowing NF. Malignant lymphoma of the testis. Br J Urol 1964;36:85–94.

119. Haddy TB, Sandlund JT, Magrath IT. Testicular involvement in young patients with non-Hodgkin's lymphoma. Am J Pediatr Hematol Oncol 1988;10:224–9.

120. Hayes DW, Bennett WA, Heck FJ. Extramedullary lesions in multiple myeloma. Review of literature and pathologic studies. Arch Pathol 1952;53:262–72.

121. Hayes MM, Sacks MI, King HS. Testicular lymphoma. A retrospective review of 17 cases. South Afr Med J 1983;64:1014–6.

122. Hsueh C, Gonzalez-Crussi F, Murphy SB. Testicular angiocentric lymphoma of postthymic T-cell type in a child with T-cell acute lymphoblastic leukemia in remission. Cancer 1993;72:1801–5.

123. Iizumi T, Shinohara S, Amemiya H, et al. Plasmacytoma of the testis. Urol Int 1995;55:218–21.

124. Jackson SM, Montessori GA. Malignant lymphoma of the testis: review of 17 cases in British Columbia with survival related to pathological subclassification J Urol 1980;123:881–3.

125. Levin HS, Mostofi FK. Symptomatic plasmacytoma of the testis. Cancer 1970;25:1193–203.

126. Martenson JA Jr, Buskirk SJ, Ilstrup DM, et al. Patterns of failure in primary testicular non-Hodgkin's lymphoma. J Clin Oncol 1988;6:297–302.

127. McDermott MB, O'Briain DS, Shiels OM, Daly PA. Malignant lymphoma of the epididymis. A case report of bilateral involvement by a follicular large cell lymphoma. Cancer 1995;75:2174–9.

128. Mehrota RM, Wahal KM, Agarwal PK. Testicular lymphoma: a clinicopathologic study of 22 cases. Ind J Pathol Microbiol 1978;21:91–6.

128a. Melicow M. Classification of tumors of the testis: a clinical and pathological study based on 105 primary and 13 secondary cases in adults, and 3 primary and 4 secondary cases in children. J Urol 1955;73:547–74.

129. Melicow MM, Cahill GF. Plasmacytoma (multiple myeloma) of testis: a report of four cases and review of the literature. J Urol 1954;71:103–13.

130. Moertel CL, Watterson J, McCormick SR, Simonton SC. Follicular large cell lymphoma of the testis in a child. Cancer 1995;75:1182–6.

131. Moller MB, d'Amore F, Christensen BE. Testicular lymphoma: a population-based study of incidence, clinicopathological correlations and prognosis. The Danish Lymphoma Study Group, LYFO. Eur J Cancer 1994;30A:1760–4.

132. Neiman RS, Barcos M, Berard C, et al. Granulocytic sarcoma: a clinicopathologic study of 61 biopsied cases. Cancer 1981;48:1426–37.

133. Nonomura N, Aozasa K, Ueda T, et al. Malignant lymphoma of the testis: histological and immunohistological study of 28 cases. J Urol 1989;141:1368–71.

134. Saxena A, Saidman B, Greenwald D, Wasik MA. Testicular extramedullary myeloid cell tumor in a patient with myelodysplastic syndrome. Arch Pathol Lab Med 1996;120:389–92.

135. Sussman EB, Hajdu SI, Lieberman PH, Whitmore WF. Maligant lymphoma of the testis: a clinicopathological study of 37 cases. J Urol 1977;118:1004–7.

136. Talerman A. Primary malignant lymphoma of the testis. J Urol 1977;118:783–6.

137. Turner RR, Colby TV, MacKintosh FR. Testicular lymphomas: a clinicopathologic study of 35 cases. Cancer 1981;48:2095–102.

137a. Unger PD, Strauchen JA, Greenberg M, Kirschenbaum A, Rabinowitz A, Parsons RB. Testicular plasmacytoma: a report of a case and a review of the literature. J Urol Pathol 1998;7:207–14.

138. Wilkins BS, Williamson JM, O'Brien CJ. Morphological and immunohistological study of testicular lymphomas. Histopathology 1989;15:147–56.

Secondary Tumors

139. Berdjis CC, Mostofi FK. Carcinoid tumors of the testis. J Urol 1977;118:777–82.

140. Bouvier DP, Fox CW Jr, Frishberg DP, Kozakowski M, Cobos E. A solitary testicular relapse of a rhabdomyosarcoma in an adult. Cancer 1990;65:2611–4.

140a. Carr NJ, Sobin LH. Unusual tumors of the appendix and pseudomyoma peritonei. Semin Diagn Pathol 1996;13:314–25.

141. Cho KR, Olson JL, Epstein JI. Primitive rhabdomyosarcoma presenting with diffuse bone marrow involvement: an immunohistochemical and ultrastructural study. Mod Pathol 1988;1:23–8.

142. Dockerty MB, Scheifley CH. Metastasizing carcinoid; report of an unusual case with episodic cyanosis. Am J Clin Pathol 1955;25:770–4.

143. Grignon DJ, Shum DT, Hayman WP. Metastatic tumours of the testes. Can J Surg 1986;29:359–61.

144. Gupta TD, Grabstald H. Melanoma of the genitourinary tract. J Urol 1965;93:607–14.

145. Hanash KA. Metastatic tumors to the testicles. In: Khoury S, ed. Progress in clinical and biological research, Vol. 203. Testicular cancer. New York: Alan R. Liss, Inc, 1985:61–7.

146. Hanash KA, Carney JA, Kelalis PP. Metastatic tumors to testicles: routes of metastasis. J Urol 1969;102:465–8.

147. Haupt HM, Mann RB, Trump DL, Abeloff MD. Metastatic carcinoma involving the testis. Clinical and pathologic distinction from primary testicular neoplasms. Cancer 1984;54:709–14.

148. Johansson JE, Lannes P. Metastases to the spermatic cord, epididymis and testicles from carcinoma of the prostate–five cases. Scand J Urol Nephrol 1983;17:249–51.

149. Johnson DE, Jackson L, Ayala AG. Secondary carcinoma of the testis. South Med J 1971;64:1128–30.

150. Kanomata N, Eble JN. Adenocarcinoma of the pancreas presently as an epididymal mass. J Urol Pathol 1997;6:159–70.

151. Kushner BH, Vogel R, Hajdu SI, Helson L. Metastatic neuroblastoma and testicular involvement. Cancer 1985;56:1730–2.

151a. Lioe TF, Biggart JD. Tumors of the spermatic cord and paratesticular tumors. A clinicopathological study. Br J Urol 1993;71:600–6.

151b. Lodato RF, Zentner GJ, Gomez CA, Nochomovitz LE. Scrotal carcinoid. Presenting manifestation of multiple lesions in the small intestine. Cancer 1991;96:664–8.

152. Lowell DM, Lewis EL. Melanospermia: a hitherto undescribed entity. J Urol 1966;95:407–11.

153. Moore JB, Law DK, Moore EE, Dean CM. Testicular mass: an initial sign of colon carcinoma. Cancer 1982;49:411–2.

154. Patel SR, Richardson RL, Kvols L. Metastatic cancer to the testes: a report of 20 cases and review of the literature. J Urol 1989;142:1003–5.

155. Pienkos EJ, Jablokow VR. Secondary testicular tumors. Cancer 1972;30:481–5.

156. Price EB, Mostofi FK. Secondary carcinoma of the testis. Cancer 1957;10:592–5.

157. Ribalta T, Ro JY, Sahin AA, Dexeus FH, Ayala AG. Intrascrotally metastatic renal cell carcinoma. Report of two cases and review of the literature. J Urol Pathol 1993;1:201–9.

158. Richardson PG, Millward MJ, Shrimankar JJ, Cantwell BM. Metastatic melanoma to the testis simulating primary seminoma. Br J Urol 1992;69:663–5.

159. Ro JY, Ayala AG, Tetu B, et al. Merkel cell carcinoma metastatic to the testis. Am J Clin Pathol 1990;94:384–9.

160. Ro JY, Sahin AA, Ayala AG, Ordonez NG, Grignon DJ, Popok SM. Lung carcinoma with metastasis to testicular seminoma. Cancer 1990;66:347–53.

161. Scully RE, Parham AR. Testicular tumors. II. Interstitial cell and miscellaneous neoplasms. Arch Pathol 1948;46:229–42.

162. Tiltman AJ. Metastatic tumors in the testis. Histopathology 1979;3:31–7.

163. Young RH, Rosenberg AE, Clement PB. Mucin deposits within inguinal hernia sacs: a presenting finding of low grade mucinous cystic tumors of the appendix. A report of two cases and review of the literature. Mod Pathol 1997;10:1228–32.

164. Young RH, Van Patter HT, Scully RE. Hepatocellular carcinoma metastatic to the testis. Am J Clin Pathol 1987;87:117–20.

8

TUMOR-LIKE LESIONS OF TESTIS, PARATESTIS, AND SPERMATIC CORD

Although the majority of masses within the scrotal sac are neoplasms, a few are the result of diverse non-neoplastic processes (4,5). The proportion of non-neoplastic mimics of neoplasms varies widely in the literature: one comprehensive review from the British Testicular Tumour Panel reported a frequency of 6 percent (1); another series from a large general hospital in the United States found that almost 30 percent of processes encountered in over 200 explorations performed for the suspicion of testicular or paratesticular cancer were non-neoplastic (Table 8-1) (3). This chapter focuses primarily on lesions that may be misinterpreted by the pathologist; certain non-neoplastic processes that are not prone to misinterpretation as preneoplastic or neoplastic are not covered, and excellent reviews of these topics are available in other sources (6). A similar comment pertains to most lesions of infectious nature (2) which are generally clinically recognized as such, although a few particular infectious processes are mentioned here.

LEYDIG CELL HYPERPLASIA AND EXTRAPARENCHYMAL LEYDIG CELLS

Leydig cell hyperplasia occurs whenever the testis is exposed to elevated levels of luteinizing hormone, as in cases of central precocity and the androgen insensitivity syndrome, or chorionic gonadotropin, which may be secreted by several types of neoplasm (Table 8-2) (7–14). Rarely, Leydig cells mature morphologically and physiologically independently of pituitary stimulation (gonadotropin-independent sexual precocity; testotoxicosis) (see page 321) (7,14a).

In testes with marked tubular atrophy and sclerosis, Leydig cells may appear hyperplastic, forming nodular aggregates or growing diffusely and occupying much of the parenchyma. Although it is uncertain if such prominence of Leydig cells

Table 8-1

NON-NEOPLASTIC DISORDERS SIMULATING NEOPLASMS

Disorder	Series A*	Series B**
Idiopathic granulomatous orchitis	16	8
Nonspecific epididymo-orchitis	5	—
Sperm granuloma	4	—
Hydrocele with marked fibrosis†	4	19
Fibrous pseudotumor	3	—
Malakoplakia	1	—
Syphilitic gumma	1	—
Tuberculous epididymo-orchitis	1	9
Inflammatory pseudotumor	1	—
Organized hematoma	1	—
Cysts	1	22
Torsion	—	3
Sarcoidosis	—	2
Cholesterol, xantho-, foreign body granuloma	—	4
TOTAL	38	67

*Series A: Non-neoplastic lesions of testis and paratestis simulating malignancy: British Testicular Tumour Panel, 1964 (5).
**Series B: Non-neoplastic lesions suspicious of cancer. Henry Ford Hospital, 1965-1985 (3).
†One case associated with mesothelial hyperplasia, another may possibly have represented resolved meconium periorchitis.
Note: Some lesions have been reclassified according to currently used terminology.

Table 8-2

CAUSES OF LEYDIG CELL HYPERPLASIA

1. Central sexual precocity.

2. Gonadotropin-independent sexual precocity.

3. Germ cell tumor, testicular or extratesticular, with hCG production.

4. Hepatocellular carcinoma with ectopic hCG production.

5. Klinefelter's and related syndromes.

6. Androgen insensitivity syndrome.

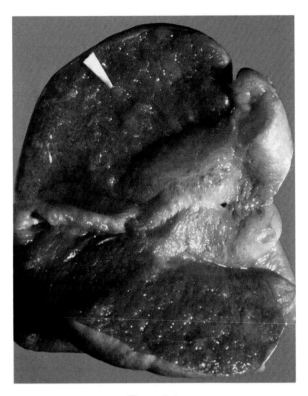

Figure 8-1
LEYDIG CELL HYPERPLASIA
Multiple, small, light tan nodules are visible within the testicular parenchyma.

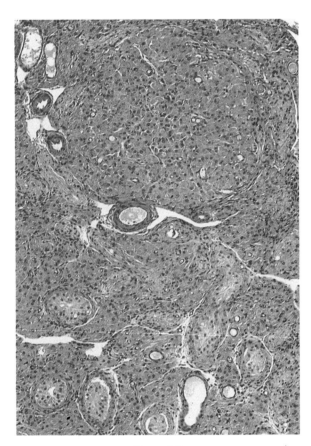

Figure 8-2
LEYDIG CELL HYPERPLASIA
Note the residual seminiferous tubules at the bottom.

reflects pseudohyperplasia secondary to tubular atrophy or true hyperplasia, it may be sufficiently striking to lead to a misdiagnosis of a neoplasm, especially in cases of Klinefelter's syndrome and related disorders.

Leydig cell hyperplasia is rarely grossly visible but can produce multiple, small, yellow-brown spots or, rarely, larger nodules (fig. 8-1). Microscopic examination shows small aggregates or nodules of Leydig cells (fig. 8-2) without effacement of underlying tubules, except occasionally over a small area. These features and the clinical background generally facilitate the distinction from a neoplasm. In atrophic testes Leydig cells may be present within the seminiferous tubules (fig. 8-3, left) (7a).

In some cases Leydig cells outside the testicular parenchyma may cause some confusion for those who are unaware that they are often present in the tunica albuginea and occasionally beyond it. In a study of almost 300 patients at autopsy (10), Leydig cells were found in the tunica albuginea in

66 percent (fig. 8-3, right), and in the paratesticular and spermatic cord soft tissue in 3 percent (fig. 8-4). A study of surgical orchiectomy specimens demonstrated extra-parenchymal Leydig cells in over 90 percent of the cases, most commonly in the testicular tunics but also in the spermatic cord in almost 15 percent (11a). These cells sometimes involve nerves (fig. 8-4) which should not be misinterpreted as indicating that they are neoplastic (7).

SERTOLI CELL NODULES

This term denotes the small clusters of immature tubules that are usually an incidental finding on microscopic examination but may be grossly visible as small, white nodules (fig. 8-5) (15). These lesions are typically encountered in cryptorchid testes, but 22 percent of descended testes in one study also harbored them (16). On

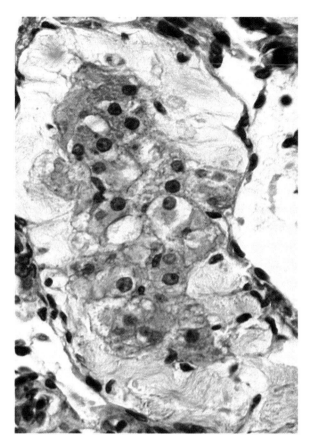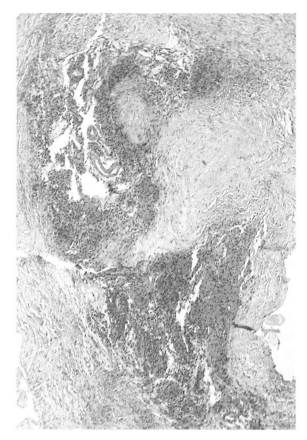

Figure 8-3
UNUSUAL LOCATIONS OF LEYDIG CELLS
Left: Leydig cells within an atrophic testicular tubule.
Right: Hyperplastic Leydig cells within the tunica albuginea.

microscopic examination, nonencapsulated aggregates of tubules lined by immature Sertoli cells typically encircle hyaline material that may resemble Call-Exner bodies or contain laminated calcific material (figs. 8-6, 8-7). The lining Sertoli cells may be associated with scattered spermatogonia in some cases, and Leydig cells are often present between the tubules (fig. 8-6). Although these lesions are often referred to in the literature as tubular adenoma, Pick's adenoma, or Sertoli cell adenoma, they are almost certainly non-neoplastic. Their characteristic morphology and usual microscopic size permit their distinction from true Sertoli or Sertoli-Leydig cell tumors. In patients with germ cell tumors, Sertoli cell nodules may be colonized by intratubular germ cell neoplasia, unclassified type (IGCNU) and thereby resemble gonadoblastoma (see fig. 5-19).

TESTICULAR "TUMOR" OF THE ADRENOGENITAL SYNDROME

General and Clinical Features. Masses composed of steroid-type cells develop in the testes of a significant number of males with untreated or inadequately treated adrenogenital syndrome (18,19,21,22,25,27). These masses, which may become evident in childhood or adult life, occur most often in patients with the salt-losing form of the disorder (21-hydroxylase deficiency). Clues to the diagnosis include clinical evidence of the adrenogenital syndrome or a family history of it, and bilateral testicular involvement. Laboratory examination shows the features of the underlying adrenogenital syndrome, including elevated plasma levels of adrenocorticotropic hormone (ACTH), androstenedione, and 17-hydroxyprogesterone, and increases

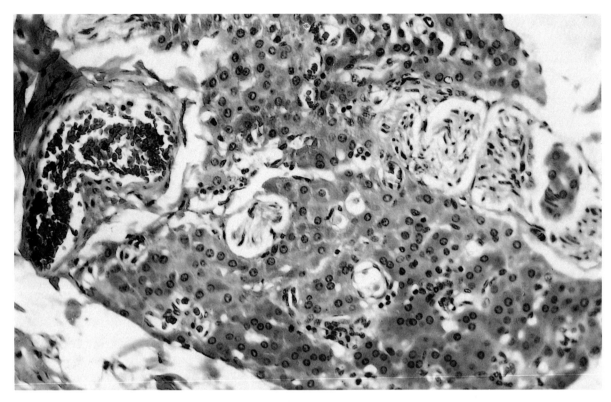

Figure 8-4
LEYDIG CELL HYPERPLASIA
Aggregates of Leydig cells are associated with nerves and blood vessels in the spermatic cord. (Fig. 83, Fascicles 31b and 32, 1st Series.)

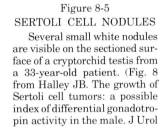

Figure 8-5
SERTOLI CELL NODULES
Several small white nodules are visible on the sectioned surface of a cryptorchid testis from a 33-year-old patient. (Fig. 8 from Halley JB. The growth of Sertoli cell tumors: a possible index of differential gonadotropin activity in the male. J Urol 1963;90:220–9.)

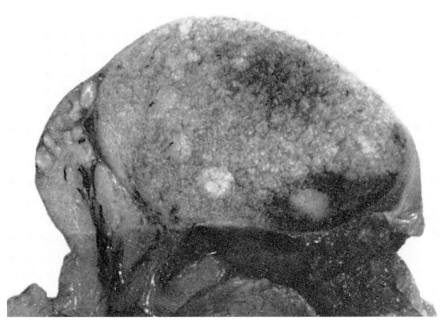

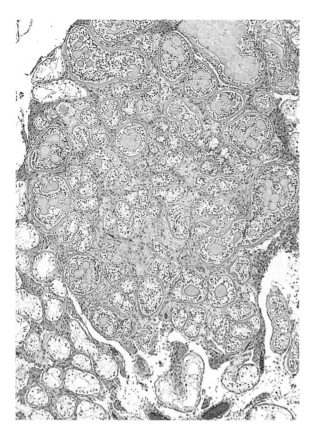

Figure 8-6
SERTOLI CELL NODULE
The periphery of the lesion is well circumscribed but somewhat irregular. Note Leydig cells in the stroma.

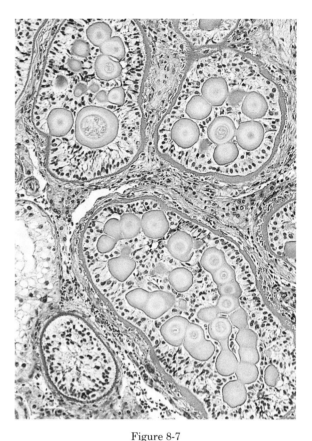

Figure 8-7
SERTOLI CELL NODULE
The annular hyaline foci, which are sometimes calcified, may suggest Call-Exner bodies or a sex cord tumor with annular tubules.

in urinary 17-ketosteroids and pregnanetriol. A persistent elevation of 17-ketosteroids in the absence of detectable metastatic disease after the removal of a "Leydig cell tumor" suggests the possibility of an underlying adrenogenital syndrome. Other characteristic features of these tumors are their enlargement and enhanced hormonal secretion after the administration of ACTH (22) and a decrease in their size and hormone output after suppression of ACTH by the administration of corticosteroids. Since they respond to ACTH suppression, surgical excision is generally considered unnecessary except for cosmetic reasons. Nonetheless, the report of one patient with the adrenogenital syndrome who developed a malignant tumor interpreted as a Leydig cell tumor (crystals of Reinke were not identified) (20) provides a cautionary note against considering all steroid cell tumors in these patients as invariably

benign. One reported case occurred in a cryptorchid testis and was admixed with a myelolipoma and had an adjacent seminoma (16a).

Gross Findings. The masses measure up to 10 cm in diameter, appear to originate in the hilar region, and extend peripherally into the parenchyma. Sectioning typically reveals multiple dark brown nodules or a single lobulated mass traversed by fibrous septa (fig. 8-8).

Microscopic Findings. Large cells that resemble Leydig cells typically grow diffusely or in large nodules (fig. 8-9). Seminiferous tubules may be encountered within the lesion, and there may be hyaline fibrosis of the stroma. The cells have abundant eosinophilic cytoplasm which typically contains a large amount of lipochrome pigment (fig. 8-9) but lacks crystals of Reinke. The nuclei may be atypical (fig. 8-10), and abnormal mitotic figures are rarely seen.

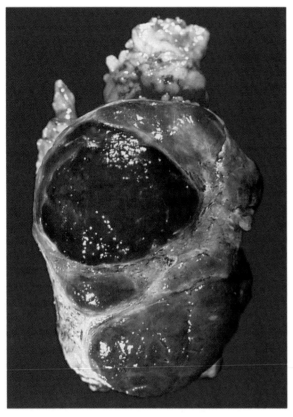

Figure 8-8
TESTICULAR "TUMOR" OF THE
ADRENOGENITAL SYNDROME

The mass is composed of multiple brown-green to almost black nodules intersected by fibrous septa. (Fig. 9.5 from Young RH, Scully RE. Testicular tumors, Chicago: ASCP Press, 1990:201.)

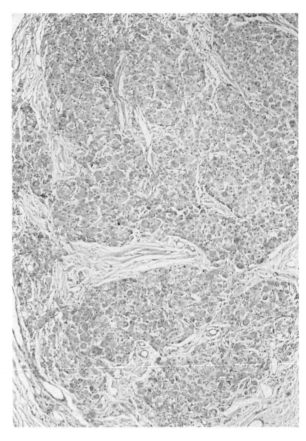

Figure 8-9
TESTICULAR "TUMOR" OF THE
ADRENOGENITAL SYNDROME

The lesional cells grow in nodular aggregates and contain large amounts of brown-yellow lipochrome pigment in their cytoplasm.

Figure 8-10
TESTICULAR "TUMOR"
OF THE ADRENOGENITAL
SYNDROME

The lesional cells have abundant, slightly granular, eosinophilic cytoplasm, and there is slight nuclear variability.

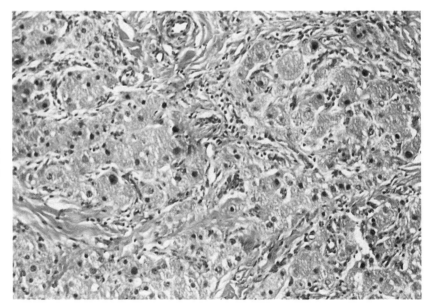

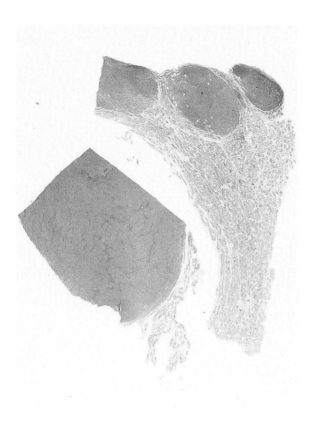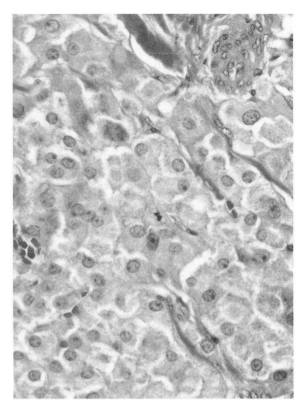

Figure 8-11
TESTICULAR "TUMOR" OF NELSON'S SYNDROME

Left: Multiple nodules of different sizes are present in the testis.

Right: The cells in the nodules have pale, eosinophilic cytoplasm and abundant lipochrome. There are scattered mitotic figures (center). (Courtesy of Dr. H. Levin, Cleveland, OH.)

Differential Diagnosis. The usual bilaterality and frequent multifocality of these masses contrasts with the usual solitary nature of Leydig cell tumors. They are typically dark brown, whereas Leydig cell tumors are more often yellow or yellow-tan. Preserved seminiferous tubules may be present within them but are found only rarely within a Leydig cell tumor. The cells tend to be larger and to have more abundant cytoplasm than those of Leydig cell tumors and contain lipochrome pigment more frequently and in greater amounts. Crystals of Reinke have not been identified within the cells but are found in at least one third of Leydig cell tumors. A recent series of three boys with precocious puberty due to the adrenogenital syndrome, each of whom had bilateral testicular tumors, emphasizes the potential for misdiagnosis, even in contemporary series, as two of the cases were initially misdiagnosed as Leydig cell tumors (25a).

STEROID CELL NODULES WITH OTHER ADRENAL DISEASES

Testicular or paratesticular nodules of steroid cells may be seen in patients with Nelson's syndrome (the rapid growth of an ACTH-secreting pituitary adenoma after bilateral adrenalectomy for Cushing's syndrome) (23,24). These lesions have biologic, biochemical, and pathologic similarities to the lesions of the adrenogenital syndrome, and they develop in the setting of elevated ACTH levels and may produce cortisol with the resultant recurrence of the Cushing's syndrome. The gross and microscopic features are as described above for the adrenogenital syndrome (fig. 8-11).

Testicular steroid cell nodules also develop in patients who have features of the syndrome described by Carney as "the complex of myxomas, spotty pigmentation, and endocrine overactivity"

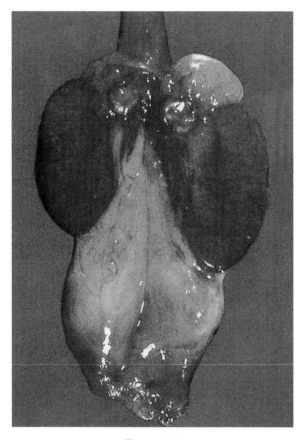

Figure 8-12
ADRENAL CORTICAL REST
A discrete, small, round, orange-yellow nodule lies between the testis and epididymis. (Fig. 9.1 from Young RH, Scully RE. Testicular tumors, Chicago: ASCP Press, 1990:199.)

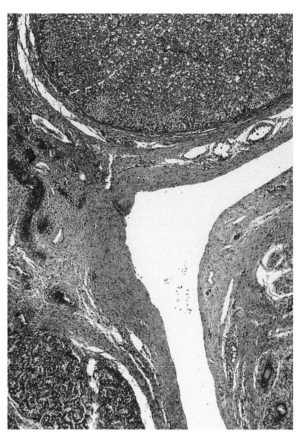

Figure 8-13
ADRENAL CORTICAL REST
A portion of the well-encapsulated nodule of adrenal cortical tissue is seen at the top, with fetal testis and epididymis at the bottom. (Courtesy of Dr. E. Lack, Washington, DC.)

(17). These patients usually have normal or low ACTH levels and primary pigmented nodular adrenocortical hyperplasia or a pituitary adenoma that secretes growth hormone. The steroid cell nodules are usually found incidentally when the patients are discovered to have a large cell calcifying Sertoli cell tumor (see page 202), the most common testicular manifestation of this unusual syndrome. Although crystals of Reinke have been identified in the steroid cell nodules in at least one of these cases, indicating a Leydig cell nature, they have not been found in the majority of them. The steroid cell nodules may be located in the hilus and may be associated with cells that appear to be mature adipocytes. A case of bilateral, small, hilar steroid cell nodules was described in a 4-year-old boy (26) with

Cushing's syndrome and adrenal nodular hyperplasia; Rutgers and associates (27) recorded a similar case. These lesions are also similar to those of the adrenogenital syndrome.

ADRENAL CORTICAL RESTS

Yellow-orange nodules of ectopic adrenocortical tissue, usually under 0.5 cm in diameter, are found in the spermatic cord, epididymis, rete testis, and tunica albuginea, and between the epididymis and testis, in approximately 10 percent of infants (fig. 8-12); they are also seen occasionally in older males (28–30). Microscopic examination reveals encapsulated nodules (fig. 8-13) that typically exhibit the zonation of the normal adrenal cortex (fig. 8-14); occasionally, the rests are unencapsulated.

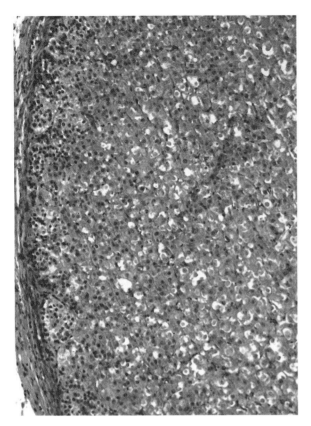

Figure 8-14
ADRENAL CORTICAL REST
Most of the cells are of the fetal cortical type. A thin layer of definitive cortex is present just beneath the capsule. (Courtesy of Dr. E. Lack, Washington, DC.)

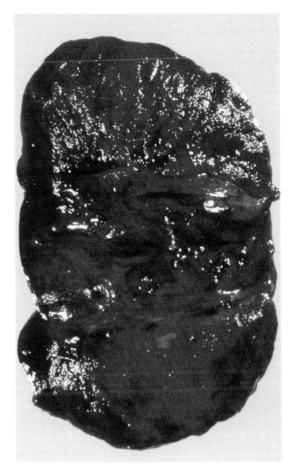

Figure 8-15
HEMORRHAGIC INFARCTION OF TESTIS

TORSION, INFARCTS, AND HEMATOMAS OF TESTIS

A testicular infarct may be caused by thrombotic vascular occlusion or torsion (36). Conditions predisposing to thrombosis include polycythemia, infections (32b), trauma, vasculitis (32c), inherited coagulation disorders, and sickle cell disease (32a). Occasionally, a testicular infarct clinically simulates a neoplasm, particularly when the infarct is remote (33). The sectioned surfaces of an infarct may be hemorrhagic (fig. 8-15) or pale (fig. 8-16). Microscopic examination shows necrotic tubules and, in most cases, varying degrees of hemorrhage. Care should be taken to exclude a necrotic tumor such as a seminoma that may possibly be mistaken for an infarct. The underlying pattern of a neoplasm, with ghost outlines of tumor cells, is still visible in such cases, and there are usually some residual, non-necrotic seminiferous tubules that may demonstrate IGCNU. Old infarcts may be associated with marked fibrosis, cholesterol clefts, and calcification (fig. 8-17). Torsion may induce prominent reactive changes in the paratesticular soft tissues that simulate an inflammatory pseudotumor (see page 313) (38).

In utero infarction of the testis, designated as either the "vanishing testis syndrome" (34a) or the "testicular regression syndrome" (36a), results in a small, fibrotic nodule that may not be readily identifiable as a testis. Patients typically present in infancy with an impalpable testis, and scrotal exploration identifies a "fibrous nubbin," usually attached to an identifiable vas deferens (fig. 8-18) (34a). The epididymis is less consistently present; Smith and coworkers (36a) identified it in 36 percent of the 77 cases they studied. The left testis is involved in about three fourths of these

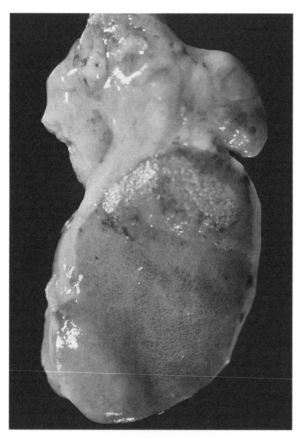

Figure 8-16
TESTICULAR INFARCT, REMOTE
The granular yellow lesion in the upper pole of the testis was clinically thought to be a neoplasm.

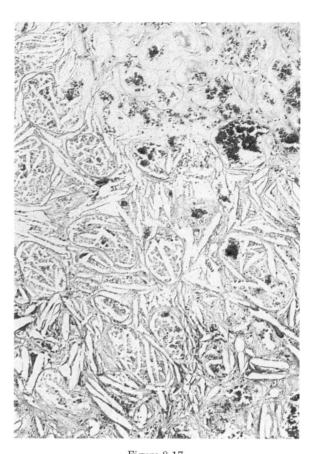

Figure 8-17
TESTICULAR INFARCT, REMOTE
There are cholesterol clefts and focal calcification, with "ghost" outlines of seminiferous tubules.

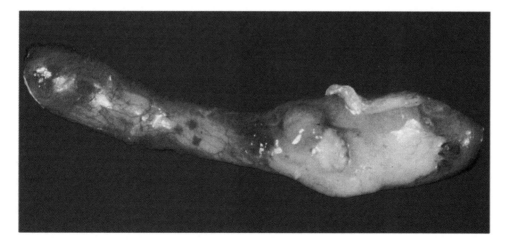

Figure 8-18
INFARCTION OF TESTIS IN UTERO
The spermatic cord terminates in a fibrous "nubbin" that represents the infarcted testis. (Courtesy of Dr. A.R. Schned, Lebanon, NH.)

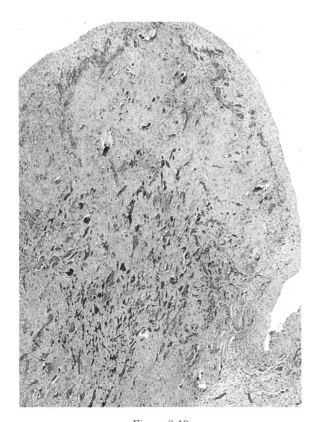

Figure 8-19
INFARCTION OF TESTIS IN UTERO
The shape of a fetal testis is recognizable, but the entire organ is infarcted with secondary fibrosis.

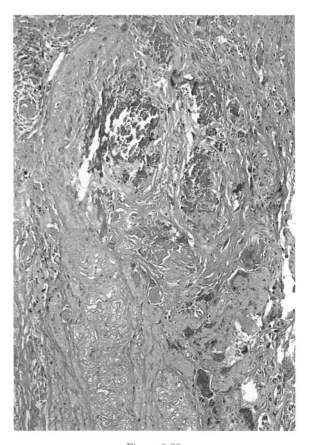

Figure 8-20
INFARCTION OF TESTIS IN UTERO
There is prominent calcification and hemosiderin deposition in a dense fibrous stroma.

cases (34a). On microscopic examination there are calcifications, often with a ring-like configuration, in a variably dense fibrous stroma with hemosiderin deposits (figs. 8-19, 8-20) and, sometimes, multinucleated giant cells. Atrophic fibers from the cremasteric muscle may mimic Leydig cells in these cases (34a). Seminiferous tubule remnants are often not apparent (34a,36a).

Although testicular hemorrhage is usually related to infarction or a malignant neoplasm, rupture of an artery secondary to arteritis (32, 35) may lead, rarely, to the formation of a large hematoma (fig. 8-21) which may be confused on gross examination with a choriocarcinoma (31a). Sometimes the inflammation and edema of testicular and paratesticular vasculitis, in the absence of a hematoma, result in a mass that clinically mimics a neoplasm (31b). Testicular and epididymal vasculitis may be accompanied or followed by evidence of systemic vasculitis, but it may also occur as an isolated phenomenon

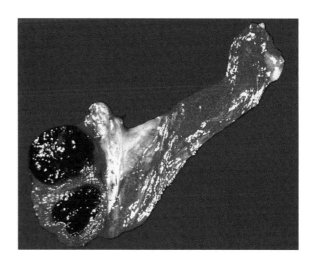

Figure 8-21
HEMATOMA OF TESTIS
The large, sharply circumscribed hematoma is secondary to a localized necrotizing arteritis with rupture. (Fig. 9.42 from Young RH, Scully RE. Testicular tumors, Chicago: ASCP Press, 1990:219.)

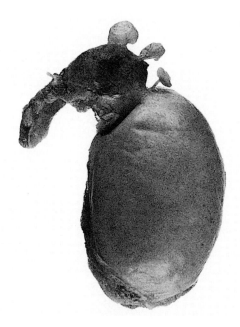

Figure 8-22
MAJOR TESTICULAR APPENDAGES
From left to right: the paradidymis (organ of Giraldes),
appendix epididymis, and appendix testis. (Fig. 104A from
Algaba F. Atlas de patologia de los tumores urogenitales.
Barcelona: Fundacion Puigvert, 1991.)

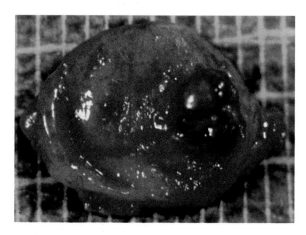

Figure 8-23
INFARCTED APPENDIX TESTIS
There is a discrete hemorrhagic nodule.

(32c,37a). In cases of periarteritis nodosa, there
is commonly paratesticular and testicular involvement, with secondary infarcts (32). Granulomatous vasculitis may also involve either the
testis or paratestis, causing a tumor-like mass
(31b). We have seen such a case associated with
Crohn's disease (33b).

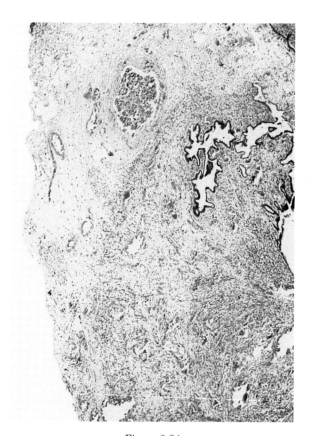

Figure 8-24
INFARCTED APPENDIX TESTIS
Some viable epithelium is visible, but the remaining
tissue is infarcted with focal calcification.

THE TESTICULAR APPENDAGES AND WALTHARD NESTS

There are five testicular appendages: the appendix testis (hydatid of Morgagni), the appendix epididymis, the paradidymis (organ of
Giraldes), and the inferior and superior aberrant
ducts (vas aberrans of Haller) (34,37). The latter
two are infrequently present and not the source
of any concern for surgical pathologists. In most
instances the paradidymis is not as striking
grossly as it is in the accompanying illustration
(fig. 8-22) in which it is seen as the most superior
of the three visible appendages, that in the middle
being the appendix epididymis and the inferior the
appendix testis with its characteristic attachment
to the anterior-superior aspect of the upper pole
of the testis (see also figs. 1-4, 1-5). Because the
latter two structures are those that are usually
grossly visible and often are pedunculated, they

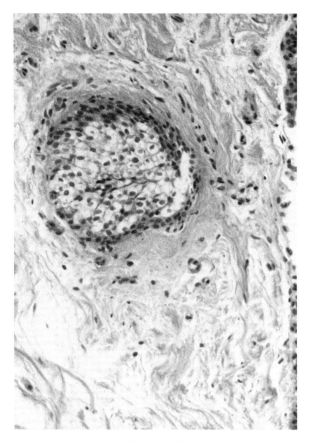

Figure 8-25
WALTHARD NEST
A discrete nest of transitional cells is present in the lining of the tunica vaginalis.

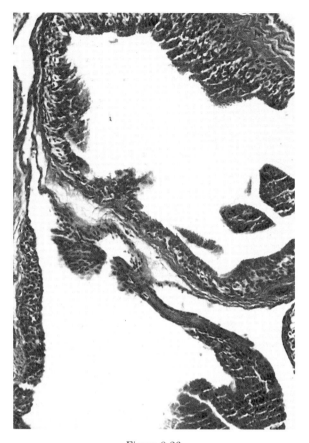

Figure 8-26
CYSTIC WALTHARD NESTS
Much of the lining epithelium is compressed, but residual transitional cells are evident, particularly at the top.

may undergo torsion and infarction (figs. 8-23, 8-24) with accompanying significant symptoms (31,33a). Identifying the characteristic structure and epithelium of the appendages is often difficult but may be important to establish the correct clinicopathologic correlation. Confusion with a neoplasm is unlikely. The classic study of Sundarasivarao (37) provides detailed information on the testicular appendages, but a brief summary follows.

The appendix testis is found in about 80 percent of carefully examined testes (37). It typically measures from 2 to 4 mm but may occasionally be larger, and contains a fibrovascular core of loose connective tissue covered by simple cuboidal to low columnar müllerian-type epithelium that merges with the mesothelium of the tunica vaginalis lateral to its base. The epithelium typically invagi-

nates into the underlying stroma, but isolated müllerian duct remnants may also be seen in the stroma, which is occasionally calcified.

The usually cystic appendix epididymis is less frequently present (about 25 percent of the cases) and arises from the anterior-superior pole of the head of the epididymis. It is lined by cuboidal to low columnar epithelium which may be ciliated and shows some secretory activity. Rarely, marked cystic change of the appendix epididymis presents as a paratesticular mass (36b).

The mesothelium of the tunica vaginalis undergoes transitional metaplasia in about 12 percent of cases (37). This results in epithelial nests (fig. 8-25) similar to the Walthard nests that commonly occur on the serosa of the fallopian tube in females, and, like them, they may undergo cystic change (fig. 8-26).

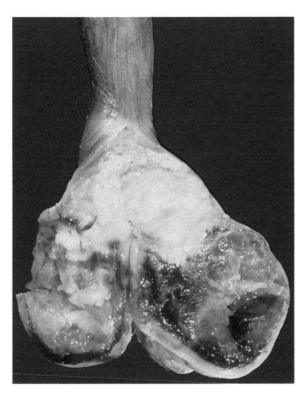

Figure 8-27
CHRONIC EPIDIDYMO-ORCHITIS
There is prominent destruction of the testicular parenchyma with cyst formation and extensive involvement of the epididymis and paratesticular soft tissues by fibrosis.

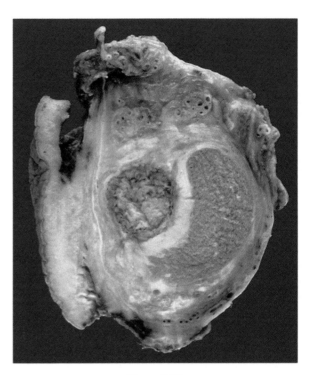

Figure 8-28
EPIDIDYMAL ABSCESS
An abscess centered in the epididymis is associated with marked fibrosis in the surrounding tissues but lacks significant extension into the testicular parenchyma.

ORCHITIS AND EPIDIDYMITIS

Bacterial Orchitis

In bacterial orchitis the epididymis is typically also affected, and the gross appearance is variable. The testis may contain abscesses or be fibrotic and adherent to adjacent tissues (fig. 8-27) which are also fibrotic. Occasionally, a neoplasm is suggested in longstanding cases (43,46). Isolated abscesses of the epididymis and testis are less frequently encountered; in chronic cases of the former, ill-defined, fibrotic paratesticular "masses" may be striking (fig. 8-28). Microscopic examination discloses varying amounts of acute and chronic inflammation, abscess formation, granulation tissue, and fibrosis, depending on the duration of the process. In some cases there is focal infarction, which may be the result of venous occlusion (44).

Viral Orchitis

The testis is involved in approximately one quarter of adult males with mumps, but in well under 1 percent of children with this disease. Testicular involvement is bilateral in almost one fifth of the cases and is accompanied by epididymitis in 85 percent of the cases (41). The testis is swollen and tender, and incision of the tunica albuginea reveals edema and, in some cases, hemorrhage. Microscopic examination discloses interstitial edema early in the course, followed by vascular dilatation and interstitial lymphocytic infiltration, sometimes accompanied by neutrophils and macrophages (41). Subsequently, interstitial hemorrhage occurs, along with inflammatory cell infiltration of the seminiferous tubules and degeneration of the germinal epithelium (fig. 8-29). Healing results in patchy hyalinization of tubules and interstitial fibrosis, with intervening unaffected areas.

The microscopic features of other rarely described forms of viral orchitis, many of which are

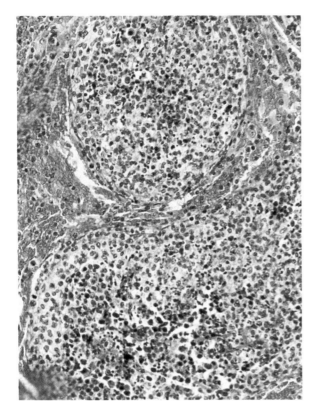

Figure 8-29
MUMPS ORCHITIS
The tubules are filled with mononuclear cells, polymorpho-
nuclear leukocytes, degenerating cells, and nuclear debris.

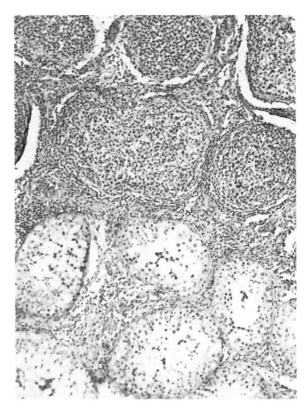

Figure 8-30
VIRAL ORCHITIS
The tubules at the top are distended by a prominent
mononuclear cell infiltrate which also involves the interstitial tissue. (Fig. 9.16 from Young RH, Scully RE. Testicular
tumors. Chicago: ASCP Press, 1990:206.)

due to coxsackie B (39), resemble those of mumps
orchitis. In the exceptional cases in which
mumps orchitis precedes parotitis or is the only
evidence of the infection, or in those cases in
which orchitis is the exclusive or major manifestation of another viral illness, the gross and
microscopic findings (figs. 8-30, 8-31) may be
confused with those of a malignant tumor, particularly a seminoma or lymphoma. However, in
orchitis the infiltrate is much more heterogenous,
and tubules are not effaced to the same degree as
in seminoma. Most importantly, cytologically malignant cells are absent, although activated lymphocytes may appear somewhat atypical.

Granulomatous Orchitis, Infectious

A vast array of infectious organisms may involve the testis and result in a granulomatous
orchitis. The list of potential pathogens includes
tuberculosis, syphilis, brucellosis, leprosy, fungi,

parasites, and rickettsia. In tuberculosis the epididymis is the primary site of genital tract involvement (fig. 8-32), and the testis is usually
affected only in the late stages (fig. 8-33) (40,47).
This sequence of involvement, the 30 percent frequency of bilaterality, and the 50 percent frequency
of an abscess or sinus tract formation are important clues to the infectious nature of the process.
Histoplasmosis (44a) or coccidioidomycosis (42a)
may selectively involve the epididymis. In cases of
syphilis, a gumma may mimic a neoplasm on
clinical and gross evaluation (fig. 8-34), but the
microscopic features (fig. 8-35) are unlike those
of any neoplasm (45). In cases of leprosy, the
testes are usually normal or decreased in size
but are occasionally enlarged. The microscopic
findings in the three stages of this disease—vascular, interstitial, and obliterative—are unlikely
to cause confusion with a neoplasm (42).

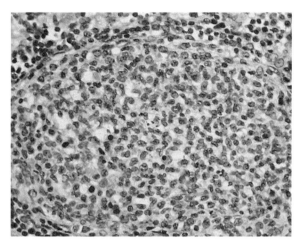

Figure 8-31
VIRAL ORCHITIS
A tubule is distended by mononuclear cells and surrounded by lymphocytes. (Fig. 9.17 from Young RH, Scully RE. Testicular tumors. Chicago: ASCP Press, 1990:207.)

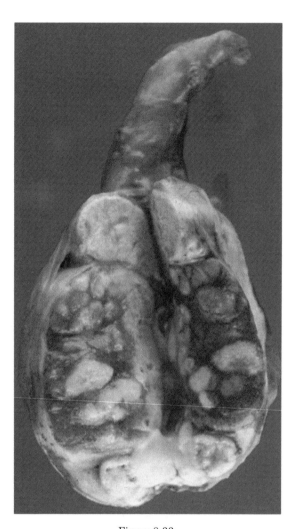

Figure 8-33
TUBERCULOSIS OF THE TESTIS
Multiple white nodules extensively involve the testicular parenchyma in this autopsy case. Note the prominent epididymal involvement. (Fig. 9.19 from Young RH, Scully RE. Testicular tumors. Chicago: ASCP Press, 190:207.)

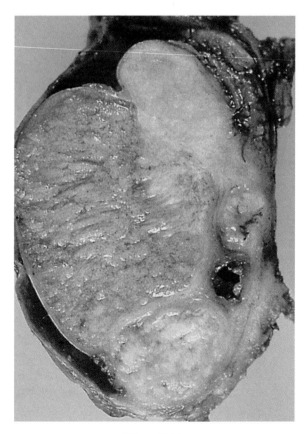

Figure 8-32
TUBERCULOUS EPIDIDYMO-ORCHITIS
There is extensive nodular involvement of the entire epididymis with secondary involvement of the testis. (Fig. 9.18 from Young RH, Scully RE. Testicular tumors. Chicago: ASCP Press, 1990:207.)

Granulomatous Orchitis, Idiopathic

General and Clinical Features. Idiopathic granulomatous orchitis accounts for 0.2 percent of testicular masses and, in the experience of the British Testicular Tumour Panel (49), is the most common non-neoplastic lesion to mimic a malignant neoplasm (Table 8-1). It usually occurs during the fifth or sixth decade (49,51), and follows a urinary tract infection with gram-negative bacilli in about two thirds of the cases. Although some cases of granulomatous orchitis may be clinically indistinguishable from a neoplasm, in

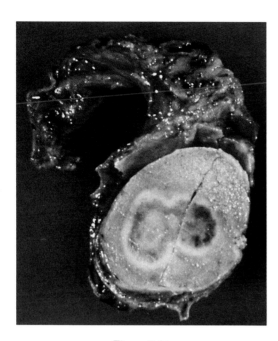

Figure 8-34
SYPHILITIC GUMMA OF TESTIS
A large area of necrotic tissue is surrounded by a thick rim of white tissue.

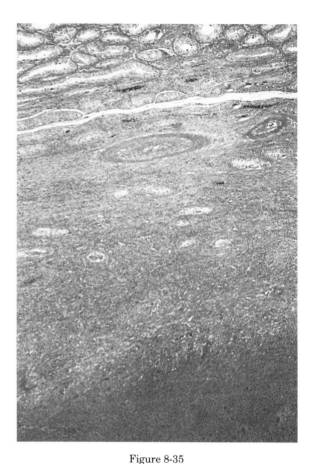

Figure 8-35
SYPHILITIC GUMMA OF TESTIS
Gummatous necrosis is bordered by a zone of fibrous tissue containing chronic inflammatory cells. (Fig. 9.21 from Young RH, Scully RE. Testicular tumors. Chicago: ASCP Press,1990:209.)

others a history of a flu-like illness, the sudden onset of testicular swelling, and the usual associated pain or tenderness suggest an inflammatory process. The testis enlarges, sometimes with pain or tenderness, which may disappear, leaving a painless mass (49). The contralateral testis is occasionally affected metachronously.

Gross Findings. Typically there is thickening of the tunica albuginea and replacement of the testicular parenchyma by homogeneous, sometimes lobulated, tan-yellow, grey, or white tissue (fig. 8-36). The process is usually diffuse but there is sometimes a localized, well-circumscribed nodule. The involved foci are often firm and rubbery and have a reduced tendency to bulge on sectioning. The epididymis and spermatic cord are involved in about half the cases, and an exudate is often present on the tunica vaginalis, which may show fibrous adhesions. Rarely, the epididymis is the site of predominant (fig. 8-37) or exclusive involvement (52) by an idiopathic granulomatous or xanthogranulomatous process (see below).

Microscopic Findings. Microscopic examination of the testis shows filling of the seminiferous tubules by inflammatory cells with a pre-

dominance of epithelioid histiocytes (fig. 8-38), but also intermixed lymphocytes and plasma cells; Langhans-type giant cells are seen in one third of the cases (fig. 8-39). The interstitial tissue contains numerous chronic inflammatory cells, including eosinophils, in most cases. In advanced stages complete obliteration of the lumens of the seminiferous tubules produces a striking follicular pattern (fig. 8-38). The process may extend to involve the epididymis.

Differential Diagnosis. The primarily intratubular location of the granulomatous process is helpful in differentiating the lesion from granulomatous orchitis of infectious origin and from sarcoidosis, in both of which the granulomas are predominantly interstitial. Necrosis within the granulomas may be seen in the infectious lesions, but is rarely, if ever, identified in idiopathic

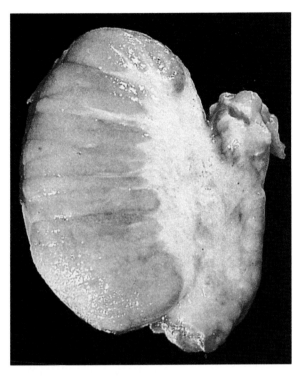

Figure 8-36
GRANULOMATOUS ORCHITIS, IDIOPATHIC
The parenchyma is replaced by lobulated, pale yellow tissue, with fibrosis in the rete and epididymis. (Fig. 9.22 from Young RH, Scully RE. Testicular tumors. Chicago: ASCP Press, 1990:209.)

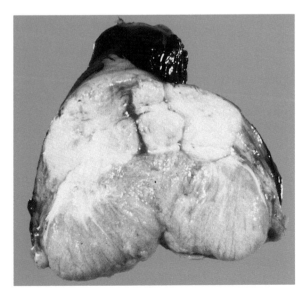

Figure 8-37
GRANULOMATOUS EPIDIDYMITIS, IDIOPATHIC
There is extensive involvement of the epididymis by an ill-defined, yellow-white mass, with lesser involvement of the testis.

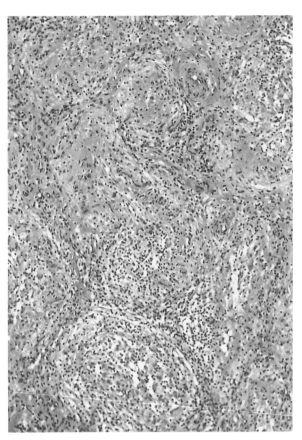

Figure 8-38
GRANULOMATOUS ORCHITIS, IDIOPATHIC
The tubules are filled with epithelioid histiocytes and chronic inflammatory cells, and the interstitium is also involved by the infiltrate.

granulomatous orchitis. Identification of organisms by smear, culture, or histochemical study of paraffin-embedded material is indicated to exclude specific forms of granulomatous orchitis. A potential pitfall in interpretation is the fact that remnants of sperm may be acid-fast positive in cases of idiopathic granulomatous orchitis. The granulomatous reaction of seminoma may cause confusion with idiopathic granulomatous orchitis but tends to have a greater interstitial rather than intratubular distribution, and seminoma cells, even if rare, can be identified.

Granulomatous Epididymitis

This rare entity is usually an incidental finding at autopsy or in surgical specimens obtained for other indications, but in one personally observed case formed a mass (fig. 8-40) that required

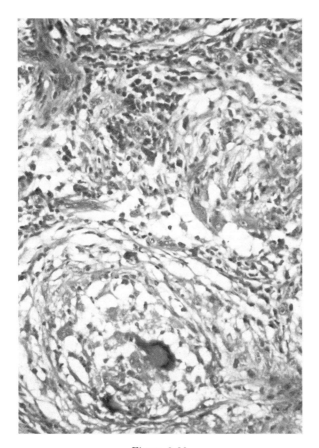

Figure 8-39
GRANULOMATOUS ORCHITIS, IDIOPATHIC
High-power view showing epithelioid histiocytes and two giant cells.

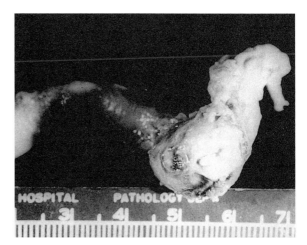

Figure 8-40
GRANULOMATOUS EPIDIDYMITIS
There is nodular thickening of the epididymis.

exploration and removal to exclude a neoplasm (52a). The patients may have a history of vascular disease, prior surgery in the region such as herniorrhaphy, or bacterial epididymitis. The reported age range is 30 to 62 years (49a). The process is unilateral, may have inconspicuous findings on gross examination, and consists of zones of necrosis centered on the efferent ducts, with a surrounding zone of granulomatous inflammation (fig. 8-41, left). Peripheral to this, and near adjacent intact ducts, a lymphocytic infiltrate occurs, but neutrophils are often inconspicuous (although in the case we have seen there was a significant intraductal neutrophilic component). Secondary changes may include sperm granulomas, ceroid granulomas, macrophage accumulation in the duct lumens, and regenerative changes of the efferent ductal epithelium including squamous metaplasia (fig. 8-41, right). An ischemic

origin is hypothesized (49a) for at least some of the cases; this appears more likely for those cases localized to the caput. Others may represent an obstructive phenomenon with duct rupture and secondary granulomatous inflammation. It is important to exclude an infectious etiology by appropriate stains and culture.

Sarcoidosis

Sarcoidosis may affect the epididymis and, rarely, the testis (50); exceptional cases with prominent testicular enlargement have provoked orchiectomy. In a review in 1993, 28 mainly black patients had epididymal involvement, with testicular involvement in 6 (50). The epididymal disease is usually unilateral, nodular (fig. 8-42), and painless, but epididymitis may be mimicked. For testicular cases, the differential diagnosis includes seminoma with massive granulomatous inflammation, but the granulomas in seminoma are typically less organized and discrete, and, although markedly obscured in some cases, seminoma cells will always be found on close scrutiny. In contrast to idiopathic granulomatous orchitis, the granulomas in sarcoidosis are interstitial.

Malakoplakia

General and Clinical Features. The testis alone is affected in about two thirds of the cases, and both the epididymis and testis in most of the remainder when all cases of testicular and adnexal

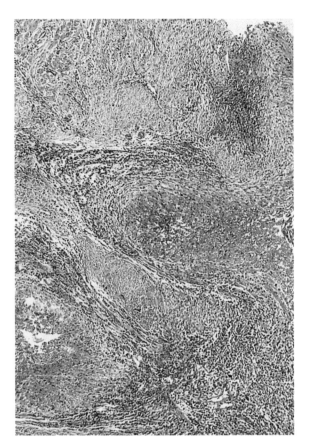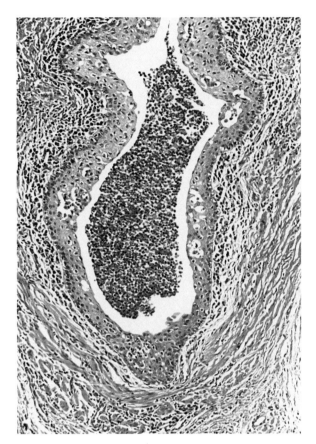

Figure 8-41
GRANULOMATOUS EPIDIDYMITIS
Left: Zones of necrosis are centered on the efferent ducts of the epididymis, with a surrounding mononuclear infiltrate.
Right: Squamous metaplasia of the epithelium of an efferent duct, with intraluminal inflammatory cells. (Both illustrations are from the case depicted in figure 8-40.)

Figure 8-42
SARCOIDOSIS OF
THE EPIDIDYMIS
The yellow-white mass simulates a neoplasm.

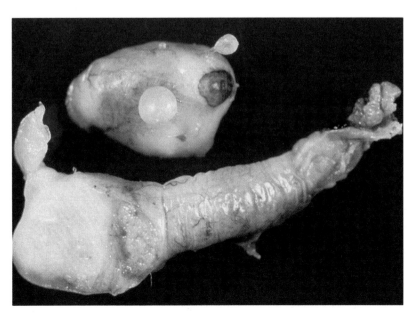

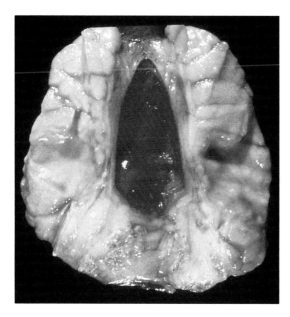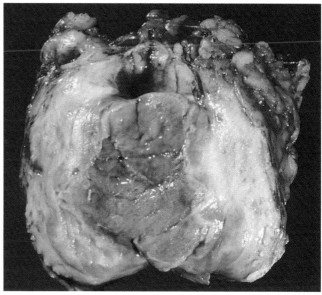

Figure 8-43
MALAKOPLAKIA OF TESTIS
Left: The testis is replaced by a lobulated yellow mass that simulates a neoplasm. There is, however, a small area of abscess formation. (Fig. 9.25 from Young RH, Scully RE. Testicular tumors. Chicago: ASCP Press, 1990:211.)
Right: In this specimen there is conspicuous abscess formation with necrotic tissue and fibrosis, more obviously indicative of an inflammatory process than the specimen on the left.

malakoplakia are considered (53,54). The right testis is more often affected than the left. Rarely, there is isolated epididymal involvement. The symptoms are nonspecific; occasionally, there is a history of a prior urinary tract infection, often with *Escherichia coli*. The testis is usually enlarged and may be difficult to remove because of fibrous adhesions to surrounding tissues. In all the reported cases, testicular enlargement was unilateral and occurred in adults.

Gross Findings. Sectioning shows replacement of all or part of the testicular parenchyma by yellow (fig. 8-43, left), tan, or brown tissue, which is often divided into lobules by bands of fibrous tissue. The consistency is usually soft, but may be firm if there is prominent fibrosis. One or more abscesses and the presence of epididymal involvement and reactive inflammatory changes in the tunics are clues to the diagnosis (fig. 8-43, right).

Microscopic Findings. Microscopic examination reveals replacement of the tubules and interstitial tissue by large histiocytes with abundant, granular, eosinophilic cytoplasm (von Hansemann cells) (fig. 8-44), some of which contain solid and targetoid, calcific, basophilic inclu-

sions of varying sizes (Michaelis-Gutmann bodies) (fig. 8-44). In occasional cases, the von Hansemann cells have a spindled configuration (fig. 8-45). Acute and chronic inflammatory cells, granulation tissue, fibrosis, and abscesses are also usually present and may obscure the characteristic features of the process, especially if Michaelis-Gutmann bodies are inconspicuous. These structures are accentuated by periodic acid–Schiff, von Kossa, and iron stains (fig. 8-46), which are positive in almost all cases. Ultrastructural studies have shown that the Michaelis-Gutmann bodies are phagolysosomes that ingest the breakdown products of bacteria of various types, most often *Escherichia coli* (54).

Differential Diagnosis. Malakoplakia is sometimes confused with a Leydig cell tumor, but the latter does not involve tubules and its cells lack the characteristic features of von Hansemann cells, including Michaelis-Gutmann bodies. Antibodies directed against histiocytic markers (CD68, KP1) and inhibin could address this differential diagnosis, with expected positive and negative results, respectively, in malakoplakia, and the opposite pattern in Leydig cell tumor.

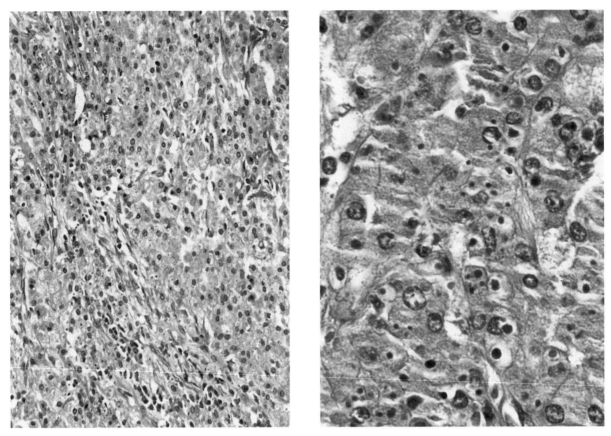

Figure 8-44
MALAKOPLAKIA OF TESTIS
Left: There is a sheet-like growth of histiocytes with eosinophilic cytoplasm (von Hansemann cells).
Right: Many eosinophilic histiocytes (von Hansemann cells) contain targetoid basophilic inclusions (Michaelis-Gutmann bodies).

Figure 8-45
MALAKOPLAKIA
OF TESTIS
The spindle-shaped cells
(left) stained for the histiocytic
marker KP1 (right).

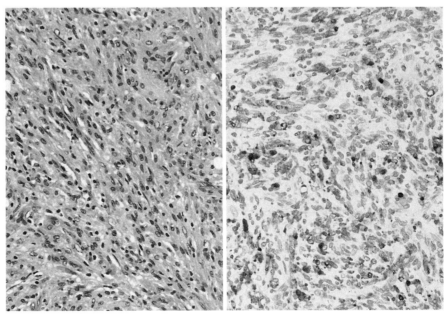

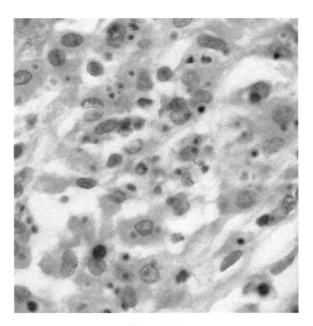

Figure 8-46
MALAKOPLAKIA OF TESTIS
Michaelis-Guttman bodies are positive with an iron stain.

ROSAI-DORFMAN DISEASE (SINUS HISTIOCYTOSIS WITH MASSIVE LYMPHADENOPATHY)

This idiopathic disease may exceptionally involve the testis and epididymis and be clinically confused with a neoplasm (54a,54b). Children or adults may be affected, and there is typically involvement at other sites, most notably lymph nodes. Testicular involvement may be bilateral (synchronous or metachronous) or unilateral. A distinct testicular or epididymal nodule may be seen, or diffuse testicular replacement may occur, with homogeneous involvement producing symmetric, firm and rubbery enlargement (fig. 8-47). On microscopic examination, the typical pale eosinophilic histiocytes, some containing lymphocytes within their cytoplasm, are distributed in the testicular interstitium (fig. 8-47) (54a). The clinical course is variable, largely depending on the extent of involvement at other sites. This process

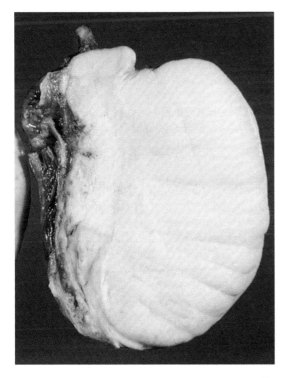
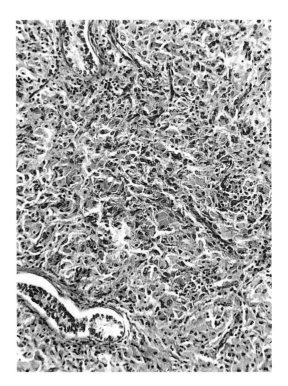

Figure 8-47
ROSAI-DORFMAN DISEASE
Left: The cut surface is homogeneous and bulging.
Right: Photomicrograph of testis depicted on the left showing plump cells with abundant cytoplasm that was eosinophilic growing between seminiferous tubules. There are also scattered chronic inflammatory cells. (Figs. 1 and 2 from Azoury FJ, Reed RJ. Histiocytosis: report of an unusual case. N Engl J Med 1966;274:928–30.) (Courtesy of Dr. R.J. Reed, New Orleans, LA.)

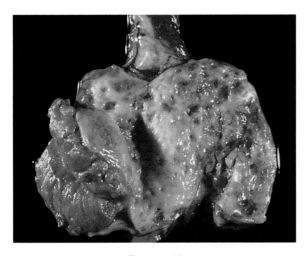

Figure 8-48
HYDROCELE SAC
There is marked, irregular thickening of the tunica vaginalis.

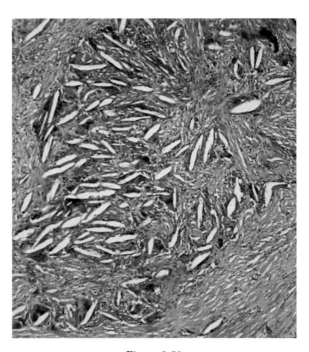

Figure 8-50
CHOLESTEROL GRANULOMA
Many cholesterol clefts are present within a fibrotic tunica vaginalis. (Courtesy of Dr. F. Algaba, Barcelona, Spain.)

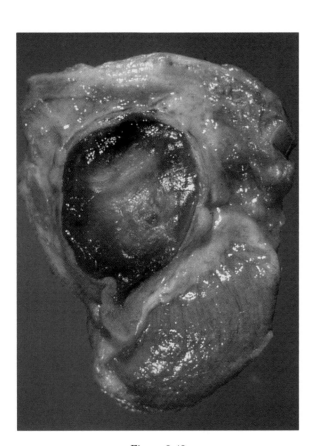

Figure 8-49
HEMATOCELE
A hydrocele sac contains an old blood clot within its lumen.

must be distinguished from true neoplastic infiltrates of histiocytic nature.

HYDROCELE-RELATED CHANGES AND MISCELLANEOUS OTHER ABNORMALITIES OF THE TUNICA VAGINALIS

In cases of simple, uncomplicated hydrocele clinical and pathologic evaluation is straightforward, but in some longstanding hydroceles there may be marked chronic inflammation and fibrosis, with tethering of the testis to the tunica such that a neoplasm is mimicked on clinical examination (fig. 8-48) (55,58). On microscopic examination, distinction from a neoplasm is straightforward. Squamous metaplasia is rarely seen (55a), providing a histogenesis for the very rare squamous cell carcinomas that complicate hydroceles (see page 271). When there is extensive hemorrhage into a hydrocele (hematocele) (fig. 8-49), thorough sectioning may be needed to exclude an underlying neoplasm. Calcification (56) and cholesterol granulomas (fig. 8-50) (57) may involve the tunica vaginalis in some cases.

INFLAMMATORY PSEUDOTUMOR (PSEUDOSARCOMATOUS MYOFIBROBLASTIC PROLIFERATION; PROLIFERATIVE FUNICULITIS)

General and Clinical Features. The spermatic cord is the most common site in the male genital tract for the lesions that are variously reported under the above and other diverse designations (59–66). They are usually incidental microscopic findings within inguinal hernia specimens, but occasionally the patient may note a mass. In some instances the appearance of an inflammatory pseudotumor in the epididymal region is an apparent reaction to testicular torsion (66) and is usually noted as an incidental microscopic finding. If not completely excised, the possibility of recurrence exists, but, by definition, these lesions are nonmetastasizing. In two cases of epididymal inflammatory pseudotumor that presented as mass lesions, in situ hybridization studies failed to detect Epstein-Barr virus RNA, unlike some inflammatory pseudotumors at other sites (58a).

Gross Findings. Typically there is an ill-defined gray-white nodule with a firm or gelatinous consistency (fig. 8-51); rarely cystic change and hemorrhage may be seen. The majority of the lesions do not exceed 3 cm in maximum dimension, but at least one measured 7 cm. Single cases of inflammatory pseudotumor occurring in the rete testis of a 26-year-old and the epididymis of a 43-year-old have been described (60,61): the first was a 1.2-cm yellow-gray mass and the second an ill-defined 1.5-cm mass at the periphery of the testis.

Microscopic Findings. There is characteristically a moderately cellular, irregular, spindle cell proliferation in a loose collagenous stroma that may be focally or conspicuously myxoid. The process is typically heterogeneous in appearance, with the cellularity differing from area to area (fig. 8-52). The overall picture varies according to the degree of associated inflammation and the nature of the stroma. In at least some cases the cellularity is more pronounced centrally (62), and there is typically a focal fascicular arrangement. The lesional mesenchymal cells (fig. 8-53) usually have plump, oval to fusiform, vesicular nuclei, and some may have conspicuous, tapering eosinophilic cytoplasm and mimic, to some degree,

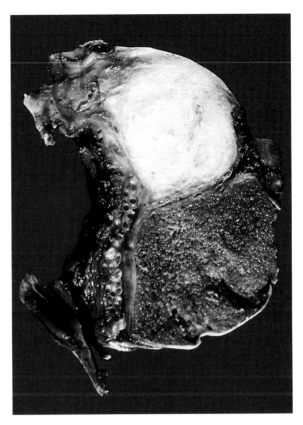

Figure 8-51
INFLAMMATORY PSEUDOTUMOR
(PROLIFERATIVE FUNICULITIS)
A solid white mass replaces much of the lower portion of the spermatic cord.

rhabdomyoblasts. In some cases the appearance of stellate cells in a myxoid background imparts a "tissue culture" appearance. Occasional cells have prominent eosinophilic nucleoli. Giant cells that are similar to those seen in proliferative fasciitis of the soft tissues may be encountered and, indeed, occasionally the appearance is indistinguishable from that of fasciitis. The mitotic rate usually does not exceed 1 per 10 high-power fields, although in two cases associated with torsion there were 3 to 10 mitotic figures per 10 high-power fields (66). Abnormal mitotic figures are characteristically absent. The lesions are typically prominently vascular and may exhibit circumferential hyaline fibrosis of blood vessel walls. Immunohistochemistry is positive for actin and vimentin, less strongly for desmin, and rarely for cytokeratin, consistent with a myofibroblastic lineage, but has no great diagnostic value.

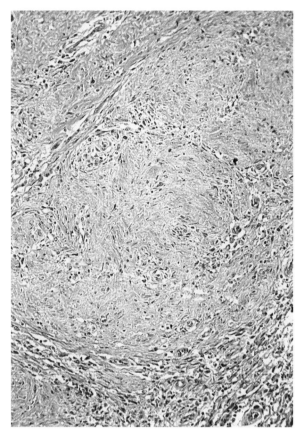

Figure 8-52
INFLAMMATORY PSEUDOTUMOR
(PROLIFERATIVE FUNICULITIS)
The lesion is characterized by myofibroblasts and inflammatory cells with marked fibrosis. (Courtesy of Dr. C.D.M. Fletcher, Boston, MA.)

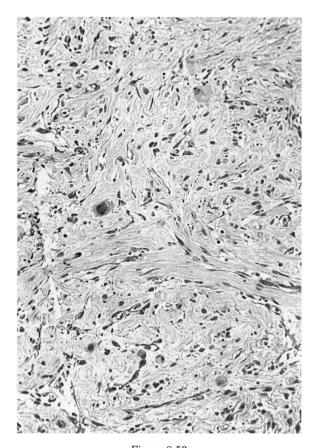

Figure 8-53
INFLAMMATORY PSEUDOTUMOR
(PROLIFERATIVE FUNICULITIS)
A high-power view shows the characteristic myofibroblastic features of the majority of the lesional cells.

Differential Diagnosis. Potentially such lesions, like inflammatory pseudotumors elsewhere, may be confused with a malignant neoplasm, but awareness that this process also occurs at these sites should avoid this pitfall. In general, inflammatory pseudotumor appears, at least focally, similar to exuberant granulation tissue, and the inflammatory, reactive appearance suggests a non-neoplastic process. Nonetheless, the consideration of a sarcoma, such as rhabdomyosarcoma, myxoid leiomyosarcoma, inflammatory variant of liposarcoma, inflammatory fibrosarcoma, or malignant fibrous histiocytoma, is not unreasonable in occasional instances. We have seen a case of inflammatory liposarcoma (60a) of the spermatic cord that closely resembled an inflammatory pseudotumor. The absence of a fascicular pattern, the presence of intermixed, noncompressed fat, hyperchromatic atypical nuclei, and atypical adipocytes are distinguishing features (60a). Inflammatory fibrosarcoma has not been described in this location, to our knowledge, but is a potential pitfall if the cytologic atypia of the lesional cells is not appreciated (59a,61a). Nevertheless, a diagnosis of sarcoma should only be made after the possibility of a reactive process is carefully evaluated by noting the inflammatory nature of the lesion, lack of other than reactive cytologic atypia, usual lack of brisk mitotic activity, and absence, in most cases, of a gross appearance suggestive of a malignant tumor.

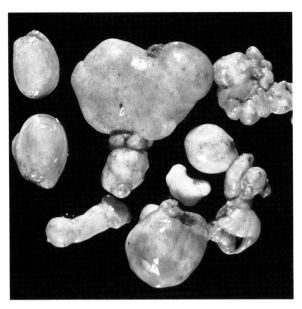

Figure 8-54
FIBROUS PSEUDOTUMOR
Multiple, discrete, free-lying masses were present in the tunica vaginalis ("corpora libera").

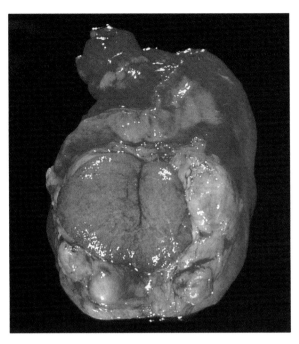

Figure 8-55
FIBROUS PSEUDOTUMOR
This lesion forms an ill-defined mass encasing the testis.

FIBROUS PSEUDOTUMOR, FIBROMATOUS PERIORCHITIS, NODULAR PERIORCHITIS

General and Clinical Features. The existence of fibromatous masses of the testicular tunics (67,69–75,77,78) and adjacent tissues has been long known, one of the earliest documented cases being referred to by Sir Astley Cooper in 1830 (68). More recently, Meyer (71) and Goodwin (70) focused on the likely non-neoplastic reactive nature of such lesions, a viewpoint widely supported in the early 1960s when three cases of "nodular periorchitis" were included in the pseudotumors of the British Testicular Tumour Panel (72). In the prior Fascicle that considered the testis, the term fibrous pseudotumor was introduced for such lesions and is now preferred for those cases that present as one or more relatively discrete masses. When the process is ill-defined, sometimes forming a plaque-like lesion coating the testis, the term fibromatous periorchitis is perhaps preferable. Although usually adjacent to the testis, occasional lesions are present in the spermatic cord.

These lesions, which are seen at essentially any age (75,78), usually present as a mass; there

may be an associated hydrocele and history of trauma or infection in some cases. A rare patient has retroperitoneal fibrosis (83a), leading to speculation that lymphatic obstruction may play a role in the genesis of the testicular lesion (73). One patient had the nevoid basal cell carcinoma syndrome (79).

Gross Findings. In the more common, localized form, single or disseminated nodules (fig. 8-54) or, less frequently, plaques may be present. They may be confluent and exceptionally encase the testis (fig. 8-55), or they may be free and numerous, lying in the tunica vaginalis (fig. 8-54). Massive examples resulting in grotesque scrotal enlargement have been described (69). In the diffuse form of this disorder, dense fibrous tissue involves the tunica vaginalis (fig. 8-56). We have seen one case that was bilateral and extended into the testes (fig. 8-57). Sectioning reveals firm, sometimes stony hard, white tissue.

Microscopic Findings. Typically, hyalinized collagen (fig. 8-58), which may be focally (fig. 8-59) or massively calcified, is seen. In some cases, which presumably represent an earlier manifestation of the more fibrotic lesion, there is greater cellularity (75), with inflammation and granulation tissue.

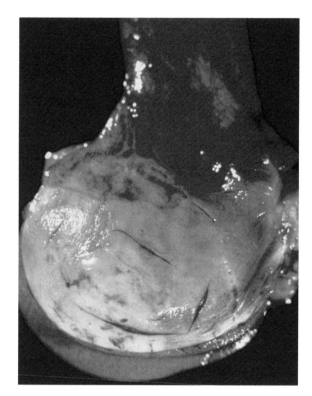

Figure 8-56
FIBROMATOUS PERIORCHITIS
A plaque-like lesion coats the testis.

Indeed, that some cases of fibrous pseudotumor represent "matured" examples of inflammatory pseudotumor is entirely plausible, as has been noted by others (67). A lesion possibly related to fibrous pseudotumor, with which we have no personal experience, is "constrictive albuginitis" (76).

Differential Diagnosis. Fibrous pseudotumor is distinguished from the rare fibroma of the tunics (see page 259) by its paucicellular nature in established cases and inflammatory appearance in earlier stages. The very rare

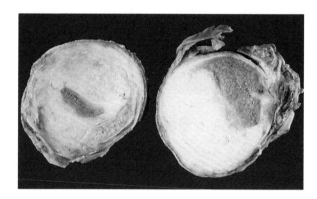

Figure 8-57
FIBROMATOUS PERIORCHITIS
The lesion is bilateral and extensively involves the testes.
(Courtesy of Dr. A. Dorado, Panama.)

Figure 8-58
FIBROMATOUS PERIORCHITIS
Three discrete nodules are present on the tunica vaginalis. (Fig. 142, Fascicle 8, 2nd Series.)

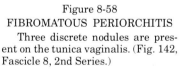

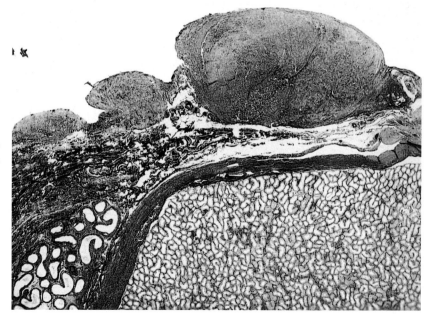

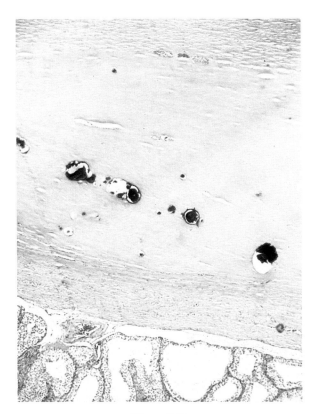

Figure 8-59
FIBROUS PSEUDOTUMOR
A hyalinized plaque with focal calcification covers the testis.

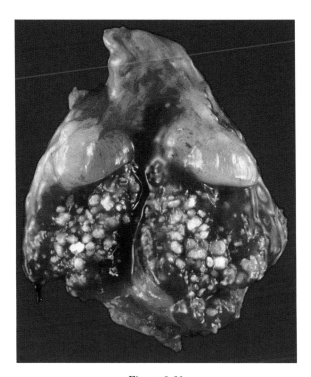

Figure 8-60
MECONIUM PERIORCHITIS
Multiple yellow nodules stud the tunica vaginalis.

fibromatosis of the paratestis is more cellular than the typical case of fibrous pseudotumor and overtly infiltrative, in contrast to the latter.

MECONIUM PERIORCHITIS

This unusual condition results from perforation of the bowel wall in utero with subsequent passage of meconium into the tunica vaginalis. In 1986, Dehner and colleagues (80) reported 4 cases, each of which was thought initially to be a neoplasm, and were able to find 20 other cases in the literature. The usual clinical presentation is a scrotal mass in the first few months of life. Occasional cases present as an "acute scrotum" in the neonatal period (81a).

The typical gross manifestation is studding of the tunica vaginalis by yellowish to green gritty tissue (fig. 8-60). On microscopic examination lobules of myxoid tissue containing spindle cells and scattered foci of calcification are seen (fig. 8-61). Scattered macrophages, nucleated and anu-

cleated squamous cells, and rare lanugo hairs may also be seen, as may mesothelial hyperplasia. Other than the macrophages, an inflammatory component is generally not striking.

The overall clinical background and rather distinctive gross appearance of meconium periorchitis should enable its recognition, provided the observer is familiar with it. Confusion with a neoplasm is furthermore unlikely if it is recollected that testicular and paratesticular tumors in neonates are quite rare, with the majority of cases representing testicular juvenile granulosa cell tumors that have a distinctly different morphology (see page 222). In utero testicular infarction results in atrophy (81) with scattered calcifications but shares none of the other features of meconium periorchitis.

MESOTHELIAL HYPERPLASIA

General and Clinical Features. This is a common form of pseudotumor that occurs in hydrocele sacs, hernia sacs (84), and diverse other testicular and adnexal specimens. It was

319

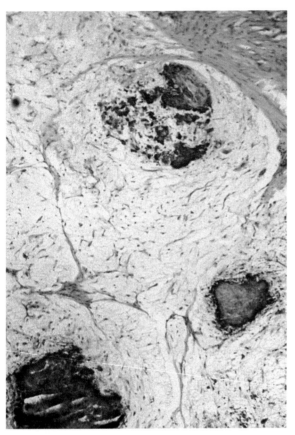

Figure 8-61
MECONIUM PERIORCHITIS
Lobules of myxoid tissue contain calcific deposits.

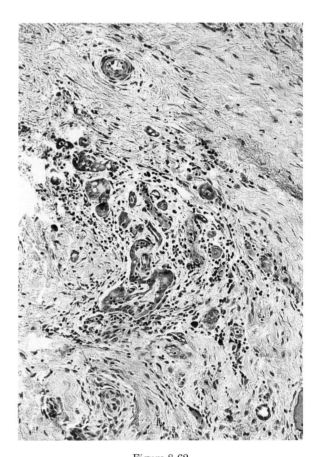

Figure 8-62
MESOTHELIAL HYPERPLASIA
Small tubules are associated with an inflammatory cell infiltrate.

seen in 14 of 18 inflamed hydroceles in the British Testicular Tumour Panel material (83a). In contrast to other pseudotumors it is almost invariably an incidental finding on microscopic examination (83) and has no distinct gross features. It is seen at essentially all ages, but is more commonly identified in older patients who more frequently undergo hydrocelectomy. In the series describing the phenomenon in hernia sacs, however, 9 of the 13 patients were children (84).

Microscopic Findings. There may be giant cells and cells that resemble strap cells, but the overall picture is usually of nonspindled mesothelial cells, in contrast to the dominant spindle cell population of the inflammatory pseudotumor. Small tubular (fig. 8-62), cord-like (fig. 8-63), and papillary patterns may be seen. The aggregates of mesothelial cells generally do not invade into underlying tissues to any apprecia-

ble degree and, if they do, have an orderly distribution; massive expansile aggregates of cells are not seen (fig. 8-64), unlike many mesotheliomas. There may be mild nuclear pleomorphism, but the overall nuclear features are bland and mitotic figures rare; an associated inflammatory background often points to a reactive process. Associated histiocytes are often present, as may be confirmed by appropriate immunohistochemical stains (83b).

Differential Diagnosis. The differential diagnosis is primarily with malignant mesothelioma, but rarely metastatic carcinoma or even sarcoma may be considered; at least one example of misdiagnosis as sarcoma is documented (84). Architectural features are important in the differential diagnosis with mesothelioma because some mesotheliomas lack significant pleomorphism or conspicuous mitotic

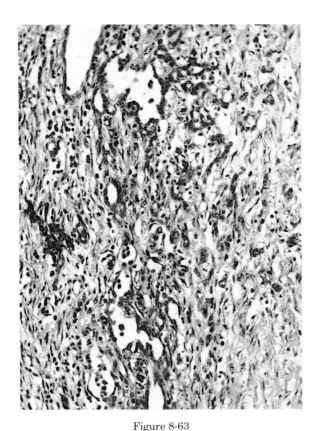

Figure 8-63
MESOTHELIAL HYPERPLASIA
Small tubules and cords are embedded in a reactive stroma. (Fig. 159, Fascicle 8, 2nd Series.)

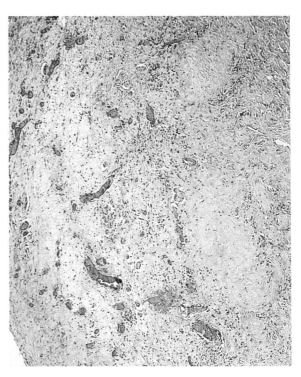

Figure 8-64
MESOTHELIAL HYPERPLASIA
This low-power view shows a lack of confluence of the small aggregates of mesothelial cells which on high-power view had bland cytologic features.

activity. Obviously if the latter is seen, a malignant diagnosis should be strongly favored; when it is absent, extensive confluence or prominent infiltration into subjacent tissues strongly favors mesothelioma. Immunohistochemical findings have recently been presented that may be of potential help, but experience is still limited (81b,82,85).

SCLEROSING LIPOGRANULOMA

A granulomatous mass may result from injection of lipids to enhance the size of the genitalia (86). The mass usually involves the scrotum and is discussed in detail in chapter 9, but occasionally it involves the spermatic cord (fig. 8-65), epididymis, or testis. Two of the 23 cases reviewed by Oertel and Johnson (86) involved the cord and another 2 the testis, with bilateral testicular involvement in 1 case.

ABNORMALITIES RELATED TO SEXUAL PRECOCITY/IDIOPATHIC HYPERTROPHY

Two lesions associated with sexual precocity can be confused with testicular tumors. The more common of these, the testicular "tumor" of the adrenogenital syndrome, has already been discussed (see page 293). A rarer lesion is so-called nodular precocious maturation of the testis in which chorionic gonadotropin secreted by an extragonadal germ cell tumor causes focal rather than diffuse stimulation of Leydig cells and tubules, forming a nodule that may be visible on ultrasound examination. In such cases, microscopic examination shows variable degrees of maturation of tubules and Leydig cells within the ill-defined nodule (fig. 8-66) and little or no maturation in the adjacent testis (90). In the rare gonadotropin-independent sexual precocity "testotoxicosis" similar focal maturation may be seen but a detectable mass has not been reported (88,89). Rarely, idiopathic testicular "hypertrophy" has been reported (87).

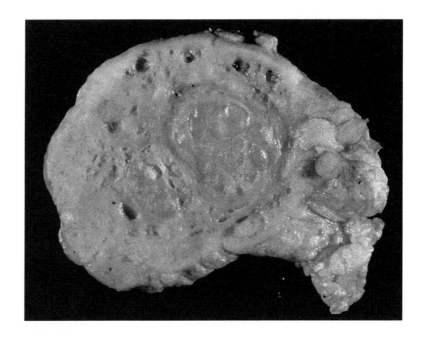

Figure 8-65
LIPOGRANULOMA
OF THE SPERMATIC CORD
Note the striking yellow color.

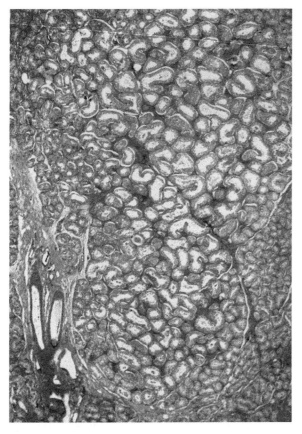

Figure 8-66
NODULAR PRECOCIOUS MATURATION

A nodule of mature testicular tissue contrasts with the normal prepubertal appearance elsewhere. This boy had an extratesticular, hCG-secreting germ cell tumor.

HYPERPLASIA AND MISCELLANEOUS OTHER BENIGN LESIONS OF THE RETE TESTIS

True hyperplasia of the rete testis is rare (91,92,94). In atrophic testes a relative prominence of the rete may suggest hyperplasia (fig. 8-67) or even carcinoma. Indeed, in some cases the decision as to whether the rete is hyperplastic or not is subjective. It is also debatable in some cases whether a lesion is a hyperplasia or a benign tumor. To designate a lesion hyperplasia it is desirable to see a complex tubulo-papillary pattern inconsistent with that of the normal rete. Occasional examples of rete hyperplasia may form a grossly visible lesion, although they usually do not: in one series of nine cases of hyperplasia the lesion was seen grossly in three (91). These lesions show no atypia, minimal mitotic activity, and no necrosis.

In some cases the rete becomes hyperplastic when invaded by a germ cell or other tumor (fig. 8-68) (94). The proliferation in these cases may exhibit solid, papillary, and microcystic patterns, with associated intracellular hyaline globules, leading to potential confusion with yolk sac tumor. In a study of 48 cases, hyperplastic epithelium with hyaline globules was found in the rete or tubuli recti in 16 of 27 cases of germ cell tumor, 1 of 5 other testicular tumors, and none

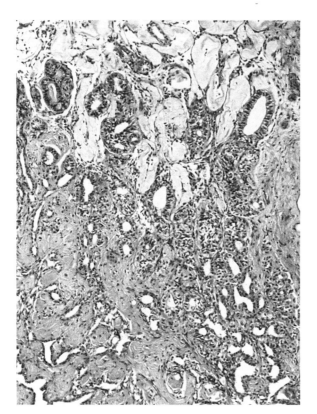

Figure 8-67
RELATIVE HYPERPLASIA OF RETE TESTIS
AND EFFERENT DUCTULES

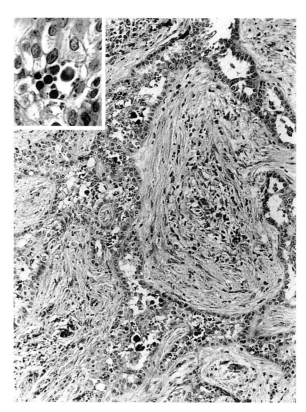

Figure 8-68
HYPERPLASIA OF RETE TESTIS

Inset shows hyaline bodies that may be seen in cases of rete hyperplasia in patients with testicular tumors. (Fig. 3 from Ulbright TM, Gersell DJ. Rete testis hyperplasia with hyaline globule formation. A lesion simulating yolk sac tumor. Am J Surg Pathol 1991;15:66–74.)

of 16 non-neoplastic lesions (94). The hyperplastic epithelium of the rete in these cases is cytologically bland, and mitoses are absent or rare. In addition, the arborizing nature of the rete is apparent, unlike the diffuse or nodular growth of yolk sac tumor involving the rete.

Srigley and Hartwick (93a) described a hamartoma of the rete testis in a 3-year-old that consisted of a disorganized collection of branching rete tubules in a fibrous stroma.

Rarely, microscopic proliferations of nodular to pedunculated connective tissue with focal calcification occur within the rete channels. These "nodular proliferations of calcifying connective tissue" are thought possibly to be related to organized blood (93).

CYSTS

Epidermoid cysts account for approximately 1 percent of testicular parenchymal masses (97, 98). Less commonly, they involve the tunica al-

buginea or the epididymis (98a). In the testis, they are most common during the second to fourth decades but may be seen at any age. They average 2 cm in diameter, are round to oval, and are composed of laminated cheesy material surrounded by a fibrous wall (fig. 8-69).

Microscopic examination shows that at least part of the cyst wall is lined by keratinizing squamous epithelium (fig. 8-70); the lining may be denuded over large areas with ulceration, fibrosis, and a foreign body giant cell reaction (fig. 8-71). It is crucial to sample epidermoid cysts extensively to exclude other elements that indicate a teratomatous nature. Extensive sampling of adjacent nonlesional tissue is also indicated because an association with intratubular germ cell neoplasia would warrant the diagnosis of teratoma. IGCNU is not identified in cases of true epidermoid cyst, and the exclusion of

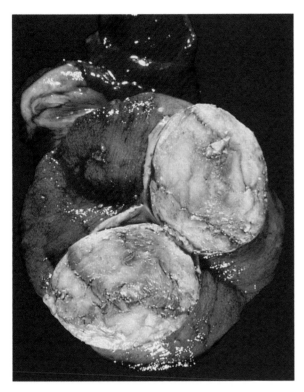

Figure 8-69
EPIDERMOID CYST OF TESTIS
The intratesticular cyst contains yellow-white material.

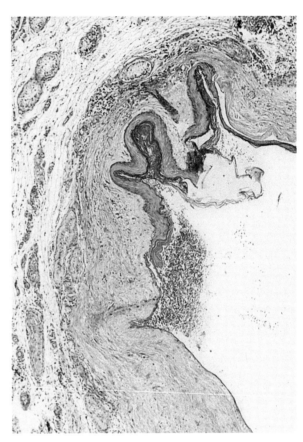

Figure 8-70
EPIDERMOID CYST OF TESTIS
Note the pure squamous lining without other elements beneath the cyst lining.

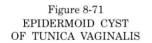

Figure 8-71
EPIDERMOID CYST
OF TUNICA VAGINALIS

The cyst ruptured and was associated with a prominent fibrotic response.

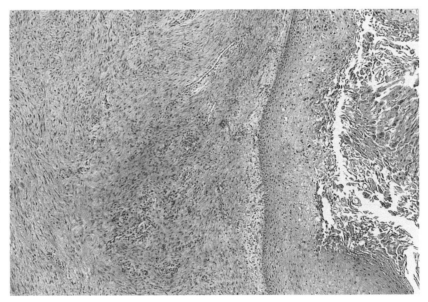

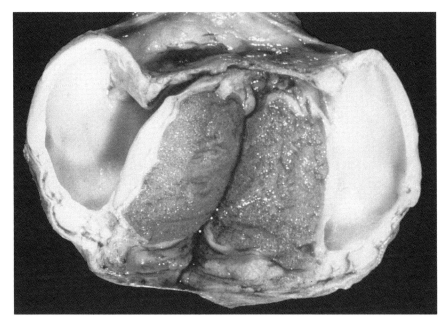

Figure 8-72
CYST OF TUNICA
ALBUGINEA
(Courtesy of Dr. F. Askin, Baltimore, MD.)

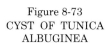

Figure 8-73
CYST OF TUNICA
ALBUGINEA

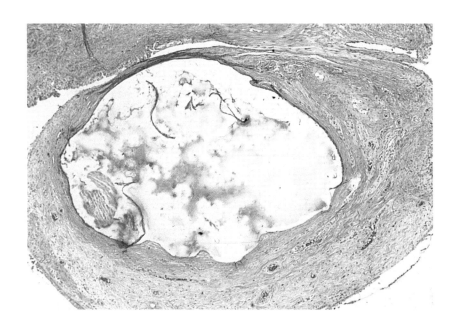

IGCNU by examination of two or more biopsy specimens of the adjacent testis permits conservative local excision (96a).

Other testicular and paratesticular cysts include those of the tunica albuginea (figs. 8-72, 8-73) (96c), rete cysts (98b) (fig. 8-74), cystic Walthard nests (see page 303), epididymal cysts (fig. 8-75), mesothelial cysts, and paratesticular dermoid cysts (fig. 8-76) (95,96,98a). A case of "multicystic

mesothelioma" of the spermatic cord has also been reported (98b), but it is controversial whether this is a low-grade neoplasm (99b) or a reactive, cystic mesothelial proliferation (96b). All of these entities are relatively uncommon. Cysts of the tunica albuginea usually do not exceed 4 cm, may be multiple, can be unilocular or multilocular, and usually contain serous fluid (96c,99a). Their lining is cuboidal or flat epithelial cells. The

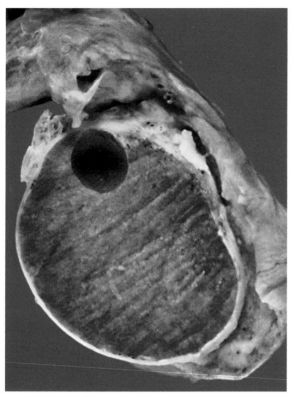

Figure 8-74
CYST OF RETE TESTIS
(Courtesy of Dr. J. Eble, Indianapolis, IN.)

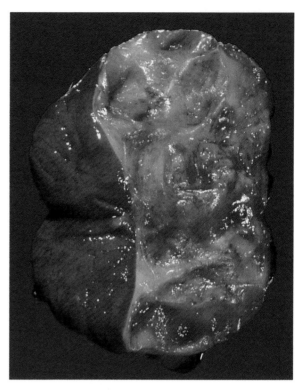

Figure 8-75
EPIDIDYMAL CYST
The multilocular cyst contained clear fluid.

distinction between a rete cyst and cystic dilatation of the rete (fig. 8-77) is imprecise but not clinically important. Simple dilatation of the rete tubules may produce a striking picture, the tubules sometimes containing a prominent eosinophilic colloid-like secretion.

True hermaphrodites who are phenotypic males may have ovotestes or very rarely an ovary in the scrotum (99). The ovarian tissue may contain cystic follicles and corpora lutea, and on occasion, ovulation causes the sudden onset of hemorrhage with pain and a mass in the scrotum, simulating a testicular tumor (fig. 8-78).

CYSTIC DYSPLASIA

This rare testicular lesion, which occurs in infants and children, is characterized by multiple anastomosing cysts of varying sizes and shapes, separated by fibrous septa (100–102a). It is associated with ipsilateral renal agenesis and renal dysplasia and, rarely, with bilateral renal dysplasia. Cystic dysplasia of the testis is bilateral in one third of the cases. Gross examination reveals a multicystic mass replacing much of the testis (fig. 8-79) or a more localized lesion based in the hilum. The process begins in the region of the rete testis and extends into the parenchyma, which may be compressed to a thin rim. The cysts are lined by a single layer of flat or cuboidal epithelial cells similar to those of the rete testis (fig. 8-80).

MICROLITHIASIS

This lesion may be found in patients without any underlying abnormality but also is associated with infertility, and, in at least one case, there was pulmonary alveolar microlithiasis (103–105). It often is initially appreciated on radiographic examination. Renshaw (104a) has discussed two forms of microlithiasis, both of

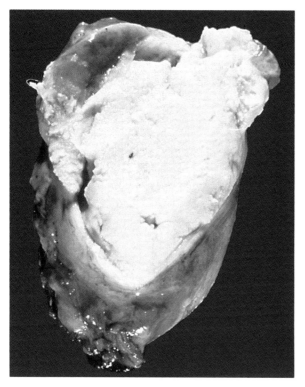

Figure 8-76
DERMOID CYST OF SPERMATIC CORD
Note grumous material that protrudes from the opened cyst.

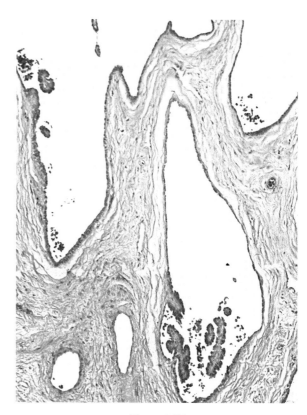

Figure 8-77
CYSTIC DILATATION OF RETE TESTIS

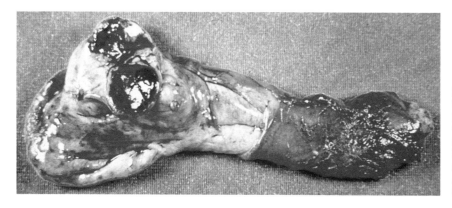

Figure 8-78
RUPTURED CORPUS
LUTEUM IN A
HERMAPHRODITE

A hemorrhagic corpus luteum is present in the upper pole of an ovotestis of a true hermaphrodite. This patient, a 14-year-old boy, presented with "testicular" pain and gynecomastia. Examination of the gonad led to the diagnosis of true hermaphroditism. (Courtesy of Dr. F. Vellios, Atlanta, GA and Dr. J. Albores-Saavedra, Dallas, TX.)

which occur in seminiferous tubules: laminated (psammomatous) (fig. 8-81) and amorphous (hematoxylin bodies). The latter is specific to usual germ cell tumors or regressed germ cell tumors, while the former occurs commonly with germ cell tumors (40 percent) but also is seen in about 4 percent of normal testes. Follow-up of childhood cases has not yet demonstrated progression to tumor, but the data are limited (103a).

SPERMATOCELE

This is an acquired, cystic lesion containing sperm that is usually caused by cystic dilatation of the efferent ductules of the head of the epididymis (106a). Less commonly, the lesion results from dilatation of the tubules of the rete testis or the aberrant ducts. The lesion may appear at any age after puberty but has a peak incidence in the

327

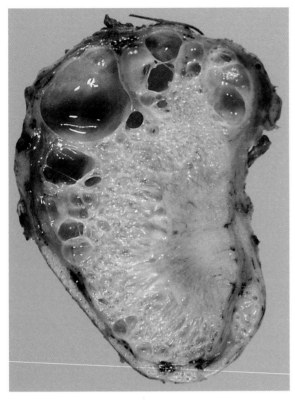

Figure 8-79
CYSTIC DYSPLASIA
Multiple cysts of varying sizes are visible. (Courtesy of
Professor W. Wegmann, Liestal, Switzerland.)

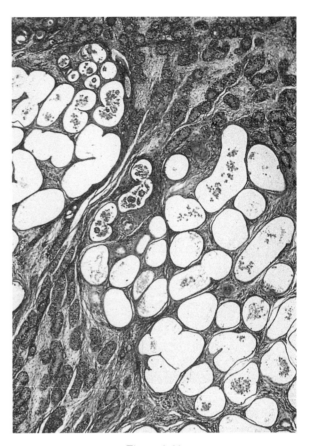

Figure 8-80
CYSTIC DYSPLASIA
Most of the cysts are dilated and lined by flattened epithe-
lium. (Courtesy of Professor W. Wegmann, Liestal, Switzerland.)

Figure 8-81
MICROLITHIASIS
Many tubules contain intralumi-
nal calcifications.

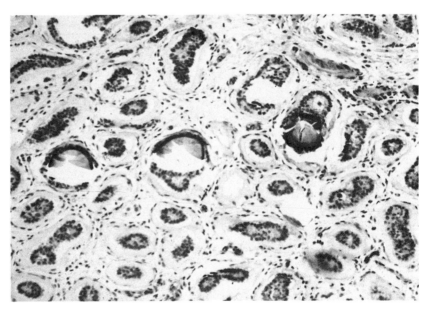

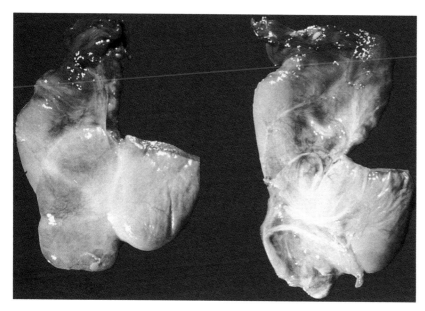

Figure 8-82
SPERMATOCELE
The thin, translucent wall of a spermatocele is apparent (left: unopened; right: opened).

fourth and fifth decades. The cysts may be unilocular or multilocular, and may attain a large size (fig. 8-82). They have a thin translucent wall and contain cloudy fluid reflecting the contents of sperm. Histologically, the fibromuscular wall is lined by a cuboidal to, rarely, pseudostratified epithelium. Rarely, spermatoceles contain mural papillary proliferations (papillomas) composed of a small papilla with a fibrovascular core lined by bland columnar epithelium. The luminal contents consist of an eosinophilic secretion containing degenerated spermatozoa. Occasionally, large spermatoceles may undergo torsion (106).

SPERM GRANULOMA

General and Clinical Features. This lesion is characterized by a granulomatous reaction to extravasated sperm that produces a nodule that is usually painful and may be clinically mistaken for a tumor (110–112,118,120). In one study of 60 cases, 8 were felt to represent a tumor of the epididymis or testis on clinical examination (112). In two large series, 1 to 5 percent of men undergoing vasectomy developed sperm granulomas (117,119), with vasitis nodosa also representing a significant complication of this procedure. Sperm granulomas are currently related to a prior vasectomy in over 40 percent of the cases. Other etiologies include trauma, infection, urinary tract obstruction, and prior surgery. About

80 percent of the patients are under 40 years of age (112). Approximately 90 percent of granulomas that follow vasectomy are in the vas deferens and the remainder in the epididymis.

Gross Findings. Sperm granulomas can measure up to 4 cm but average about 0.7 cm (112). They are typically firm nodules but may have small, soft, yellow to white foci on sectioning (fig. 8-83). They may be focally cystic due to associated obstruction and dilatation of the epididymal ducts associated with the lesion.

Microscopic Findings. The appearance varies according to the stage of the process. In the initial phase there is an infiltrate of neutrophils, which is gradually replaced by epithelioid histiocytes; the histiocytes and occasional giant cells surround the sperm, resulting in the most characteristic appearance of the lesion (figs. 8-84, 8-85); calcification is occasionally seen. In the later stages, there is progressive fibrosis and hyalinization, and deposition of lipochrome pigment may be prominent. Sperm granulomas occurring in the vas deferens are associated with vasitis nodosa in approximately one third of the cases.

Differential Diagnosis. There are limited considerations. Some cases reported under the heading of "sperm granuloma" appear more typical of idiopathic granulomatous orchitis because of an absence or paucity of associated sperm and the history of a febrile illness.

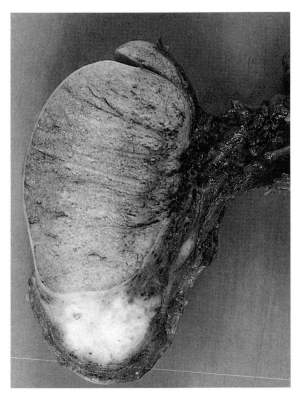

Figure 8-83
SPERM GRANULOMA
A firm, white nodule with foci of necrosis involves the lower pole of the epididymis. (Fig. 1 from Glassy FJ, Mostofi FK. Spermatic granulomas of the epididymis. Am J Clin Pathol 1956; 26:1303–13.)

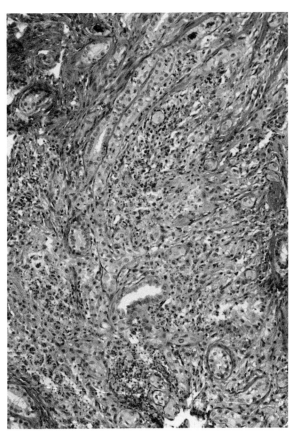

Figure 8-84
SPERM GRANULOMA
Darkly staining sperm are associated with epithelioid histiocytes. Several small tubules representing associated vasitis nodosa are visible.

Figure 8-85
SPERM GRANULOMA
Langhans-type giant cells are conspicuous.

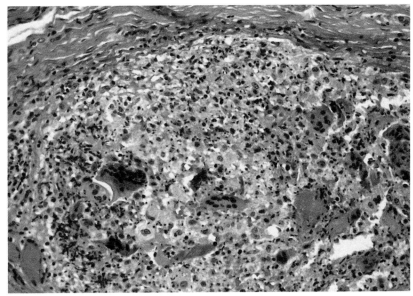

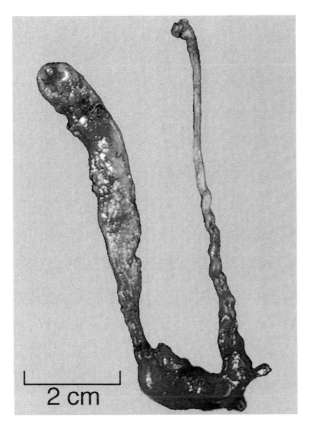

Figure 8-86
VASITIS NODOSA

Nodular thickening is apparent in the mid-portion (bottom) of the vas deferens. (Fig. 12-9A from Bostwick DG. Spermatic cord and testicular adnexa. In: Bostwick DG, Eble JN, eds. Urologic surgical pathology. St. Louis: Mosby, 1997:646–73.)

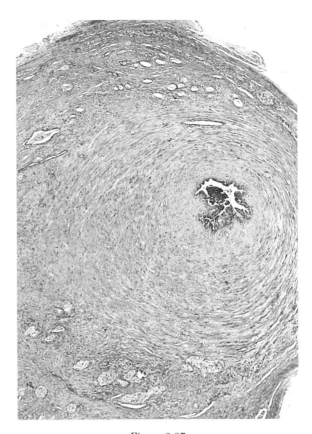

Figure 8-87
VASITIS NODOSA

Tubules involve the outer aspect of the wall of the vas deferens.

VASITIS NODOSA

General and Clinical Features. Benjamin et al. (108) coined the term vasitis nodosa because of similarity to salpingitis isthmica nodosa. It is usually encountered at the time of a vasovasostomy, and therefore typically occurs in young men with a mean age of 36 years and an interval from vasectomy to vasovasostomy of 1 to 15 (mean, 7) years (115). There may be associated pain, but most patients are asymptomatic. An analogous epididymal lesion, epididymitis nodosa (121), also occurs. Stout (122) described possibly similar pseudoneoplastic proliferations of the epididymis in response to inflammation.

Gross Findings. The lesions are typically firm nodules in the scrotal portion of the vas deferens, 5 to 6 cm above the testis (fig. 8-86), corresponding to the frequent site of vasectomy

(109). They usually measure up to just over 1 cm and typically have a white cut surface that may exude milky fluid.

Microscopic Findings. Microscopic examination reveals small, gland-like structures lined by cuboidal epithelium in the wall of the vas deferens and the surrounding adventitia (figs. 8-87, 8-88). The tubules have an irregular distribution, and perineural invasion may be observed (figs. 8-89, 8-90) (107,113,116). There are coexistent sperm granulomas in many cases, 70 percent in one series (115). The tubules may also contain histiocytes, some with ceroid pigment. Pagetoid spread of a seminoma to vasitis nodosa is described (114).

Differential Diagnosis. The usual presence of sperm in the tubal lumens is important in distinguishing the tubules from the glands of adenocarcinoma, as is the lack of any significant cytologic atypia or mitotic activity, although nucleoli may be prominent.

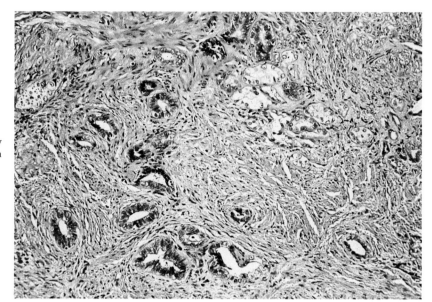

Figure 8-88
VASITIS NODOSA
The small tubules are irregularly disposed causing potential confusion with adenocarcinoma.

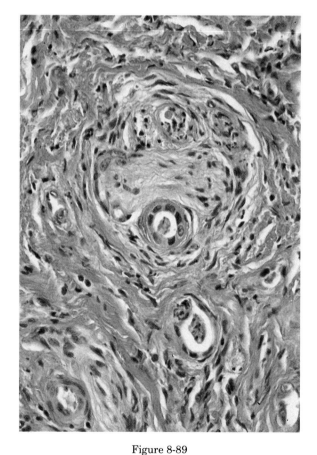

Figure 8-89
VASITIS NODOSA
The small tubules show perineural invasion. (Courtesy of Dr. K. Balogh, Boston, MA.)

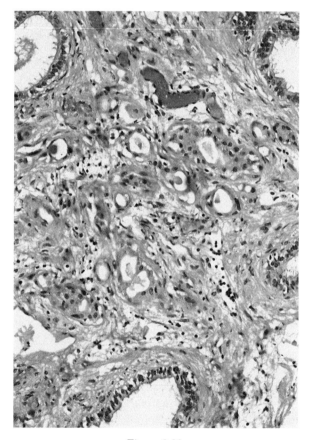

Figure 8-90
EPIDIDYMITIS NODOSA
A cluster of small tubules, resembling those of vasitis nodosa, is present between epididymal tubules.

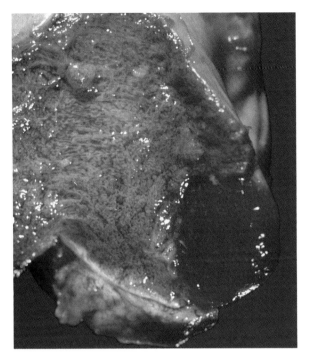

Figure 8-91
SPLENIC-GONADAL FUSION
Beefy red tissue consistent with spleen is located within the lower pole of the testis. (Fig. 9.37 from Young RH, Scully RE. Testicular tumors. Chicago: ASCP Press, 1990:217.)

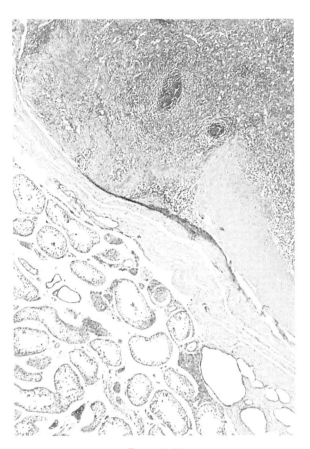

Figure 8-92
SPLENIC-GONADAL FUSION
Splenic tissue is separated from testicular tissue by a fibrous band.

SPLENIC-GONADAL FUSION

This condition, in which splenic and gonadal tissues become adherent and fuse during early intrauterine development, is seen in both sexes but has a strong male predilection (123,124). The left side is almost invariably involved. The abnormality occurs in two forms, continuous and discontinuous. In the former a cord connects the normal splenic tissue to the testis, while in the latter no connection to the normally positioned spleen is present. Small aggregates of splenic tissue may be found in the fibrous cord as it traverses the peritoneal cavity, or the cord may be composed entirely of splenic tissue. Almost one third of the patients with the continuous form have severe defects of the extremities (peromelia), sometimes associated with micrognathia. In patients without associated congenital abnormalities, the clinical presentation is in the form of a scrotal or inguinal mass, typically discovered during an operation for either an inguinal hernia (which is present in over one third of the cases) or an undescended testis (present in one sixth of the cases). Two patients had scrotal pain during attacks of malaria.

The splenic tissue typically forms a discrete mass that is almost always fused to the upper pole of the testis or the head of the epididymis, but occasionally is attached to the lower pole and rarely is intratesticular. It is usually small but may be over 10 cm and has the characteristic gross (fig. 8-91) and microscopic features of normal spleen (fig. 8-92).

TUMOR-LIKE ASPECTS OF NORMAL HISTOLOGY

There are two normal histologic features of the epididymis that occasionally cause confusion with a dysplastic or neoplastic process (125a). The first is a prominent cribriform pattern of the

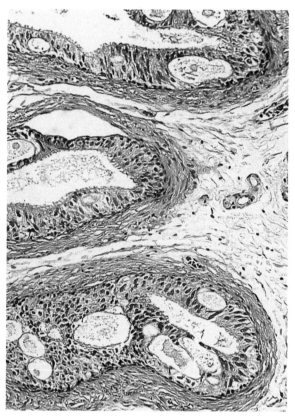

Figure 8-93
NORMAL EPIDIDYMIS
The cribriform appearance of the tubules may cause confusion with adenocarcinoma.

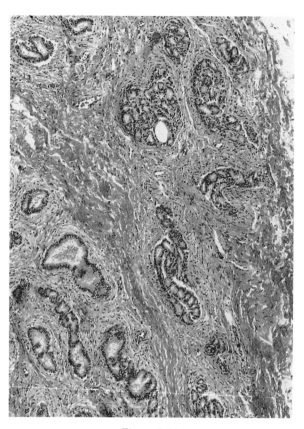

Figure 8-94
CRIBRIFORM HYPERPLASIA
OF EFFERENT DUCTULES
There is a vaguely lobular arrangement of cribriform structures adjacent to identifiable efferent ductules.

epididymal tubules that is occasionally seen (fig. 8-93). The lack of invasion and absence of neoplastic-type cytologic atypia of the epithelial cells, and awareness of the phenomenon, should help avoid a misdiagnosis of carcinoma. Rarely, a similar cribriform process may involve the efferent ductules, sometimes showing the cytoplasmic lipofuscin characteristic of those structures (fig. 8-94).

In the second normal variant, bizarre nuclear atypicality, similar to that more commonly identified in the seminal vesicle, may be seen in the efferent ductules and, to a lesser extent, in the epididymis proper (fig. 8-95). It was found in 28 percent of specimens in one study (125), apparently caused by fusion of several nuclei to form single, large, bizarre nuclei. The degenerative appearance of the nuclei, the focality of the process, and the lack of mitotic activity should facilitate recognition of this phenomenon.

MISCELLANEOUS OTHER LESIONS

One unique tumor-like lesion of müllerian nature in the paratesticular region was a uterus-like structure composed of endometrial-type glands and stroma surrounded by bundles of smooth muscle (fig. 8-96) (138). This lesion arose in an 82-year-old man who had received diethylstilbestrol for carcinoma of the prostate gland.

Other uncommon to rare tumor-like lesions include: smooth muscle hyperplasia of the adnexa (126), prostatic glands in the epididymis (126a), osseous metaplasia of the epididymis (135), several cases of a spermatic cord mass caused by a necrotic, granulomatous reaction induced by the injection of a sclerosing agent ("alparene no. 2") for the treatment of inguinal hernia (131a), at least one case each of an ossified calcific nodule (137) and fatty metaplasia (131),

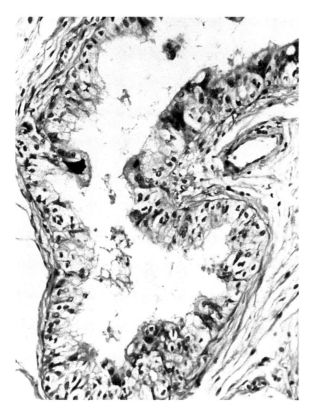

Figure 8-95
NORMAL EPIDIDYMIS
Degenerative nuclear features similar to those often seen in the seminal vesicles are present.

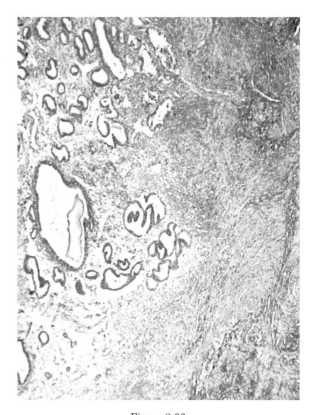

Figure 8-96
ENDOMETRIOSIS ADJACENT TO EPIDIDYMIS
Endometrial-type glands and stroma with adjacent smooth muscle.

talc or starch granulomas causing masses (130, 133), congenital testicular lymphangiectasis (132), secondary oxalosis associated with a sperm granuloma that formed a mass (127), and a granulomatous nodule in the vas deferens with stromal and epithelial atypia attributed to contrast medium (136). Examination of unexplained granulomatous lesions, particularly of the paratesticular region, by polarized light is crucial in elucidating the nature of those due to foreign material. Amyloidosis may also rarely cause testicular enlargement (129).

We have seen one example of metanephric dysplastic hamartoma (128) that occurred as an epididymal mass discovered at the time of surgery for a hernia repair in an 18-month-old boy. Microscopic examination showed scattered blastema with papillae, glomeruloid formations, and dysplastic tubules (fig. 8-97). Our personal experience with this process is limited to this one case which was seen in consultation by Dr. Louis P.

Dehner. Although the exact nature of this process is uncertain, its small size and the scattered presence of the immature elements without the usual confluence of a Wilms' tumor are features that favor a peculiar, apparently benign process, rather than an extrarenal Wilms' tumor.

We have seen a case of radiation injury to the testis that imparted a white, fibrotic tumor-like aspect (fig. 8-98) and also a case of testicular edema that mimicked a neoplasm on clinical examination, prompting orchiectomy. The edema was probably related to a coexistent hydrocele. Finally, atypical mononucleate or multinucleate stromal cells of fibroblastic or myofibroblastic nature may be seen in the testis (fig. 8-99) (127a,134). In one series these were found in about 40 percent of cases at autopsy, with no clear etiology (127a). In the most striking case we have seen they were associated with idiopathic granulomatous orchitis (fig. 8-99).

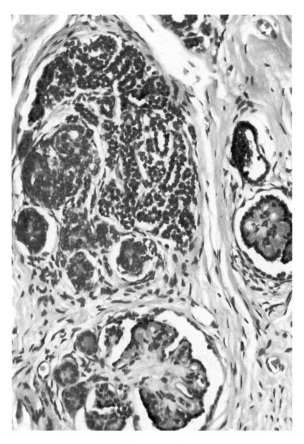

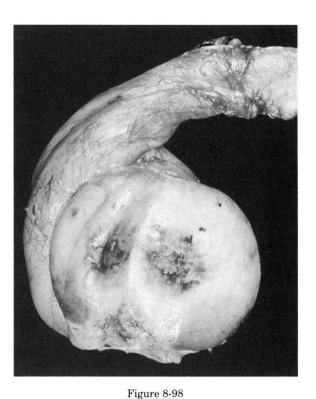

Figure 8-98
RADIATION FIBROSIS
Most of the testis is firm and white, potentially simulating a neoplasm.

Figure 8-97
METANEPHRIC DYSPLASTIC
HAMARTOMA OF EPIDIDYMIS
Immature tissue of renal type formed an epididymal mass.

Figure 8-99
ATYPICAL STROMAL CELLS
Some cells are mononucleate and others are multinucleate. Nucleoli are conspicuous. A portion of a seminiferous tubule is seen at the top left.

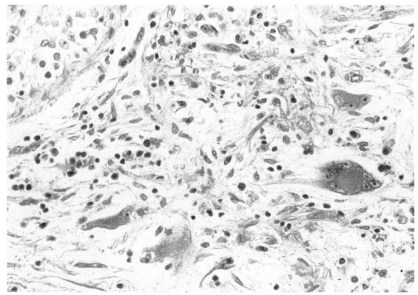

REFERENCES

General References

1. Collins DH, Pugh RC. Classification and frequency of testicular tumors. Br J Urol 1964;36 (Suppl):1–11.
2. Connor DH, Chandler FW, Schwartz DA, Manz HJ, Lack EE. Pathology of infectious diseases. Norwalk CT: Appleton Lange, 1997.
3. Haas GP, Shumaker BP, Cerny JC. The high incidence of benign testicular tumors. J Urol 1986;136:1219–20.
4. Mikuz G, Damjanov I. Inflammation of the testis, epididymis, peritesticular membranes and scrotum. Pathol Annu 1982;17(Pt. I):101–28.

4a. Morgan AD. Inflammation and infestation of the testis and paratesticular structures. In: Pugh RC, ed. Pathology of the testis. Oxford: Blackwell Scientific, 1976:79–138.
5. Morgan AD. Inflammatory lesions simulating malignancy. Br J Urol 1964;36 (Suppl):95–102.
6. Nistal M, Paniagua R. Non-neoplastic diseases of the testis. In: Bostwick DG, Eble JN, eds, Urologic surgical pathology. St. Louis: Mosby-Year Book, 1997.

Leydig Cell Hyperplasia

7. Gondos B, Egli CA, Rosenthal SM, Grumbach MM. Testicular changes in gonadotropin-independent familial male sexual precocity. Familial testotoxicosis. Arch Pathol Lab Med 1985;109:990–5.
7a. Halley JB. The infiltrative activity of Leydig cells. J Pathol Bacteriol 1961;81:347–53.
8. Jemerin EE. Hyperplasia and neoplasia of the interstitial cells of the testicle. Arch Surg 1937;35:967–98.
9. Mark GJ, Hedinger CH. Changes in remaining tumor-free testicular tissue in cases of seminoma and teratoma. Virchows Arch Pathol Anat Physiol Klin Med 1965;340:84–92.
10. McDonald JH, Calams JA. A histological study of extraparenchymal Leydig-like cells. J Urol 1958;79:850–8.
11. Nelson AA. Giant interstitial cells and extraparenchymal interstitial cells of the human testis. Am J Pathol 1938;14:831–41.

11a. Park YW, Ro JY, Kim CH, Shah V, Amin MB, Ayala G. Location, distribution, pattern, and quantity of testicular adnexal Leydig cells (TALC) [Abstract]. Mod Pathol 1998;11:92A.
12. Schedewie HK, Reiter EO, Beitins IZ, et al. Testicular Leydig cell hyperplasia as a cause of familial sexual precocity. J Clin Endocrinol Metab 1981;52:271–8.
13. Umiker W. Interstitial cell hyperplasia in association with testicular tumors: a study of its relationship to urinary gonadotrophins, testicular atrophy and histological type of tumor. J Urol 1954;72:895–903.
14. Warren S, Olshausen KW. Interstitial cell growths of the testicle. Am J Pathol 1943;19:307–31.
14a. Wierman ME, Beardsworth DE, Mansfield MJ, et al. Puberty without gonadotropins. A unique mechanism of sexual development. N Engl J Med 1985;312:65–72.

Sertoli Cell Nodules

15. Halley JB. The growth of Sertoli cell tumors: a possible index of differential gonadotrophin activity in the male. J Urol 1963;90:220–9.

16. Hedinger CE, Huber R, Weber E. Frequency of so-called hypoplastic or dysgenetic zones in scrotal and otherwise normal human testes. Virchows Arch Pathol Anat Physiol Klin Med 1967;342:165–8.

Testicular "Tumors" of the Adrenogenital Syndrome and Steroid Cell Nodules with Other Adrenal Diseases

16a. Adesokan A, Adegboyega PA, Cowan DF, Kocurek J, Neal DE Jr. Testicular "tumor" of the adrenogenital syndrome: a case report of an unusual association with myelolipoma and seminoma in cryptorchidism. Cancer 1997;80:2120–7.
17. Carney JA, Gordon H, Carpenter PC, Shenoy BV, Go VL. The complex of myxomas, spotty pigmentation, and endocrine overactivity. Medicine 1985;64:270–83.
18. Carpenter PC, Wahner HW, Salassa RM, Duick DS. Demonstration of steroid-producing gonadal tumors by external scanning with the use of NP-59. Mayo Clin Proc 1979;54:332–4.
19. Chrousos GP, Loriaux DL, Sherins RJ, Cutler GB Jr. Unilateral testicular enlargement resulting from inapparent 21-hydroxylase deficiency. J Urol 1981;126:127–8.
20. Davis JM, Woodroof J, Sadasivan R, Stephens R. Case report: congenital adrenal hyperplasia and malignant Leydig cell tumor. Am J Med Sci 1995;309:63–5.
21. Franco-Saenz R, Antonipillai I, Tan SY, McCorquodale M, Kropp K, Mulrow PJ. Cortisol production by testicular tumors in a patient with congenital adrenal hy-

perplasia (21-hydroxylase deficiency). J Clin Endocrinol Metab 1981;53:85–90.
22. Hamwi GJ, Gwinup G, Mostow JH, Besch PK. Activation of testicular adrenal rest tissue by prolonged excessive ACTH production. J Clin Endocrinol Metab 1963;23:861–9.
23. Johnson RE, Scheithauer B. Massive hyperplasia of testicular adrenal rests in a patient with Nelson's syndrome. Am J Clin Pathol 1982;77:501–7.
24. Krieger DT, Samojlik E, Bardin CW. Cortisol and androgen secretion in a case of Nelson's syndrome with paratesticular tumors: response to cyprohepatadine therapy. J Clin Endocrinol Metab 1978;47:837–44.
25. Miller EC, Murray HL. Congential adrenocortical hyperplasia: case previously reported as "bilateral interstitial cell tumor of the testicle." J Clin Endocrinol Metab 1962;22:655–7.
25a. Rich MA, Keating MA, Levin HS, Kay R. Tumors of the adrenogenital syndrome: an aggressive conservative approach. J Urol 1998;160:1838–41.

26. Rose EK, Enterline HT, Rhoads JE, Rose E. Adrenal cortical hyperfunction in childhood. Report of a case with adrenocortical hyperplasia and testicular adrenal rests. Pediatrics 1952;9:475–84.

27. Rutgers JL, Young RH, Scully RE. The testicular "tumor" of the adrenogenital syndrome. A report of six cases and review of the literature on testicular masses in patients with disorders of the adrenal glands. Am J Surg Pathol 1988;12:503–13.

Adrenal Cortical Rests

28. Dahl EV, Bahn RC. Aberrant adrenal cortical tissue near the testis in human infants. Am J Pathol 1962;40:587–98.

29. Delmas V, Dauge MC. Accessory adrenal glands in the spermatic cord. Report of two cases. Ann Urol 1986;20:261–4.

30. Nelson AA. Accessory adrenal cortical tissue. Arch Pathol 1939;27:955–65.

Torsion, Infarcts, Hematomas, Testicular Appendages, Walthard Nests

31. Arcadi JA. Torsion of the appendix epididymis: an unusual urological entity. J Urol 1963;89:467–9.

31a. Belville WD, Insalaco SJ, Drexner ML, Buck AS. Benign testis tumors. J Urol 1982;128:1198–200.

31b. Corless CL, Daut D, Burke R. Localized giant cell vasculitis of the spermatic cord presenting as a mass lesion. J Urol Pathol 1997;6:235–42.

32. Dahl EV, Baggenstoss AH, DeWeerd JH. Testicular lesions of periarteritis nodosa with special reference to diagnosis. Am J Med 1960;28:222–8.

32a. Gofrit ON, Rund D, Shapiro A, Pappo O, Landau EH, Pode D. Segmental testicular infarction due to sickle cell disease. J Urol 1998;160:835–6.

32b. Hourihane DO'B. Infected infarcts of the testis: a study of 18 cases preceded by pyogenic epididymo-orchitis. J Clin Pathol 1975;23:668–75.

32c. Levine TS. Testicular and epididymal vasculitides. Is morphology a help in classification and prognosis? J Urol Pathol 1994;2:81–8.

33. Nayal W, Brassett C, Singh L, Boyd PJ. Segmental testicular ischaemia mimicking testicular tumor. Br J Urol 1996;78:318–9.

33a. Nöske HD, Kraus SW, Altinkilic BM, Weidner W. Historical milestones regarding torsion of the scrotal organs. J Urol 1998;159:13–6.

33b. Palmer-Toy DE, McGovern F, Young RH. Granulomatous orchitis and vasculitis with testicular infarction complicat-

ing Crohn's disease: a hitherto undescribed tumor-like lesion of the testis. J Urol Pathol (in press).

34. Rolnick D, Kawanoue S, Szanto P, Bush IM. Anatomical incidence of testicular appendages. J Urol 1968;100:755–6.

34a. Schned AR, Cendron M. Pathologic findings in the vanishing testis syndrome. J Urol Pathol 1997;6:95–107.

35. Shurbaji MS, Epstein JI. Testicular vasculitis: implications for systemic disease. Hum Pathol 1988;19:186–9.

36. Skoglund RW, McRoberts JW, Ragde H. Torsion of the spermatic cord: a review of the literature and an analysis of 70 new cases. J Urol 1970;104:604–7.

36a. Smith NM, Byard RW, Bourne AJ. Testicular regression syndrome—a pathologic study of 77 cases. Histopathology 1991;19:269–72.

36b. Srigley JR, Hartwick RW. Tumors and cysts of the paratesticular region. Pathol Annu 1990;25(Pt. 2):51–108.

37. Sundarasivarao D. The Müllerian vestiges and benign epithelial tumors of the epididymis. J Pathol Bacteriol 1953;66:417–32.

37a. Womack C, Ansell ID. Isolated arteritis of the epididymis. J Clin Pathol 1985;38:797–800.

38. Yamashina M, Honma T, Uchijima Y. Myofibroblastic pseudotumor mimicking epididymal sarcoma. A clinicopathologic study of three cases. Pathol Res Pract 1992;188:1054–9.

Orchitis (Infectious)

39. Craighead JE, Mahoney EM, Carver DH, Naficy K, Fremont-Smith P. Orchitis due to Coxsackie virus group B types. Report of a case with isolation of virus from the testis. N Engl J Med 1962;267:498–500.

40. Ferrie BG, Rundle JS. Tuberculous epididymo-orchitis. A review of 20 cases. Br J Urol 1983;55:437–9.

41. Gall EA. The histopathology of acute mumps orchitis. Am J Pathol 1947;23:637–51.

42. Grabstald H, Swan LL. Genitourinary lesions in leprosy, with special reference to the problem of atrophy of the testes. JAMA 1952;149:1287–91.

42a. Haddad FS. Coccidioidomycosis of the genitourinary tract with special emphasis on the epididymis and the prostate. J Urol Pathol 1996;4:205–11.

43. Honore LH. Nonspecific peritesticular fibrosis manifested as testicular enlargement. Clinicopathological study of nine cases. Arch Surg 1978;113:814–6.

44. Hourihane DO'B. Infected infarcts of the testis: a study of 18 cases preceded by pyogenic epididymo-orchitis. J Clin Pathol 1970;23:668–75.

44a. Kanomata N, Eble JN. Fungal epididymitis caused by Histoplasma capsulatum. J Urol Pathol 1997;5:229–34.

45. Menninger WC. Congenital syphilis of the testicle. With report of twelve autopsied cases. Am J Syphilis 1928;12:221–34.

46. Morgan AD. Inflammatory lesions simulating malignancy. Br J Urol 1964;36(Suppl):95–102.

47. Wechsler H, Westfall M, Lattimer JK. The earliest signs and symptoms in 127 male patients with genitourinary tuberculosis. J Urol 1960;83:801–3.

Granulomatous Orchitis (Nonspecific) and Epididymitis (Including Sarcoidosis)

48. Amenta PS, Gonick P, Katz SM. Sarcoidosis of testis and epididymis. Urology 1981;17:616–7.
49. Morgan AD. Inflammatory lesions simulating malignancy. Br J Urol 1964;36(Suppl):95–102.
49a. Nistal M, Mate A, Paniagua R. Granulomatous epididymal lesion of possible ischemic origin. Am J Surg Pathol 1997;21:951–6.
50. Ryan DM, Lesser BA, Crumley LA, et al. Epididymal sarcoidosis. J Urol 1993;149:134–6.
51. Spjut H, Thorpe J. Granulomatous orchitis. Am J Clin Pathol 1956;26:136–45.
52. Wiener LB, Riehl PA, Baum N. Xanthogranulomatous epididymitis: a case report. J Urol 1987;138:621–22.
52a. Yantiss RK, Young RH. Idiopathic granulomatous epididymitis: report of a case and review of the literature. J Urol Pathol 1998;8:171–9.

Malakoplakia

53. McClure J. Malakoplakia. J Pathol 1983;140:275–330.
54. McClure J. Malakoplakia of the testis and its relationship to granulomatous orchitis. J Clin Pathol 1980;33:670–8.

Sinus Histiocytosis with Massive Lymphadenopathy

54a. Azoury FJ, Reed RJ. Histiocytosis. Report of an unusual case. N Engl J Med 1966;274:928–30.
54b. Foucar E, Rosai J, Dorfman R. Sinus histiocytosis with massive lymphadenopathy (Rosai-Dorfman disease): review of the entity. Semin Diag Pathol 1990;7:19–73.

Hydrocele-Related Changes

55. Honoré LH. Nonspecific peritesticular fibrosis manifested as testicular enlargement. Arch Surg 1978;113:814–6.
55a. King ES. Squamous epithelium in encysted hydrocele of the cord. NZ J Med 1951;20:265–71.
56. Kokotas N, Kontogeorgos L, Kyriakidis A. Calcification of the tunica vaginalis. Br J Urol 1983;55:128.
57. Lowenthal SB, Goldstein AM, Terry R. Cholesterol granuloma of tunica vaginalis. Urology 1981;18:89–90.
58. Morgan AD. Inflammatory lesions simulating malignancy. Br J Urol 1964;36(Suppl):95–102.

Inflammatory Pseudotumor

58a. Chan KW, Chan KL, Lam KY. Inflammatory pseudotumor of epididymis and Epstein-Barr virus: a study of two cases. Pathology 1997;29:100–1.
59. Hollowood K, Fletcher CD. Pseudosarcomatous myofibroblastic proliferations of the spermatic cord ("proliferative funiculitis"). Histologic and immunohistochemical analysis of a distinctive entity. Am J Surg Pathol 1992;16:448–54.
59a. Hollowood K, Fletcher CD. Soft tissue sarcomas that mimic benign lesions. Semin Diag Pathol 1995;12:87–97.
60. Khalil KH, Ball RY, Eardley I, Ashken MH. Inflammatory pseudotumor of the rete testis. J Urol Pathol 1996;5:39–43.
60a. Kraus MD, Guillou L, Fletcher CD. Well-differentiated inflammatory liposarcoma: an uncommon and easily overlooked variant of a common sarcoma. Am J Surg Pathol 1997;21:518–27.
61. Lam KY, Chan KW, Ho MH. Inflammatory pseudotumor of the epididymis. Br J Urol 1995;75:255–7.
61a. Meis JM, Enzinger FM. Inflammatory fibrosarcoma of the mesentery and retroperitoneum: a tumor closely simulating inflammatory pseudotumor. Am J Surg Pathol 1991;15:1146–56.
62. Melamed MR, Farrow GM. Fibromyxomatous pseudotumor of the spermatic cord. In: Urologic neoplasms, Proceedings of the 50th Annual Anatomic Pathology Slide Seminar of the American Society of Clinical Pathologists, Chicago: ASCP Press, 1997:124–7.
63. Morgan AD. Inflammatory lesions simulating malignancy. Br J Urol 1964;36(Suppl):95–102.
64. Nishimura T, Akimoto M, Kawai H, Ohba S, Ohto S. Peritesticular xanthogranuloma. Urology 1981;18:189–90.
65. Piscioli F, Polla E, Pusiol T, Failoni G, Luciani L. Pseudomalignant cytologic presentation of spermatic hydrocele fluid. Acta Cytol 1982;27:666–70.
66. Yamashima M, Honma T, Uchijima Y. Myofibroblastic pseudotumor mimicking epididymal sarcoma. A clinicopathologic study of three cases. Pathol Res Pract 1992;188:1054–9.

Fibrous Pseudotumor, Fibromatous Periorchitis, Nodular Periorchitis

67. Bégin, LR, Frail D, Brzezinski A. Myofibroblastoma of the tunica testis: evolving phase of so-called fibrous pseudotumor? Hum Pathol 1990;21:866–8.
68. Cooper A. Observations on the structure and diseases of the testis. London, 1830.
69. Elem B, Patil PS, Lambert TK. Giant fibrous pseudotumor of the testicular tunics in association with schistosoma haematobium infection. J Urol 1988;141:376–7.
70. Goodwin WE. Multiple, benign, fibrous tumors of tunica vaginalis testis. J Urol 1946;56:438–47.

71. Meyer AW. Corpora libera in the tunica vaginalis testis. Am J Pathol 1928;4:445–55.
72. Morgan AD. Inflammatory lesions simulating malignancy. Brit J Urol 1964;36(Suppl):95–102.
73. Nistal M. Paniagua R, Torres A, Hidalgo L, Regadera J. Idiopathic peritesticular fibrosis associated with retroperitoneal fibrosis. Eur Urol 1986;12:64–8.
74. Parveen T, Fleischmann J, Petrelli M. Benign fibrous tumor of the tunica vaginalis testis. Arch Pathol Lab Med 1992;116:277–80.
75. Sen S, Patterson D, Sandoval O Jr, Wold L. Testicular adnexal fibrous pseudotumors. Urology 1984;23:594–7.

76. Shafik A. Constrictive albuginitis: report of 3 cases. J Urol 1979;122:269–71.
77. Thompson JE, Van Der Walt JD. Nodular fibrous proliferation (fibrous pseudotumor) of the tunica vaginalis testis. A light, electron microscopic and immunocytochemical study of a case and review of the literature. Histopathology 1986;10:741–8.
78. Vates TS, Ruemmler-Fisch C, Smilow PC, Fleisher MH. Benign fibrous testicular pseudotumors in children. J Urol 1993;150:1886–8.
79. Watson RA, Harper BN. Paratesticular fibrous pseudotumor in a patient with Gorlin's syndrome: nevoid basal cell carcinoma syndrome. J Urol 1992;148:1254–5.

Meconium Periorchitis

80. Dehner LP, Scott D, Stocker JT. Meconium periorchitis: a clinicopathologic study of four cases with a review of the literature. Hum Pathol 1986;17:807–12.
81. Forouhar F. Meconium peritonitis. Pathology, evolution, diagnosis. Am J Clin Pathol 1982;78:208–13.

81a. Stokes S III, Flom S. Meconium filled hydrocele sacs as a cause of acute scrotum in a newborn. J Urol 1997;158:1960–1.

Mesothelial Hyperplasia

81b. Daya D, McCaughey WT. Pathology of the peritoneum: a review of selected topics. Semin Diag Pathol 1991;8:277–89.
82. Lee JS, Nam JH, Lee MC, Park CS, Juhng SW. Immunohistochemical panel for distinguishing between carcinoma and reactive mesothelial cells in serous effusions. Acta Cytol 1996;40:631–6.
83. McCaughey WT, Al-Jabi M. Differentiation of serosal hyperplasia and neoplasia in biopsies. Pathol Annu 1986;(Pt. I)21:271–93.
83a. Morgan AD. Inflammation and infestation of the testis and paratesticular structures. In: Pugh RC, ed. Pathology of the testis. Oxford: Blackwell Scientific, 1976:79–138.

83b. Ordonez NG, Ro JY, Ayala AG. Lesions described as nodular mesothelial hyperplasia are primarily composed of histiocytes. Am J Surg Pathol 1998;22:285–92.
84. Rosai J, Dehner LP. Nodular mesothelial hyperplasia in hernia sacs. A benign reactive condition simulating a neoplastic process. Cancer 1975;35:165–75.
85. Singh HK, Silverman JF, Berns L, Haddad MG, Park HK. Signficance of epithelial membrane antigen in the work-up of problematic serous effusions. Diagn Cytopathol 1995;13:3–7.

Sclerosing Lipogranuloma

86. Oertel YC, Johnson FB. Sclerosing lipogranuloma of male genitalia. Review of 23 cases. Arch Pathol Lab Med 1977;101:321–6.

Abnormalities Related to Sexual Precocity-Idiopathic Hypertrophy

87. Nisula BC, Loriaux DL, Sherins RJ, Kulin HE. Benign bilateral testicular enlargement. J Clin Endocrinol Metab 1974;38:440–5.
88. Rosenthal SM, Grumbach MM, Kaplan SL. Gonadotropin-independent familial sexual precocity with premature Leydig and germinal cell maturation (familial testotoxicosis): effects of a potent luteinizing hormone-releasing factor

agonist and medroxyprogesterone acetate therapy in four cases. J Clin Endocrinol Metab 1983;57:571–9.
89. Wierman ME, Beardsworth DE, Mansfield MJ, et al. Puberty without gonadotropins. A unique mechanism of sexual development. N Engl J Med 1985;312:65–72.
90. Young RH, Scully RE. Testicular tumors. Chicago: ASCP Press, 1990.

Hyperplasia and Other Benign Lesions of the Rete

91. Hartwick RW, Ro JY, Srigley JR, Ordonez NG, Ayala AG. Adenomatous hyperplasia of the rete testis. A clinicopathologic study of nine cases. Am J Surg Pathol 1991;15:350–7
92. Nistal M, Paniagua R. Adenomatous hyperplasia of the rete testis. J Pathol 1988;154:343–6.

93. Nistal M, Paniagua R. Nodular proliferation of calcifying connective tissue in the rete testis: a study of three cases. Hum Pathol 1989;20:58–61.
93a. Srigley JR, Hartwick RW. Tumors and cysts of the paratesticular region. Pathol Annu 1990;25(Pt. 2):51–108.
94. Ulbright TM, Gersell DJ. Rete testis hyperplasia with hyaline globule formation. A lesion simulating yolk sac tumor. Am J Surg Pathol 1991;15:66–74.

Cysts

95. Eason AA, Spaulding JT. Dermoid cyst arising in testicular tunics. J Urol 1977;117:539.

96. Ford J, Singh S. Paratesticular dermoid cyst in 6-month-old infant. J Urol 1988;139:89–90.

96a. Heidenreich A, Zumbe J, Vorreuther R, Klotz T, Vietsch H. Testicular epidermoid cyst; orchiectomy or enucleation resection? (German) Urologe A 1996;35:1–5.

96b. McFadden DE, Clement PB. Peritoneal inclusion cysts with mural mesothelial proliferation: a clinicopathologic analysis of six cases. Am J Surg Pathol 1986;10:844–54.

96c. Nistal M, Iniguez L, Paniagua R. Cysts of the testicular parenchyma and tunica albuginea. Arch Pathol Lab Med 1989;113:902–6.

97. Price EB. Epidermoid cysts of the testis: a clinical and pathologic analysis of 69 cases from the testicular tumor registry. J Urol 1969;102:708–13.

98. Shah KH, Maxted WC, Chun B. Epidermoid cysts of the testis: a report of three cases and analysis of 141 cases from the world literature. Cancer 1981;47:577–82.

98a. Srigley JR, Hartwick RW. Tumors and cysts of the paratesticular region. Pathol Annu 1990;25(Pt. 2):51–108.

98b. Tejada E, Eble JN. Simple cyst of the rete tetis. J Urol 1988;139:376–7.

98c. Tobioka H, Manabe K, Matsuoka S, Sano F, Mori M. Multicystic mesothelioma of the spermatic cord. Histopathology 1995;27:479–81.

99. Van Niekerk WA. True hermaphroditism. Pediatr Adolesc Endocrinol 1981;8:80–99.

99a. Warner KE, Noyes DT, Ross JS. Cysts of the tunica albuginea testis: a report of three cases with a review of the literature. J Urol 1984;132:131–2.

99b. Weiss SW, Tavassoli FA. Multicystic mesothelioma: an analysis of pathologic findings and biologic behavior in 37 cases. Am J Surg Pathol 1988;12:737–46.

Cystic Dysplasia

100. Nistal M, Regardera J, Paniagua R. Cystic dysplasia of the testis. Light and electron microscopic study of three cases. Arch Pathol Lab Med 1984;108:579–83.

101. Tesluk H, Blankenberg TA. Cystic dysplasia of testis. Urology 1987;23:47–9.

102. Wegmann W, Illi O, Kummer-Vago M. Zystische Hodendysplasie mit ipsilateraler nierenagenesie. Schweiz Med Wschr 1984;114:144–8.

102a. Wojcik LJ, Hansen K, Diamond DA, et al. Cystic dysplasia of the rete testis: a benign congenital lesion associated with ipsilateral urological anomalies. J Urol 1997;158:600–4.

Microlithiasis

103. Coetzee T. Pulmonary alveolar microlithiasis with involvement of the sympathetic nervous system and gonads. Thorax 1970;25:637–42.

103a. Furness PD, Husmann DA, Brock JW, et al. Multi-institutional study of testicular microlithiasis in childhood: a benign or premalignant condition? J Urol 1998;160:1151–4.

103b. Mullins TL, Sant GR, Ucci AA, Doherty FJ. Testicular microlithiasis occurring in postorchiopexy testis. Urol 1986;27:144–6.

104. Priebe CJ, Garret R. Testicular calcification in a 4-year-old boy. Pediatrics 1970;46:785–8.

104a. Renshaw AA. Testicular calcifications: incidence, histology, and proposed pathological criteria for testicular microlithiasis. J Urol 1998;160:1625–8.

105. Weinberg AG, Currarino G, Stone IC Jr. Testicular microlithiasis. Arch Pathol 1973;95:312–4.

Spermatocele

106. Jassie MP, Mahmood P. Torsion of spermatocele: a newly described entity with 2 cases. J Urol 1985;125:47–50.

106a. Wakely CP. Cysts of the epididymis, the so-called spermatocele. Br J Surg 1943;31:165–71.

Sperm Granuloma, Vasitis Nodosa

107. Balogh K, Travis WD. The frequency of perineurial ductules in vasitis nodosa. Am J Clin Pathol 1984;82:710–3.

108. Benjamin JA, Robertson TD, Cheetham JG. Vasitis nodosa: a new clinical entity simulating tuberculosis of the vas deferens. J Urol 1943;49:575–82.

109. Civantos F, Lubin J, Rywlin AM. Vasitis nodosa. Arch Pathol 1972;94:355–61.

110. Cullen TH, Voss HJ. Sperm granulomata of the testis and epididymis. Brit J Urol 1966;37:202—7.

111. Friedman NB, Garske GL. Inflammatory reactions involving sperm and the seminiferous tubules: extravasation, spermatic granulomas and granulomatous orchitis. J Urol 1949;62:363–74.

112. Glassy FJ, Mostofi FK. Spermatic granulomas of the epididymis. Am J Clin Pathol 1956;26:1303–13.

113. Goldman RL, Azzopardi JG. Benign neural invasion in vasitis nodosa. Histopathology 1982;6:309–15.

114. Heaton JM, Maclennan KA. Vasitis nodosa—a site of arrest of malignant germ cells. Histopathology 1986;10:981–9.

115. Kiser GC, Fuchs EF, Kessler S. The significance of vasitis nodosa. J Urol 1986;136:42–4.

116. Kovi J, Agbata A. Benign neural invasion in vasitis nodosa [Letter]. JAMA 1974;228:1519.

117. Leader AJ, Alexrad SD, Frankowski R. Mumford SD. Complications of 2711 vasectomies. J Urol 1974;111:365–9.

118. Morgan AD. Inflammatory lesions simulating malignancy. Brit J Urol 1964;36(Suppl):95–102.

119. Schmidt SS, Technics and complications of elective vasectomy. The role of spermatic granuloma in spontaneous recanalization. Fertil Steril 1966;17:467–82.

120. Schmidt SS. Morris RR. Spermatic granuloma: the complication of vasectomy. Fertil Steril 1973;24:941–7.

121. Schned AR, Selikowitz SM. Epididymitis nodosa. An epididymal lesion analogous to vasitis nodosa. Arch Pathol Lab Med 1986;110:61–4.

122. Stout AP. Conditions of the epididymis simulating carcinoma. Proc New York Path Soc 1917;17:129–37.

Splenic-Gonadal Fusion

123. Putschar WG, Manion WC. Splenic-gonadal fusion. Am J Pathol 1956; 32:15-33.

124. Walter MM, Trulock TS, Finnerty DP, Woodard J. Splenic gonadal fusion. Urology 1988;32:521–4.

Atypical Epithelial Cells in Epididymis

125. Kuo TT, Gomez LG. Monstrous epithelial cells in human epididymis and seminal vesicles. A pseudomalignant change. Am J Surg Pathol 1981;5:483–90.

125a. Shah VI, Ro JY, Amin MB, Mullick S, Nazeer T, Ayala AG. Histologic variations in the epididymis: findings in 167 orchiectomy specimens. Am J Surg Pathol 1998;22:990–6.

Miscellaneous Lesions

126. Barton JH, Davis CJ, Sesterhenn IA, Mostofi FK. Smooth muscle hyperplasia of the testicular adnexa clinically mimicking neoplasia. Clinicopathologic study of sixteen cases. Am J Surg Pathol 1999;23:903–9.

126a. Bromberg WD, Kozlowski JM, Oyasu R. Prostate-type gland in the epididymis. J Urol 1991;145:1273–4.

127. Coyne J, Al-Nakib L, Goldsmith D, O'Flynn K. Secondary oxalosis and sperm granuloma of the epididymis. J Clin Pathol 1994;47:470–1.

127a. Coyne JD, Dervan PA. Multinucleated stromal giant cells of testis. Histopathology 1997;31:381–3.

128. Cozzutto C, Stracca-Pansa V, Salano F. Renal dysplasia of the sacral region: Metanephric dysplastic hamartoma of the sacral region. Virchows Arch [A] 1983;402:99–106.

129. Handelsman DJ, Yue DK, Turtle JR. Hypogonadism and massive testicular infiltration due to amyloidosis. J Urol 1983;129:610–2.

130. Healey GB, McDonald DF. Talc granuloma presenting as a testicular mass. J Urol 1977;118:122.

131. Honoré LH. Fatty metaplasia in a postpubertal undescended testis: a case report. J Urol 1979;122:841–2.

131a. Kaplan L. Granulomas due to "alparene no. 2" used in injection treatment of hernia. JAMA 1953;151:1188–90.

132. Nistal M, Paniagua R. Congenital testicular lymphangiectasia. Virchows Arch [A] 1977;377:79–84.

132a. Payan HM, Mendoza C Jr, Ceraldi A. Diffuse leiomyomatous proliferation in the epididymis. A cause of pain in hydrocele. Arch Surg 1967;94:427–9.

133. Pugh JI, Stringer P. Glove-powder granuloma of the testis after surgery. Brit J Surg 1973;60:240–2.

134. Schofield JB, Evans DJ. Multinucleate giant stromal cells in testicular atrophy following estrogen therapy. Histopathology 1990;16:200–1.

135. Srigley JR, Hartwick RW. Tumors and cysts of the paratesticular region. Pathol Annu 1990;25(Pt. 2):51–108.

136. Talerman A. Granulomatous lesions in the vas deferens caused by injection of radiopaque contrast medium. J Urol 1972;107:818-820.

137. Yoneda S. Kagawa S, Kurokana K. Dystrophic calcifying nodule with osteoid metaplasia of the testis. Brit J Urol 1979;51:413.

138. Young RH, Scully RE. Testicular and paratesticular tumors and tumor-like lesions of ovarian common epithelial and Müllerian types. A report of 4 cases and review of the literature. Am J Clin Pathol 1986;86:146–52.

9
THE SCROTUM

A wide variety of epithelial and stromal tumors of the scrotum have been reported (Table 9-1), but all of them are uncommon or rare. In this chapter we briefly review the normal anatomic and histologic features important to understanding the spectrum of scrotal lesions and the pathologic staging system for neoplasms, followed by a discussion of the salient clinicopathologic features of the disparate tumors and tumor-like lesions that may involve the scrotum. Only selected dermatological lesions, including skin appendage tumors and mesenchymal tumors that are seen with any appreciable frequency in the scrotum, are discussed. The entities included in this chapter are those involving the scrotum as defined below in the anatomy section, rather than those considered scrotal because they are in the scrotal sac. Lesions reported in the literature as "scrotal" often occur within the sac and are described in the chapters on paratesticular tumors (chapter 7) and tumor-like lesions of the testis and adnexa (chapter 8). Most standard textbooks of anatomy do not consider the tunica vaginalis part of the scrotum (1), although some sources consider it the innermost layer of the scrotum (2). We use the former approach here.

NORMAL ANATOMY AND HISTOLOGY

Embryologically, the scrotum is derived from the genital swellings or labioscrotal folds which, under the influence of 5-alpha-dihydrotestosterone, enlarge and fuse in the midline to form the scrotal sac (6).

The scrotum is a cutaneous fibromuscular sac that contains the testes, epididymes, and the lower part of the spermatic cord (3). The surface of the scrotum is divided into right and left halves by a midline cutaneous raphe, which continues ventrally to the inferior penile surface and dorsally along the perineum to the anus. The scrotum consists of: 1) skin, 2) the dartos muscle, 3) external spermatic fascia, 4) cremasteric muscle, and 5) internal spermatic fascia; it is partitioned in the midline by a fibrous septum (fig. 9-1) (1). The scrotal skin is thin, corrugated, and

Table 9-1

TUMORS AND TUMOR-LIKE LESIONS OF THE SCROTUM

I. Primary Tumors

Epithelial

  Premalignant
    Carcinoma in situ
  Other
    Bowenoid papulosis

  Malignant
    Squamous cell carcinoma
    Basal cell carcinoma
    Paget's disease
    Merkel cell carcinoma
    Carcinomas of skin adnexal-type

  Benign
    Tumors of epidermal origin
    Tumors of skin adnexal-type

Mesenchymal

  Malignant
    Leiomyosarcoma
    Liposarcoma
    Malignant fibrous histiocytoma
    Others
  Benign
    Hemangioma and angiokeratoma
    Lymphangioma and cystic hygroma
    Leiomyoma
    Myxoma and angiomyxoma
    Others

Hematopoietic
  Malignant lymphoma
  Others

Malignant melanoma

II. Secondary Tumors

III. Tumor-Like Lesions
  Condyloma acuminatum
  Verruciform xanthoma
  Idiopathic scrotal calcinosis and epidermoid cyst
  Sclerosing lipogranuloma (paraffinoma)
  Post-traumatic spindle cell nodule
  Hamartoma including "accessory scrotum" and elastoma
  Fat necrosis
  Scrotal edema
  Polymorphic reticulosis of genital skin
  Inflammatory and infectious diseases

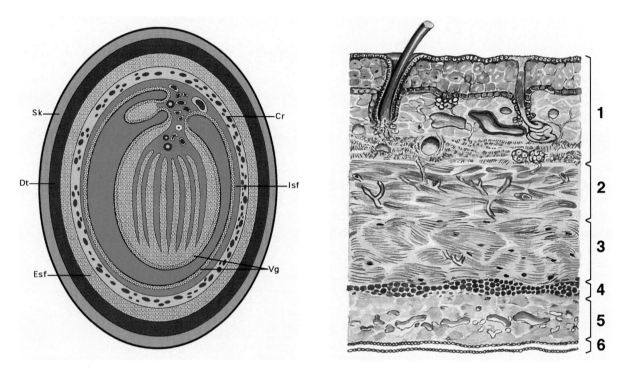

Figure 9-1
SCROTAL ANATOMY AND HISTOLOGY
Schematic diagrams of a cross section of the scrotal wall: 1) skin (Sk); 2) dartos (Dt); 3) external spermatic fascia (Esf); 4) cremasteric muscle (Cr); 5) internal spermatic fascia (Isf). The internal spermatic fascia is attached to the monolayered tunica vaginalis (Vg). (Courtesy of Dr. A. Cubilla, Asunción, Paraguay.)

pigmented, and contains a full complement of adnexal structures including hair follicles and sebaceous and sweat glands. Subcutaneous adipose tissue is absent although scattered fat cells may be present. The amount of fat varies between individuals, with more in obese men (7). Numerous nerve endings responsive to thermal and mechanical stimuli are also present. The dartos muscle consists of two coherent plexuses of smooth muscle cells. The superficial layer contains scattered individual cells (which are ultrastructurally myofibroblasts) and small ramifying bundles of smooth muscle which inhabit the papillary and upper reticular dermis (fig. 9-2, top) (4). Thicker bundles of smooth muscle, which stand out from the surrounding connective tissue, lie in the deep reticular dermis and subcutis (fig. 9-2, bottom) (4). The muscle contracts in the cold or during sexual stimulation and relaxes in warm temperatures. The external spermatic fascia continues from the external oblique aponeurosis. The skeletal mus-

cle bundles of the cremasteric muscle form the scrotal wall in the upper part and represent a continuation of the internal oblique muscle. The internal spermatic fascia continues from the transversalis fascia and is loosely attached to the monolayered, mesothelial lined parietal layer of the tunica vaginalis (8).

The scrotum derives its blood supply from the external pudendal artery (supplying chiefly the anterior scrotum), the scrotal branches of the internal pudendal artery, and a cremasteric branch of the inferior epigastric artery. Additional vascular supply comes from the testicular artery. The anterior scrotal wall is innervated by ilioinguinal and genitofemoral nerves while the posterior wall is supplied by branches of the pudendal nerve. Cutaneous nerve branches from the posterior femoral nerve contribute to the innervation of the scrotal skin. Although lymphatics from both halves of the scrotal wall anastomose across the midline raphe, the scrotal lymphatics drain into the ipsilateral inguinal lymph nodes (5).

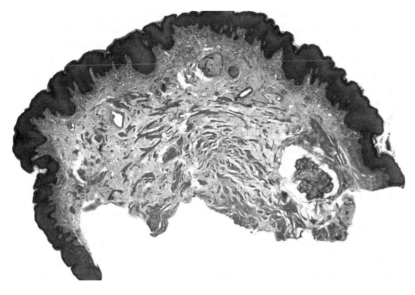

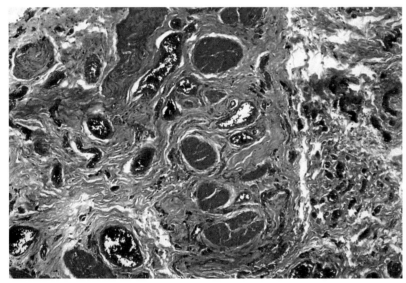

Figure 9-2
DARTOS MUSCLE
Top: Muscle bundles of the dartos are seen beneath the keratinized squamous epithelium.
Bottom: Thick bundles of conspicuous smooth muscle in the deep reticular dermis.

MALIGNANT EPITHELIAL TUMORS

Squamous Cell Carcinoma

General and Clinical Features. Over the past half century the incidence of squamous cell carcinoma, the most common malignant tumor of the scrotum, has dramatically decreased. Recent large series of cases from tertiary care centers in the United States including Memorial Sloan-Kettering Cancer Center (35), M.D. Anderson Cancer Center (30), Mayo Clinic (9), and Johns Hopkins Hospital (28) all averaged only one patient every 2 to 3 years.

This tumor is of great historical interest as it was the first cancer to be directly linked to occupational exposure (31). Carcinoma of the scrotum is said to have been prevalent among nomadic tribes of Persia because they carried pots with burning charcoal under their robes to keep warm (32). Over two and a half centuries ago, the tumor was described in Great Britain by Bassius (1731) and Treyling (1740) but received most attention when in 1775 Sir Percivall Pott, a surgeon at St. Bartholomew's Hospital in London, reported it to be a common occurrence in chimney sweeps (19,34). Over the next two centuries this tumor generated considerable interest as it has been linked to numerous industrial and occupational carcinogens (Table 9-2).

Pott conjectured that soot embedded in scrotal rugae caused the cancer, but it was only in 1922 that the alkaline ether extract of chimney soot was demonstrated to be the carcinogen (33). In 1875 Volkmann found an association of scrotal cancer in coal tar workers and the next year Bell reported the disease in paraffin and shale oil workers (19). In the early part of this century Southam and Wilson (38) noted this cancer in mule spinners in the cotton industry, an occupational hazard that persists. Further reports in the past several decades have shown a strong causal relationship between industrial oils and scrotal cancer. Occupations at risk have included machine operators in engineering, screw-making workers, automatic lathe operators, and petroleum wax pressmen (10,14,16,42). It appears that exposure to carcinogens in soot, tar, oils, and oil mist are unequivocally associated with an increased risk of scrotal cancer (22,25).

Kennaway and Kennaway (23) showed that, after excluding cases with occupational exposure to carcinogens, social class was an important predisposing factor, and no case in their series of 1029 patients was seen in white collar workers and professional classes. They attributed the incidence in laborers to lack of hygiene. Scrotal cancer is approximately eight times more common in the United Kingdom than in the United States in men over 25 years of age (20). The incidence was higher in an industrialized town (Birmingham, U.K.), 1 per 100,000, versus a college town (Oxford, U.K.), 0.2 per 100,000 (16). Race has not been extensively studied, but this disease appears less frequent in blacks (32). Combinations of psoralens and ultraviolet irradiation (PUVA) have been shown to be associated with malignant tumors of the male genital system (39); the risk to the genitalia (penis and scrotum) for squamous cell carcinoma is 5 to 15 times greater than for other regions at similar dosage levels of exposure (40,41). The increased risk of squamous cell carcinoma in patients with psoriasis treated with PUVA is dose dependent (15,40,41). Another recently documented risk factor is human papillomavirus infection. Of 14 patients with scrotal cancer with long-term follow-up from the Mayo Clinic files, 45 percent had documented human papillomavirus infection (9). A

Table 9-2

PROBABLE CAUSATIVE AGENTS AND OCCUPATIONS AT RISK FOR SCROTAL SQUAMOUS CELL CARCINOMA

Chimney sweepers
Coal tar workers
Paraffin and oil workers
"Mule-spinners" (cotton)
Textile workers
Machine engineers
Petroleum wax pressman
Screw-making industry
Automatic lathe operators
Coal tar, oils, soot
Psoralens and ultraviolet A radiation (PUVA)
Human papillomavirus

recent study reported integration of human papillomavirus type 16 into the tumor cell genome (32a). Finally, patients with multiple "epitheliomas" are susceptible to develop scrotal cancer; 3 of 14 patients from the Mayo Clinic series had a history of such lesions (9). Currently, most cases reported in the United States are not associated with occupational exposure (37,44). The epidemiologic and etiologic factors of scrotal cancer have recently been reviewed by Lowe, and readers desiring more detailed information may refer to his excellent review (29).

Squamous cell carcinoma is usually a solitary lesion involving men in their fifties (9,19,28,30, 35). In patients with occupational exposure, the left side and anterolateral aspect of the scrotum are more commonly involved; however, this proclivity is not significant when cases with occupational exposure are excluded (35). Mechanical irritation as workers continually brush against the greased machinery is the most likely explanation for left-sided scrotal involvement (11).

Gross Findings. The lesions present as slow-growing nodules, "warts," or pimples which persist for several months before ulcerating (figs. 9-3, 9-4) (35,38). At diagnosis, most are ulcerated, with raised rolled edges and an indurated base displaying a seropurulent discharge. Advanced lesions show invasion of the testis or penis (38). Approximately 50 percent of the patients have palpable

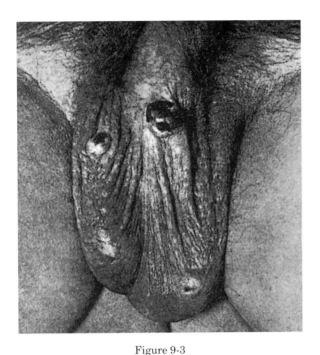

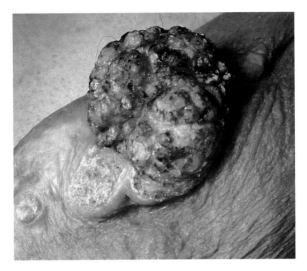

Figure 9-4
SQUAMOUS CELL CARCINOMA OF SCROTUM
Large bosselated mass. (Courtesy of Dr. S. F. Cramer, Rochester, NY.)

Figure 9-3
SQUAMOUS CELL CARCINOMA AT THE
JUNCTION OF SCROTUM AND PENIS
A second smaller lesion is seen on the right scrotum. The patient was a corkstone maker. (Fig. 128 from Fascicles 31b and 32, 1st Series.)

ipsilateral inguinal lymphadenopathy at presentation, and half of these will have metastasis in their lymphadenectomy specimen (29,35).

Microscopic Findings. The neoplasm is usually well to moderately differentiated, keratinizing, and identical to conventional cutaneous squamous cell carcinoma (fig. 9-5). Rare variants such as verrucous carcinoma may be seen (26). The epidermis adjacent to the ulcerated neoplasm may show dysplastic changes and is frequently acanthotic with hyperkeratosis. Squamous cell carcinoma in situ (Bowen's disease) accounted for 6 of 14 cases of scrotal squamous cell carcinoma in one series; human papillomavirus related changes were seen in 4 of these (9). The lesion may be heavily pigmented and is histologically characterized by a full-thickness involvement of the epidermis by atypical cells. The underlying stroma characteristically shows chronic inflammation and vascular proliferation (43). Bowenoid papulosis, a multicentric lesion that frequently affects younger men and which may have an indolent clinical course, is histologically very similar to Bowen's disease or may be

indistinguishable from it. Most cases of bowenoid papulosis involving the scrotum also involve the penis (21). In contrast to Bowen's disease, some cases of bowenoid papulosis may show greater maturation of keratinocytes.

Differential Diagnosis. The clinical differential diagnosis is wide and includes a variety of lesions including nevus, epidermoid cysts, eczema, psoriasis, folliculitis, tuberculosis, syphilis, hemangioma, lymphangioma, and other malignant tumors such as basal cell carcinoma, malignant melanoma, Paget's disease, and sarcoma. These entities are not likely to pose serious diagnostic difficulties on microscopic examination. Distinction from pseudoepitheliomatous hyperplasia depends on criteria similar to those discussed in the Fascicle on non-melanocytic lesions of the skin (31a).

Prognosis and Staging. The six patients with carcinoma in situ mentioned above had no evidence of disease at last follow-up (mean follow-up, 8.8 years)(9). The association of Bowen's disease and visceral malignancies remains controversial but must be borne in mind (12,13, 17,18). Due to the few analyzed cases, the prognostic significance of histologic grade is not known. The most commonly used staging system is Lowe's modification (27) of the system proposed by Ray and Whitmore (35). It is based on the extent of local disease and level of metastasis

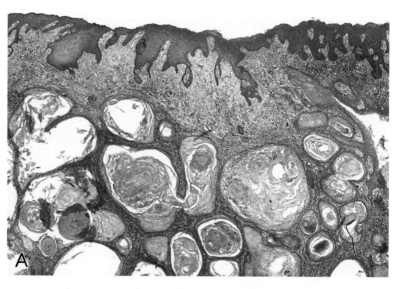

Figure 9-5
SQUAMOUS CELL
CARCINOMA OF SCROTUM

Histologic spectrum of differentiation.
Well differentiated (A), moderately differentiated (B), and poorly differentiated (C).
(A and C courtesy of Dr. A. Cubilla, Asunción, Paraguay.)

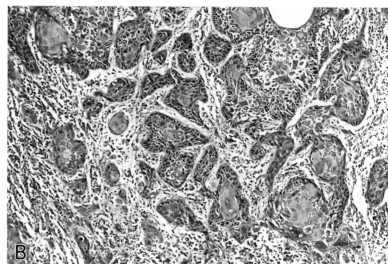

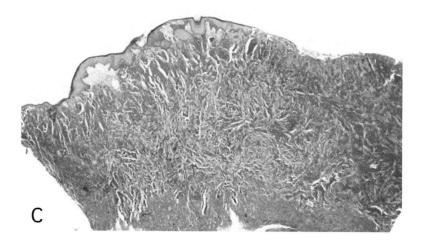

Table 9-3

STAGING SYSTEM FOR SCROTAL CARCINOMA*

Stage	Description
A1	Disease localized to the scrotum
A2	Locally extensive tumor invading adjacent structures such as testis, spermatic cord, penis, pubic bone, and perineum
B	Metastatic disease involving inguinal lymph nodes only
C	Metastatic disease involving pelvic lymph nodes without evidence of distant spread
D	Metastasis beyond the pelvic lymph nodes, to involve distant organs

*From Lowe FC. Squamous cell carcinoma of the scrotum. J Urol 1983;130:423–7.

(Table 9-3). Data regarding survival are limited, but overall the outcome is poor for invasive carcinoma: 2- and 5-year survival rates in the reported series vary from 65 to 76 percent and 22 to 52 percent, respectively (14,29,42). More recent studies by Ray and Whitmore (1977) (35) and McDonald (1982) (30) have shown a correlation of advanced stage with adverse outcome. Patients with localized (stage A1) disease in one study remained disease free while all patients with stage C disease died of widespread cancer (9). In a study of scrotal cancers in metal workers from Connecticut, Roush (36) noted that patients older than 65 years of age usually had nonlocalized cancers, with a 17 percent 5-year survival rate, while younger patients usually had localized cancer, with a 75 percent 5-year survival rate.

Basal Cell Carcinoma

Less than 30 cases of this neoplasm have been reported (45–48,50–52). The cause of basal cell carcinoma in non-sun exposed areas is unknown. Polymerase chain reaction to detect human papillomavirus infection has failed to link viral infection to the tumor (50). One case in India occurred in a jute-mill worker who was constantly exposed to mineral oil, but occupational carcinogens have not been incriminated otherwise (49).

The average patient age is 65 years (range, 42 to 82 years) (50). The lesion usually presents as plaques or ulcerated nodules. Histologically the lesions have typical features. Nodular, superficial, and superficial multicentric types have

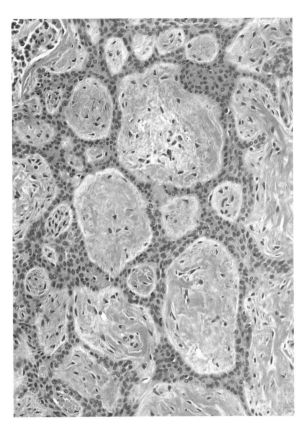

Figure 9-6
BASAL CELL CARCINOMA OF SCROTUM, FIBROEPITHELIOMA OF PINKUS-TYPE

been reported; we have personally seen a case of fibroepithelioma of Pinkus involving the scrotal skin (fig. 9-6). The proliferating nests and cords of basaloid cells show the characteristic peripheral palisading with occasional central squamous differentiation, microcyst formation, and retraction spaces. The stroma may be inflammatory or desmoplastic.

Basal cell carcinoma of the scrotum appears to be more aggressive than its nongenital cutaneous counterpart. The follow-up period of the reported cases has ranged from 5 months to 11 years (45,46,48,50,51). Three of 24 patients (13 percent) had lymph nodal or visceral metastasis and one patient died of disease (45,46,48,50,51).

Wide local excision with negative margins probably constitutes adequate therapy; the role of inguinal lymph node dissection is controversial (45,50). Radiation therapy has been administered in up to 15 percent of cases, usually in combination with surgery.

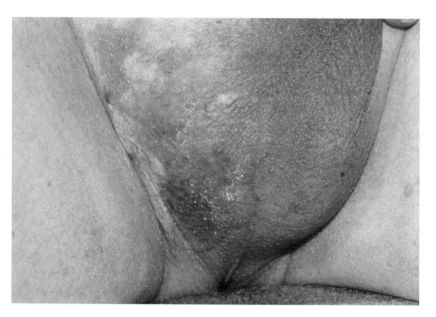

Figure 9-7
PAGET'S DISEASE OF SCROTUM
An ill-defined eczematous, scaly lesion involves a large portion of the scrotal skin. (Courtesy of Dr. D. Bell, Halifax, Nova Scotia, Canada.)

Paget's Disease

General and Clinical Features. In 1888, 14 years after Paget described the lesion of the breast (64), Crocker (56) described a case of Paget's disease of the scrotum, the first report of extramammary Paget's disease. Extramammary Paget's disease occurs chiefly in apocrine gland–bearing skin and involves anogenital regions more commonly in females than males. In 1937, Weiner (66) accepted only 15 of 58 previously reported cases as extramammary Paget's disease; in 4 the scrotum was involved. In 1985, Chandra (55) reviewed a 20-year experience with Paget's disease and identified 18 cases arising in the penis, scrotum, and groin. A few more case reports have been published since (54,60,63,64). The histogenesis of extramammary Paget's disease remains speculative but some of the lesions are believed to originate in the epidermis from cells programmed for apocrine differentiation and can be regarded as an intraepidermal adenocarcinoma with potential to invade the dermis. However, like mammary Paget's disease, the lesion in the scrotum may also be a consequence of epidermotropic spread from an underlying colorectal, urogenital, or cutaneous adnexal malignancy. Many patients have synchronous or metachronous visceral malignancy (57–59,61). Prostatic adenocarcinoma and apocrine gland carcinoma have coexisted with scrotal Paget's disease (61). Two cases of scrotal Paget's disease had widespread metastases without documented invasion at the primary site (53,65). The lesion presents as an erythematous or eczematous scaly lesion, occasionally associated with weeping serous fluid (fig. 9-7). A clinical misdiagnosis of eczema or dermatitis may delay appropriate therapy (64).

Microscopic Findings. Microscopically there are large, pale, vacuolated cells predominantly in the basal portion of the epidermis, often above an attenuated basal cell layer (fig. 9-8A). Single cells, nests, and occasional glands may be present, with migration of atypical cells to the superficial epidermis. The epidermis is usually acanthotic, often with hyperkeratosis and parakeratosis. There is frequent involvement of acrosyringeal adnexal structures. Focal microinvasion or frank invasion may be present but is rare. The abundant clear or vacuolated cytoplasm may stain with mucicarmine, colloidal iron, and alcian blue (fig. 9-8B). To aid in the differential diagnosis between malignant melanoma and Bowen's disease, immunohistochemical stains for carcinoembryonic antigen (CEA) (fig. 9-8C), cytokeratin, epithelial membrane antigen (EMA), S-100 protein, and HMB-45 may be performed, the latter two being negative in Paget's disease (54,62).

Treatment and Prognosis. Treatment of Paget's disease of the scrotum is wide surgical excision. Combinations of radiation and topical

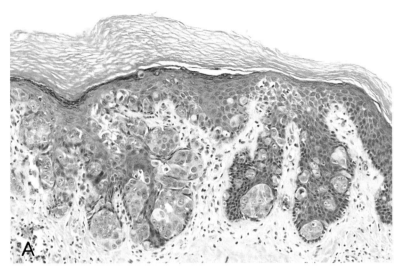

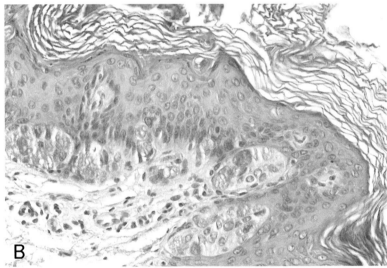

Figure 9-8
PAGET'S DISEASE OF SCROTUM
Intraepidermal nests of large vacuolated cells are situated predominantly in
the basal portion of the epidermis (A). Alcian blue stain (B) and immunohistochemical stain for carcinoembryonic antigen (C).

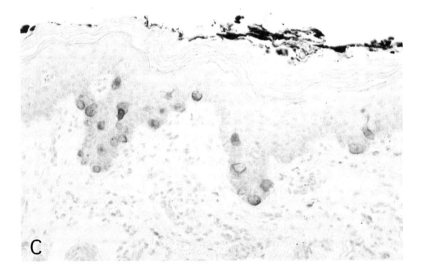

chemotherapy may also be administered (54). The outcome for patients depends on the extent of local disease and evolution of associated malignancy (55).

Merkel Cell Carcinoma

A single scrotal example of this cutaneous tumor has been described in an 84-year-old who presented with a rapidly enlarging dermal mass of the left hemiscrotum (67). The tumor measured 6 cm, and histologically consisted of small cells with oval hyperchromatic nuclei and scant cytoplasm. Numerous mitoses and foci of necrosis were present. The tumor was immunoreactive for neuron-specific enolase and ultrastructural studies showed poorly formed desmosomes and scattered membrane-bound, electron-dense neurosecretory granules. The patient died after 16 months with widespread metastases (67).

Miscellaneous Malignant Tumors of Skin Adnexal-Type

Since the scrotum is a cutaneous-lined fibromuscular sac, neoplasms of the skin adnexa such as apocrine gland adenocarcinoma and malignant syringoadenoma papilliferum may occur. Their features are as seen elsewhere.

MALIGNANT MESENCHYMAL TUMORS

A wide range of tumors in this category, mainly leiomyosarcomas and liposarcomas, have been reported, but all are rare. Reported other tumors include rhabdomyosarcoma (84), fibrosarcoma (75), neurogenic sarcoma (83), and Kaposi's sarcoma (71,86).

Leiomyosarcoma

Approximately 27 leiomyosarcomas of the scrotum have been reported (69,70,72,73,79–82, 84,87). In a review of 14 cases, the mean patient age was 57 years (range, 35 to 89 years) and the mean tumor size was 10.5 cm (range, 2.5 to 60 cm). One occurred in a man who received scrotal irradiation as a child (70). These tumors may arise from the arrector pili muscle of the dermis, the smooth muscle of vessel walls, or the smooth muscle of the dartos muscle.

Microscopic examination shows the typical interdigitating fascicles of spindle cells with oval

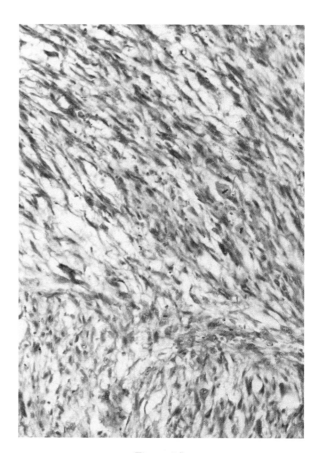

Figure 9-9
LEIOMYOSARCOMA OF SCROTUM
Interlacing fascicles of malignant spindle cells. (Courtesy of Dr. A. Cubilla, Asunción, Paraguay.)

to cigar-shaped nuclei and moderate to abundant eosinophilic fibrillar cytoplasm (fig. 9-9). The most reliable criterion of malignancy is mitotic activity. Based on the largest series of six cases reported by Newman and Fletcher (81), any mitotic activity (similar to cutaneous or subcutaneous leiomyosarcoma) in a scrotal lesion should be regarded as worrisome for a possible malignant course. Four of the tumors in their series were high grade with many mitoses and marked pleomorphism and two were low grade.

Leiomyosarcoma of the scrotum has a potential for both local recurrence and distant metastasis. Of the 14 patients reviewed by Moon et al. (79), 5 of 9 had metastases (3 with initial local recurrence), 3 had no evidence of disease, and 1 died of other causes (follow-up, 1 to 24 years). In the Newman and Fletcher series (81) only one patient with high-grade tumor developed metastasis and subsequently died of disease. Prolonged clinical surveillance is necessary as metastases may develop after many years (85).

Liposarcoma

Many of the cases reported in the literature as "liposarcoma of the scrotum" are actually paratesticular (spermatic cord) neoplasms presenting as an intrascrotal mass. Six liposarcomas of the scrotal wall have been reported (68, 76,77). Clinical examination and imaging studies have shown a large scrotal mass separate from the testis and spermatic cord (68). Histologic subtyping into well differentiated, myxoid, round cell, and pleomorphic categories, as for liposarcomas of the extremities and retroperitoneum, should be done and may have prognostic implications (68).

Malignant Fibrous Histiocytoma

Three cases of malignant fibrous histiocytoma involving the scrotal wall have been reported (74,78,88). The tumors usually present as a mass of several centimeters with variable hemorrhage and necrosis. The prognosis has been poor, with the longest survival period 27 months (74).

MALIGNANT LYMPHOMA

A case of malignant lymphoma of the scrotum, diagnosed as a "reticulum cell sarcoma," was reported in 1972 (90). The patient had concurrent inguinal lymphadenopathy and subsequently developed a scrotal recurrence and pulmonary lesions. A more recent case (1994) of primary scrotal lymphoma of T-cell phenotype occurred in a 64-year-old human immunodeficiency virus (HIV)-negative homosexual male (89). Thorough staging evaluation revealed no other lesions. This histologically high-grade tumor was treated with local surgical excision and multiple cycles of chemotherapy. At 26 months the patient was in clinical remission after a relapse in the skin of the hand (89).

MALIGNANT MELANOMA

One of the earliest, possibly the earliest, case of malignant melanoma of the scrotum, was described in the classic treatise on the diseases of the

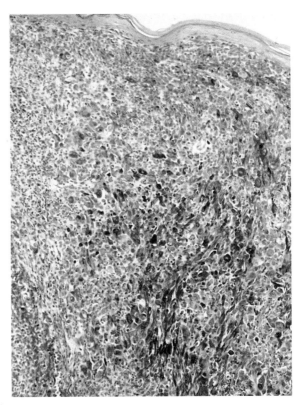

Figure 9-10
MALIGNANT MELANOMA OF SCROTAL SKIN
Infiltrating atypical melanocytes which demonstrate nuclear pleomorphism and heavy pigmentation are present in the dermis. (Courtesy of Dr. A. Cubilla, Asunción, Paraguay.)

testes, spermatic cord, and scrotum by Curling in 1856 (90a). Six additional malignant melanomas of the scrotum have been reported in the more contemporary literature (91–96). The mean age of the patients was 53 years (range, 43 to 68 years), and they presented with an ulcerated red papule or a pigmented elevated lesion. Histologically, the lesions were superficial spreading or nodular types (fig. 9-10). Three patients had inguinal lymphadenopathy, two of whom later developed systemic metastases. The three other patients survived for long periods (5, 17, and 18 years) (93).

BENIGN TUMORS

Almost all benign tumors of the scrotum are of mesenchymal derivation and a plethora of histologic subtypes may occur. A few benign epithelial tumors of skin adnexal type have also been described. They appear as they do elsewhere in the body.

Benign Epithelial Tumors

A typical sebaceous trichofolliculoma of the scrotum and penis was reported in a 22-year-old (97). No other cutaneous lesions were present. Other cutaneous adnexal tumors of apocrine, eccrine, or hair follicle origin may also involve the scrotal skin.

Benign Mesenchymal Tumors

Vascular Tumors. These lesions arise within the dermis and may be classified as hemangioma, angiokeratoma, lymphangioma, or cystic hygroma.

Hemangioma. Less than 50 cases of hemangioma have been documented although we suspect the frequency may be higher than that reflected in published reports (99,110,114,138). They may clinically mimic scrotal carcinoma. Gibson (114) noted that genital hemangiomas of the skin were usually of capillary type and those of subcutaneous tissue were cavernous hemangiomas. The lesions may be congenital or acquired, the former being more common. The neoplastic nature of these lesions is subject to debate as some may represent arteriovenous malformations, and a history of trauma has been recorded in some cases. Hemangiomas frequently present in the first two decades of life as a painless enlargement. The overlying skin may have a bluish or red hue. Pain, heaviness, bleeding, and ulceration are less frequent. Many of the lesions in children involute with age, but some remain stable or enlarge as the child grows. Histologically, the lesions are as seen elsewhere and can be distinguished from scrotal arteriovenous malformations which exhibit numerous arterioles and thick-walled veins without an intervening capillary bed (143).

Angiokeratoma. This distinctive vascular lesion of the scrotum is histologically characterized by multiple, blood-filled, capillary-sized vascular spaces that bulge into the overlying hyperplastic epithelium (122). In 1896 Fordyce (113) first reported a case of angiokeratoma of the scrotum which he regarded as being distinct from the angiokeratoma described by Mibelli in 1889 (129) and which had a proclivity for the bony prominences of young females with a history of chilblains (an inflammatory process that develops secondary to exposure to cold). Since then the clinical spectrum of angiokeratoma has

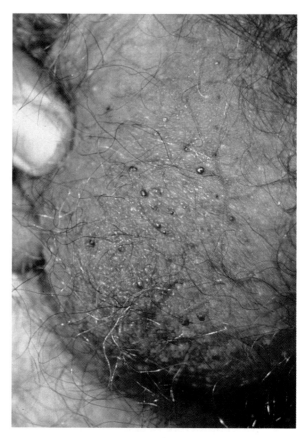

Figure 9-11
ANGIOKERATOMAS OF SCROTUM
Multiple, small red lesions are visible. (Fig. 18.1 from Weiss MA, Mills SE. Atlas of genitourinary tract disorders, Philadelphia: Lippincott-Raven, 1988:18.2.)

considerably widened and scrotal angiokeratoma is regarded as a variant of angiokeratoma distinct from diffuse systemic angiokeratoma corporis diffusum (associated with Fabry's disease), angiokeratoma of Mibelli, solitary papillary angiokeratoma, and plaque-like angiokeratoma circumscriptum (103).

Angiokeratomas of Fordyce are the most common angiokeratomas and are clinically evident as 1- to 4-mm, red to blue, soft, compressible lesions which are usually multifocal (fig. 9-11) in middle-aged to elderly patients. The lesions may present as early as late adolescence, but become progressively more common with increasing age (123). Three fourths of patients are symptomatic, with complaints of soreness, itchiness, or bleeding. Conditions resulting in increased venous pressure are felt to be predisposing factors and include

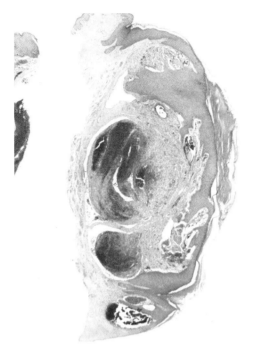 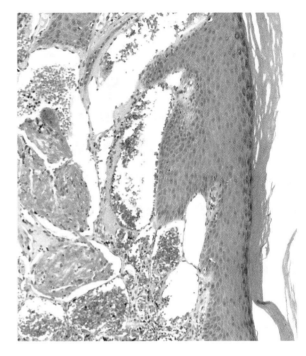

Figure 9-12
ANGIOKERATOMA OF SCROTUM
Left: A low-power view shows marked vascular dilatation in the papillary dermis with thrombi.

varicocele, hernia, thrombophlebitis, prostatitis, and genitourinary malignancies (122). Fordyce believed that senility predisposed to loss of vascular support, atrophy of the dartos muscle, and degeneration of elastic tissue. In the series of Imperial and Helwig (122), 69 percent had one of the associated predisposing conditions mentioned above, supporting the role of elevated venous pressure. Agger and Osmundsen (98) documented a case in which surgical correction of a varicocele resulted in regression. A more recent study, however, questions the association of varicocele and angiokeratoma of the scrotum, with only coincidental occurrence in 435 soldiers (135). Nonetheless, in patients seeking attention for angiokeratoma of the scrotum, a search for a potential predisposing factor is in order.

A study of 35 cases of angiokeratoma reported by the Armed Forces Institute of Pathology (122) provides a classic histologic description of these lesions: 1) marked dilation of the papillary dermal vasculature with or without thrombi (fig. 9-12); 2) acanthosis and elongation of rete ridges forming a collarette partly or circumferentially engulfing vascular lacunae; 3) hyperkeratosis

which may be moderate to marked (66 percent); 4) parakeratosis (20 percent); 5) a direct communication between the cystic vascular spaces and underlying dilated veins in the deep dermis; and 6) dermal fibrotic and mild chronic inflammatory changes, atrophy of the dartos muscle, and degeneration of elastic tissue.

Lymphangioma. Guenkdjian (118) recorded 16 cases of scrotal lymphangiomas seen from 1929 to 1955, and about 25 have been added subsequently (120a,125,131,137,140). Lymphangiomas may also be acquired secondary to filariasis (120). Cystically dilated lymphangiomas (cystic hygromas) also rarely involve the scrotum (fig. 9-13) and characteristically occur in children with a mean age of 3 years (120a). Many not only involve the scrotal soft tissues but extend into the deep perineum and/or inguinal region, making complete excision difficult and predisposing to recurrence (120a). Histologically, lymphangiomas are devoid of blood but have delicate valves and frequently contain lymphocytes which may also percolate into the adjacent loose connective tissue. A disorganized smooth muscle wall may be present.

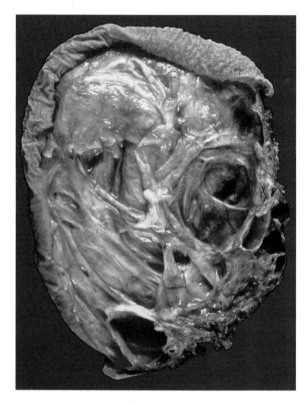

Figure 9-13
LYMPHANGIOMA OF SCROTUM
A multiloculated cystic lesion. (Courtesy of Dr. C. Galliani, Birmingham, AL.)

Leiomyoma. Leiomyomas of the scrotum may be subclassified as *leiomyoma cutis* and *dartoic leiomyoma*. The former may be further classified on the basis of a presumed origin as pilar leiomyoma (from adnexal smooth muscle) or angioleiomyoma (from vascular smooth muscle). All are exceeding rare and usually range from 0.2 to 3.0 cm, but may be larger. Less than 50 cases have been described, most as case reports, but three series report 4, 4, and 10 cases each (101,111,116,119,121,127,128,130,132,133, 136,141,141a,142,144,145). Clinically, the lesions are firm to hard rubbery masses which may be fixed to the overlying skin. In almost all cases the diagnosis of leiomyoma was not made on clinical grounds. Two cases of pedunculated leiomyoma have been reported (104,105).

Histologically, the tumors are unencapsulated but circumscribed proliferations of spindle-shaped cells arranged in fascicles within the dermis, with or without involvement of subcutaneous tissue (fig. 9-14, left). The overlying skin is atten-

uated but not ulcerated. The smooth muscle fascicles are separated by variably collagenized stroma (fig. 9-14, right). Myxoid change is unusual and rarely lymphoid aggregates may be present at the periphery. Bizarre and degenerate-appearing "symplastic" changes have been described (106,133). The criteria that help separate benign from malignant tumors are discussed on page 352. An unusual case of a 35-year-old with an "egg-size" mass of the scrotum which was initially histologically benign and which recurred on several occasions has been reported; the lesion ultimately showed features of leiomyosarcoma. The patient had received postoperative radiation after excision of the first mass; 15 years later he developed metastasis to the liver and died of disease (141). The authors concluded from their experience with 11 cases that surgical excision was curative, recurrence an ominous sign, and radiation contraindicated.

Other Benign or Locally Aggressive Mesenchymal Tumors. Several cases of scrotal and intrascrotal lipoma have been reported, but many are probably paratesticular rather than true scrotal wall lesions (see page 259). In large lesions it is frequently impossible to know the site of origin (112,117,139).

Fibromas, including the so-called giant fibroma (126) and giant pendulous fibroma of the scrotum (124); fibrolipoma; myxoma; and myxofibroma are all rare scrotal tumors. They are histologically bland and clinically indolent. Other even rarer tumors that have been documented include infantile fibromatosis of external genitalia (102) and giant cell fibroblastoma (fig. 9-15) (107,108), a nonmetastasizing, locally recurring tumor of childhood and youth. Angiomyofibroblastomas and aggressive angiomyxomas arise in paratesticular soft tissues and are discussed in chapter 7.

A lesion distinct from angiomyofibroblastoma is superficial angiomyxoma or cutaneous myxoma (110a). Four cases involving the scrotum have been reported, all presenting as a slowly growing, painless mass of 2 months to at least 4 years duration. The lesions varied from 1 to 6 cm and presented as well-demarcated, nodular or multinodular masses. The cut section was typically mucoid, gelatinous, and semitranslucent, reflecting the myxoid nature of the lesion. Histologically, all lesions contained abundant myxoid

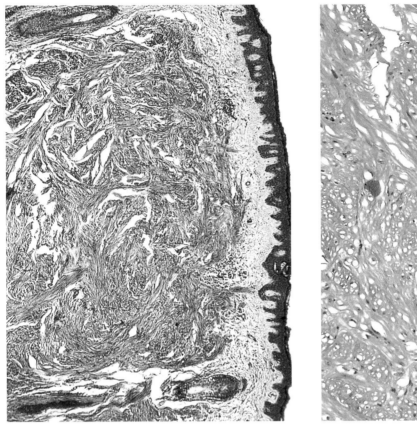
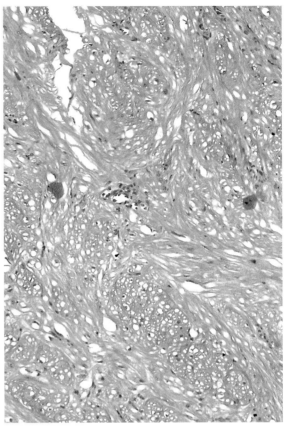

Figure 9-14
LEIOMYOMA OF DARTOS

Left: Low-power view.
Right: High-power view of another case showing smooth muscle bundles separated by abundant collagenized stroma.

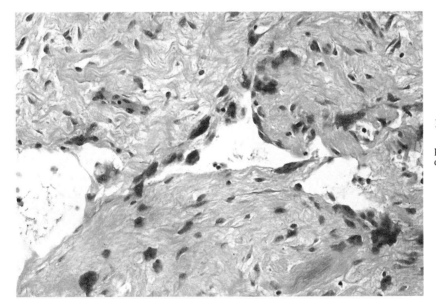

Figure 9-15
GIANT CELL
FIBROBLASTOMA OF SCROTUM
Multinucleated giant cells lining a pseudovascular space, with spindle cells in a hyalinized stroma.

matrix that formed pools in the dermis or subcutis. The lesional cells were bipolar and stellate shaped with occasional multinucleated cells. The vascularity varied from hypovascular to prominent with a complex arborizing pattern. No recurrence was reported in the two cases in which follow-up was available (91 and 240 months) (110a).

Benign neural tumors reported to involve the scrotum include schwannoma (109), neurofibroma (134,146), and granular cell tumors; no reported neurofibromas were associated with von Recklinghausen's disease (146).

Juvenile xanthogranuloma (solitary reticulohistiocytic granuloma) has been reported in the scrotum (100,115). The lesions occur in children or young adults, may involute spontaneously, and appear unrelated to Langerhans' granulomatosis (histiocytosis X) (100,115).

SECONDARY TUMORS

Cutaneous scrotal metastases from carcinomas of the prostate, colon, stomach, and kidney (fig. 9-16) have been reported (147–151). The clinical history, usually advanced age of the patient, multiplicity of lesions, presence of tumor in vascular/lymphatic spaces, and adenocarcinoma histology of most points towards a secondary origin of these tumors.

TUMOR-LIKE LESIONS

Condyloma Acuminatum

Condyloma acuminatum is more common on the penis but may also involve the peno-scrotal junction and scrotum. The lesions are usually papillomatous, pedunculated or sessile growths with a roughened keratotic surface (condyloma acuminatum), but on occasion may be flat (condyloma plana) and clinically inapparent until detected by enhancement with 3 to 5 percent acetic acid. Most lesions are single and less than 2 cm, but multiple lesions may occur (fig. 9-17A,B) and coalesce to form a mass of several centimeters (giant condyloma). Most condylomas occur in young males but when seen in children (fig. 9-17C) should raise the possibility of sexual abuse or transmission from the mother at delivery (170). The histologic features are identical to condylomatous lesions of the penis

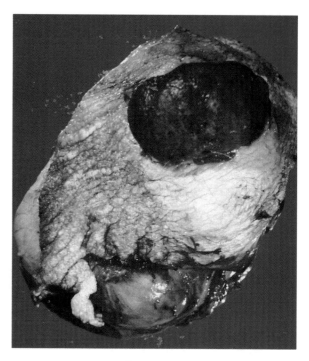

Figure 9-16
METASTATIC RENAL CELL CARCINOMA
INVOLVING SCROTAL SKIN

and more detailed descriptions may be found in the Fascicles on nonmelanocytic skin tumors (172a) and uterine cervix (165a).

Verruciform Xanthoma

Verruciform xanthoma is a rare entity of uncertain nature occurring primarily in the oral mucosa but infrequently also arising in the skin at several sites, notably the anogenital region (165,172,173,181). One penile and three scrotal cases were recently reported (172). The mean age of the patients was 52 years. The lesions were solitary, varying in size from 0.2 to 1.8 cm, and were clinically slow growing.

On microscopic examination the surface is verrucoid, papillary, or crater shaped (fig. 9-18). The epidermis displays acanthosis, papillomatosis, and hyperkeratosis; the granular layer is absent. Parakeratosis is prominent between the papillae, and is associated with a variably intense but prominent neutrophilic infiltrate at the junction of the parakeratotic layer and stratum spinosum. The epidermis lacks koilocytotic atypia. Besides the verrucoid appearance, the

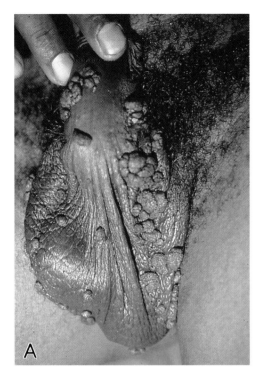

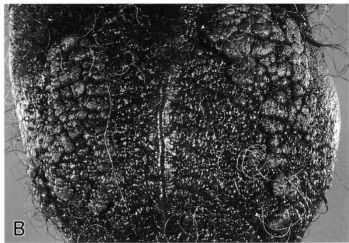

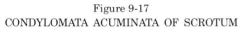

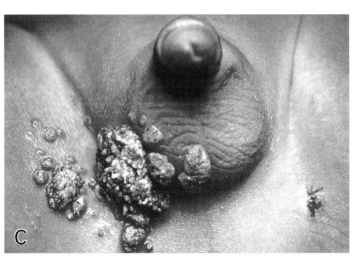

Figure 9-17
CONDYLOMATA ACUMINATA OF SCROTUM
Numerous, discrete and confluent lesions involve the scrotal skin (A–C). The extensive disease required radical excision of the entire scrotal skin in one of the illustrated cases (B). Numerous lesions in a child involve the scrotal skin and skin of inner thigh (C). (A is fig. 18.19 from Weiss MA, Mills SE. Atlas of genitourinary tract disorders. Philadelphia: Lippincott-Raven, 1988:18.18.) (B, C are figs. 17.2 and 17.1 from Ro JY, Grignon DG, Amin MB, Ayala AG. Atlas of surgical pathology of the male reproductive tract. Philadelphia: W.B. Saunders Co., 1997:202.)

hallmark of this lesion is the presence of plump, round, foamy histiocytes which fill the papillary dermis between and at the tips of papillae (fig. 9-18). A band-like lymphoplasmacytic infiltrate may be present at the base (172).

The etiology of this lesion remains elusive. Due to its peculiar occurrence in the oral cavity and genital skin, the possible role of a transmittable viral infection like human papillomavirus has been considered. However, no human papillomavirus was detected by DNA in situ hybridization with an omniprobe against 14 viral types. More sensitive tests, including polymerase chain reaction and whole-genomic probe to RNA of human papilloma types 6, 11, and 16, were also negative (172).

The differential diagnosis includes verrucous lesions of the genital skin, particularly condyloma acuminatum which lacks the distinctive xanthomatous infiltrate. A Grocott stain may be valuable to rule out fungal infection as we have personally seen a case of candida infection closely mimic verruciform xanthoma.

Porokeratosis of Mibelli

Porokeratosis of Mibelli presenting exclusively on genital skin is extremely rare; much more commonly it involves the genitalia as part of a generalized widespread eruption. A 27-year-old had a 2-year history of asymptomatic marginated lesions on his penis, scrotum, and natal cleft (166).

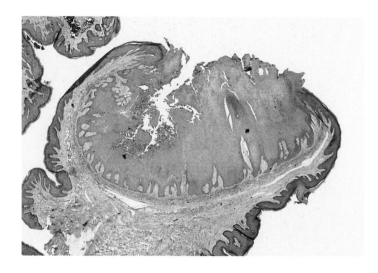

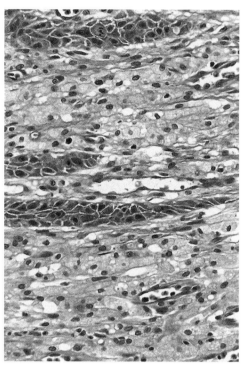

Figures 9-18
VERRUCIFORM XANTHOMA OF SCROTUM
Above: Low power shows a crater-shaped verrucoid lesion.
Right: High-power view showing numerous foamy macrophages between elongated rete ridges.

The three scrotal lesions measured 1 cm each, and were characterized by a hyperkeratotic epidermis and coronoid lamellae containing parakeratotic nuclei. The etiology remains unknown but has a genetic component with an autosomal dominant pattern mostly affecting males (166).

"Idiopathic" Scrotal Calcinosis and Epidermoid Cysts

Scrotal calcinosis is an uncommon disorder characterized by the progressive development of calcific nodules in the scrotal skin which if untreated may result in dramatic distortion and destruction of the scrotum (154,171,183,187,189). The lesions first appear in childhood or early adulthood (90 percent occur before 40 years of age), and may be solitary or multiple with a tendency to slowly enlarge. The etiology of this lesion has been debated. In most patients the lack of a clinical history of hyperparathyroidism, advanced renal failure, or systemic sarcoidosis fails to support metastatic calcification as a mechanism (187). Dystrophic calcification is currently favored. Dare and Axelsen (154) have shown small cysts lined by stratified squamous epithelium in three of four cases. The cysts were deemed to be eccrine duct

milia because of 1) communication with eccrine ducts; 2) ultrastructural differentiation towards eccrine duct in one case; and 3) immunohistochemical positivity for carcinoembryonic antigen, a marker for eccrine sweat glands. These findings have been supported by Song et al. (183) who histologically studied 51 lesions in a 29-year-old male with a 2-year history of subcutaneous nodules which sometimes discharged chalky material. They noted that some nodules were intact cysts that were histologically of epidermoid, pilar, or, because of extensive calcification of indeterminate nature, hybrid (183). Similar observations were made by Michl et al. (171) and Melo et al. (169). It is, therefore, plausible that idiopathic scrotal calcinosis represents an end stage of numerous "old" epidermal cysts. Dare and Axelsen conclude that because the evidence strongly suggests a dystrophic rather than idiopathic origin for this disease, the term idiopathic be dropped from the nomenclature. It is unclear why some cysts show a predilection for calcification and others do not.

The lesions vary in size from a few millimeters to larger, nodular, bosselated masses (fig. 9-19); one remarkable example was 26 x 15 x 8 cm. The lesions are nontender and usually asymptomatic but may be associated with discharge of

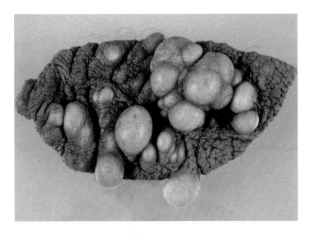

Figure 9-19
IDIOPATHIC SCROTAL CALCINOSIS
Multiple variably sized nodules extensively involve the scrotal skin. (Courtesy of Dr. J. Watts, Royal Oak, MI.)

chalky white material from ulcerated lesions, or may be pruritic.

Histologically, the lesions are characterized by granules and globules of basophilic calcific material in the dermis (fig. 9-20). A foreign body giant cell granulomatous reaction may be present and infrequently a recognizable cyst wall lining is seen. By infrared spectrophotometry the dermal deposits consist of calcium phosphate (52 percent) and magnesium ammonium phosphate (48 percent) (163).

The differential diagnosis includes dystrophic calcification due to parasites. Four patients from Africa who were infected with *Onchocerca volvulus* had scrotal calcinosis, and in two individuals dead nematodes were demonstrated in the calcific masses (153). Clinically well-delineated, noncoalescent dermal nodules which histologically show characteristic features of epidermoid cysts, including keratinizing squamous epithelium and keratinaceous material, should be regarded as such (fig. 9-21).

Most cases of scrotal calcinosis are managed effectively by local excision; however, large lesions with marked destruction of the scrotum have required partial to total scrotectomy (187,189).

Sclerosing Lipogranuloma (Paraffinoma)

Oertel and Johnson (174) found 23 cases of this lesion in the files of the Armed Forces Institute of Pathology, 14 of them involving the scrotum. Their findings and those of most others

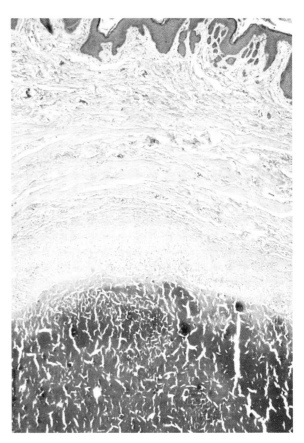

Figure 9-20
IDIOPATHIC SCROTAL CALCINOSIS
Basophilic calcific material is seen in the deep dermis.

suggest that the lesions are secondary to injections or topical application of oil-based substances such as paraffin, silicone, oil, or wax, either for cosmetic (enlargement of genitals) or therapeutic use. While most penile lipogranulomas are secondary to injections of oils, scrotal lipogranulomas may additionally be due to trauma and cold weather. Takihara et al. (186) reported two cases of "primary" scrotal lipogranuloma, histologically identical to most lipogranulomas, in which lipid analysis showed no exogenous fatty elements.

Most lesions are seen in men less than 40 years of age who complain of a localized plaque or mass which may be tender and indurated. The mass is usually a few centimeters in diameter but may be massive and replace the scrotal wall (fig. 9-22). Biopsy, excision, or both are mandatory to exclude a neoplasm, especially in the absence of a clinical history of injection. The gross specimens are often fragmented because the

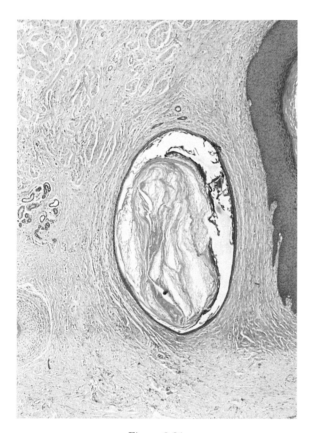

Figure 9-21
EPIDERMOID CYST OF SCROTUM

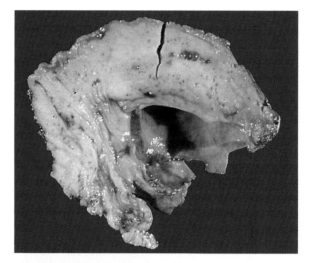

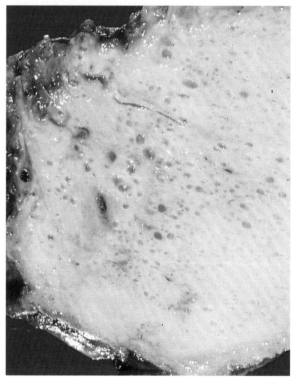

Figure 9-22
LIPOGRANULOMA OF SCROTAL WALL
Low-power view (top) shows replacement of entire scrotal wall
by solid yellow-white tissue with interspersed cysts (bottom).

lesion is removed in pieces due to its location and ill-defined margins, but rarely intact specimens are encountered (fig. 9-22, top). The tissue is usually firm, yellow to grayish white, and solid or solid and cystic (fig. 9-22, bottom). On microscopic examination lipid vacuoles of varying sizes are embedded in a variably sclerotic stroma. Considerable variation in vacuole size is a useful diagnostic feature; some vacuoles are barely larger than an erythrocyte while others are large, corresponding to grossly visible cysts. The cysts lack an epithelial lining but may be lined by multinucleated giant cells (fig. 9-23, left). The inflammatory response is variable; a histiocytic or foreign body granulomatous infiltrate, with or without lymphocytes and eosinophils, is usually present (167,168,182). The diagnosis is not difficult in most cases and may be confirmed by lipid stains. Sections from frozen tissue show positivity for oil red O (fig. 9-23, right); osmium tetroxide fails to blacken the lipid which is characteristic of par-

affin hydrocarbons (174). Infrared spectrophotometry has demonstrated paraffin hydrocarbons in most cases (174).

The histologic differential diagnosis may include signet-ring cell carcinoma or sclerosing liposarcoma, but distinction from these should be

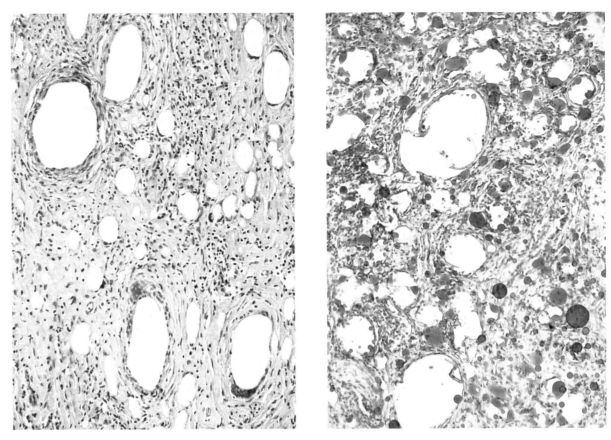

Figure 9-23
LIPOGRANULOMA OF SCROTAL WALL

Left: Numerous, variably sized vacuolated spaces often lined by giant cells are separated by a fibroinflammatory stroma.
Right: Oil red O stain.

straightforward because the vacuoles in the former are due to accumulation of mucin, and foreign body giant cells are lacking in the two neoplasms.

Post-Traumatic Spindle Cell Nodule

Postoperative spindle cell nodules of the male genital system usually occur in the prostate, but rarely a similar lesion occurs in the scrotum because of trauma. Papadimitriou and Drachenberg (175) described two "post-traumatic spindle cell nodules" in the scrotum of two patients, 22 and 67 years of age. One lesion was circumscribed and measured 2.5 cm, while the other presented as progressive enlargement and irregular nodular thickening of the scrotal sac. Histologically, haphazardly arranged fascicles of spindle cells were admixed with a dense collagenous matrix. There were few mitoses and no cytologic atypia. The testis and epididymis were not in-

volved. The history, the bland cytology, and an awareness of the entity aid in the differential diagnosis with leiomyosarcoma.

Other lesions reactive to trauma may also form a scrotal nodule but have an obvious non-neoplastic inflammatory pseudotumor-like nature on microscopic examination (100a).

Scrotal Hamartoma Including "Accessory Scrotum"

Accessory scrotum is distinct from "ectopic scrotum," which is defined by the presence of scrotal tissue including scrotal corrugated skin in a location other than the normal (97a,108a). Ectopic scrotum is frequently associated with testicular ectopia. Accessory scrotum occurs with normally developed scrotal sacs and testes. The term accessory scrotum has been loosely applied in the literature to include perineal lesions containing fat. Another term used is "perineal lipoma with accessory scrotum" (105a,130a,131a,143a). The overlying skin of the perineal fat-containing lesions is simple and noncorrugated, and the adipose tissue is histologically normal.

Amann et al. (99a) described three patterns of accessory scrotum in which the lesion is lined by corrugated scrotal skin: type 1, in which the mass is vaguely defined, with or without continuity with the scrotum; type 2, in which the accessory scrotum is evident as a tiny nodule or skin tag; and type 3, in which the lesion presents as an incompletely separated, distinct additional nodule covered by rugated skin. Histologically, the lesions have features more in keeping with a hamartomatous proliferation, with varying degrees and combinations of fat and smooth muscle. The histology overlaps with that of smooth muscle hamartoma (see below).

Fibrous Hamartoma of Infancy

Fibrous hamartoma of infancy is an uncommon benign myofibroblastic proliferation typically occurring in the first year of life and most commonly occurring in the axillary or shoulder region of male infants. Popek et al. (178) described 15 cases from the Armed Forces Institute of Pathology files involving the genital region of 13 males and 2 females. Five lesions involved the scrotum. The tumors ranged in size from 0.5 to 6.0 cm and grossly appeared fibroma-like or lipoma-like with ill-defined margins extending into adjacent soft tissues. Histologically, the lesions were composed of three components: adipose tissue, spindled myofibroblasts, and round mesenchymal cells, all arranged haphazardly and in varying amounts (fig. 9-24). The adipose tissue occurred in well-delineated lobules while the spindled cells had a fascicular organization. The small mesenchymal cells formed scattered perivascular whorls. Immunohistochemical studies support a fibroblastic/myofibroblastic derivation (vimentin, actin, desmin, CD68, and factor XIIIa positivity); the adipocytes stain for S-100 protein (159,178,184,185). Angiomyofibroblastoma of the paratesticular soft tissues may enter in the differential diagnosis, however, the older age of the patient, the well-demarcated nature of angiomyofibroblastoma, and the alternating hypercellular and edematous hypocellular areas, vascu-

lar proliferation, and perivascular accentuation of mesenchymal cells, help distinguish it from fibrous hamartoma (see page 263).

Smooth Muscle Hamartoma of Dartos

Smooth muscle hamartoma is a rare benign skin lesion containing a random proliferation of dermal smooth muscle bundles. It may be congenital or acquired, or seen in association with Becker's nevus (162,188). A distinct variant associated with muscular arterioles and prominent nerve branches embedded in a densely collagenized stroma has recently been described (fig. 9-25) (179). The epidermis was acanthotic and similar to that seen in angiokeratoma.

Isolated Exophytic Elastoma

Fork et al. (158) described a new type of connective tissue nevus: isolated exophytic elastoma involving the scrotum of a 64-year-old male. The lesion persisted for 35 years, growing slowly over time, and presented as four grape-like clusters of 1 to 3 cm. Histologically, the polypoid lesions showed a papillomatous architecture with paucicellular expansion of the reticular dermis. Elastic tissue stains highlighted numerous tortuous elastic fibers and homogenous elastic material.

Scrotal Fat Necrosis

Scrotal fat necrosis is frequently bilateral and occurs in obese prepubertal boys, presenting as a swollen scrotum which is firm and tender (160, 177). The testis is not involved. Most cases are conservatively managed once a diagnosis is achieved but exploration may be necessary if the diagnosis is not clear clinically. The lesion may appear as an ill-defined gray-yellow mass which histologically shows the typical features of fat necrosis with associated inflammation. The etiology is unknown but hypothermia as produced by swimming in very cold water may play a role.

Scrotal Edema

Scrotal edema is usually characterized by minimally painful swelling due to subcutaneous fluid. The findings of a normal testis and spermatic cord enable clinical distinction from other acute scrotal swellings such as traumatic hydrocele, torsion of testis, incarcerated hernia, and

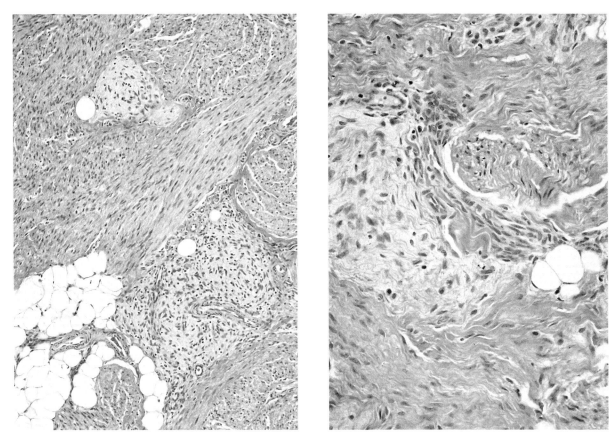

Figure 9-24
FIBROUS HAMARTOMA OF INFANCY
Left: A haphazard arrangement of the three lesional components—adipose tissue, spindled myofibroblasts, and round mesenchymal cells—are seen.
Right: High-power view.

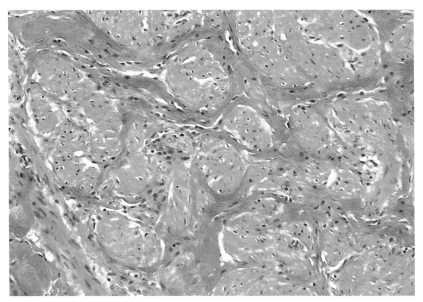

Figure 9-25
SMOOTH MUSCLE
HAMARTOMA OF THE DARTOS
(Courtesy of Dr. T. Quinn, Boston, MA.)

torsion of appendix testis. Several etiologies have been postulated including streptococcal cellulitis, trauma, perianal infection, and allergic processes. Evans and Snyder (157) conclude on the basis of their 8-year experience with 30 patients that the process may be a localized allergic phenomenon similar to angioneurotic edema. The disease is characterized by diffuse subcutaneous edema that does not need excision and hence is rarely histologically evaluated. Failure to respond to conservative therapy, persistent pain, and cosmetic considerations may result in surgical intervention, as in the case illustrated in figure 9-26 in which the process was considered due to lymphatic obstruction secondary to postsurgical scarring.

Polymorphic Reticulosis of Genital Skin

A case of polymorphic reticulosis (idiopathic midline destructive disease) involving the genital skin of the penis, scrotum, and perineum is reported (152). There is controversy as to whether this lesion represents an inflammatory process or an Epstein-Barr virus–positive T-cell lymphoma. The histology showed abundant mature lymphoid cells without angiocentricity. The destructive process involved the entire ventral surface of the penis, with ulceration extending to the anal region. Radiotherapy and chemotherapy were ineffective and radical excisional surgery was required which was successful in limiting disease with no recurrence for 7 years.

Inflammatory and Infectious Diseases

A wide range of inflammatory and infectious diseases may affect the scrotum and clinically resemble a neoplastic process. Elephantiasis of the scrotum, a disease rare in Western countries but still relatively common in tropical and subtropical developing countries and the Pacific islands, may produce dramatic and grotesque enlargement of the scrotum. The scrotal involvement is frequently accompanied by edema of the lower extremities (unilateral or bilateral), and is the result of longstanding filarial infection which alters the lymphatic drainage resulting in blockage of lymphatics and stagnation of lymph, with transudate and secondary cellular proliferation in the connective tissue. Histologically, the lymphatic walls show a cellular proliferation (obliterative

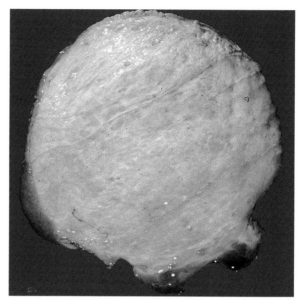

Figure 9-26
MASSIVE SCROTAL EDEMA

endolymphangitis); calcified adult worms may be present in the scrotal soft tissues (166a).

Cutaneous granulomatous diseases such as sarcoidosis (164) and fungal infection may rarely be encountered but are usually part of a more generalized disease process (180). Sexually transmitted diseases such as syphilis (fig. 9-27), herpes simplex, lymphogranuloma venereum, chancroid, and granuloma inguinale (fig. 9-28) may involve the scrotal skin, although they more commonly involve the penis where trauma during sexual intercourse serves as a portal of entry for the organisms.

Fournier's Gangrene

This idiopathic form of necrotizing fasciitis of the subcutaneous tissue and skeletal muscle of the genital tract and perineum frequently involves the scrotum (156,176). The lesions form reddish plaques with sloughing, necrosis, and ulceration, with or without scrotal emphysema (fig. 9-29). There are associated systemic symptoms, including pain and fever, and the diagnosis is usually evident on clinical evaluation although grossly a necrotizing neoplastic process might be a consideration. The disease probably results from infection by staphylococcal or streptococcal

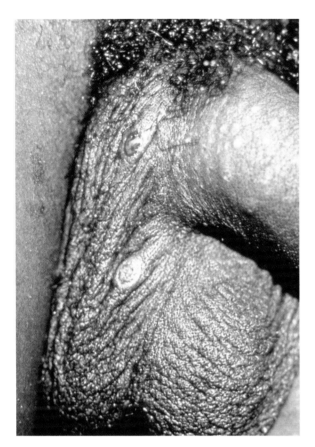
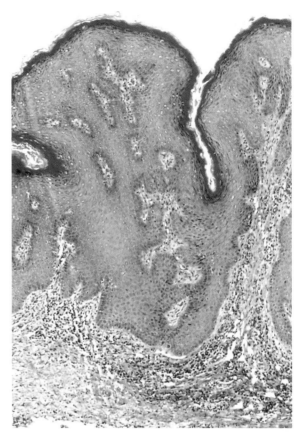

Figure 9-27
SYPHILITIC CONDYLOMATA LATA

Two well circumscribed, minimally elevated lesions with sharp borders and necrotic centers are present (left). Histologically the lesion is characterized by acanthosis and a dense perivascular lymphoplasmacytic infiltrate in the dermis (right). (Figs. 8.13 and 8.15 from Weiss MA, Mills SE. Atlas of genitourinary tract disorders. Philadelphia: Lippincott-Raven, 1988:18.8.)

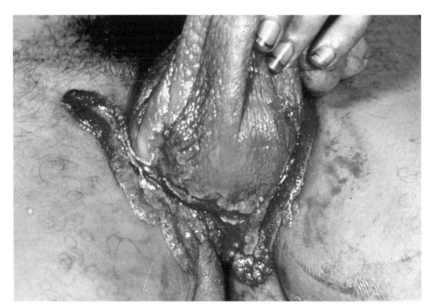

Figure 9-28
GRANULOMA INGUINALE INVOLVING THE SKIN OF THE SCROTUM AND INNER THIGH
(Fig. 18.17 from Weiss MA, Mills SE. Atlas of genitourinary tract disorders. Philadelphia: Lippincott-Raven, 1988:18.10.)

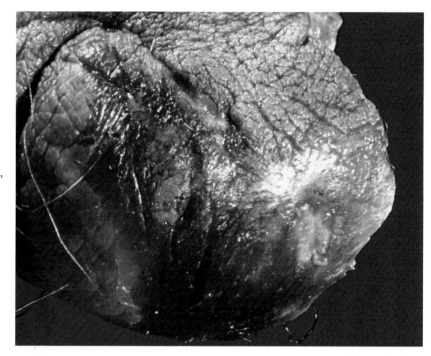

Figure 9-29
FOURNIER'S GANGRENE
Extensive sloughing, ulceration,
and necrosis of the scrotal skin.

organisms, which may be pure or, more commonly, mixed with anaerobic and other gram-negative bacteria. Awareness of Fournier's gangrene is important because it is a serious life-threatening condition that requires prompt diagnosis and intensive therapy (155,156,158a,176).

REFERENCES

Normal Anatomy and Histology

1. Bannister LH, Dyson M. Reproductive system. In: Williams PL, ed. Gray's anatomy. The anatomical basis of medicine and surgery. New York: Churchill Livingstone, 1995:1848–77.
2. Campbell MF. Surgical anatomy of the genitourinary tract. In: Retik AB, Stamey TA, Vaughn ED, Walsh PC, eds. Campbell's urology. Philadelphia: WB Saunders, 1992:3–69.
3. Herbut PA. Urological pathology. Philadelphia: Lea & Febiger, 1952:1196–222.

4. Holstein AF, Orlandini GE, Baumgarten HG. Morphological analysis of tissue components in the tunica dartos of man. Cell Tiss Res 1974;154:329–44.
5. Morley J, Manch CM. The lymphatics of the scrotum: in relation to the radical operation for scrotal epithelioma. Lancet 1911;2:1545.
6. Sadler TW. Urogenital system. In: Langman's medical embryology. Baltimore: Williams & Wilkins, 1990:260–96.
7. Shafik A, Olfat S. Scrotal lipomatosis. Br J Urol 1981;53:50–4.
8. Trainer TD. Histology of the normal testis. Am J Surg Pathol 1978;11:797–809.

Squamous Cell Carcinoma

9. Andrews PE, Farrow GM, Oesterling JE. Squamous cell carcinoma of the scrotum: long-term follow-up of 14 patients. J Urol 1991;146:1299–304.
10. Avellan L, Breine U, Jacobsson B, Johanson B. Carcinoma of scrotum induced by mineral oil. Scand J Plast Reconstr Surg 1967;1:135–40.
11. Brockbank EM. Mule-spinner's cancer. Br Med J 1941;1:622–4.

12. Callen JP, Headington JT. Bowen's and non-Bowen's squamous intraepithelial neoplasia of the skin: relationship to internal malignancy. Arch Dermatol 1980;116:422–6.
13. Chuang TY, Tse J, Reizner GT. Bowen's disease (squamous cell carcinoma in situ) as a skin marker for internal malignancy: a case control study. Am J Prev Med 1990;6:238–43.
14. Cruickshank CN, Squire JR. Skin cancer in engineering industry from use of mineral oil. Br Ind Med 1950;7:1–11.

15. de la Brassinne M, Richert B. Genital squamous cell carcinoma after PUVA therapy. Dermatology 1992;185:316–408.

16. Doll R, Payne P, Waterhouse J. In: Waterhouse J, ed. Cancer incidence in five continents. Lyon: International Agency for Research on Cancer, 1976:584.

17. Graham JH, Helwig EB. Bowen's disease and its relationship to systemic cancer. Arch Dermatol 1961;83:738–58.

18. Graham JH, Helwig EB. Erythroplasia of Queyrat. A clinico-pathologic and histochemical study. Cancer 1973;32:1396–414.

19. Graves RC, Flo S. Carcinoma of the scrotum. J Urol 1940;43:309–32.

20. Henry SA. The study of fatal cases of cancer of scrotum from 1911 to 1935 in relation to occupation, with special reference to chimney sweeping and cotton mule spinning. Am J Cancer 1937;31:28–57.

21. Iwai Y, Someya K, Moriya K, Kobayakawa H, Ohyama T, Horii A. A case of bowenoid papulosis of the penis. Hinyokika Kiyo 1989;35:517–21.

22. Karube H, Aizawa Y, Nakamura K, et al. Oil mist exposure in industrial health—a review. Sangyo Eiseigaku Zasshi 1995;37:113–22.

23. Kennaway EL, Kennaway NM. The social distribution of cancer of the scrotum and cancer of the penis. Cancer Res 1946;6:49–53.

24. Kickham CJ, Dufresne M. An assessment of carcinoma of the scrotum. J Urol 1967;98:108–10.

25. Lee WR. Occupational aspects of scrotal cancer and epithelioma. Ann NY Acad Sci 1976;271:138–42.

26. Lopez AE, Aliaga RM, Martinez MJ, et al. Scrotal verrucous carcinoma. Actas Urol Esp 1995;19:169–73.

27. Lowe FC. Squamous cell carcinoma of the scrotum. J Urol 1983;130:423–7.

28. Lowe FC. Squamous cell carcinoma of the scrotum. Urology 1985;25:63–5.

29. Lowe FC. Squamous cell carcinoma of the scrotum. Urol Clin North Am 1992;19:397–405.

30. McDonald MW. Carcinoma of scrotum. Urology 1982;19:269–74.

31. Melicow MM. Percivall Pott (1713-1788): 200th anniversary of first report of occupation-induced cancer of scrotum in chimney sweepers (1775). Urology 1975;6:745–9.

31a. Murphy GF, Elder DE. Non-melanocytic tumors of the skin. Atlas of Tumor Pathology, 3rd Series, Fascicle 1. Washington, D.C.: Armed Forces Institute of Pathology, 1991.

32. Oesterling JE, Lowe FC. Squamous cell carcinoma of the scrotum. Am Urol Assoc Update Series 1990;9:178–83.

32a. Orihuela E, Tyring SK, Pow-Sang M, et al. Development of human papillomavirus type 16 associated squamous cell carcinoma of the scrotum in a patient with Darier's disease treated with systemic isotretinoin. J Urol 1995;153:1940–3.

33. Passey RD. Experimental soot cancer. Br Med J 1922;2:1112.

34. Pott P. Cancer scroti. In: Hawes L, Clarke W, Collins R, eds. Chirurgical observations relative to the cataract, the polypus of the nose, the cancer of the scrotum, the different kinds of ruptures and the mortification of toes and feet. London: Longerman, 1775:63.

35. Ray B, Whitmore WF. Experience with carcinoma of the scrotum. J Urol 1977;117:741–5.

36. Roush GC, Kelly JA, Meigs JW, Flannery JT. Scrotal carcinoma in Connecticut metal workers: sequel to a study of sinonasal cancer. Am J Epidemiol 1982;116:76–85.

37. Schellhammer PF, Jordan GH, Robey EL, Spaulding JT. Premalignant lesions and nonsquamous malignancy of the penis and carcinoma of the scrotum. Urol Clin North Am 1992;19:131–42.

38. Southam AH, Wilson SR. Cancer of the scrotum: the etiology, clinical features, and treatment of the disease. Br Med J 1922;2:971.

39. Stern RS. Genital tumors among men with psoriasis exposed to psoralens and ultraviolet A radiation (PUVA) and ultraviolet B radiation. The photochemotherapy follow-up study. N Engl J Med 1990;322:1093–7.

40. Stern RS, Laird N, Melski J, et al. Cutaneous squamous-cell carcinoma in patients treated with PUVA. N Engl J Med 1984;310:1156–61.

41. Stern RS, Lange R. Non-melanoma skin cancer occurring in patients treated with PUVA five to ten years after first treatment. J Invest Dermatol 1988;91:120–4.

42. Tourenc R. Le cancer du scrotum chez les decolleteurs (a propos de 21 cas). Presse Med 1964;72:2009–12.

43. Wagner RF Jr, Grande DJ. Solitary pigmented Bowen's disease of the scrotum. J Dermatol Surg Oncol 1986;12:1114–5.

44. Weinstein AL, Howe HL, Burnett WS. Sentinel health event surveillance: skin cancer of the scrotum in New York state. Am J Public Health 1989;79:1513–5.

Basal Cell Carcinoma

45. Greider HD, Vernon SE. Basal cell carcinoma of the scrotum: a case report and literature review. J Urol 1982;127:145–6.

46. Grossman HB, Sogani PC. Basal cell carcinoma of the scrotum. Urology 1981;17:241–2.

47. Ho WS, King WW, Chan WY, et al. Basal cell carcinoma of the scrotum. N Med J Ind 1995;8:195.

48. McEleney DA. Basal cell carcinoma of the scrotum. Cutis 1976;18:227.

49. Murthy KV. Primary cutaneous carcinoma of the scrotum. J Occup Med 1993;35:888–9.

50. Nahass GT, Blauvelt A, Leonardi CL, Penneys NS. Basal cell carcinoma of the scrotum: report of three cases and review of the literature. J Am Acad Dermatol 1992;26:574–8.

51. Parys BT. Basal cell carcinoma of the scrotum—a rare clinical entity. Br J Urol 1991;68:434–5.

52. Richter VG. Subpleurale lungenmetastasen bei sog. Basalzellencarcinom Hautarzt 1957;8:215–9.

Paget's Disease

53. Balducci L, Athar M, Smith GF, Khansur T, McKenzie D, Crawford ED. Metastatic extramammary Paget's disease: dramatic response to combined modality treatment. J Surg Oncol 1988;38:38–44.

54. Bewley AP, Bracka A, Staughton RC, et al. Extramammary Paget's disease of the scrotum: treatment with topical 5-fluorouracil and plastic surgery. Br J Dermatol 1994;131:445–6.

55. Chandra JJ. Extramammary Paget's disease: prognosis and relationship to internal malignancy. J Am Acad Dermatol 1985;13:1009–14.

56. Crocker HR. Paget's disease affecting the scrotum and penis. Trans Pathol Soc London, 1888;40:187.

57. Grimes OF. Extramammary Paget's disease. Surgery 1959;45:569.

58. Hamm H, Vroom TM, Czarnetzki BM. Extramammary Paget's cells: further evidence of sweat gland derivation. J Am Acad Dermatol 1986;15:1275–81.

59. Hoch WH. Adenocarcinoma of the scrotum (extramammary Paget's disease): case report and review of the literature. J Urol 1984;132:137–9.

60. Koh KB, Nazarina AR. Paget's disease of the scrotum: report of a case with underlying carcinoma of the prostate. Br J Dermatol 1995;133:306–7.

61. Michimoto O, Buzou S, Nakashima K. Simultaneous prostatic and genital Paget's disease associated with subjacent adenocarcinoma. Br J Urol 1979;51:49.

62. Ordonez NG, Awalt H, Mackay B. Mammary and extramammary Paget's disease: an immunocytochemical and ultrastructural study. Cancer 1987;59:1173–83.

63. Payne WG, Wells KE. Extramammary Paget's disease of the scrotum. Ann Plast Surg 1994;33:669–71.

64. Reedy MB, Morales CA, Moliver CL, Boman DA, Dudrey EF. Paget's disease of the scrotum: a case report and review of current literature. Tex Med J 1991;87:77–9.

65. Satoh Y, Kanbayashi H, Azuma A, Asahina S, Nakamura K. An autopsy case of Paget's disease of the scrotum with general metastasis. Jpn J Cancer Clin 1987;33:1294–301.

66. Weiner HA. Paget's disease of the skin and its relation to carcinoma of the apocrine sweat glands. Am J Cancer 1937;31:373–403.

Merkel Cell Carcinoma

67. Best TJ, Metcalfe JB, Moore RB, et al. Merkel cell carcinoma of the scrotum. Ann Plast Surg 1994;33:83–5.

Malignant Mesenchymal Tumors

68. Bauer JJ, Sesterhenn IA, Costabile RA. Myxoid liposarcoma of the scrotal wall. J Urol 1995;153:1938–9.

69. Collier DS, Pain JA, Hamilton-Dutoit SJ. Leiomyosarcoma of the scrotum. J Surg Oncol 1987;34:176–8.

70. Dalton DP, Rushovich AM, Victor TA, Larson R. Leiomyosarcoma of the scrotum in a man who had received scrotal irradiation as a child. J Urol 1988;139:136–8.

71. Johnson DE, Chica J, Rodriguez LH, Luna M. Kaposi's sarcoma presenting as scrotal ulcerations. Urology 1977;9:686–8.

72. Johnson S, Rundell M, Platt W. Leiomyosarcoma of the scrotum: a case report with electron microscopy. Cancer 1978;41:1830–5.

73. Koh KB, Joyce A, Boon AP. Leiomyosarcoma of the scrotum. Br J Urol 1994;73:717–8.

74. Konety BR, Campanella SC, Hakam A, et al. Malignant fibrous histiocytoma of the scrotum. J Urol Pathol 1996;5:51–5.

75. Lane D. Fibrosarcoma of the scrotum. Aust N Z J Surg 1958;28:139.

76. Lewis DJ, Moul JW, Williams SC, Sesterhenn IA, Colon E. Perirenal liposarcoma containing extramedullary hematopoiesis associated with renal cell carcinoma. Urology 1994;43:106–9.

77. Lissmer L, Kaneti J, Klain J, et al. Liposarcoma of the perineum and scrotum. Int Urol Nephrol 1992;24:205–10.

78. Maeno K, Enami N, Miyabe N, et al. Malignant fibrous histiocytoma of the scrotal wall—a case report. Gan No Rinsho 1988;34:825–8.

79. Moon TD, Sarma DP, Rodriguez FH. Leiomyosarcoma of the scrotum. J Am Acad Dermatol 1989;20:290–2.

80. Naito S, Kaji S, Kumazawa J. Leiomyosarcoma of the scrotum. Case report and review of literature. Urol Int 1988;43:242–4.

81. Newman PL, Fletcher CD. Smooth muscle tumours of the external genitalia: clinicopathological analysis of a series. Histopathology 1991;18:523–9.

82. Ozeki S, Yasuda M, Nakano M, et al. Leiomyosarcoma of the scrotum: a case report. Acta Urol Jpn 1996;42:229–31.

83. Peters KM, Gonzalez JA. Malignant peripheral nerve sheath tumor of the scrotum: a case report. J Urol 1996;155:649–50.

84. Ray B, Huvos AG, Whitmore WF Jr. Unusual malignant tumors of the scrotum: review of 5 cases. J Urol 1972;108:760–6.

85. Siegal GP, Gaffey TA. Solitary leiomyomas arising from the tunica dartos scroti. J Urol 1976;116:69–71.

86. Vyas S, Manabe T, Herman JR, Newman HR. Kaposi's sarcoma of scrotum. Urology 1976;8:82–5.

87. Washecka RM, Sidhu G, Surya B. Leiomyosarcoma of scrotum. Urology 1989;34:144–6.

88. Watanabe K, Ogawa A, Komatsu H, Yamashita T, Ho N. Malignant fibrous histiocytoma of the scrotal wall: a case report. J Urol 1988;140:150–2.

Malignant Lymphoma

89. Doll DC, Diaz-Arias AA. Peripheral T-cell lymphoma of the scrotum. Acta Haematol 1994;91:77–9.

90. Ray B, Huvos AG, Whitmore WF Jr. Unusual malignant tumors of the scrotum: review of 5 cases. J Urol 1972;108:760–6.

Malignant Melanoma

90a. Curling PB. Carcinoma of the scrotum. A practical treatise on the diseases of the testis and of the spermatic cord and scrotum. Philadelphia: Blanchard and Lee, 1856:407–9.

91. Davis NS, Kim CA, Dever DP. Primary malignant melanoma of the scrotum: case report and literature review. J Urol 1991;145:1056–7.

92. Higgins CC, Warden JG. Cancer of the scrotum. J Urol 1949;62:250–6.
93. Konstadoulakis MM, Ricaniadis N, Karakousis CP. Malignant melanoma of the scrotum: report of 2 cases. J Urol 1994;151:161–2.
94. Moul JW, Ho CK, McLeod DG. Primary malignant melanoma of the scrotum. Int Urol Neph 1992;24:641–3.

95. Ray B, Huvos AG, Whitmore WF Jr. Unusual malignant tumors of the scrotum: review of 5 cases. J Urol 1972;108:760–6.
96. Sasaki H, Ishihara K. Clinical symptoms and prognosis in malignant melanoma of the pubic region. Jpn J Cancer Chemo 1989;6:1721–7.

Benign Epithelial Tumors

97. Nomura M, Hata S. Sebaceous trichofolliculoma on scrotum and penis. Dermatology 1990;181:68–70.

Benign Mesenchymal Tumors

97a. Adair EL, Lewis EL. Ectopic scrotum and diphallia. Report of a case. J Urol 1960;84:115–7.
98. Agger P, Osmundsen PE. Angiokeratoma of the scrotum (Fordyce). A case report on response to surgical treatment of varicocele. Acta Dermatol (Stockholm) 1970;50:221–4.
99. Alter GJ, Trengove-Jones G, Horton CE Jr. Hemangioma of penis and scrotum. Urology 1993;42:205–8.
99a. Amann G, Berger A, Rokitansky A. Accessory scrotum or perineal collision-hamartoma. A case report to illustrate a misnomer. Pathol Res Pract 1996;192:1039–43.
100. Anaguchi S, Sinomiya S, Kinebuchi S, et al. Solitary reticulohistiocytic granuloma—a report of three cases and a review of literature. Jpn J Dermatol 1991;101:735–42.
100a. Bartoletti R, Costanzi A, Messerini L, Palomba A, Dominici A, Di Cello V. Early stage inflammatory scrotal pseudotumor. J Urol 1997;157:1844.
101. Benson CD, Webster JD, McDonald JR. Leiomyoma of tunica dartos scroti. A case report. J Mich Med Soc 1961;60:1553–4.
102. Brock JW, Jones C. Infantile fibromatosis of the external genitalia: diagnosis and management strategy. J Urol 1993;149:357–8.
103. Bruce DH. Angiokeratoma circumscriptum and angiokeratoma scroti. AMA Arch Dermatol 1960;81:84–9.
104. Chang SG, Lee SC, Park YK, et al. Pedunculated leiomyoma of scrotum. J Korean Med Sci 1991;6:284–6.
105. Das AK, Bolick D, Little NA, Walther PJ. Pedunculated scrotal mass: leiomyoma of scrotum. Urology 1992;39:376–9.
105a. Daut WW, Daut RV. Accessory scrotum, posteriorly located: review of the literature and report of one case. J Iowa Med Soc 1949;39:194.
106. De Rosa G, Boscaino A, Giordano V, et al. Symplastic leiomyoma of the scrotum. A case report. Pathologica 1996;88:55–7.
107. DeSanctis DP, Maglietta R, Miranda R, et al. Giant cell fibroblastoma of the scrotum. A case report. Tumori 1993;79:367–9.
108. Dymock RB, Allen PW, Gilbert EF, Thornberg JM. Giant cell fibroblastoma. A distinctive, recurrent tumor of childhood. Am J Surg Pathol 1987;11:263–71.
108a. Elder JS, Jeffs RD. Suprainguinal ectopic scrotum and associated anomalies. J Urol 1982;127:336–8.
109. Fernandez MJ, Martino A, Khan H, Considine TJ, Burden J. Giant neurilemoma: unusual scrotal mass. Urology 1985;30:74–6.
110. Ferrer FA, McKenna PH. Cavernous hemangioma of the scrotum: a rare benign genital tumor of childhood. J Urol 1995;153:1262–4.

110a. Fetsch JF, Laskin WB, Tavassoli FA. Superficial angiomyxoma (cutaneous myxoma): a clinicopathologic study of 17 cases arising in the genital region. Int J Gynecol Pathol 1997;16:325–34.
111. Fisher WC, Helwig EB. Leiomyomas of the skin. Arch Dermatol 1963;88:510–20.
112. Florante J, Leyson J, Doroshow LW, et al. Extratesticular lipoma: report of 2 cases and a new classification. J Urol 1976;116:324–6.
113. Fordyce JA. Angiokeratoma of the scrotum. J Cutan Genitourin Dis, 1896;14:81–7.
114. Gibson TE. Hemangioma of the scrotum. Urol Cutan Rev 1937;41:843–5.
115. Goulding FJ, Traylor RA. Juvenile xanthogranuloma of the scrotum. J Urol 1983;129:841–2.
116. Grace DA. Leiomyoma of the scrotum: a case report and review of the literature. J Urol 1964;91:396–9.
117. Greeley DJ Jr, Sullivan JG, Wolfe GR. Massive primary lipoma of the scrotum. Am Surg 1995;61:954–5.
118. Guekdjian SA. Lymphangioma of the groin and scrotum. J Int Coll Surg 1955;24:159–70.
119. Habuchi T, Okagaki T, Miyakawa M. Leiomyoma of the scrotum: a case report and sonographic findings. Acta Urol Japon 1990;36:959–62.
120. Hagiwara K, Toyama K, Miyazato H, et al. A case of acquired lymphangioma due to a suspected old filariasis and review of literature. J Dermatol 1994;21:358–62.
120a. Hurwitz RS, Shapiro E, Hulbert WC, Diamond DA, Casale AJ, Rink RC. Scrotal cystic lymphangioma: the misdiagnosed scrotal mass. J Urol 1997;158:1182–5.
121. Iloreta AT, Bekirov H, Newman HR. Leiomyoma of scrotum. Urology 1977;10:48–9.
122. Imperial R, Helwig EB. Angiokeratoma of the scrotum (Fordyce type). J Urol 1967;98:379–87.
123. Isaki M. Angiokeratoma of the scrotum (Fordyce). Keio J Med 1952;1:61–8.
124. Kitajima T, Okuwa T, Imamura S. Giant pendulous fibroma with unusual clinical appearance arising on the scrotum. Clin Exp Dermatol 1994;19:278–9.
125. Kurimoto S, Yamazaki S, Eguchi M, et al. Cystic lymphangioma of the scrotum. Apropos of a case. J Urol (Paris) 1993;99:186–8.
126. Lakey D, Mihailescu E, Stepanescu D. Giant fibroma of the scrotal tunica vaginalis. Morphol Embryol 1977;23:203–5.
127. Livne PM, Nobel M, Savir A, et al. Leiomyoma of the scrotum. Arch Dermatol 1983;119:358–9.
128. Marrese M, Ribeiro C, Nudel JE. Leiomyoma of the scrotum. Rev Paul Med 1979;94:38–9.

129. Mibelli V. Di una nuova forma di cheratosi "angiokeratoma." Gior Ital Mal Ven 1889;30:285–301.

130. Montgomery H, Winkelmann RK. Smooth muscle tumors of the skin. Arch Dermatol 1959;79:32–40.

130a. Morita T, Yasukawa S, Matsumoto M, Shinka T, Ohkawa T. Congenital perineal lipoma with accessory scrotum: a case report. Acta Urol Jpn 1991;37:647–9.

131. Mulcahy JJ, Schileru M, Donmezer MA, et al. Lymphangioma of scrotum. Urology 1979;14:64–5.

131a. Nagano S, Takaha M, Ikoma F. Accessory scrotum: report of a case. Acta Urol Jpn 1971;17:766–8.

132. Newman PL, Fletcher CD. Smooth muscle tumours of the external genitalia: clinicopathological analysis of a series. Histopathology 1991;18:523–9.

133. Nishiyama N, Hibi H, Yanaoka M, et al. A case of bizarre leiomyoma of the scrotum. Acta Urol Jpn 1987;33:961–3.

134. Ogawa A, Watanabe K. Genitourinary neurofibromatosis in a child presenting with an enlarged penis and scrotum. J Urol 1986;135:755–7.

135. Orvieto R, Alcalay J, Leibovitz I, Nehama H. Lack of association between varicocele and angiokeratoma of the scrotum (Fordyce). Milit Med 1994;159:523–4.

136. Palacios J, Fiter L, Regadera J, et al. Leiomyoma of the scrotum: presentation of 2 cases. Arch Esp Urol 1987;40:45–7.

137. Rao PL. Lymphangioma of scrotum [Letter]. Ind Pediatr 1993;30:551–2.

138. Ray B, Clark SS. Hemangioma of scrotum. Urology 1976;8:502–5.

139. Shafik A, Olfat S. Scrotal lipomatosis. Br J Urol 1981;53:50–4.

140. Sheth S, Nussbaum A, Hutchins GM, et al. Cystic hygromas in children: sonographic-pathologic correlation. Radiology 1987;162:821–4.

141. Siegal GP, Gaffey TA. Solitary leiomyomas arising from the tunica dartos scroti. J Urol 1976;116:69–71.

141a. Slone S, O'Connor D. Scrotal leiomyomas with bizzare nuclei: a report of three cases. Mod Pathol 1998;11:282–7.

142. Stout AP. Solitary cutaneous and subcutaneous leiomyoma. Am J Cancer 1937;29:435–69.

143. Sule JD, Lemmers MJ, Barry JM. Scrotal arteriovenous malformation: case report and literature review. J Urol 1993;150:1917–9.

143a. Sule JD, Skoog SJ, Tank ES. Perineal lipoma and the accessory labioscrotal fold: an etiological relationship. J Urol 1994;151:475–7.

144. Tomera KM, Gaffey TA, Goldstein IS, et al. Leiomyoma of scrotum. Urology 1981;18:388–9.

145. Wolf DI. Solitary nodule of the scrotum. Leiomyoma. Arch Dermatol 1989;125:418–22.

146. Yoshimura K, Maeda O, Saiki S, et al. Solitary neurofibroma of scrotum. J Urol 1990;143:823.

Secondary Tumors

147. Kawanishi N, Koyama S, Hotta S, et al. A recurrent gastric carcinoma found by metastasis to the scrotum. Jpn J Can Clin 1990;36:101–4.

148. Ray B, Sharifi R, Clark SS. Massive scrotal and occult preputial metastases from carcinoma of the prostate. Br J Urol 1978;50:143.

149. Shetty MR, Khan F. Carcinoma of the rectum with scrotal metastases. Br J Urol 1988;62:612.

150. Ward A, Soni N. An unusual presentation of renal carcinoma. Br J Urol 1978;50:141.

151. Zalev AH, Baker JP, Gardiner GW. Linitis plastica of the alimenary tract and scrotum. Gastrointest Radiol 1990;15:72–5.

Tumor-like Lesions

152. Bostwick DG, Guthman DA, Letendre L, et al. Polymorphic reticulosis (idiopathic midline destructive disease) of the penis, scrotum, and perineum. J Urol Pathol 1996;5:57–63.

153. Browne SG. Calcinosis circumscripta of the scrotal wall: the etiological role of Onchocerca volvulus. Br J Dermatol 1962;74:136–40.

154. Dare AJ, Axelsen RA. Scrotal calcinosis: origin from dystrophic calcification of eccrine duct milia. J Cutan Pathol 1988;15:142–9.

155. de Roos WK, van Lanschot JJ, Bruining HA. Fourniers gangrene: the need for early recognition and radical surgical debridement. Neth J Surg 1991;43:184–8.

156. Ecker KW, Derouet H, Omlor G, Mast GJ. Fournier's gangrene. Chirurgia 1993;64:58–62.

157. Evans JP, Snyder HM. Idiopathic scrotal edema. Urology 1977;9:549–51.

158. Fork HE, Sanchez RL, Wagner RF, et al. A new type of connective tissue nevus: isolated exophytic elastoma. J Cutan Pathol 1991;18:457–63.

158a. Gibson TE. Idiopathic gangrene of the scrotum with report of a case and review of literature. J Urol 1930;23:125–53.

159. Groisman G, Kerner H. A case of fibrous hamartoma of infancy in the scrotum including immunohistochemical findings. J Urol 1990;144:340–1.

160. Hollander JB, Begun FP, Lee RD. Scrotal fat necrosis. J Urol 1985;134:150–1.

161. Holscher AH, Rahlf G, Zimmerman A. Sclerosing lipogranuloma of male genitalia. Urologe 1979;18:106–8.

162. Hsiao GH, Chen JS. Acquired genital smooth-muscle hamartoma. A case report. Am J Dermatopathol 1995;17:67–70.

163. Irisawa C, Hashimoto T, Matsuoka H, et al. A case of idiopathic calcinosis of the scrotum. Acta Urol Jpn 1991;37:1731–3.

164. Kataoka M, Nakata Y, Ejiri T, et al. Sarcoidosis of scrotum: A case report. Jpn J Thorac Dis 1988;26:1201–6.

165. Kimura S. Verruciform xanthoma of the scrotum. Arch Dermatol 1984;120:1378–9.

165a. Kurman RJ, Norris HJ, Wilkinson E. Tumors of the cervix, vagina, and vulva. Atlas of Tumor Pathology, 3rd Series, Fascicle 1. Washington, D.C.: Armed Forces Institute of Pathology, 1992.

166. Levell NJ, Bewley AP, Levene GM. Porokeratosis of Mibelli on the penis, scrotum and natal cleft. Clin Exp Dermatol 1994;19:77–8.

166a. Manson-Bahr PE, Apted FI. Filariases. In: Masson's tropical diseases, 18th ed. London: Bailliere Tindall, 1983:148–80.

167. Matsuchima M, Tajima M, Maki A, et al. Primary lipogranuloma of the male genitalia. Urology 1988;31:75–7.

168. Matsuda T, Shichiri Y, Hida S, et al. Eosinophilic sclerosing lipogranuloma of the male genitalia not caused by exogenous lipids. J Urol 1988;140:1021–4.

169. Melo CR, Schmitt FC, Melo IS, Vaca J, Lucia Caetano A, Souza F. Calcinosis of the scrotum. Report of a case associated with epidermoid cysts. Med Cut Ibero-Lat-Am 1988;16:355–8.

170. Menton M, Neeser E, Walker S, et al. Condylomata acuminata in pregnancy. Is there an indication for cesarean section? Geburtshilfe Frauenheilkunde 1993;53:681–3.

171. Michl UH, Gross AJ, Loy V, et al. Idiopathic calcinosis of the scrotum—a specific entity of the scrotal skin. Scan J Urol Nephrol 1994;28:213–7.

172. Mohsin SK, Lee MW, Amin MB, Stoller MH, et al. Cutaneous verruciform xanthoma: a report of five cases investigating the etiology and nature of xanthomatous cells. Am J Surg Pathol 1998;22:479–87.

172a. Murphy GF, Elder DE. Non-melanocytic tumors of the skin. Atlas of Tumor Pathology, 3rd Series, Fascicle 1. Washington, D.C.: Armed Forces Institute of Pathology, 1991.

173. Nakamura S, Kanamuri S, Nakayama K, et al. Verruciform xanthoma on the scrotum. J Dermatol 1989; 16:397–401.

174. Oertel YC, Johnson FB. Sclerosing lipogranuloma of male genitalia. Review of 23 cases. Arch Pathol 1977;101:321–6.

175. Papadimitriou JC, Drachenberg CB. Posttraumatic spindle cell nodules. Immunohistochemical and ultra-structural study of two scrotal lesions. Arch Pathol Lab Med 1994;118:709–11.

176. Paty R, Smith AD. Gangrene and Fournier's gangrene. Urol Clin N Am 1992;19:149–62.

177. Peterson LJ, Whitlock NW, Odom RB, Ramirez RE, Stutman RE, Mcaninch JW. Bilateral fat necrosis of the scrotum. J Urol 1976;116:825–6.

178. Popek EJ, Montgomery EA, Fourcroy JL. Fibrous hamartoma of infancy in the genital region: findings in 15 cases. J Urol 1994;152:990–3.

179. Quinn TR, Young RH. Smooth muscle hamartoma of the tunica dartos of the scrotum: report of a case. J Cutan Pathol 1997;24:322–6.

180. Sarosdy MF, Brock WA, Parsons CL. Scrotal actinomycosis. J Urol 1979;121:256–7.

181. Shindo Y, Mikoshiba H, Okamoto K, Morohashi M. Verruciform xanthoma of the scrotum. J Dermatol 1985;12:443–8.

182. Smetana HF, Bernhard W. Sclerosing lipogranuloma. Arch Pathol 1950;50:296–325.

183. Song DH, Lee KH, Kang WH. Idiopathic calcinosis of the scrotum: histopathologic observations of fifty-one nodules. Erythroderma Immunohistol 1988;19:1095–101.

184. Sotelo-Avila C, Bale PM. Subdermal fibrous hamartoma of infancy: pathology of 40 cases and differential diagnosis. Pediatr Pathol 1994;14:39–52.

185. Stock JA, Niku SD, Packer MG, Krous H, Kaplan GW. Fibrous hamartoma of infancy: a report of two cases in the genital region. Urology 1995;45:130–1.

186. Takihara H, Takahashi M, Ueno T, Ishihara T, Naito K. Sclerosing lipogranuloma of the male genitalia: analysis of the lipid constituents and histological study. Br J Urol 1993;71:58–62.

187. Theuvenet WJ, Nolthenius-Puylaert TN, Juraha ZL, et al. Massive deformation of the scrotal wall by idiopathic calcinosis of the scrotum. Plast Reconstr Surg 1984;74:539–43.

188. Urbanek RW, Johnson WC. Smooth muscle hamartoma associated with Becker's nevus. Arch Dermatol 1978;114:104–6.

189. Zamora S, Betkerur V, Guinan P. Calcific dystrophy of scrotal skin. Br J Urol 1982;54:198.

INDEX*

Aberrant ducts, inferior and superior (vas aberrans of Haller), 5, **5**, 302
Abscess
    in granulomatous orchitis, 305
    in malakoplakia, 311
Accessory scrotum, 363
ACTH, 293, 295, 297
Actin
    in angiomyofibroblastoma, 264
    in fibrous hamartoma of infancy, scrotum, 364
    in granulosa cell tumor of adult and juvenile types, 229
    in inflammatory pseudotumor, 315
    in leiomyosarcoma, 268
    in myoid cells of testicular interstitium, 8
    negativity in spermatocytic seminoma, 90
    in rhabdomyosarcoma, 266
    in teratoma, 159
    in tumors in the fibroma-thecoma group, 226, 229
    in unclassified sex cord-stromal tumor, 227
Adenocarcinoma
    clear cell
        of epididymis, 255, **256**
        of testis, 235
    endometrioid, 235, **237**
    metastatic, 281, **281–285**
        to epididymis, 284, **284**
    mucinous, 235, **238**
    rete testis, 240, **242**
    serous, 235, **235–237**
    vs. mesothelioma, 238
        vs. rete testis adenocarcinoma, 243
Adenoma, Sertoli cell, 30, 293; *see also* Cystadenoma
Adenomatoid tumor
    differential diagnosis, 246
    general and clinical features, 243
    gross findings, 243, **243**, **244**
    microscopic findings, 243, **244–247**
    vs. malignant mesothelioma, 252
    vs. Sertoli cell tumor, 208
Adrenal cortical rests, 298, **298**, **299**
Adrenocorticotropic hormone, *see* ACTH
Adrenogenital syndrome "tumors," 211, 293, 321
    differential diagnosis, 297
    general and clinical features, 293
    gross findings, 295, **296**
    microscopic findings, 295, **296**
    vs. Leydig cell tumor, 218
Adult-type granulosa tumor, *see* Granulosa cell tumor, adult type
Alpha-fetoprotein
    absence of elevation in seminoma, 60
    in embryonal carcinoma, 103, 110, 116
    in polyembryoma, 177
    prognostic significance, 117
    in teratoma, 148, 159
    in yolk sac tumor, 119, 131, **132**, 136, 246

Alpha-1-antitrypsin staining
    in seminoma, 80
    in yolk sac tumor, 131
Alveolar rhabdomyosarcoma, 266
American Joint Committee on Cancer (AJCC) staging system, 20, **21**
Amyloidosis, 335
Anatomy
    normal scrotum, 343, **344**, **345**
    normal testis, 4, **5–7**
Androblastoma, *see* Sertoli cell tumor and Sertoli-Leydig cell tumor
Androgen insensitivity syndrome
    hamartomatous nodules of the testis in, 30
    intratubular germ cell neoplasia, unclassified in, 30
    Leydig cell hyperplasia in, 30
    Sertoli cell tumors in, 30, 193
Angiokeratoma, scrotum, 354, **354**, **355**
Angioma, *see* Hemangioma and Lymphangioma
Angiomyofibroblastoma
    scrotum, 356
    testis, 262, **264**, **265**
Angiomyxoma
    scrotum, 356
    testis, 262, **264**
    vs. liposarcoma, 268
Appendages of testis, 4, 5, **4**, **5**, 302, **302**
Appendix epididymis, 4, **4**, 5, **5**, 302, **302**
Appendix testis (hydatid of Morgagni), 4, 5, 302
Appendix, vermiform, mucinous tumor of
    spread to hernia sac, 285, **285**
Argentaffin cells
    in carcinoid tumor, 161, **162**
Argyrophil cells
    in teratoma, 161
Arteritis, *see* Vasculitis
Artery, testicular, 5, **7**
Artifactual "invasion" of blood vessels, 23, 110
Atrophy, testis, 29
    with relative prominence of rete testis, 322, **323**
Atypical epithelial cells in epididymis, 13, **14**, 334, **335**
Autoimmune hemolytic anemia, 31

B72.3, 238, 243, 251, 252
Bacterial orchitis, *see* Orchitis, bacterial
B-cell lymphoma, 274
Basal cell carcinoma, scrotum, 349, **349**
Beckwith-Wiedemann syndrome, 185
Ber-H2, *see* CD30
Bilateral testicular tumors, 29
Bile duct carcinoma, metastatic to testis, 283
Borderline tumors, ovarian types, 235, **235**, **236**
Brenner tumor, 235, **239**
British Testicular Tumour Panel, 15, 103, 160
    classification, 15, **17**
Burkitt's lymphoma, 274

---

*Numbers in boldface indicate table and figure pages.

"Burnt-out" germ cell tumor, 181

Calcification
  idiopathic, 326, **328**
  in appendix testis, **302**, 303
  in calcifying fibrous pseudotumor, 264
  in fibrous pseudotumor/fibromatous periorchitis, 260,
      317, **319**
  in gonadoblastoma, 186, **186**
  in hydrocele, 314
  in infarcts, 299, **300**
  in intratubular embryonal carcinoma, 51, 110
  in intratubular germ cell neoplasia, 48
  in large cell calcifying Sertoli cell tumor, 203, **204, 205**
  in malakoplakia, 311, **312**
  in meconium periorchitis, 268, 319, **320**
  in microlithiasis, 326, **328**
  in nodular proliferation of calcifying connective tissue
      of rete, 323
  in regressed germ cell tumor, 184, **185**
  in scrotal calcinosis, 360, **361**
  in seminoma, **70**, 72
  in serous tumor, **237**
  in Sertoli cell nodules, 207, 293
  in Sertoli cell tumor with Peutz-Jeghers syndrome, **205**
  in sperm granuloma, 329
  in "vanishing testis" syndrome, 299, **301**
Calcifying fibrous pseudotumor, testis, 262
Calcinosis, scrotum, 360, **361**
Call-Exner bodies
  in granulosa cell tumors, 220, **221**
  in Sertoli cell nodules, 293
Carcinoid tumor
  carcinoid syndrome in, 31, 160
  metastatic
      to epididymis, 284
      to testis, 283
  primary
      differential diagnosis, 161
      general and clinical features, 160
      gross findings, 160, **161**
      microscopic findings, 161, **162**
      special diagnostic studies, 161
      treatment and prognosis, 161
Carcinoma, basal cell, scrotum, 349, **349**
Carcinoma, clear cell
  of epididymis, 255, **256**
  of testis, 235
Carcinoma, embryonal, testis
  appliqué pattern, 106, **107**, 146
  cytologic findings, 116, **116**
  definition, 103
  differential diagnosis, 116
  general features, 103
  glandular pattern, **109, 115**
  gross findings, 103, **104, 105**
  immunohistochemical findings, 110, **112, 113**
  intratubular, 51, **53**, 110, **111**
  microscopic findings, 104, **105–111**
  papillary pattern, **106, 107**
  solid pattern, **105**
  special diagnostic techniques, 113

treatment and prognosis, 117
ultrastructural findings, 113, **114, 115**
vascular invasion, 110, **111**
vs. anaplastic large cell lymphoma, 276
vs. seminoma, 83
vs. spermatocytic seminoma, 93
Carcinoma, epididymis
  differential diagnosis, 255
  general, clinical, and gross features, 255
  microscopic findings, 255, **256**
  vs. clear cell adenocarcinoma of ovarian type, 239
Carcinoma in situ, 45
Carcinoma, Merkel cell, scrotum, 352
Carcinoma, metastatic, 281
Carcinoma, mucinous, 235, **238**
Carcinoma, rete testis
  differential diagnosis, 241
  general and clinical features, 240
  gross findings, 241, **242**
  microscopic findings, 241, **242**
  vs. malignant mesothelioma, 252
  vs. serous tumors, 238
Carcinoma, scrotum, secondary, 358, **358**
Carcinoma, serous
  paratesticular, **236**
  testicular, **237**
Carcinoma, squamous cell, scrotum, 345
  differential diagnosis, 347
  general and clinical features, 345, **346**
  gross findings, 346, **347**
  microscopic findings, 347, **348**
  prognosis and staging, 347, **349**
Carcinoma, squamous cell, testis, 271
Carcinosarcoma, 272, **272**
Carney's syndrome, 194, 202, 297
CD30, 78
  in anaplastic large cell lymphoma, 117, 276
  in embryonal carcinoma, 112, **113**
  in embryonal carcinoma vs. seminoma, 80, 83
  in embryonal carcinoma vs. yolk sac tumor, 116, 132, 136
  in spermatocytic seminoma, 90
CD45, *see* Leukocyte common antigen
Cellular fibroma, 226, **226**
Chancroid, 366
Charcot-Böttcher filaments, 9, **10**, 205
Choriocarcinoma, 18
  clinical features, 138
  definition, 138
  differential diagnosis, 145
  general features, 138
  gross findings, 139, **139**
  immunohistochemical findings, **142, 143, 144, 145**
  microscopic findings, 139, **139–143**
  monophasic, 140, **142**
  spread and metastasis, 146
  syndrome, 147
  treatment and prognosis, 146
  ultrastructural findings, 144, **145**
  vs. appliqué pattern of embryonal carcinoma, 116
  vs. seminoma with syncytiotrophoblast cells, 84

Chorionic gonadotropin production
    in choriocarcinoma, 138, 144
    in embryonal carcinoma, 103, 116
    gynecomastia association, 31
    in seminoma, 59, 60, 76, 78, **79**, 85
    thyrotoxicosis association, 31
Chromogranin
    in carcinoid tumor, 161
    in Sertoli cell tumor, 161
Chromosomal anomalies in germ cell tumors, 41, 82, 113, 134, 159
c-kit proto-oncogene, immunostaining for the protein product of
    in intratubular germ cell neoplasia, unclassified, 50
    in seminoma, 80
Classification
    scrotal tumors, 343
    testicular tumors, 15, **17**
Clear cell carcinoma
    of epididymis, 255, **256**
    of testis, 235
Clinical aspects of testicular cancer, general, 31
Colorectal carcinoma
    metastatic to epididymis, 284
    metastatic to testis, 283
Condyloma acuminatum, 358, **359**
    vs. verruciform xanthoma, 359
Condylomata lata, **367**
Corpus luteum, in scrotum of hermaphrodite, 326, **327**
Cribriform appearance, normal epididymis, 13, **15**, 333, **334**
Crohn's disease, with vasculitis and infarct, 302
Cryptorchidism, 27, 59
Crystals of Reinke, 11, **11, 12**, 212, **216, 217**, 295
Cushing's syndrome, 31, 272, 297
Cyst, scrotum, epidermoid, 361, **362**
Cyst
    dermoid, 148, **149**, 152, **154**, 325, **327**
    epidermoid, 23, 159, 323, **324**, 360, **362**
    epididymal, **326**
    "multicystic mesothelioma," 325
    rete testis, **326**
    tunica albuginea, **325**
    vs. teratoma, 159
Cystadenoma
    mucinous, 235
    papillary of epididymis, 254, **254, 255**
        vs. epididymal carcinoma, 255
    rete testis, 239, **240**
Cystic dysplasia, 326, **328**
Cytokeratin
    in adenomatoid tumor vs. histiocytoid hemangioma, 262
    in adenomatoid tumor vs. Leydig cell tumor, 247
    in carcinoid tumor, 161
    in choriocarcinoma, 144
    in desmoplastic small round cell tumor, 253
    in desmoplastic small round cell tumor vs. lymphoma, 254
    in embryonal carcinoma, 112, **112**
    in embryonal carcinoma vs. lymphoma, 117, 276
    in embryonal carcinoma vs. seminoma, 83
    in embryonal carcinoma vs. spermatocytic seminoma, 94
    in gonadoblastoma, 187
    in granulosa cell tumor, 229, adult type, 220

    in inflammatory pseudotumor, 315
    in Leydig cell tumor, 229
    in malignant mesothelioma, 251
    in Paget's disease vs. malignant melanoma, 350
    in retinal anlage tumor, 257
    in seminoma, 78
    in Sertoli cell tumor, 229
    in Sertoli cell tumor vs. Leydig cell tumor, 208
    in Sertoli cell tumor vs. seminoma, 208
    in spermatocytic seminoma, 92
    in trophoblast cells, 78
    in unclassified sex cord-stromal tumor, 229
    in yolk sac tumor, 127, 132
    in yolk sac tumor vs. embryonal carcinoma, 132
    in yolk sac tumor vs. juvenile granulosa cell tumor, 225
    in yolk sac tumor vs. Leydig cell tumor, 218
    in yolk sac tumor vs. seminoma, 84
    in yolk sac tumor vs. unclassified sex cord-stromal tumor, 137
Cytologic examination, 23

Dermoid cyst, 148, **149**, 152, **154, 327**
    vs. teratoma, 159
Desmin
    in angiomyofibroblastoma, 264
    in desmoplastic small round cell tumor, 253, 254
    in fibrous hamartoma of infancy, scrotum, 364
    in granulosa cell tumor, 229
    in inflammatory pseudotumor, 315
    in leiomyosarcoma, 268
    in myoid cells of testicular interstitium, 8
    negativity in fibromatous tumors, 229
    negativity in spermatocytic seminoma, 90
    in retinal anlage tumor, 257
    in rhabdomyosarcoma, **158**, 266
    in seminoma, 79
    in teratoma, **158**, 159
    in tumors in the fibroma-thecoma group, 226
Desmoplastic small round cell tumor
    clinical features, 253
    differential diagnosis, 253
    gross findings, 253, **253**
    immunohistochemical findings, 253
    microscopic findings, 253, **254**
    vs. primitive neuroectodermal tumor, 164
Diethylstilbestrol, 334
Diffuse embryoma, 181, **182**
Distribution of germ cell tumors, **44**
Down's syndrome, 27, 147
Drash syndrome, 222
Ductuli efferentes (efferent ductules), 4, **4**, 5, **5**, 11, **14, 15**, 334, **334**
Dysgenesis, gonadal, 30
Dysplasia, cystic, 326, **328**
Dystrophic calcification, 72

Ectopic scrotum, 363
Edema, scrotal, 364, **366**
Efferent ductules (ductuli efferentes), 4, **4**, 5, **5**, 11, **14, 15**, 334, **334**
Elastoma, exophytic, scrotum, 364
Elephantiasis, 366

Embryo-like bodies ("embryoid bodies"), **179**, 180, **180**
Embryology, normal testis, 1, **2**, **3**, **4**
Embryoma, diffuse, 181, **182**
Embryonal carcinoma
    appliqué pattern, 106, **107**, 146
    cytologic findings, 116, **116**
    definition, 103
    differential diagnosis, 116
    general features, 103
    glandular pattern, **109**, **115**
    gross findings, 103, **104**, **105**
    immunohistochemical findings, 110, **112**, **113**
    intratubular, 51, **53**, 110, **111**
    microscopic findings, 104, **105–111**
    papillary pattern, **106**, **107**
    solid pattern, **105**
    special diagnostic techniques, 113
    treatment and prognosis, 117
    ultrastructural findings, 113, **114**, **115**
    vascular invasion, 110, **111**
    vs. anaplastic large cell lymphoma, 276
    vs. seminoma, 83
    vs. spermatocytic seminoma, 93
Embryonal rhabdomyosarcoma, 265
    vs. desmoplastic small round cell tumor, 253
Endodermal sinus tumor, *see* Yolk sac tumor
Endometrioid adenocarcinoma, 235, **237**
Endometriosis, 334, **335**
Epidemiology, 23
Epidermoid cyst
    scrotum, 360, **362**
    testis, 23, 159, 323, **324**
Epididymal carcinoma
    differential diagnosis, 255
    general, clinical, and gross features, 255
    microscopic findings, 255, **256**
    vs. clear cell adenocarcinoma of ovarian type, 239
Epididymis
    adenomatoid tumor of, 243, **243–247**
    atypical cells in, 13, **14**, 334, **335**
    carcinoma of, 255, **256**
    normal findings, 5, 13, **14**, 334, **335**
    papillary cystadenoma of, 254, **254**, **255**
    retinal anlage tumor of, 256, **256–259**
    sperm granuloma of, 329, **330**
Epididymitis, granulomatous, 308, **309**, **310**
Epididymitis nodosa, **332**
Epithelial cells, atypical of epididymis, 13, **14**, 334, **335**
Epithelial membrane antigen, staining for
    in adenocarcinoma vs. Sertoli cell tumor, 208
    in anaplastic large cell lymphoma, 117
    in choriocarcinoma, 144
    in desmoplastic small round cell tumor, 253
    in embryonal carcinoma, 112
    in Leydig cell tumor, 229
    in malignant mesothelioma, 251
    in Paget's disease of scrotum, 350
    in plasmacytoma, 279
    in retinal anlage tumor, 257
    in seminoma, 79
    in Sertoli cell tumor, 229

in yolk sac tumor, 132
Epithelial tumors, scrotum, 345
Epstein-Barr virus, 25, 27
Etiology, 25
Examination
    cytologic, 23
    frozen section, 23
    gross, 20
Exophthalmos, in patients with seminoma, 31, 59
Extragonadal germ cell tumors, 2

Familial cancer, testicular, 29
Fat necrosis, scrotum, 364
Ferritin, staining for
    in embryonal carcinoma, 112
    in intratubular germ cell neoplasia, unclassified, 50
    in seminoma, 79
    in teratoma, 159
    in yolk sac tumor, 132
Fibroblastoma, giant cell, scrotum, 356, **357**
Fibroepithelioma of Pinkus, 349, **349**
Fibrolipoma, scrotum, 356
Fibroma-thecoma tumors, testis
    clinical findings, 226
    differential diagnosis, 226
    gross findings, 226
    immunohistochemical findings, 229
    microscopic findings, 226, **226**
Fibromas
    giant pendulous, 356
    scrotum, 356
    testicular, tunics and paratestis, 259, **260**, **261**
        vs. fibroma of sex cord-stromal type, 226
        vs. fibrous pseudotumor, 318
Fibromatosis, 265
Fibromatous periorchitis, 317, **318**
Fibrosarcoma, 270
    vs. cellular fibroma, 226
Fibrous hamartoma of infancy, scrotum, 364
Fibrous histiocytoma, *see* Malignant fibrous histiocytoma
Fibrous pseudotumor, *see* Pseudotumor, fibrous
Fibrous tumor, solitary, 260
Flow cytometry
    in carcinoid tumor, 161
    prognostic value, 118
    use in predicting metastases, 117
Fournier's gangrene, 366, **368**
Frozen section examination, 23

Genetic susceptibility, 29
Genital ridges, 2, **2**
Germ cell neoplasia, intratubular, *see* Intratubular germ
    cell neoplasia
Germ cell-sex cord-stromal tumor, 184
    "collision" tumor, 190
    differential diagnosis, 188
    unclassified, 188, **189**
        vs. gonadoblastoma, 187
Germ cell tumor, mixed
    clinical features, 175
    components, **175**

definition, 175
diffuse embryoma, 181, **182**
general features, 175, **175**
gross findings, 175, **176, 177**
microscopic findings, 175, **177–182**
polyembryoma, 176, **179**, **180**
treatment and prognosis, 181
Germ cell tumor, nonseminomatous, 103; *see also:*
  Choriocarcinoma, Embryonal carcinoma, Mixed
  germ cell tumor, Placental site trophoblastic tumor,
  Teratoma, Yolk sac tumor
Germ cell tumor, regressed ("burnt-out"), 31, 47
general features, 31, 181
gross findings, **183,** 184, **184**
microscopic findings, 184, **184**, **185**
Germ cell tumor, testicular
bilateral, 29
frequency, **44**
histogenesis, 41, **42**, **43**
intratubular, 45, *see also* Intratubular germ cell
  neoplasia, unclassified type
Glial fibrillary acidic protein, in retinal anlage tumor, 257
Glutathione-S-transferase, staining for in intratubular
  germ cell neoplasia, unclassified, 50
Glycolipid globotriaosylceramide, staining for in intratubular germ cell neoplasia, unclassified, 50
Gonadal dysgenesis, 30, 185
Gonadoblastoma, 30, 72
differential diagnosis, 187, **188**
general features, 185
gross findings, 186
immunohistochemical findings, 187
microscopic findings, 186, **186**, **187**
treatment and prognosis, 188
Gonadotropin, human chorionic
in choriocarcinoma, 138, 144
in embryonal carcinoma, 103, 116
gynecomastia association, 31
in seminoma, 59, 60, 76, 78, **79**, 85
thyrotoxicosis association, 31
Granular cell tumor, scrotal, 358
Granulocytic sarcoma, testis
differential diagnosis, 279
general and clinical features, 279
gross findings, 279, **280**
microscopic findings, 279, **280**, **281**
Granuloma inguinale, **367**
Granuloma, solitary reticulohistiocytic, scrotum, 358
Granuloma, sperm
differential diagnosis, 329
general and clinical features, 329
gross findings, 329, **330**
microscopic findings, 329, **330**
Granulomatous orchitis, 306, **308, 309**
Granulosa cell tumor, testis, 219
adult type, 219
  clinical features, 219, **220**
  differential diagnosis, 220
  gross findings, 220, **220**
  immunohistochemical findings, 229
  microscopic findings, 220, **221**, **222**
  prognosis and treatment, 222

vs. juvenile granulosa cell tumor, 225
vs. Sertoli cell tumor, 207
juvenile type, 222
  confusion with Sertoli cell tumor, 193
  differential diagnosis, 225
  general and clinical features, 222
  gross findings, 222, **223**
  immunohistochemical findings, 229
  microscopic findings, 222, **223–225**
  vs. Sertoli cell tumor, 207
  vs. yolk sac tumor, 136
Granulosa-stromal cell tumors, testis, 219
Gross examination, 20
Growing teratoma syndrome, 160
Gumma, syphilitic, 305, **307**
Gynecomastia, 31, 59, 103, 138, **138**, 185, 194, 209, 211,
  211, 219, **220**, 227

Hamartoma, melanotic, *see* Retinal anlage tumor
Hamartoma, metanephric dysplastic, 335, **336**
Hamartoma of dartos smooth muscle, 364, **365**
Hamartoma of infancy, fibrous, scrotal, 364, **365**
Hamartoma, scrotal, 363
Hamartomatous nodules, testis, in androgen insensitivity
  syndrome, 30
HCG, *see* gonadotropin, human chorionic
Hemangioma
  scrotum, 354
  testis, 260, **262**, **263**
Hematocele, 314, **314**
Hematoma, testis, 299, **301**
Hematopoietic tumors, testis, 272
Hemorrhagic infarction, 299, **299**
Hepatocellular carcinoma, metastatic
  to epididymis, 285
  to testis, 283
Hermaphrodite, 30, 326, **327**
Herpes simplex, 366
Histiocytoid hemangioma, 260
  vs. adenomatoid tumor, 247
Histiocytoma, malignant fibrous
  paratestis, 270
    vs. liposarcoma, 268
  scrotum, 353
Histiocytosis, *see* Rosai-Dorfman disease
Histogenesis of germ cell tumors, 41
Histology, normal, testis, 7, **7–15**
Hodgkin's disease, 274
HPL, *see* Human placental lactogen
Human placental lactogen, 76, 112, 144
  in choriocarcinoma, 144
  in embryonal carcinoma, 112
  in placental site trophoblastic tumor, 144, **145**
  in seminomas with trophoblast cells, 76
Hydroceles, 314, **314**, 335
Hygromas, cystic, 355, **356**
Hypercalcemia, 31, 59
Hyperplasia
  Leydig cell, 291, **292–294**
  mesothelial, 319, **320, 321**
  rete testis, 137, 322, **323**
  Sertoli cell, 292, **294, 295**

steroid cell, 293, 297, **296, 297**
Hyperthyroidism, 31, 139
Hypertrophy of testis, 321

Idiopathic granulomatous orchitis, *see* Orchitis,
    granulomatous
Immunohistochemistry
    germ cell tumors, 78
    sex cord-stromal tumors, 229
Incidence of testicular cancer, 24, **24, 26**
Infarction
    in utero, 299, **300, 301**
    of testicular appendages, 302, **302**
    of testis, 299, **299–301**
    vs. choriocarcinoma, 145
Infectious granulomatous orchitis, *see* Orchitis,
    granulomatous
Infertility, 30, 59
Inflammatory pseudotumor, *see* Pseudotumor, inflam-
    matory
Inhibin, 229
    in gonadoblastoma, 187
    in juvenile granulosa cell tumor vs. yolk sac tumor, 136
    in Leydig cell tumor, 218
    in Leydig cell tumor vs. Sertoli cell tumor, 208
    in Sertoli cell tumor vs. carcinoid, 161
    in Sertoli cell tumor vs. endometrioid adenocarcinoma, 208
    in Sertoli cell tumor vs. metastatic adenocarcinoma, 209
    in Sertoli cell tumor vs. seminoma, 84, 208
    in Sertoli cell tumor with heterologous elements vs.
    in syncytiotrophoblast cells, 113, 144
International Union Against Cancer, 20, **21**
Intersex syndromes, 30, 222, 326
Intestinal carcinoma, metastatic to testis, 283
Intratubular embryonal carcinoma, 51, **53**, 110, **111**
Intratubular germ cell neoplasia, 45, **47–53**
Intratubular germ cell neoplasia, unclassified type
    in androgen insensitivity syndrome, 46
    in atrophic testes, 46
    biopsy detection, 46
    chromosomal changes, 50
    contralateral to a germ cell tumor, 29, 46
    in cryptorchidism, 28, 46
    differential diagnosis, 51, **51–53**
    general features, 45, **46**
    in gonadal dysgenesis, 46
    gross findings, 47
    histogenesis role, 41
    immunohistochemical findings, 49, **50**
    in infertility, 30, 46
    microscopic findings, 47, **47–50**
    other forms, 53
    pagetoid spread of, 48
    ploidy, 46
    screening for, 47
    special diagnostic techniques, 50
    in teratoma, 147
    treatment and prognosis, 53, **54**
    ultrastructural findings, 50
Intratubular seminoma, **51, 52**
Intratubular spermatocytic seminoma, 51, **52**
Intravascular tumor, 110, **111**

Juvenile granulosa cell tumor, 222
    confusion with Sertoli cell tumor, 193
    differential diagnosis, 225
    general and clinical features, 222
    gross findings, 222, **223**
    immunohistochemical findings, 229
    microscopic findings, 222, **223–225**
    vs. Sertoli cell tumor, 207
    vs. yolk sac tumor, 136
Juvenile xanthogranuloma, 358

Kaposi's sarcoma of the testis, 270, **271**
Keratin, *see* Cytokeratin
Ki-1, *see* CD30
Ki-1 positive lymphoma, 274, **275, 276**
Kidney carcinoma, metastatic
    to epididymis, 284
    to scrotum, 358, **358**
    to testis, 283
Kiel classification, 274
Klinefelter's syndrome, 27, 147, 211, 292

Laminin, stains for in yolk sac tumor, 132
Large cell calcifying Sertoli cell tumor, *see* Sertoli cell
    tumor, large cell calcifying type
Leiomyoma
    paratestis/testis, 259
        vs. fibroma, 226
        vs. leiomyosarcoma, 270
    scrotum, 356
        dartoic, 356, **357**
        leiomyoma cutis, 356
Leiomyosarcoma
    paratestis, 270, **270**
        vs. embryonal rhabdomyosarcoma, 268
    scrotum, 352, **352**
Leprosy, 305
Leu-7
    in embryonal carcinoma, 112
    in retinal anlage tumor, 257
    in seminoma, 79
    in yolk sac tumor, 132
Leukemia, 279
Leukocyte common antigen
    in anaplastic large cell lymphoma vs. embryonal
        carcinoma, 117
    in lymphoma, testicular, 276
    in lymphoma vs. seminoma, 84
    in lymphoma vs. spermatocytic seminoma, 94
Leu-M1
    negativity in mesothelioma, 251
    in papillary serous tumors vs. mesothelioma, 238
    in rete carcinoma vs. mesothelioma, 243
Leydig cells, 3, 7, 11, **11–13**
    extraparenchymal, 11, **13**, 292, **293**
Leydig cell hyperplasia, 30, 31, 291, **291–294**
    vs. Leydig cell tumor, 216
Leydig cell tumor, testis
    differential diagnosis, 216
    general and clinical features, 210, **211**
    gross findings, 211, **212**

immunohistochemical findings, 218, **218**, 229
microscopic findings, 211, **213–216**
prognosis and treatment, 219
ultrastructural findings, 216, **217**
vs. adenomatoid tumor, 247
vs. adrenogenital syndrome "tumor," 297
vs. malakoplakia, 311
vs. plasmacytoma, 279
vs. Sertoli cell tumor, 207
Li-Fraumeni syndrome, 29
Limbic encephalopathy, 31
Lipoblastoma, paratestis, 259
Lipogranuloma, sclerosing
    paratestis/testis, 321, **322**
        vs. liposarcoma, 268
    scrotum, 361, **362**, **363**
Lipomas
    paratestis, 259
    scrotum, 356
Liposarcoma
    paratestis, 268, **269**
    scrotum, 353
Liver carcinoma, metastatic
    to epididymis, 285
    to testis, 283
Lung carcinoma, metastatic to testis, 281
Lutein cells, in sex cord-stromal tumors, 190, **222**
Lymph node, distribution of metastases in testicular
    cancer, 18, **19**
Lymphangiectasis, congenital testicular, 335
Lymphangioma, scrotum, 355, **356**
Lymphatics, scrotum, 344
Lymphogranuloma venereum, 366
Lymphoma, malignant, testis
    anaplastic large cell type, 274, **275**, **276**
    differential diagnosis, 276
    general and clinical features, 272
    gross findings, 272, **273**
    microscopic findings, 272, **273–276**
    prognosis, 276
    vs. desmoplastic small round cell tumor, 254
    vs. embryonal carcinoma, 116
    vs. embryonal rhabdomyosarcoma, 268
    vs. granulocytic sarcoma, 279
    vs. Leydig cell tumor, 218
    vs. plasmacytoma, 278
    vs. seminoma, 84
    vs. spermatocytic seminoma, 94
Lymphoma, scrotal, 353

Malakoplakia, testis
    differential diagnosis, 311
    general and clinical findings, 309
    gross findings, 311, **311**
    microscopic findings, 311, **312**, **313**
    vs. Leydig cell tumor, 216
Malignant fibrous histiocytoma
    paratestis, 270
        vs. liposarcoma, 268
    scrotum, 353
Malignant melanoma

metastatic to testis, 281, **283**
    vs. Leydig cell tumor, 219
of scrotum, 353
Malignant mesothelioma, *see* Mesothelioma, malignant
Marfan's syndrome, 27
Meconium periorchitis, 268, 319
    vs. rhabdomyosarcoma, 268
Mediastinum testis, 5, **6**
Melanoma, malignant, scrotum, 353, **353**
    vs. Paget's disease, 350
Melanoma, metastatic to testis, 281, **283**
    vs. Leydig cell tumor, 219
Melanospermia, 283
Melanotic hamartoma, *see* Retinal anlage tumor
Melanotic neuroectodermal tumor, *see* Retinal anlage tumor
Melanotic progonoma, *see* Retinal anlage tumor
Meninges in teratoma, 149, **153**
Merkel cell carcinoma, scrotum, 352
Merkel cell tumor, metastatic to testis, 283, **284**
Mesenchymal tumors, scrotum, 352
Mesothelial hyperplasia
    differential diagnosis, 320
    general and clinical features, 319
    microscopic findings, 320, **320**, **321**
    vs. malignant mesothelioma, 251
Mesothelioma, malignant
    differential diagnosis, 251
    general and clinical features, 247
    gross findings, 248, **248**
    immunohistochemical findings, 251
    microscopic findings, 248, **249–252**
    multicystic, 325
    prognosis and treatment 253
    vs. adenomatoid tumor, 246
    vs. mesothelial hyperplasia, 320
    vs. rete testis carcinoma, 243
    vs. serous tumors, 238
Metanephric dysplastic hamartoma of epididymis, 335, **336**
Metastases to epididymis, 284
Metastases to spermatic cord, 285
Metastases to testis, 281
Metastatic spread, 18
Michaelis-Gutmann bodies, 311, **312**, **313**
Microlithiasis, 326, **328**
Mimics of neoplasms, 291
Mixed germ cell-sex cord-stromal tumor, *see* Germ cell-
    sex cord-stromal tumor
Mixed germ cell tumors
    clinical features, 175
    components, **175**
    definition, 175
    diffuse embryoma, 181, **182**
    general features, 175
    gross findings, 175, **176**
    microscopic findings, 175, **177–183**
    polyembryoma, 176, **179**, **180**
    treatment and prognosis, 181
Monodermal testicular tumors, 160, *see also* Carcinoid tumor
    others, 164
    primitive neuroectodermal tumor, 163, **163**
Mucinous adenocarcinoma, 235, **238**
Mucinous borderline tumor, 235

Multiple myeloma
    clinical features, 277
    differential diagnosis, 278
    gross findings, 277, **277, 278**
    microscopic findings, 277, **278**
    vs. granulocytic sarcoma, 279
Mumps orchitis, 304, **305**
Mural papilloma in spermatocele, 329
    vs. papillary cystadenoma of epididymis, 255
Myeloma, multiple, *see* Multiple myeloma
Myxoma, *see* Aggressive angiomyxoma

Nelson's syndrome, "tumors" in, 297, **297**
    vs. Leydig cell tumor, 218
Nephroblastoma, 152, **156**, 271, 283, 335
Neuroectodermal tumor, primitive, 156, 163, **163**
Neurofibroma, scrotal, 358
Neuron-specific enolase, staining for
    in carcinoid tumor, 161
    in desmoplastic small round cell tumor, 253
    in seminoma, 79
Nodular periorchitis, 317
Nodular precocious maturation, 321, **322**
Nodule, Sertoli cell, 187, **188**, 292, **294, 295**
Nonseminomatous germ cell tumors, *see* Germ cell
    tumors, nonseminomatous

Oncogenes, 82, 113
Orchidopexy, 28
Orchitis
    bacterial, 304, **304**
    vs. lymphoma, 276
    viral, 304, **305**
Orchitis, granulomatous
    idiopathic, 306
        differential diagnosis, 307
        general and clinical features, 306
        gross findings, 307, **308**
        microscopic findings, 307, **308, 309**
    infectious, 305, **306, 307**
        vs. idiopathic granulomatous orchitis, 307
Osseous metaplasia, 334
Osteosarcoma, in carcinosarcoma, 272
Ovarian-type epithelial tumors
    differential diagnosis, 238
    general and clinical features, 235
    gross findings, **235**, 236, **236, 239**
    microscopic findings, 236, **236–239**
    prognosis and treatment, 239
Ovotestis, 326, **327**
Oxalosis, secondary, 335

p53
    in choriocarcinoma, 144
    in embryonal carcinoma, 112
    in germ cell tumors, 29
    in intratubular germ cell neoplasia, unclassified, 50
    in seminoma, 82
    in yolk sac tumor, 132
Paget's disease, scrotum
    general and clinical features, 350, **350**

microscopic findings, 350, **351**
    treatment and prognosis, 350
Pampiniform plexus, 6, **7**
Pancreas, carcinoma metastatic
    to epididymis, 284, **284**
    to testis, 283
Paneth cell-like metaplasia, epididymis, 13, **15**
Papillary cystadenoma of epididymis, 254, **254, 255**
Paradidymis (organ of Giraldes), 5, **5**, 302, **302**
Paraffinoma, scrotum, 361
Paraganglioma, 271
Periarteritis nodosa, 302
Periorchitis
    fibromatous, 317, **318**
    meconium, 319, **319, 320**
    nodular, 317
Peutz-Jeghers syndrome, 194, 202, 205, **206, 207**
Pheochromocytoma, *see* Paraganglioma
Pick's adenoma, 293
Pilomatrixoma, testis, 152
Pituitary gonadotropin-independent sexual precocity, 321
Placental lactogen, human, 76, 112, 144
    in choriocarcinoma, 144
    in embryonal carcinoma, 112
    in placental site trophoblastic tumor, 144, **145**
    in seminomas with trophoblast cells, 76
Placental-like alkaline phosphatase
    in choriocarcinoma, 144
    in embryonal carcinoma, 112, vs. large cell lymphoma, 117
    in embryonic germ cells, 1
    in gonadoblastoma, 187
    in intratubular germ cell neoplasia, unclassified, 28,
        49, **50**
    in seminoma, 60, 78, **79**, vs. granulomatous inflam-
        mation, 84, vs. lymphoma, 84, vs. Sertoli cell
        tumor, 84, 208
    in teratoma, 159
    in yolk sac tumor, 132
Placental site trophoblastic tumor, 144, **144, 145**
PLAP, *see* Placental-like alkaline phosphatase
Plasmacytoma
    clinical features, 277
    differential diagnosis, 278
    gross findings, 277, **277, 278**
    microscopic findings, 277, **278**
    vs. granulocytic sarcoma, 279
Ploidy of germ cell tumors, 41, 92, 113, 135, 159
Polycythemia, 31
Polyembryoma, 176, **179, 180**
Polymorphic reticulosis, 366
Porokeratosis of Mibelli, 359
Post-traumatic spindle cell nodule, scrotum, 363
Pott, Sir Percivall, 345
Precocious maturation, nodular, 321, **322**
Primitive neuroectodermal tumor, 156, 163, **163**
Progonoma, melanotic, *see* Retinal anlage tumor
Proliferative funiculitis, 315, **315, 316**
    vs. fibroma, 260
Prostatic adenocarcinoma, metastatic
    to epididymis, 284
    to testis, 281, **281, 282**
Pseudoendodermal sinus pattern, 106

Pseudohermaphroditism, 30
Pseudohyperplasia of rete testis, 322, **323**
Pseudoinvasion of blood vessels, 23, 110
Pseudoprecocity, 31, 211
Pseudosarcomatous myofibroblastic proliferation, 315
Pseudotumor, fibrous
    differential diagnosis, 318
    general and clinical findings, 317
    gross findings, 317, **317, 318**
    microscopic findings, 317, **318, 319**
    vs. fibroma, 260
Pseudotumor, inflammatory, testis and epididymis
    differential diagnosis, 316
    general and clinical features, 315
    gross findings, 315, **315**
    microscopic findings, 315, **316**

Radiation fibrosis, 335, **336**
Ras proto-oncogenes, 29, 82, 113
Regression of germ cell tumors, 181
Reinke crystals, 11, **11, 12**, 212, **216, 217**
Renal cell carcinoma, metastatic
    to epididymis, 284
    to scrotum, 358, **358**
    to testis, 283
Rete testis, 11, **13**
    benign tumors, 239, **240, 241**
    carcinoma, 240
        differential diagnosis, 241
        general and clinical features, 240
        gross findings, 241, **242**
        microscopic findings, 241, **242**
        vs. malignant mesothelioma, 252
        vs. serous tumors, 238
    cystadenoma, **240**
    hamartoma, 323
    hyperplasia, 137, 322, **323**
    pseudohyperplasia, 322, **323**
Rete testis cords, 3, **3**
Retiform pattern, in Sertoli cell tumor, 195, **198**
Retinal anlage tumor
    differential diagnosis, 257
    clinical features, 256
    gross findings, 256, **256, 257**
    immunohistochemical findings, 257
    microscopic findings, 256, **257–259**
Retinal-type epithelium in teratoma, 149, **152**
Rhabdoid tumor, 265
Rhabdomyoma, paratestis, 259
Rhabdomyosarcoma, 156, **158**, 265, **265–267**, 352
    immunohistochemical findings, 266
    spindle cell type, 265, **266, 267**
    vs. juvenile granulosa cell tumor, 225
    vs. liposarcoma, 268
Rosai-Dorfman disease, 313, **313**

S-100 protein
    absence of reactivity in angiomyofibroblastoma, 264
    in fibrous hamartoma of infancy of scrotum, 364
    in granulosa cell tumor, 229
    in large cell calcifying Sertoli cell tumor, 229
    in Leydig cell tumor, 219, 229
    in malignant melanoma vs. Paget's disease, 350
    in retinal anlage tumor, 257
    in Sertoli cell tumor, NOS, 229
    in unclassified sex cord–stromal tumor, 227, 229
Sarcoidosis, 309, **310**
Sarcomas, 265, *see also:* Fibrosarcoma, Granulocytic
    sarcoma, Kaposi's sarcoma, Leiomyosarcoma,
    Liposarcoma, Malignant fibrous histiocytoma,
    and Rhabdomyosarcoma
    neurogenic, scrotum, 352
    vs. inflammatory pseudotumor, 316
    with spermatocytic seminoma, 90, **91**
Scar, testis, in regressed germ cell tumor, 184, **184, 185**
Schiller-Duval body, 122, **122, 123**
Schwannoma, scrotal, 358
Sclerosing lipogranuloma, scrotum, 361
    testis, 321
Scrotal calcinosis, "idiopathic," 360, **361**
Scrotal fat necrosis, 364
Scrotum
    anatomy, 343, **344**
    histology, 344, **344, 345**
Sebaceous trichofolliculoma, scrotum, 354
Secondary tumors
    scrotal, 358
    testis
        general and clinical features, 281
        gross findings, **281**, 283, **284**
        microscopic findings, **282–284**, 283
Seminiferous tubules, 7, **7, 8**
Seminoma, "anaplastic," 74
Seminoma, intratubal, 51, **51, 52**, 69, **72**
Seminoma, spermatocytic
    "anaplastic," 90, **91**
    clinical features, 86
    definition, 85
    differential diagnosis, 93, **95**
    general features, 85
    gross findings, 86, **86**
    immunohistochemical findings, 90
    microscopic findings, 86, **87–92**
    sarcomatous change in, 90, **91, 92**
    special diagnostic techniques, 92
    treatment and prognosis, 94
    ultrastructural findings, 92, **93, 94**
    vs. plasmacytoma, 279
Seminoma, typical
    clinical features, 59
    cryptorchidism association, 28
    cytologic findings, 82, **83**
    definition, 59
    differential diagnosis, 83
    general features, 59
    gonadoblastoma association, 185
    gross findings, 60, **61–63**
    histogenetic role, 41
    immunohistochemical findings, 78, **78, 79**
    microscopic findings, 61, **64–77**
    special diagnostic methods, 81
    syncytiotrophoblast cells in, 76, **77**, 146
    treatment and prognosis, 84

ultrastructural findings, 80, **80, 81**
  vs. idiopathic granulomatous orchitis, 308
  vs. lymphoma, 276
  vs. plasmacytoma, 279
  vs. sarcoidosis, 309
  vs. Sertoli cell tumor, 208
  vs. spermatocytic seminoma, 93, **95**
Serous borderline tumor, 235, **235, 236**
Serous carcinoma, 235, **236, 237**
Sertoli cell, 8, **9, 10**
Sertoli cell adenoma, 30, 293
Sertoli cell nodule, 187, **188,** 292, **294, 295**
  vs. gonadoblastoma, 187
  vs. Sertoli cell tumor, 205
Sertoli cell tumor
  general and clinical features, 193
  gross findings, 194, **194, 195**
  immunohistochemical findings, 229
  microscopic findings, 195, **195–202**
  prognosis and treatment, 202
  sclerosing type, 193, **194,** 199, **201**
  ultrastructural findings, 199, **201**
  vs. adenomatoid tumor, 247
  vs. carcinoid, 161
  vs. seminoma, 84
Sertoli cell tumor, large cell calcifying type, 202
  benign vs. malignant, 209, **209**
  differential diagnosis, 205
  gross findings, 202, **203**
  microscopic findings, 203, **204, 205**
  prognosis and treatment, 209, **209**
  ultrastructural features, 205, **206**
Sertoli-Leydig cell tumor, 209
  differential diagnosis, 210
  gross findings, 209
  microscopic findings, 210, **210**
Sex cords, 1, **2**
Sex cord-stromal tumors, 31, 193, **193**
  vs. Sertoli cell tumor, 207
Sex cord-stromal tumor, mixed and unclassified
  differential diagnosis, 227
  general and clinical features, 227
  gross findings, 227, **227**
  immunohistochemistry, 229
  microscopic findings, 227, **228**
  prognosis, 229
  vs. fibroma, 226
  vs. sarcomas, 271
  vs. sarcomatoid yolk sac tumor, 137
  vs. spindle cell Leydig cell tumor, 219
Sex cord tumor with annular tubules, 205
Sinus histiocytosis with massive lymphadenopathy, 313
Smooth muscle hamartoma of dartos, 364, **365**
Smooth muscle hyperplasia, 334
Soft tissue tumors, 259
  benign, 259
Solitary fibrous tumor, 260
Sperm granuloma
  differential diagnosis, 329
  general and clinical features, 329
  gross findings, 329, **330**

  microscopic findings, 329, **330**
Spermatids, **8,** 10
Spermatocele, 327, **329**
Spermatocytes, **8,** 9
Spermatocytic seminoma, *see* Seminoma, spermatocytic
Spermatogenesis, **8,** 9
Spermatogonia, **8,** 9
Spindle cell nodule, post-traumatic, 363
Splenic-gonadal fusion, 333, **333**
Squamous cell carcinoma
  scrotum, 345
    differential diagnosis, 347
    general and clinical features, 345, **346**
    gross findings, 346, **347**
    microscopic findings, 347, **348**
    prognosis and staging, 347, **349**
  testis, 156, 271
Staging, testicular tumors, 20, **21**
Steroid cell nodules, 297, **297**
Stomach carcinoma, metastatic
  to epididymis, 284
  to testis, 283
Struma testis, 149, **153,** 164
Swyer's syndrome, 30
Syncytiotrophoblast cell
  in choriocarcinoma, 138, 139, **140–143**
  in embryonal carcinoma, 103, 113
  in polyembryoma, 180, **180**
  in seminoma, 42, 60, 76, **77,** 78, **79,** 84
Syphilis
  scrotum 366, **367**
  testis, 305, **307**

T-cell lymphoma, 274
Teratoma
  clinical features, 148
  definition, 147
  dermoid cyst, **149,** 152, **154**
  differential diagnosis, 159
  general features, 147
  grading, 158
  gross findings, 148, **148, 149**
  immature, 152, **154–157**
  immunohistochemical findings, 159
  mature, 149, **149–153**
  microscopic findings, 149, **150–158**
  other monodermal, 164
  retinal type, **152**
  secondary malignant component, 156, **158**
  special diagnostic techniques, 159
  spread and metastasis, 159
  treatment and prognosis, 160
  vs. glandular yolk sac tumor, 136
Testicular cancer, incidence, 24, **24, 26**
Testicular feminization syndrome, *see* Androgen
  insensitivity syndrome
Testicular infarction, 299, **299–302**
Testicular parenchyma, 5
Testicular regression syndrome, 299
Testis cords, 3, **3, 4**
Testotoxicosis, 291, 321

Thecoma, 226
TNM staging, 21
Torsion
    of appendix testis, **302**
    of testis, 31, 299, **299**
Trophoblastic neoplasia, 138, **143–145**
Tuberculosis, 305, **306**
Tubular adenomas, 293
Tubuli recti, 5, 11
Tumor staging, 21
Tunica albuginea, 3, **3**, 4, 60, 325, **325**
Tunica vaginalis, 4
    abnormalities, 314

Vanishing testis syndrome, 299
Varicocele, 7
Vascular invasion, 110, **111**
Vascular supply, testis, **7**
Vascular tumors, *see also* Angiokeratoma, Hemangioma,
        Cystic hygroma, Lymphangioma
    scrotum, 354
    testis, 260, **262, 263**
Vasculitis, 299, 301
Vasitis nodosa
    differential diagnosis, 331
    general and clinical features, 331
    gross findings, 331, **331**
    microscopic findings, 331, **331, 332**
Venous drainage, 6, **7**
Verruciform xanthoma, 358, **360**
Viral orchitis, 304, **305**
Von Hansemann cells, 311, **312**
Von Hippel-Lindau disease, 254

Waldeyer's ring, 272
Walthard nests, 302, **303,** 325
Wiedemann-Beckwith syndrome, 185

Wilms' tumor, 152, **156**, 271, 283, 335
    in teratoma, 152, **156**
Working Formulation classification, 274
World Health Organization (WHO), 15, 16

Xanthogranuloma, juvenile, scrotum, 358
Xeroderma pigmentosa, 147

Yolk sac tumor
    clinical features, 119
    cytologic findings, 136
    definition, 119
    differential diagnosis, 136
    endodermal sinus pattern, 122, **122, 123**
    general features, 119
    glandular pattern, 124, **125, 126, 135**
    gross findings, 119, **120**
    hepatoid pattern, 129, **129, 130**
    immunohistochemical findings, 131, **132**
    microcystic and macrocystic patterns, **120, 121, 123,**
            125, 126, 128, 129, 131
    microscopic findings, 119, **120–131**
    myxomatous pattern, **121**, 127, **130**
    papillary pattern, 122, **123**
    parietal pattern, 129, **130,**
    polyvesicular vitelline pattern, 128, **128, 129**
    reticular pattern, 120, **120, 121, 123**
    sarcomatoid pattern, 127, **128**
    solid pattern, 122, **124, 133**
    special diagnostic techniques, 134
    treatment and prognosis, 137
    ultrastructural findings, 132, **133–135**
    vs. adenomatoid tumor, 246
    vs. embryonal carcinoma, 116
    vs. juvenile granulosa cell tumor, 225
    vs. Leydig cell tumor, 218
    vs. seminoma, 83

❖❖❖